PRIMARY PREVENTIVE DENTISTRY

4th Edition

PRIMARY PREVENTIVE DENTISTRY

4th Edition

Norman O. Harris, DDS, MSD, FACD
Professor (Retired), Department of Community Dentistry
University of Texas Dental School at San Antonio
San Antonio, Texas

Arden G. Christen, DDS, MSD, MA, FACD
Professor and Chairman of Preventive Dentistry
Indiana University School of Dentistry
Indianapolis, Indiana

APPLETON & LANGE
Stamford, Connecticut

Copyright © 1995 by Appleton & Lange
Paramount Publishing Business and Professional Group
Copyright © 1991 by Appleton & Lange
A Publishing Division of Prentice Hall
Copyright © 1987 by Appleton & Lange
Copyright © 1982 by Reston Publishing Company, Inc.

96 97 98 / 10 9 8 7 6 5 4 3

Prentice Hall International (UK) Limited, *London*
Prentice Hall of Australia Pty. Limited, *Sydney*
Prentice Hall Canada, Inc., *Toronto*
Prentice Hall Hispanoamericana, S. A., *Mexico*
Prentice Hall of India Private Limited, *New Delhi*
Prentice Hall of Japan, Inc., *Tokyo*
Simon & Schuster Asia Pte. Ltd., *Singapore*
Editora Prentice Hall do Brasil Ltda., *Rio de Janeiro*
Prentice Hall, *Englewood Cliffs*, *New Jersey*

Library of Congress Cataloging-in-Publication Data
Primary preventive dentistry / [edited by] Norman O. Harris, Arden G.
  Christen.—4th ed.
      p. cm.
    Rev. ed. of: Primary preventive dentistry / Norman O. Harris,
  Arden G. Christen. 3rd ed. c1991.
    Includes bibliographical references and index.
    ISBN 0-8385-8000- 9
    1. Preventive dentistry.   2. Preventive dentistry—Examinations,
  questions, etc.   I. Christen, Arden G., 1932–   II. Harris,
  Norman O. Primary preventive dentistry.
    [DNLM: 1. Preventive Dentistry.   2. Primary Prevention. WU 113
  P9522 1994]
  RK60.7.H37   1994
  617.6'01—dc20
  DNLM/DLC   94-19930
  for Library of Congress   CIP

Acquisitions Editor: Cheryl Mehalik
Production Editor: Sondra Greenfield
Designer: Libby Schmitz

PRINTED IN THE UNITED STATES OF AMERICA

ISBN 0-8385-8000-9

90000

9 780838 580004

Contributors

David W. Banting, DDS, DDPH, MSc, PhD
Professor and Associate Academic Dean
University of Western Ontario Faculty
   of Dentistry
London, Ontario, Canada

Bradley B. Beiswanger, DDS
Professor, Preventive/Community
   Dentistry
Oral Health Research Institute
415 Lansing Street
Indianapolis, Indiana

Eros S. Chaves, DDS, MS
Assistant Professor in Periodontics
University of Alabama at Birmingham
School of Dentistry
Birmingham, Alabama

Arden G. Christen, DDS, MSD, MA., FACD
Professor and Chairman of Preventive
   Dentistry/Community Dentistry
Indiana University School of Dentistry
Indianapolis, Indiana

D. Christopher Clark, BSc, DDS, MPH
Associate Professor and Chair
Division of Preventive and
   Community Dentistry
University of British Columbia
   Faculty of Dentistry
Vancouver, British Columbia, Canada

Leonard A. Cohen, DDS, MPH, MS
Professor and Chairman
Department of Oral Health Care Delivery
Baltimore College of Dental Surgery
Dental School, University of Maryland
   at Baltimore
Baltimore, Maryland

Laurence P. Crigger, DDS, MSD
Commander, 381st Dental Training
   Squadron, School of Health Care
   Sciences
Sheppard AFB, Texas

Marsha A. Cunningham-Ford, RDH, BS, MS
Associate Professor, Department of
   Preventive and Community Dentistry
University of Iowa College of Dentistry
Iowa City, Iowa

Michael W. J. Dodds, BDS, PhD
Assistant Professor
University of Texas Health Science Center
   at San Antonio
San Antonio, Texas

Stuart L. Fischman, DMD
Professor of Oral Medicine
State University of New York at Buffalo
   School of Dentistry
Buffalo, New York

Jacquelyn L. Fried, RDH, MS
Associate Professor
University of Maryland Dental School
Baltimore, Maryland

Franklin García-Godoy, DDS
Professor
Department of Pediatrics
University of Texas Health Science Center
   at San Antonio
San Antonio, Texas

Harold S. Goodman, DMD, MPH
Director, Dental Public Health Residency
   Program
Department of Veterans Affairs
VA Medical Center, Dental Service
Perry Point, Maryland

Norman O. Harris, DDS, MSD, FACD
Professor, Department of Community
   Dentistry (Retired)
University of Texas Dental School
   at San Antonio
San Antonio, Texas

Clifford A. Katz, DDS, PhD
Management Consultant
The Katz Company
Austin, Texas

F. Morell MacKenzie BDS, DDPH
Principal Dental Officer,
   Health Care Otago
Dunedin, New Zealand

Bruce A. Matis, DDS, MSD, FACD
Associate Professor
Department of Restorative Dentistry
Indiana University School of Dentistry
Indianapolis, Indiana

Michael T. Montgomery, DDS
Chairman of Hospital Dentistry
University of Texas Dental School
   at San Antonio
San Antonio, Texas

Roseann Mulligan, DDS, MS
Associate Professor and Chairman
   of Department of Dental Medicine
   and Public Health, Section of Geriatric
   and Special Patient Dentistry
University of Southern California
   School of Dentistry
Los Angeles, California

**Hubert N. Newman, B Dent Sci, FRC
   Path, MA, PhD, ScD**
Professor of Periodontology
   and Preventive Dentistry
Vice Dean (Teaching) and Head,
   Electron Microscopy Unit
British Postgraduate Medical Federation,
   Institute of Dental Surgery
London, England

Carole A. Palmer, EdD, RD
Associate Professor and Cochair
Division of Nutrition and Preventive
   Dentistry
Tufts University School of Dental Medicine
Boston, Massachusetts

**Kichuel K. Park, DDS, MSD, DDPH,
   PhD**
Professor
Department of Preventive Dentistry
Indiana University School of Dentistry
Indianapolis, Indiana

Mirren Peterson, Dental Therapist
Health Care Otago
Dunedin, New Zealand

Maureen C. Rounds, MEd, RDH
Associate Clinical Professor and Cochair
Division of Nutrition and Preventive
   Dentistry
Tufts University School of Dental Medicine
Boston, Massachusetts

Stephen Sobel, DDS
Assistant Professor of
    Clinical Dentistry
Department of Dental Medicine
    and Public Health,
Section of Geriatric and Special Patient
    Dentistry
University of Southern California School
    of Dentistry
Los Angeles, California

George K. Stookey, MSD, PhD
Associate Dean for Research
Professor of Preventive Dentistry
Director, Oral Health Research Institute
Indiana University School of Dentistry
Indianapolis, Indiana

Terri S. I. Tilliss, RDH, MS
Associate Professor
University of Colorado School of Dentistry
Department of Oral Hygiene
Denver, Colorado

James S. Wefel, BS, PhD
Associate Director of Dows Institute for
    Dental Research
The Iowa University School of Dentistry
Iowa City, Iowa

Donald E. Willmann, DDS
Associate Professor
Department of Periodontics
University of Texas Dental School
    at San Antonio, Texas
San Antonio, Texas

Samuel L. Yankell, MS, PhD
Research Professor, Department
    of Periodontics
University of Pennsylvania School
    of Dentistry
Philadelphia, Pennsylvania

Janet Yellowitz, DMD, MPH, RDH
Director, Geriatric Dentistry
University of Maryland Dental School
Baltimore, Maryland

Contents

Preface

The useful lifetime of much knowledge is finite. As new discoveries are made or as old diseases are gradually conquered, new priorities emerge. Because textbooks are a major source of information used in the education of a health professional, it is urgent that they be as current as possible.

The first three editions chronicled a great number of changes in preventive dentistry practices between 1978 and 1989; this fourth edition updates that information to 1993. One of the most troublesome problems with each successive edition has been the need to drop many older references to find space for the new. Every effort was made to retain citations from past landmark research that is still the basis for today's laboratory and clinical achievements. Major revisions have been made throughout the book to reflect the increasing emphasis on periodontal disease, patient education, use of pit and fissure sealants, remineralization of teeth, and geriatric dentistry. Thirty-one authors and coauthors from 21 teaching institutions have participated in the rewriting of the chapters to help ensure inclusion of the most current knowledge. Canadian, British, and New Zealand writers are now represented among the authors, reflecting the rich contributions to preventive dentistry from these nations.

In anticipation of the inclusion of dentistry in a U.S. national health program, we completely revised five chapters with these closely related topics: fluoride, public health dentistry, school oral health programs, hospital dentistry, and the clinical applications of primary prevention. In addition, a short concluding section entitled "Hot Topics" was added to summarize areas of emerging interest: geriatric dentistry, smoking cessation, the New Zealand School Dental Service, and antiplaque agents.

Although the facts contained in the book were greatly upgraded, the format of presentation remains the same. The text is written in an easy, narrative style that facilitates learning. Each chapter begins with a list of learning objectives, is followed by embedded and self-evaluation questions, and includes an extensive list of references. With these elements, a teacher can develop mastery learning or remedial programs, and the student can continually monitor progress. In short, the authors have earnestly striven to produce a "user-friendly," instructive and up-to-date book for the student and the dental health professional. We hope we fulfilled the words of Amos Bronson Alcott: "That is a good book which is opened with expectations, and closed with delight and profit."

Acknowledgments

Thanks must go to those who put up with us and those who helped us. In the former category are our wives, Grace and Joan, who many times patiently watched us write when it meant giving up other more enjoyable avocations. In the latter group are many of the book's authors and coauthors, as well as fellow scientists, clinicians, and teachers who contributed photographs, facts, and figures that have greatly improved the teaching capabilities of the text. Special thanks must go to Dr. William R. Grigsby of the School of Dentistry at Iowa State University for aid in preparation, editorial review, and pictorial contributions to Chapter 2. And finally, few books reach their maximum potential without the intercession of the copy editor. In this case, that laborious and meticulous task was accomplished in exemplary fashion by Linda Davoli.

It is our hope that these combined efforts by others will help contribute to a greater knowledge of and a higher level of practice of primary preventive dentistry in our profession and for our people.

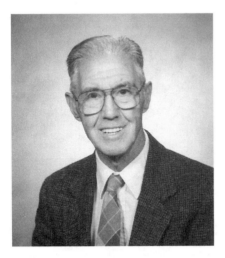

Norman O. Harris
DDS, MSD, FACD

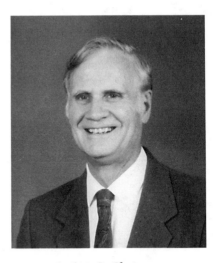

Arden G. Christen
DDS, MSD, MA, FACD

Chapter 1

Introduction to Primary Preventive Dentistry

Norman O. Harris

Objectives

At the end of this chapter it will be possible to

1. Define the following key terms—*health, primary prevention, secondary prevention*, and *tertiary prevention*—and provide specific examples of each.
2. Name four convenient categories that aid in classifying dental disease and in planning oral disease prevention and treatment programs.
3. Name five general approaches to prevention of dental caries or periodontal disease.
4. Cite two *early* actions that are essential for arresting the progression of disease once primary preventive measures have failed.
5. Analyze and explain why effective plaque control programs can prevent periodontal disease yet not be effective in preventing more than two thirds of all oral carious lesions.
6. Explain how the planned application of current preventive dentistry concepts and practices, including remineralization, when coupled with early detection and immediate treatment of the plaque diseases, can result in a zero or near zero annual extraction rate.

Introduction

First, it is necessary to define a few key words. *Health* is what we want to preserve, so the word must be defined. Health can be defined as "a state of complete *physical, mental,* and *social* well-being, and not merely the absence of disease or infirmity." For instance, some individuals may actually be in excellent health but believe for some reason, logical to them, that they have cancer. In such cases they do not have mental well-being and will continue to worry until they are somehow convinced that they indeed are healthy. Another person may be functionally healthy, although facially disfigured; such an individual could be socially shunned throughout life. Thus health can at times be what the patient thinks, not the condition of the body.

Even the phrase *preventive dentistry* has different meanings to different people. As a result, preventive dentistry has been broken down into three different levels. (1) *Primary prevention* employs techniques and agents to *forestall* the onset of disease, to *reverse* the progress of the initial stages of disease, or to *arrest* the disease process before treatment becomes necessary. (2) *Secondary prevention* employs routine treatment methods to *terminate* a disease process and to *restore* tissues to as near normal as possible. (3) *Tertiary prevention* employs measures necessary to *replace* lost tissues and to *rehabilitate* patients to the point that function is as near normal as possible after the failure of secondary prevention (Fig 1–1).

Question 1. Which of the following statements, if any, are correct?

A.   The absence of a disease or infirmity is a good sign of physical health but not of mental and social well-being.

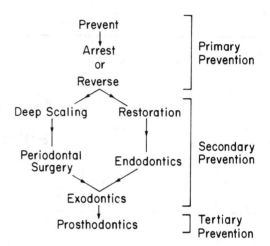

Figure 1–1. From natural teeth to denture teeth in three not-so-easy stages.

B.   A professional football player who looks well, has no physical infirmities, but continually worries about his $1,000,000 contract can be considered in excellent health.

C.   An amalgam restoration that is placed in a carious occlusal pit of a molar is an excellent example of *tertiary* prevention.

D.   The avoidance of an etiologic factor for a specific disease is an example of *primary* prevention.

E.   Preventive dentistry embodies primary, secondary, and tertiary prevention.

In going from primary to tertiary prevention, the cost of health care increases, and patient satisfaction decreases. An excellent example is the care of a poliomyelitis victim. The cost of the polio vaccine is only a few dollars; the use of this vaccine to prevent the onset of disease is inexpensive and effective. For someone not adequately immunized, the cost of polio rehabilitation, after the damage is done, approximates $35,000 or more. Yet the individual receiving the $35,000 worth of tertiary preventive treatment is certainly not as happy as one who received only a few dollar's worth of primary preventive care. Another appropriate example is the fluoridation of drinking water. This costs approximately fifty cents[1] per year per individual, yet it reduces the incidence of dental caries in the community by 20% to 40%.[2] If this primary preventive measure is not instituted, the necessary restorative dentistry (secondary prevention) costs far more—100 times more—or about $50.00 per restoration.[3] Finally, if restorative dentistry fails, as it often does, prosthetic appliances must be constructed at an even greater cost. This disparity between the lower cost of prevention and the much higher cost of treatment must be seriously considered if the United States is to develop an affordable national health program in which dentistry is represented.

From these examples it should be possible to understand that the health sciences professions are concerned with preventing not only the *onset* of disease but also the *extension* of the damage resulting from disease, once disease is inevitable. This text emphasizes the former objective, that is, *primary* prevention, and specifically focuses on primary prevention as it applies to the control of dental caries and periodontal disease. On the other hand, it must be recognized that primary prevention often fails for many reasons. When such failure occurs, two actions are absolutely essential to contain the damage: (1) *early identification* of the lesion and (2) *immediate treatment* of the lesion, once identified.

CATEGORIES OF ORAL DISEASE

For planning purposes dental disease can be conveniently grouped into four categories: (1) *dental caries*, (2) *periodontal disease*, (3) *acquired oral conditions* other than dental caries and periodontal disease, and (4) *hereditary disorders*.

Caries and periodontal disease account for most of the dental treatment bill of $34 billion spent in 1991 by the estimated 40% to 50% of the public who regularly visit the dentist.[4-6] Both of these dental diseases are due to the presence of dental plaque and hence are known as the *plaque diseases*. Any major reduction in the incidence of these disease processes will release resources for the investigation and treatment of conditions included in the third and fourth categories. The *ideal*, or *long-range*, planning objectives for treating both dental caries and periodontal disease should be the development of a delivery system and methods to attain a zero, or near zero, disease *incidence*[a] for a target population. However, a more *realistic and feasible, short-term goal* is the attainment of a zero, or near zero, rate of *tooth loss* from these diseases. Because of the varied etiology of the third and fourth categories, that is, other acquired conditions and hereditary disorders, the planning for the control of each of these disease areas must be accomplished individually and placed within the priorities of any overall health plan developed.

Question 2. Which of the following statements, if any, are correct?

  A. The *total* spectrum of *preventive dentistry* includes only the use of primary preventive techniques or agents.

  B. The *broad concept* of preventive dentistry places major emphasis on primary preventive care but also considers the need for secondary and tertiary preventive care.

---

[a] Incidence: The amount of disease that occurs in a given period.

C. Because dental caries and periodontal disease are infectious diseases (true), they are *acquired* conditions.

D. The *ideal*, or *long-range*, objective for dentistry is a zero annual extraction loss; the more *realistic, short-range*, objective is the development of primary preventive measures to prevent the onset of *any* pathology.

E. Acquired conditions (other than caries and periodontal disease) and hereditary disease account for the *great proportion* of income derived by the dental profession.

STRATEGIES TO PREVENT PLAQUE DISEASES

Before providing an overview of the methods used to implement primary prevention programs, it is important to point out that *both* dental caries and periodontal disease are *infectious* processes caused by the bacteria of the dental plaque. Any infectious disease can be initiated only if the *challenge organisms* are in sufficient numbers to overwhelm the combined *body defense* and *repair* capability. For this reason all strategies to prevent, arrest, or reverse the plaque diseases are based on (1) reducing the number of challenge oral pathogens, (2) building up the tooth's defenses, and (3) enhancing the repair processes.

For both caries and periodontal disease, *visible* incipient (beginning) lesions, if identified at the time of the dental examination, can be easily reversed with primary preventive strategies. For caries, the incipient lesion is a "*white spot*," which occurs on the surface of the enamel as a result of acid-induced *demineralization* occurring *under the plaque*. For periodontal disease, the incipient lesion is *gingivitis* (ie, an inflammation of the gingiva), which occurs along the

gingiva that is *in contact with the plaque*. In both cases, it should be noted that if dental plaque did not exist, or if the adverse effects of its microbial inhabitants could be negated, the decrease in the incidence of the plaque diseases would be dramatic. Based on these facts, it is understandable why plaque control is so important in an oral health program.

To control the plaque diseases with available methods and techniques, major emphasis has been directed in five general areas: (1) *mechanical and chemical plaque control*, (2) use of *fluorides*, (3) *sugar discipline*, (4) use of *pit and fissure sealants*, and (5) *education*. A brief review of each of these primary preventive procedures serves as a basis for the more detailed information presented in later chapters.

Plaque Control

Dental plaque is composed of *salivary* proteins that adhere to the teeth plus *bacteria* and *end products of bacterial metabolism*. The organic acids, which are the end products and are in close contact with the *tooth surface*, are responsible for dental caries. Still other damaging end products of bacterial metabolism that are in contact with the *soft tissues* immediately surrounding the tooth are the cause of periodontal disease. Dental plaque, with its microbial constituents, is found mainly (1) along the *margin of the gingiva*, (2) *beneath the gingiva* in the gingival sulcus, which surrounds the teeth, (3) in the *interproximal* areas, (4) in the *deep pits and fissures*, and (5) on *exposed roots*. Plaque accumulates at these specific sites because *none* of these locations is optimally exposed to the normal self-cleansing action of the saliva, the abrasive action of foods, or the muscular action of the cheeks and tongue.

The plaque is usually found in greater quantity just above the gingiva on all four sides of the tooth. It decreases in thickness as the incisal or occlusal surface is approached. Little plaque is found on the occlusal surface except in the pits and fissures. Here the amount is greatest where the fissures are deep and narrow. In the gingival sulcus between the gingiva and the tooth, little or no plaque occurs until gingival inflammation begins, at which time the bacterial population increases in quantity and complexity as the disease state intensifies. Plaque forms more profusely on malposed teeth or on teeth with orthodontic appliances, where brushing is often inadequate.

It is important to differentiate between the *supragingival* and the *subgingival* plaques. The supragingival plaque can be seen above the gingival margin; the subgingival plaque is found in periodontal pockets below the gingival margin, where it is not visible. The supragingival plaque harbors bacteria that can cause *supragingival caries;* the subgingival plaque microbiota is mainly responsible for *periodontal problems* and *root caries.* The bacterial populations of each of these plaques differ qualitatively and quantitatively in health and disease.[7] The pathogenicity of each of the plaques can vary independently of the others. For example, it is possible to have periodontal disease with or without caries, to have neither, or to have a shifting status of caries or periodontal disease or both.

In many cases plaque is difficult for a patient to identify. This problem is overcome—at least in the case of the supragingival plaque—by the use of *disclosing agents*, which are harmless dyes such as the staining agent FD&C Red #28, which stains plaque red. The dyes may be in *solution* and painted on the teeth with a cotton applicator, or they may be *tablets*, which are chewed, swished around the mouth, and then expectorated. Once disclosed, most of the supragingival plaque can be easily re-

moved by the individual by the daily use of a toothbrush (Fig 1–2) and dental floss (Fig 1–3). It can also be removed at appropriate intervals by a dental hygienist or a dentist as part of an *oral prophylaxis*, a procedure that has as its objective the mechanical removal of all soft and hard deposits on the teeth. However, because *daily* removal of the plaque is most effective, it is the individual—*not* the hygienist or the dentist—who is vital in preserving dental health.

There is one site where neither the dentist nor an individual can successfully remove all the plaque; neither can the flow of saliva nor the muscular action of cheeks and tongue greatly influence the eventual development of caries. That site is in the depth of *pits and fissures* of occlusal surfaces where the orifices are too small for the toothbrush bristle to penetrate (see Fig 10–2).

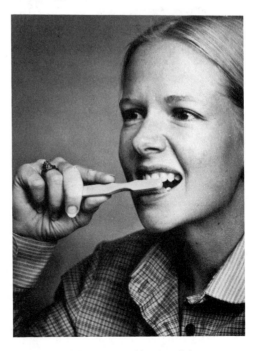

Figure 1–2. Plaque control is essential.

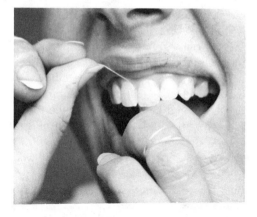

Figure 1–3. Flossing gets down under the gingiva.

As soon as the plaque is removed from any tooth, it *immediately* begins to build up again. This should not be unexpected, since by definition dental plaque is composed of salivary residue, bacteria, and their end products, all of which are always present in the mouth. Thus a good plaque control program must be *continuous*. It must be a daily commitment over a lifetime.

Question 3. Which of the following statements, if any, are correct?

A. The five general areas that form the basis for *primary* prevention of dental diseases are (1) plaque control, (2) fluorides, (3) sealants, (4) restorations, and (5) education.

B. Plaque is found *only* on the smooth surfaces of the enamel.

C. Plaque removal *requires instrumentation* employed by a dentist or a hygienist.

D. Good flossing and toothbrushing techniques remove the dental plaque from all tooth surfaces.

E. The *daily* removal of plaque by an individual is more effective than its semiannual removal by the dental hygienist.

Not only does the daily removal of the dental plaque reduce the possibility of *dental caries*; equally important, it also reduces the possibility of the onset and progression of *periodontal disease*. The toxic metabolic end products of bacteria that are contained in the plaque can be irritating to the adjacent gingival tissues, producing *inflammation*, that is, gingivitis. If the inflammation continues, bleeding (hemorrhage) can be expected following even minimal pressure. This inflammation can be *prevented* or *reversed* in the early stages by proper flossing and brushing habits.

The plaque concentrates mineralizing ions such as calcium, phosphate, magnesium, and carbonates from the saliva to provide the chemical environment for the precipitation and formation of *calculus*, a concretion that adheres firmly to the tooth. If the plaque is not removed by flossing and brushing *before* the calculus begins to form, the resultant mineralized mass provides a greater surface area for even more damaging plaque accumulation. This additional mass of plaque covering the rough surface of the calculus is responsible for damage to the periodontal tissues overlying the deposits. However, the hard, irregular calculus deposits pressing against the soft tissues probably augment the inflammation caused by the bacteria alone. Thus the daily removal of plaque can successfully abort or markedly retard the buildup of calculus. Once the calculus forms, the toothbrushing and flossing usually used for plaque control do *not* remove the deposits. At this time the hygienist or dentist must intercede to remove the calculus by instrumentation.

At this early point it should be apparent that an individual participating in an effective daily plaque control program can greatly reduce the need for treatment of those conditions for which professional dental care is most sought—cavities (dental caries), bleeding gums (gingivitis), and cleaning (calculus removal). The only exceptions are the carious lesions developing in the deep pits and fissures, where effective plaque control methods are not possible.

To this point, only mechanical plaque control (ie, use of a toothbrush and dental floss) has been highlighted. Rapidly growing in importance as a *supplement* to mechanical plaque control (*but not a replacement for it*), however, is chemical plaque control. This approach utilizes mouth rinses containing antimicrobial agents that are effective in controlling the plaque bacteria and in reducing gingivitis. Currently, the most promising rinse is *chlorhexidine.* In Europe, where *varnishes*[b] with 40% chlorhexidine have been painted on the teeth, the growth of mutans streptococci has been totally suppressed for 2 to 5 months.[8,9]

Fluorides

The use of fluorides has provided exceptionally effective reduction in the incidence of dental caries. Because of the presence of fluoride in water, dentifrices, and mouth rinses, dental caries is declining throughout the industrialized world.[10] In the United States this decline over the past 7 years has approximated 35%. The placement of fluoride in communal water supplies has repeatedly resulted in an approximate 20% to 40% reduction in caries incidence in the population[2] (Fig 1–4). This protection is greatest on the smooth surfaces of the teeth; it is least effective in protecting the pits and fissures of the teeth. Approximately 126 million individuals in the United States consume *fluoridated water* through com-

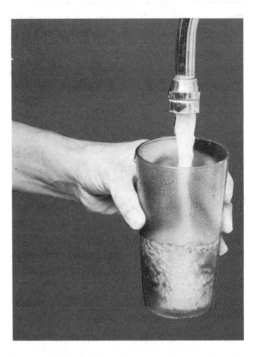

Figure 1–4. Water fluoridation reduces cavities in the population by 20% to 40%.

munal water supplies and another 9 million are drinking naturally fluoridated water—together, making up approximately 65% of the U.S. population.[11] Many times during the past years it has not been possible to fluoridate city water supplies due to *political, technical,* or *financial* considerations. In such cases it is still possible to receive the systemic benefits of fluorides by the installation of small fluoridation units in school water supplies. Dietary supplements can be given in the form of fluoride tablets or drops. It is also possible to apply fluoride directly to the teeth by use of cotton pledgets, therapeutic dentifrices, gels, or mouth rinses. Such applications to the surface of the teeth are referred to as *topical applications.* Generally speaking, the extent of caries control achieved through topical applications is directly related to the number of times the fluoride is applied and the

---

[b] Chlorhexidine varnishes are not sold in the United States. As a prescription item, it is only sold as a 1.2% mouth rinse of chlorhexidine gluconate, manufactured by Procter & Gamble under the trade name, Peridex.

length of time the fluoride is in contact with the teeth. Also, research data indicate that it is better to apply lower concentrations of fluoride to the teeth more often than to apply higher concentrations at longer spaced intervals. This is one reason for advocating the daily use of fluoridated water, dentifrices and mouth rinses.

Question 4. Which of the following statements, if any, are correct?

   A. Plaque control aids in the control of *both* caries and periodontal disease.

   B. Even after calculus becomes attached to the tooth, it can *still* be removed by good home plaque control programs.

   C. The addition of fluoride to communal water supplies is accompanied by only a 20% to 40% decrease in caries incidence.

   D. The application of *higher* concentrations of fluoride at *longer* time intervals is more effective than *lower* concentrations of fluorides at *shorter* intervals.

   E. A *topical application* of fluoride can only be accomplished by a dentist or a dental hygienist.

The action of topically applied fluoride in preventing dental caries is not completely understood. It is believed that it has several actions: (1) it may enter the dental plaque and there *affect the bacteria* by depressing their production of acid and thus reduce the possibility of demineralization of the tooth; (2) it reacts with the mineral elements on the surface of the tooth to make the *enamel more insoluble* to the acid end products of bacterial metabolism; and (3) it *facilitates the remineralization* (repair) of teeth that have been slightly demineralized by acid end products.[12,13] The source of minerals needed for remineralization is the saliva.

Sugar and Diet

The development of dental caries depends on four interrelated factors: (1) *diet*, (2) inherent factors of *host resistance*, (3) the *bacteria* located in the dental plaque, and (4) *time* (Fig 1–5). Without bacteria no caries can develop. For the bacteria in the plaque to live, they must have the same amino acids, monosaccharides, fatty acids, vitamins, and minerals that are required for all living organisms. Because these nutrients are also required by the cells of the body, the food that is ingested by the host or that later appears in the saliva in a metabolized form provides adequate nutrients for bacterial survival and reproduction. With three *well-balanced* meals per day, however, the usual plaque bacteria probably cannot release a sufficient quantity of metabolic acids to cause caries development (Fig 1–6). They continue to live even though their

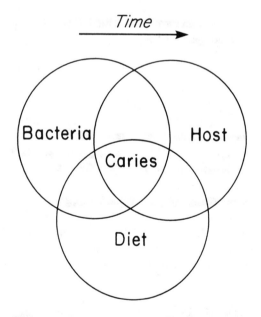

Figure 1–5. Caries is a *multifactorial* disease caused by bacteria, a supporting host diet of refined carbohydrates, decreased host resistance, and time for the cavity to develop.

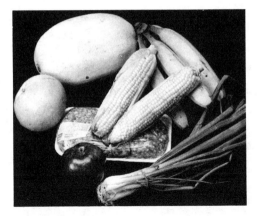

Figure 1–6. This balanced meal does not provide the bacteria with enough energy to produce acids.

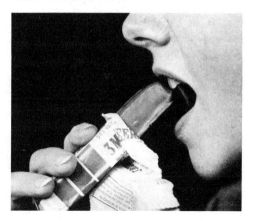

Figure 1–7. Snacks such as this expose teeth to bacterial acids.

reproduction is probably not as prolific. As soon as *sugar and sugar products* are included in the diet of the host, bacterial metabolism markedly increases. With this rapid increase of activity, the release of the acid end products that are the major factor in caries initiation and development also increases.[14] Probably of more importance than the *total* intake of refined carbohydrates are the *frequency* of intake and the *consistency* of the sugar-containing foods.[15] The continuous snacks of refined carbohydrates that characterize modern living result in the teeth being constantly exposed to bacterial acids (Fig 1–7). Similarly, prolonged adherence of sugar products to the teeth, such as that experienced after eating taffies and hard candy, results in an excessive production of the plaque acids. Thus if caries incidence is to be reduced, all three factors—total intake, frequency of intake, and the consistency of the potentially cariogenic foods—should be controlled.

Possibly one of the most promising means of reducing caries incidence in the United States has been the wide-scale acceptance of the sugar substitute aspartame (NutraSweet) as a sweetening agent. The

ingestion of this sweetener does not result in bacterial proliferation and acidogenesis. Recently another sweetener, acesulfame-K (Sunette), has been placed on the market, and will presumably further reduce sugar (sucrose) consumption.

Pit and Fissure Sealants

Approximately two thirds or more of all the carious lesions in the mouth occur on the occlusal surfaces of the posterior teeth.[16] These surfaces represent only 12% of the total number of tooth surfaces, so the occlusal surfaces are approximately eight times as vulnerable as all the other smooth surfaces. The availability of sealants offers considerable promise in reducing this problem. With their use, a thin layer of an epoxy plastic, called Bis-GMA,[c] is flowed into the deep pits and fissures of teeth not having open carious lesions, effectively isolating those areas from the oral environment (Fig 1–8). No pain or discomfort accompanies sealant placement. Following the placement of the sealant in the deep fissures, the

---

[c] Bisphenol A-glycidyl methacrylate.

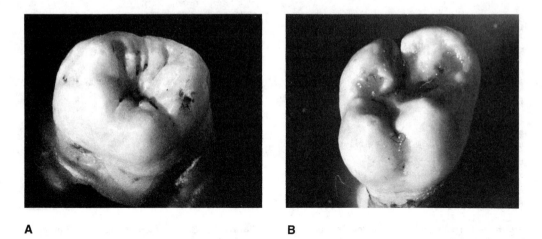

A   **B**

Figure 1–8. Molar **A.** without and **B.** with a clear plastic sealant to protect the deep occlusal fissures.

newly created shallow fossae can be cleaned very effectively with a toothbrush.

As long as the sealants are retained, no bacteria or bacterial acids can affect the sealed areas. If they are not retained, no damage to the teeth results from the treatment. The lost sealant can be easily replaced. One 10-year study demonstrated a 57% retention of the original sealants.[17] In another, approximately 95% retention occurred over 2 years.[18] With these performances the average life of a sealant is comparable to that of the 10 years projected for an amalgam.[19] It should be emphasized that sealant placement should be followed by use of topical fluorides, because the fluorides are most effective on the smooth surfaces of teeth and least effective on the occlusal surfaces—a situation that is the reverse of the results expected of the sealants.

Question 5. Which of the following statements, if any, are correct?

A. Fluorides make the mineral phase (calcium and phosphate salts) of the surface of the enamel *more resistant* to acids as well as *depress* the ability of the plaque bacteria to release acid end products.

B. If a limited amount of calcium and phosphorous is lost from the tooth surface through demineralization, it *can* be replaced by remineralization.

C. The development of dental caries depends on *four* factors: (1) *diet*; (2) inherent factors of *host resistance*; (3) *bacteria*; and (4) *time*.

D. Refined carbohydrates *alone* provide sufficient nutrition for cariogenic bacteria.

E. Plastic sealants are most effective in preventing *smooth* surface caries, whereas *fluorides* are most effective in preventing caries in the deep occlusal *pits* and *fissures*.

Public Education

If the profession of dentistry can control caries effectively through *plaque control*, the *systemic* (ingested) and *topical* (local application) use of *fluorides, dietary control*, and the use of plastic *sealants*, two important questions need to be asked:

1. Why do we not have a more effective dental caries control program in the United States and elsewhere in the world?
2. If daily toothbrushing and flossing of teeth remove plaque, why are these simple procedures not used effectively to control *both* caries and periodontal disease?

Probably the best answer to these questions is that people must first know that they need to do something as well as how it is to be done. Unfortunately the public has relatively little information about the tremendous potential of primary preventive dentistry for reducing the ravages of the plaque diseases. Without this information it is difficult to convince people that they can greatly control their own dental destiny. Instead, people think of dentistry as a treatment-oriented profession that specializes in periodontal treatment, restorations, endodontics, exodontics, and prosthetics. Thus an expanded public education program is essential to ensure the success of any preventive dentistry program in which an individual or a community is asked to participate.

In dentistry, a one-to-one relationship between the patient and the health professional is still the basic approach to patient education and motivation. This approach makes the task impossible because there are 250 million people in the United States and only approximately 143,000 practicing dentists, plus 47,000 dental hygienists and 175,000 assistants.[20,21] The main thrust of public dental health education is provided by the various dentifrice manufacturers advocating a daily toothbrushing routine and biannual visits to the dentist for a checkup.

Unfortunately, knowing facts and applying the information are two separate processes. The application of knowledge by an individual *requires* a personal commitment; it is at this point of personal commitment that most primary preventive dentistry programs fail.[3] For instance, if people embraced the daily use of mechanical and chemical plaque control, risk of caries and gingivitis would be minimal. Similarly, exercising sugar discipline would further reduce the possibility of caries. Conversely, if individuals rejected the use of cigarettes as well as smokeless tobacco, oral cancer would be a very rare disease. Clearly, self-discipline, motivation, and behavior modification are a part of enjoying good oral health.

A sound, well-planned program of dental health education is lacking in the curriculum of the great majority of primary and secondary schools. Few people can discuss the advantages and possible disadvantages of fluoride. Few have any detailed information about dental plaque and the disease-inducing potentialities of this bacterial film. Few know *why* sugar is cariogenic. Finally, few people know the cause of periodontal disease.

Ideally, school-based and public education programs should exist to help people to help themselves in applying primary preventive procedures. The same programs should teach all individuals to recognize the presence of oral disease. With proper instruction, which can be provided by school teachers, individuals can be taught to understand that they must assume major responsibility for their own oral health. Only the individual can seek immediate treatment when pain occurs or disease is obvious. Public dental health education might benefit if a consumer organization—an American Oral Health Association existed—that could promote oral health education, much like what the American Cancer Society and the American Heart Association accomplish in their domains. Besides education, a method is needed to ensure continual screening of the population to identify disease *early* and to refer afflicted individuals for *immediate*, definitive diagnosis and treatment.

An example of the great potential of such early identification and treatment in reducing extractions in a school population, is the New Zealand school dental nurse program. In the New Zealand School Dental Service, a *dental nurse* visits every primary and secondary school in New Zealand at approximately 6-month intervals. At that time all the children receive a dental examination. If necessary the dental nurse then restores the carious teeth, removes visible calculus, or refers the child to a dentist for more complex treatment requirements.

As a result of this program, the average rate of extractions dropped from 19 per 100 in 1960, to 2 per 1000 in 1979.[22] From 1973 until 1992, the average decayed, missing, or filled permanent teeth (DMFT) for 12- to 14-year-old children plummeted from 10.7 to 1.88 per child. (See Chapter 22, New Zealand School Dental Service.)[3] Approximately 96% of all New Zealand school children are enrolled in this program. Unfortunately relatively few comprehensive primary preventive dentistry programs are being conducted in U.S. school systems. With the implementation of a well-planned prevention, identification, treatment, and education program, it *should be possible to achieve rapidly a zero or near zero tooth loss among school children resulting from either caries or periodontal disease.*

Question 6. Which of the following statements, if any, are correct?

A. A primary preventive technique is more likely to be accomplished at home by individuals who know *how* to do it and *why* they are doing it.

B. Once people know *how* and *why* they are to use a preventive proce-

dure, they are then completely *motivated* to use such a procedure.

C. There are enough dentists and dental auxiliaries in the United States to give approximately 1 hour a year of education lectures to each of the 250 million inhabitants of the nation.

D. *Many aspects* of oral health care can be taught equally well (or better) by a well-trained school teacher as by a dentist or hygienist.

E. School programs routinely emphasize primary preventive dentistry information and programs as part of the curriculum.

Prognostic and Diagnostic Tests

Up to this point several methods for preventing the onset or progress of caries and periodontal disease have been discussed. Because it is impossible to apply vigorously all the preventive procedures all the time to all the people, it would be desirable to have some tests to indicate the extent of caries and periodontal disease susceptibility of an *individual* at any given time. This need is highlighted by the fact that an estimated 60% of all carious lesions in school children occur in 20% of pupils.[23] It would be highly desirable to be able to identify this 20% of high-risk students without having to examine an entire population. Although no tests are 100% correlated with the extent of caries activity or periodontal disease, several test procedures are sufficiently well correlated with either condition to be of interest. Such a screening test should be simple to accomplish, economical, require a minimum of equipment, be easy to evaluate, and be compatible with mass handling techniques.

Several microbiologic *caries activity tests* are available to estimate the *presumptive* caries status of an individual. For example, Alban's test, which is a *colorimetric* test is easily adaptable to an office practice.[24] In this test a sample of saliva is placed in a tube of selective bacteriologic medium and incubated. If the sample is taken from individuals with a large number of carious lesions, usually the high number of cariogenic bacteria grow rapidly. In the process, the bacteria release acids that cause the color indicator (a dye) in the media to change rapidly from the initial greenish blue to yellow. On the other hand, bacteria normally found in a mouth exhibiting a low caries incidence grow much more slowly in the acid environment, thus producing little, if any, change in the color of the media.

Laboratory methods also exist for *counting* the number of bacteria in the saliva. Again, if the mutans streptococci or lactobacilli counts are high, the individual from whom the sample was taken can be *presumed* to have a higher risk for dental caries, whereas a low count permits the opposite assumption. The results of both the colorimetric test and the bacterial counts are *statistically* correlated with the caries status of *groups* of people from whom the samples originated. However, attempting to apply the test findings to predict future caries status on an *individual* basis is rather precarious. How to cope with this problem of individual variation will be discussed in Chapter 12.

A second general method for estimating caries susceptibility is by use of *dietary analysis* to (1) evaluate the patient's overall diet with special attention to food preferences and amounts consumed and (2) determine if the intake of refined carbohydrates is excessive in quantity or frequency (see Chapter 15). A well-balanced diet is assumed to *raise host resistance* to all disease processes, whereas the frequent and excessive intake of refined carbohydrates (ie, sugar) has been associated with a *high risk of caries development*. The dietary analysis

is most effective when used as a guide for patient education.

The onset of periodontal disease is much more visible than the early demineralization that occurs in caries. The first indication of impending periodontal disease is an inflammation of the gingiva (gingivitis), which can be localized at one site or generalized around all the teeth. Red, bleeding, swollen, or sore gingiva are readily apparent to dentist and patient alike.

The Phase Microscope

The diverse oral microbial population seen in health or disease seen in the mouth is known as the *oral flora*. The bacteria of the flora can be readily observed by the use of a phase microscope,[25] which allows for the visualization of the number and variety of *living, unstained* organisms in a sample of plaque. Usually, in health, relatively few nonmotile cocci and rods occur. A sample of saliva taken from an inflamed site, however, demonstrates a dense, teeming, and highly motile bacterial microcosm. Rapidly vibrating small organisms; majestic, twirling spirochetes; long, rod-shaped bacteria, and large ameboid organisms move in and out of the microscope field. After the inflammation has been successfully treated, repeat specimens again show normal flora with only occasional cells moving slowly into view.

Question 7. Which of the following statements, if any, are correct?

A. Caries activity tests are 100% *specific* for indicating the susceptibility or nonsusceptibility of an *individual*.

B. Two methods used to estimate *caries* susceptibility or nonsusceptibility are Alban's test and the use of the phase microscope.

C. A high and frequent intake of refined carbohydrates are expected to be accompanied by the *greenish blue* color end point of the Alban's test.

D. A phase microscope provides a convenient way to study the *living*, unstained bacterial population of the gingival pocket.

E. Both the quantity and the frequency of intake of sugar and sugar products should be considered in a dietary analysis.

Remineralization of Teeth

Both demineralization and remineralization occur during caries development. Carious lesions develop when the rate of acid-induced demineralization of teeth exceeds the capability of the saliva to remineralize the damaged enamel components. Following the intake of sugar, a localized demineralization of the enamel occurs as a result of the acid produced by the plaque bacteria. This negative mineral balance, if continually repeated, eventually results in a carious lesion. It often requires months, or even years, for the lesion to develop.[26] During this time, under proper conditions, a compensatory remineralization of the damaged area can occur by mineral components in the saliva. There is a precedent for such a mineralization potential. Immediately after eruption of the teeth, the outer layer of the enamel is not completely mineralized; the maturing (mineralization) of this outer layer occurs within the first year as a result of being bathed in the saliva.[27]

The point at which the developing lesion is no longer reversible is not known, but clinical experience indicates that as long as the lesion is incipient (ie, with no cavitation) remineralization is possible.[28] The need to exploit this possibility is emphasized by Koulourides' statement that "there is a wide gap between current practices of many dental clinicians and the potential applica-

tion of present scientific knowledge to arrest and reverse incipient carious lesions."[29] The outstanding research contributions of Silverstone, which have led to a better understanding of the demineralization and remineralization processes, offer the possibility of substituting early biologic remineralization for later amalgam restorations.[13] Missing at the present time is an accurate predictive test that would permit the targeting of individuals experiencing early caries development.

The conditions for optimum remineralization are the *same* as for preventing the initiation of a lesion: (1) plaque control to reduce the negative effects of bacterial acidogenesis, (2) sugar discipline to minimize the number of acidogenic episodes, and (3) the use of fluorides that potentiate the remineralization process. Thus with the same primary preventive dentistry routines, an individual can simultaneously protect teeth into the *future* and compensate for limited *past* damage.

Question 8. Which of the following statements, if any, are correct?

A. Caries develops over a period of time when the cumulative negative mineral balance of the tooth exceeds the capacity for remineralization.

B. Once cavitation is present, remineralization *is still a feasible alternative* to restorative dentistry.

C. Plaque control, sugar discipline, and topical fluoride therapy not only are effective in preventing demineralization but also can arrest and reverse the carious process.

D. The concept of natural *mineralization* of teeth following eruption is more accepted than the biologic repair of teeth by natural (or fluoride induced) *remineralization*.

E. Dental auxiliaries can carry out the techniques for preventing demineralization and for facilitating remineralization of teeth.

SUMMARY

Each year more than $34 billion is spent in the United States for dental care, mostly for the treatment of dental caries and periodontal disease or their sequelae, yet manpower, money, and techniques now exist (1) that could greatly aid in *preventing the onset* of caries or periodontal disease or (2) that *prevent the loss* of the teeth by early *identification* and expeditious *treatment* of the incipient disease process. The five general approaches to the control of both caries and periodontal disease involve (1) plaque control, (2) use of fluorides, (3) use of plastic pit and fissure sealants, (4) sugar discipline, and (5) education. The zeal and thoroughness with which these preventive measures should be prescribed and used are often indicated by the information obtained from the oral examination, a dietary analysis, and caries activity testing.

If at the time of the dental examination, emphasis was placed on searching out the incipient lesions for caries (the white spot) and for periodontal disease (gingivitis), preventive strategies could be applied that would induce a reversal of either disease process. It is essential that both the *profession* and the *public* realize that biologic "repair" of incipient lesions is a viable alternative to later treatment.

Even if these primary preventive dentistry procedures fail, tooth loss can still be avoided. In practice, the early identification and expeditious treatment of caries and periodontal disease greatly minimize the loss of teeth. When such routine diagnostic and treatment services are linked with a dynamic preventive dentistry program, tooth loss can realistically be expected to reduce to zero or near zero.

This introductory chapter pointed out the means by which the dental profession can make primary preventive dentistry its hallmark. The remaining chapters provide the detailed background through which the dental health professional can make this challenge a reality.

ANSWERS AND EXPLANATIONS

1. A, D, E
   B—incorrect. With salaries going up in professional sports, maybe the poor fellow has something to worry about; the correct answer is that continued worry is not healthy.
   C—incorrect. A *restoration* is an excellent example of *secondary* prevention—not tertiary.
2. B, C
   A—incorrect. Preventive dentistry applies to any step taken to prevent, arrest, repair, or rehabilitate.
   D—incorrect. Vice versa; it probably takes many years to develop the chemical or immunologic means to prevent oral disease; we already have the means to reduce the extraction rate greatly by use of primary and secondary preventive means.
   E—incorrect. Caries and periodontal disease (and their sequelae) provide the financial basis for the dental profession.
3. E
   A—incorrect. Number 4 should not be in the list of options; because restorations are a result of operative intervention, they are considered as secondary prevention.
   B—incorrect. Plaque is found on all surfaces of the crown, including the occlusal

surfaces that have pits and fissures (which are not smooth surfaces); it is also found on the root (cementum).

C—incorrect. Plaque removal requires nothing more than a toothbrush and dental floss in the hands of an individual interested in his or her own dental health.

D—incorrect. Deep pits and fissures are often the protected sanctuaries for cariogenic organisms.

4. A, C

B—incorrect. Once calculus becomes attached to the teeth, the toothbrush and the floss are inadequate for removing it.

D—incorrect. The frequency of application is more important than the concentration.

E—incorrect. After all, fluoride dentifrices and mouth rinses are examples of topical applications.

5. A, B, C

D—incorrect. Bacteria need carbohydrates, but they also need fats, proteins, vitamins, and minerals.

E—incorrect. Vice versa; the sealants protect the deep irregular pits and fissures on the occlusal surfaces.

6. A, D

B—incorrect. Knowledge and action are two different things. For instance, people who *know* that their overeating will lead to obesity often do not reduce their food input.

C—incorrect. A one-to-one relationship requires about 1700 hours per year for every dentist; there are only about 1800 working hours in the year. Very few patients could be seen for other than education.

E—incorrect. The teaching of dental health in schools is *minimal*. It usually is restricted to a few lessons on sugar discipline (as part of nutrition) and mention of brushing and flossing.

7. D, E

A—incorrect. This is a hope of the profession; not a reality.

B—incorrect. The phase microscope provides a means of estimating the number and general types of bacteria present; it does not indicate their ability to cause caries (although periodontal involvement can be implied if a large number of spirochetes occur).

C—incorrect. Alban's medium starts with a greenish blue; acid production causes it to turn yellow.

8. A, C, D, E

B—incorrect. Once cavitation occurs, the lesion has progressed to the point that restorative dentistry is indicated.

SELF-EVALUATION QUESTIONS

1. *Health* is defined as _____.
2. If primary prevention fails, the two sequential actions necessary to minimize *progression* of a disease process are _____ and _____.
3. For planning purposes, oral disease can be grouped into four general categories: (1) _____, (2) _____, (3) _____, and (4) _____. Of these four, the following two are the plaque diseases: _____ and _____.
4. The five general agents or techniques used to attain primary prevention in caries control are: _____, _____, _____, _____, and _____.
5. Of the five general methods for caries control, the two that are also valuable in periodontal disease control are: _____ and _____.
6. Plaque control in a home environment requires the following two essential

items or devices: _____ and
_____.

7. Sodium fluoride in the water supply reduces caries by _____ percent.

8. When fluoride is topically applied to the teeth, it has three major actions that aid in the control of dental caries: _____, _____, and _____.

9. Caries development depends on four interrelated factors: _____, _____, _____, and _____. Of these four, _____ (one factor) is absolutely necessary for caries development.

10. Fluoride is most effective in preventing caries on (smooth) (occlusal) surfaces of the teeth, whereas plastic sealants are most effective in preventing caries on (smooth) (occlusal) surfaces of the teeth.

11. Which of the following statements, if any, are correct?
    a. All motivated people are educated.
    b. All educated people are motivated.
    c. All individuals who are motivated to submit to secondary and tertiary preventive methods are motivated to accomplish primary preventive techniques.

12. "Biologic repair" of a tooth results from a positive mineral balance at the enamel surface; the process of replacing the ions lost in demineralization is known as _____.

13. Which of the following statements, if any, are correct?
    a. When using a phase microscope to observe bacteria taken from the gingival pocket, it is necessary to stain the organisms.
    b. Properly spaced examination schedules and the initiation of immediate treatment procedures can reduce

extraction rates, even though they may not reduce caries incidence.
    c. The oral flora includes only those organisms found during oral health.

REFERENCES

1. US Department of Health and Human Services, US Public Health Service. *Report of the ad hoc Subcommittee to Coordinate Environmental Health and Related Programs. Review of Fluoride Benefits and Risks.* Washington, D.C. 1991.
2. Newbrun E. Effectiveness of water fluoridation. *Public Health Dent.* 1989; 49:279–289.
3. Blair KP. Fluoridation in the 1990s. *J Am Coll Dent.* 1992; 59:3.
4. Furino A. Balancing dental service requirements and supplies: The economic evidence. *J Am Dent Assoc.* 1990; 121:685–692.
5. Waldman HB. Dentists and dentistry: We need to tell the whole story. *J Am Coll Dent.* 1990; 57:46–54.
6. US Public Health Service, Centers for Disease Control and Prevention. Health care spending for 1990/1992. *MMWR.* 41/21: 372–381.
7. Listgarten MA. Structure of the microbial flora associated with periodontal health and disease in man. *J Periodont.* 1976; 47: 1–17.
8. Shaeken MJ, Van Der Hoeven JS, Hendrix JC. Effect of varnishes containing chlorhexidine on the human dental plaque flora. *J Dent Res.* 1989; 68:1786–1789.
9. Hildebrandt GH, Pape HR Jr, Syed SA, et al. Effect of slow-release chlorhexidine mouthguards on the levels of selected salivary bacteria. *Caries Res.* 1992; 26:268–274.
10. Kaminsky LS, Mahoney MC, Leach J, et al. Fluoride: Benefits and risks of exposure. *Crit Rev Oral Biol Med.* 1990; 1:261–281.
11. Department of Health and Human Services. US Public Health Service, Centers for Disease Control and Prevention. Letter: FL-139, May 1992.

12. Gron P, Amdur BH. The effect of topically applied fluoride on enamel remineralization in vitro. *Arch Oral Biol.* 1975; 20: 223–224.

13. Silverstone LM. Significance of remineralization in caries prevention. *J Canad Dent Assoc.* 1984; 50:157–166.

14. Knox KW, Schamshula RG. Role of plaque in dental caries. *Aust Dent J.* 1976; 21:48–53.

15. Gustafsson BE, Quensel CE, Lanke LS, et al. The Vipeholm dental caries study. *Acta Odont Scand.* 1954; 11:232–364.

16. National Institute of Dental Research. *Oral Health of United States Children. The National Survey of Dental Caries in U.S. School Children, 1986–1987.* DHHS Publication No. (NIH) 89-2247. Bethesda, MD: US Department of Health and Human Services, 1989.

17. Simonsen RJ. Retention and effectiveness of a single application of white sealant after 10 years. *J Am Dent Assoc.* 1987; 115:31–36.

18. Mertz-Fairhurst EJ, Shuster GS, Fairhurst CW. Arresting caries by sealants: results of a clinical study. *Am Dent Assoc.* 1986; 112: 194–203.

19. Qvist J, Qvist V, and Mjor IA. Placement and longevity of amalgam restorations in Denmark. *J Dent Res. (Spec Iss)* 1990; 69: 236, Abst 1018.

20. Waldman HB. Dentists and dentistry changed in the 1980s. *J Am Coll Dent.* 1989; 56:4–13.

21. US Department of Health and Human Services. Health Resources and Services Administration Bureau of Health Professions. Report to the President and Congress on the Status of Health Personnel in the United States. Volume 1, 1984.

22. Nash J. The New Zealand system. *J Am Dent Assoc.* 1980; 100:660. Letter to the editor.

23. Bohannan HM, Disney JA, Graves RC, et al. *Caries Prevalence in the National Preventive Dentistry Demonstration Program. P-6625,* Santa Monica, Calif: The Rand Corporation; 1981.

24. Alban A. An improved Snyder test. *J Dent Res.* 1970; 49:641.

25. Arnim SS. Microcosm of the human mouth. *J Tenn State Dent Assoc.* 1959; 39:3–28.

26. Backer-Dirks O. Longitudinal dental caries study in children 9–15 years of age. *Arch Oral Biol Supp.* 1961; 6:94–108.

27. Backer-Dirks O. Posteruptive changes in dental enamel. *J Dent Res.* 1966; 45:503–511.

28. de Liefde B. Dental caries: Diagnosis and treatment planning. *New Zealand Dent J.* 1980; 76:12–15.

29. Koulourides TI. To what extent is the incipient lesion of dental caries reversible? In: Rowe NH, ed. Proceedings of symposium on incipient lesions of enamel. University of Michigan School of Dentistry; Ann Arbor, MI, November 11–12, 1977; pp 51–68.

Chapter 2

The Development of Dental Plaque: From Preeruptive Primary Cuticle to Acquired Pellicle to Dental Plaque to Calculus Formation

Hubert N. Newman

Objectives

At the end of this chapter, it will be possible to

1. Differentiate between the *primary enamel cuticle*, the *acquired pellicle*, and the *dental plaque*.
2. Explain why the dental plaque is not unique among naturally occurring microbial layers.
3. Discuss some of the mechanisms proposed to explain *bacterial adhesion* to the acquired pellicle.
4. Distinguish between *primary* and *secondary* bacterial colonizers in dental plaque, and cite examples of each.
5. Describe some of the metabolic activities associated with plaque bacteria.
6. Identify the prime sites of calculus formation, explain how calculus forms, and detail the differences between supragingival and subgingival calculus.
7. State how the acquired pellicle, bacterial dental plaque, and dental calculus are related to caries and chronic inflammatory periodontal disease.

Introduction

The dental profession has to deal with the most widespread of all human diseases, (1) dental caries (tooth decay) and (2) chronic inflammatory diseases of the periodontium (ie, the supporting tissues of the teeth) such as chronic gingivitis (Figure 2–1). These bacterial infections, which to a greater or lesser extent affect most humans, are not caused by a single pathogenic microbe as with such infections as tuberculosis.[1,2] Instead, both are due to accumulations of many different bacteria on teeth that form what is termed the *dental plaque*. (Figure 2–2) Dental plaque *cannot* be removed by rinsing but *can* be removed by brushing and flossing. The *proportions* of different bacteria found in the plaque from a healthy mouth are different from those in a mouth with caries, and both are different from the dental plaque of an individual with chronic inflammatory periodontal disease.

If the role of oral microflora or dental plaque in causing dental caries and inflammatory periodontal disease is to be under-

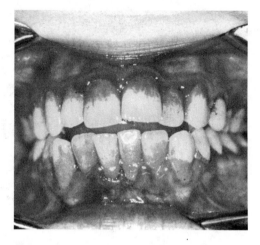

Figure 2–2. The dental plaque on these teeth has been stained with a disclosing solution and rinsed. Note the presence of plaque interproximally and adjacent to the gingiva, but relatively absent closer to the incisal edge. (*Courtesy of Dr WK Grigsby, University of Iowa College of Dentistry.*)

stood, the logical place to start is by examining how dental plaque forms and, in later chapters, how changes in the proportions of different bacteria of the dental plaque lead to oral disease.

Dental Plaque as One of Many Microbial Biofilms

Few surfaces in nature do not have their own coating of microorganisms, each highly adapted to its individual habitat. The features of dental plaque formation are by no means unique to the oral microflora and merely reflect a single instance of a natural phenomenon. In each case, the bacteria are highly adapted for survival in their individual environment. One of the first known examples of life to appear in geological formations were *stromatolites*, which are mineralized bacteria or algae[3,4] found in rocks from the Precambrian era. These formations from antiquity are quite similar to dental calculus. The same physiochemical forces of electrostatic charge, hydrogen bonding, hydrophobic interactions, or some

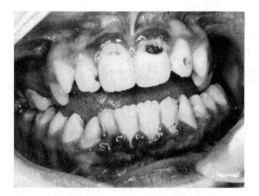

Figure 2–1. A 13-year-old female with dental caries on the facial of the maxillary incisors and swollen, discolored gingival tissues around the mandibular incisors, characteristic of chronic gingivitis. (*Courtesy of Dr WK Grigsby, University of Iowa College of Dentistry.*)

combination of these forces that underlie bacterial adhesion elsewhere in nature are the same as those observed in bacterial colonization of teeth to form dental plaque.[5] For example, all living cells, including bacterial cells, have a *net negative charge* and can be attracted to oppositely charged surfaces on such things as rocks in a stream, skin, or teeth. As with some dental plaque bacteria, bacterial organisms in other environments can produce structures, such as extracellular coatings or slime layers, or a variety of surface fibrils or appendages extending from their cell walls to provide an organic layer that may mediate their attachment to the host surface.[6]

BACTERIAL COLONIZATION OF THE MOUTH

Microorganisms initially colonize the mouth during birth, being naturally acquired from the *mother*. Thereafter, bacteria come to reside in the mouth from sources, such as the atmosphere, food, human contact, and from other animal contacts such as pets. Similarly, the interfaces between the saliva and the soft oral tissues such as the tongue, cheeks, and other surfaces, as well as the alimentary tract are colonized by bacteria, as are teeth subsequent to eruption. Mucosal surfaces, such as that of the tongue, may serve as a reservoir for dental plaque-forming organisms, including those related to disease.[7] With gingival recession due to trauma, such as from toothbrushing, or to periodontitis, exposed tooth cementum is colonized, as is the dentin in the event of tooth wear or decay.

When the tooth begins to erupt, it is exposed to saliva. At this point the formation of the dental plaque begins. This development occurs in two phases: (1) *acquired pellicle formation*, and (2) *dental plaque formation*.

The Acquired Pellicle

Bacteria rarely come into direct contact with the mineralized portion of the tooth surface. The first contact bacterial cells may have with an erupting tooth is the organic, preeruptive *enamel cuticle*, which is a residue of the enamel-forming organ.[8] Soon after eruption, the enamel cuticle is lost[9] in areas where it is either abraded from the tooth surface, or digested by colonizing bacteria.

Within seconds after saliva first contacts the external tooth surface, a coating of salivary materials, called the *acquired pellicle*, begins to develop on the tooth.[10,11] This organic layer is acquired after tooth eruption and is an acellular, mainly glycoprotein[a] layer of salivary origin that is *continually* deposited on those surfaces of the tooth exposed to the oral cavity (Figure 2–3). The saliva not only flows over the external surface of the tooth forming the pellicle, but it also occupies the millions of microscopic voids caused by surface imperfections and by acid demineralization. Collectively, these organic fingerlike projections, termed the *subsurface pellicle*, are important because they connect the protein components of the pellicle with the protein matrix network that occupies approximately 13% of the volume of the enamel. Through this matrix network, surface fluids and small-sized molecules can slowly diffuse throughout the enamel. If the pellicle is displaced by prophylaxis, it begins to reform immediately.[12,13] In approximately 2 hours the reformation of the pellicle is complete and even bacterial products may contribute to its structure.[14-16]

An acquired pellicle also forms on artificial surfaces, such as dental restorations and dentures. These organic coatings are similar to the pellicles on natural teeth and are subsequently colonized by bacteria.[17-19]

---

[a] A glycoprotein is a protein molecule that includes an attached carbohydrate component.

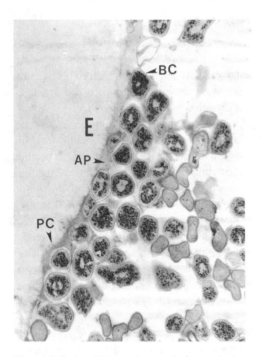

Figure 2–3. An electron micrograph demonstrates remnants of the preeruptive cuticle (PC) and the acellular acquired pellicle (AP) between the enamel (E) surface and the bacterial cells (BC) of the dental plaque. (*Electron micrograph courtesy of HN Newman, Eastman Dental Institute, London, UK*)

Finally, the bacterial colonization of the acquired pellicle can be beneficial for the bacteria because the pellicle components can serve as nutrients.[20] For example, proline-rich salivary proteins may be degraded by bacterial collagenases,[21] releasing peptides, and amino acids, whereas some salivary mucins may enhance the growth of dental plaque organisms, such as actinomycetes and spirochetes.[22]

The carbohydrate portions on some salivary glycoprotein molecules *in the pellicle* may serve as receptors for bacterial binding proteins and may contribute to bacterial adhesion to the tooth.[23,24] There is competition for the binding sites on the pellicle, not only by receptors on the *bacteria*, but also from *host proteins*, such as

immunoglobulins (ie, antibodies); proteins of the complement system; and the enzyme, lysozyme. These host proteins originate from the saliva and the gingival crevicular fluid.[25,26] Once a pellicle site is occupied by one of the competing entities, occupancy by another is interdicted.[27] Not only does competition arise for occupancy of binding sites, but an antagonistic relationship often exists between different types of bacteria occupying the binding sites. For example, it has been shown that some streptococci synthesize and release *bacteriocins*, which can inhibit some strains of *Actinomyces*.[28]

Question 1. Which of the following statements, if any, are correct?

A. The acquired pellicle is a layer of cells on the external surface of the clinical crown of a tooth.

B. The saliva, especially the salivary glycoproteins, is a major source of organic materials in the acquired pellicle.

C. Bacteria produce enzymes that may degrade some of the acquired pellicle components such as proteins.

D. It usually takes several days before the acquired pellicle is reformed after it is removed from the tooth.

E. The presence of immunoglobulins in the acquired pellicle guarantees the acquired pellicle will remain free from bacterial colonization.

Dental Plaque Formation

All bacteria that initiate plaque formation come in contact with the organically coated tooth surface fortuitously. Forces exist that tend to allow bacteria to accumulate on teeth or to remove them, and shifts in these forces determine whether more or less plaque accumulates at a given site on a tooth. Many factors influence the buildup of plaque,[29] ranging from simple factors, such as mechanical displacement, stagnation (ie, colonization in a sheltered or undisturbed environment), and availability of nutrients, to complex factors, such as interactions between the microbes and the host's inflammatory–immune systems. Bacteria tend to be removed from the teeth during mastication of foods, by the tongue, and by toothbrushing and other oral hygiene activities. For this reason, bacteria tend to accumulate on teeth in sheltered, undisturbed environments (risk sites), such as the occlusal fissures, the surfaces apical to the contact point between adjacent teeth, and at the tooth–gingiva interface.

Initial plaque formation begins on the clinical crown of a tooth and may take as long as 2 hours.[30] Binding sites and individual strain affinity for a given surface varies considerably.[31,32] The colonization process usually begins as a series of isolated colonies, often confined to abrasion lines and pits on the teeth.[15] With the aid of nutrients contained in the saliva and host food, the colonizing bacteria begin to reproduce and metabolize actively. About 2 days are then required for the plaque to double in mass, during which time, the bacterial colonies have been coalescing.[33] The most rapid change occurs during the first 4 or 5 days[34,35] and then appears to decelerate and become relatively stable by around the 21st day.[36] During this time, the bacterial and intercellular phases of the plaque are continually remodeled.[37] At the same time, the increasing thickness of the plaque limits the diffusion of oxygen to the entrapped original, oxygen-tolerant populations. As a result, the organisms that survive in the deeper parts of the plaque are either facultative or obligate[b] anaerobes.

During the formation of the plaque, the forming colonies are rapidly covered by an amorphous layer of saliva. When seen with the scanning electron microscope, the colonies protrude from the surface of the plaque as *domes*, giving the appearance of a cluster of igloos beneath new-fallen snow. Soon they are completely covered, and new domes appear over the old (Figure 2–4).

In individuals with poor oral hygiene, a further outer layer of material can cover the supragingival dental plaque. This layer, from its color, is called *materia alba* (literally, "white matter") and includes food debris which, unlike plaque, is usually removed easily by *rinsing* with water.[38] At times, the plaque demonstrates staining, with the discoloration being due to such sources as tea, iron salts, drugs, and possible chromogenic bacteria.

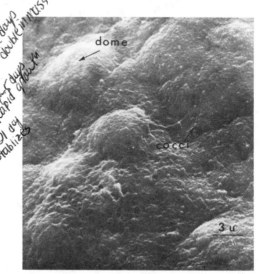

Figure 2–4. Scanning electromicrograph of dome formation in the plaque. (*From Brady JM. A plaque-free zone on human teeth—Scanning and transmission electron microscopy. J Periodontol. 1973; 44:416–428.*)

---

[b] Facultative anaerobes can exist in an environment, with or without oxygen; obligate anaerobes cannot exist in an environment with oxygen.

Molecular Mechanisms of Bacterial Adhesion

Members of the oral flora possess specific cell surface-associated adhesion proteins responsible for initiating colonization.[39] The initial bacterial attachment to the organic coating (eg, the acquired pellicle) on a tooth is thought to involve interactions such as hydrophobic bonding[40-42] (Figure 2–5A) among molecules or portions of molecules, such as the side chains of the amino acids phenylalanine and leucine. It has been suggested that the hydrophobicity of some streptococci is due to cell wall-associated molecules such as *glucosyltransferase*, an enzyme that converts the glucose portion of the sugar, sucrose, to extracellular polysaccharide. Some glucosyltransferases have been designated as *hydrophobins*, which are surface structures promoting hydrophobicity.[43]

Another molecular mechanism of bacterial adhesion may be the phenomenon termed *calcium bridging*,[44-46] which links *negatively* charged bacterial cell surfaces

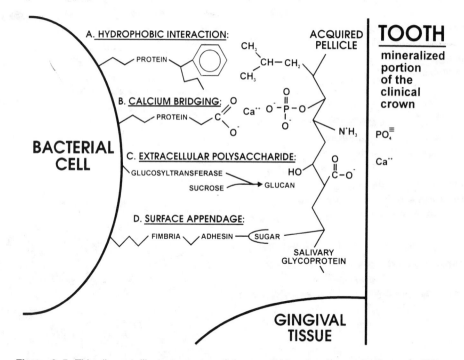

Figure 2–5. This diagram illustrates some of the possible molecular mechanisms mediating bacterial attachment to teeth during dental plaque formation. **A.** A side chain of a phenylalanine component of a bacterial protein interacts via hydrophobic bonding with a side chain of a leucine component of a salivary glycoprotein in the acquired pellicle. **B.** The negatively charged carboxyl group of a bacterial protein is attracted to a positively charged calcium ion (ie, electrostatic attraction), which in turn is attracted to a negatively charged phosphate group of a salivary phosphoprotein in the acquired pellicle. **C.** The host's dietary sucrose is converted by the bacterial enzyme, glucosyltransferase, to the extracellular polysaccharide, glucan, which has many hydroxyl groups and can interact with amino acid side-chain groups, such as serine, tyrosine, and threonine. **D.** The fimbrial surface appendage extends from the bacterial cell to permit the terminal adhesin portion to bind to a sugar component of a salivary glycoprotein in the acquired pellicle.

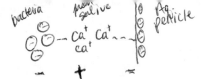

to the *negatively* charged acquired pellicle (Figure 2–5B) via *interposed, positively* charged divalent calcium ions from the saliva. Calcium bridging may only be important in early plaque formation, because recently formed plaque is readily disrupted by exposure to a calcium complexing agent (ie, chelate) such as ethylenediaminetetraacetic acid (EDTA).[47]

Some of the streptococci in plaque use the enzyme, glucosyltransferase, to synthesize *extracellular polysaccharides* (ECP). Among these are some "sticky" *glucans* that, through hydrogen bonding, are thought to contribute to the mediation of bacterial adhesion (Figure 2–5C).[48] Once the bacteria adhere, they are often entombed as additional glucan is produced.[49]

Bacteria also exhibit external cell surface proteins termed *adhesins*,[50] which have lectinlike[c] activity as they can bind to saccharide or sugar components of glycoproteins.[51,52] Some researchers have suggested that adhesins may be positioned on bacterial *surface appendages*, or *fimbriae*[53] (Figure 2–5D) and may facilitate bacterial colonization. Fimbria-associated adhesins probably mediate bacterial adhesion by ionic or hydrogen bond interactions. The adhesins and fimbriae may function together to facilitate bacterial attachment to pellicle-coated surfaces. For example, *pilin*, a structural protein that constitutes the bulk of some fimbriae, is hydrophobic due to its amino acid content.[54] These surface appendages in the form of fibrillar elements extend from the bacterial surface and may *reduce* or *mask* the repelling effect of the negative surface charges.

After having proposed the previously discussed four mechanisms for bacterial adhesion, it must be emphasized that there is

still a *lack of evidence* about the actual linking molecules in plaque, or between plaque and cuticle or pellicle.

Bacteria in the Dental Plaque

The bacteria in dental plaque vary in number and proportions from time to time and from site to site within the mouth of any one individual. The diversity is even greater among individuals and among races.[55] This difference in bacterial populations is also seen between the supra- and subgingival plaques.[56] The only abundant bacteria found almost universally in the mouths of humans and animals are streptococci and actinomycetes.

The bacteria that colonize the plaque arrive in a reasonably *predictable* sequence. The first to adhere to the tooth are called the *primary colonizers*, whereas those that arrive later as the plaque matures are termed the *secondary colonizers*. Generally speaking, the primary colonizers are not in sufficient numbers to be pathogenic. If the plaque is allowed to remain undisturbed, the early secondary colonizers can become associated with caries, chronic gingivitis, and ultimately chronic periodontitis.

The earliest colonizers are overwhelmingly cocci (ie, spherical cells),[57,58] especially streptococci, which constitute 47% to 85% of the cultivable cells found during the first four hours after professional tooth cleaning.[59] These tend to be followed by short rods. Usually the most abundant colonization is on the *interproximal surfaces*, in the *fissures* of teeth and along the *interface* between the tooth and gingiva.[60]

Cocci are probably the first to adhere because they are small and round and therefore, have a smaller energy barrier to overcome than other bacterial forms.[61] The first or primary colonizers tend to be *aerobic* (ie, oxygen-tolerant) bacteria such as *Neisseria* and *Rothia*. The streptococci, the

---

[c] Lectins are plant proteins with receptor sites that bind specific sugars.

Gram-positive facultative rods, and the actinomycetes, are the *main* organisms in both early fissure and interproximal plaque.[61-63] As the oxygen levels in the plaque fall, the Gram-*negative* rods such as the fusobacteria, and the Gram-*negative* cocci such as the veillonellae tend to increase. Of the early colonizers, *Streptococcus sanguis* often appears first,[64] followed later by *S mutans*. They depend for their growth on a sheltered environment and the presence of an excess of extracellular carbohydrate (eg, sucrose) from which they synthesize extracellular polysaccharides and gain an internal source of energy.[65,66] The polysaccharides coat the cell and help protect the cells from bursting from the *osmotic* effects of the sucrose. Also, the polysaccharide coating reduces the effect of *end products*, such as lactic acid and toxins, that can inhibit bacterial metabolism.

Whereas nonmotile cells such as the streptococci and actinomycetes come into contact with the tooth randomly, motile cells such as the spirochetes are likely to be attracted by *chemotactic* factors such as nutrients. Surface receptors probably provide a means of attachment for secondary colonizers *onto the initial bacterial layer.*[67] Thereby, bacteria that cannot adhere easily to the tooth initially via the acquired pellicle can probably attach by strong lectinlike, cell-to-cell interactions *with similar or dissimilar bacteria* that are already attached (ie, the primary colonizers).[68,69]

Gram-*negative* species are thought to predominate in the plaque during later inflammatory periodontal disease development,[70] but they are also present in early plaque, particularly the rods, *Actinobacillus, Porphyromonas, Prevotella,* and *Fusobacterium*. There is evidence that oxygen does not penetrate more than 0.1 mm into the dental plaque,[71,72] which helps to explain the presence of these *anaerobic* (ie, oxygen-intolerant) bacteria in early plaque.

Question 2. Which of the following statements, if any, are correct?

A. An important criterion for successful bacterial colonization of teeth is the availability of an unoccupied binding site.

B. Sites on teeth at risk for dental plaque formation include the occlusal fissures, interproximal surfaces apical to the contact point between adjacent teeth, and the tooth–gingiva interface.

C. An operational definition for materia alba is "the adherent material on tooth surfaces that is removed by *rinsing.*"

D. The negative charge on bacterial cells is attracted to the negative charge of the acquired pellicle as part of the initial formation of dental plaque.

E. The observation that calcium complexing agents release recently formed dental plaque from the teeth supports the argument for *calcium bridging*.

Dental Plaque Matrix

Because of the great variability of factors that may determine the accumulation of bacteria on teeth, dental plaque does not have a uniform structure in which the different species of bacteria are uniformly distributed. Dental plaque frequently exhibits "palisades" (ie, columns of cells) of cocci, rods, or filaments positioned perpendicular to the tooth surface[73] with other microcolonies distributed throughout an *intercellular plaque matrix* (Figure 2–6).[47] Saliva and fluids from the gingival sulcus may contribute to the dental plaque matrix, but

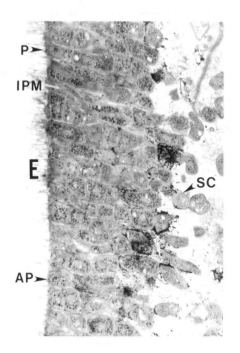

Figure 2–6. An electron micrograph showing palisades (P) of bacteria perpendicular to the enamel (E) surface, bacteria cells that are probably secondary colonizers (SC), the intercellular plaque matrix (IPM), and the acquired pellicle (AP). (*Photomicrograph courtesy of HN Newman, Eastman Dental Institute, London, UK*)

much of this material is *derived from the bacteria* and may be involved in their essential activities.

The organisms in the external, most recently formed plaque layer tend to be irregularly arranged with abundant matrix. The variety of bacterial interconnections extending through the matrix is wide and includes arrangements of cocci (*"corn cob figures"*[74]) and rods (*"test-tube brushes"*[2]) radiating from a central rod or filament (Figure 2–7).[37,75] Carbohydrate-binding adhesins (or lectinlike proteins) have been shown to link actinomycetes to streptococci in early dental plaque formation.[76,77]

Dental Plaque Metabolism

For metabolism to occur, a source of energy is required. For *Streptococcus mutans* and many other acid-forming organisms, this energy source can be *sucrose*.[78] Almost *immediately* following exposure of these organisms to sucrose, they produce (1) acid, (2) an *intra*cellular polysaccharide (ICP), which provides a reserve source of energy for each bacterium, much like glycogen does for human cells,[79] and (3) the *extra*cellular polysaccharides, glucan (eg, dextran)[80] and fructan (levan).[81] Glucans can be viscid substances that help anchor the bacteria to the pellicle, as well as stabilize the plaque mass. On the other hand, the fructans can act as an energy source for any bacteria having the enzyme, levanase, to use fructose as an energy source.[82,83] Quantitatively, the glucans constitute up to approximately 20% in dry weight of the plaque, the levans about 10%, and bacteria the remaining 70% to 80%. The glucans and fructans, along with other polymers (eg, salivary and bacterial proteins) and bacterial end products that are external to and between the cells, contribute to the *intercellular plaque matrix*.[84]

Plaque organisms are faced with a difficult environment in which extremes of pH, ionic strength, or nutrient levels may exist and in which antagonistic elements, such as competitor organisms and the host inflammatory–immune response may figure. To cope with this hostile environment, the plaque organisms must find a safe haven in relation to their neighbors and the oral environment. Such a favorable location is termed an *ecologic niche*.[85] Normally, once the niches are established, the bacteria of the microflora coexist with the host and the surrounding microcosm. This symbiosis results in a resistance to colonization by subsequent *nonindigenous* organisms.[86]

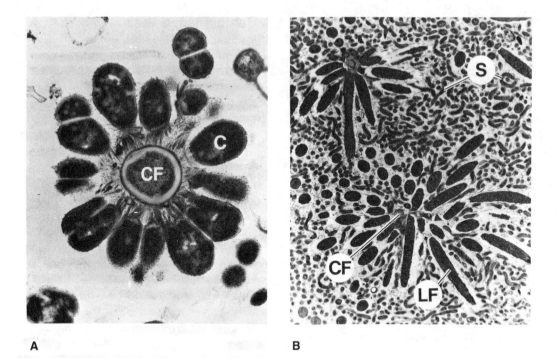

Figure 2–7. A. Cross section of "corn cob" from 2-month-old plaque. A coarse fibrillar material attaches the cocci (C) to the central filament (CF). Original magnification ×22,500. (*From List-garten MA, Mayo HE, Tremblay RJ. Development of dental plaque on epoxy crowns in man. J Periodontol. 1975; 46:10–26.*) **B.** Coarse "test tube brush" formations consisting of central filament (CF) surrounded by large, peritrichously flagellated filamentous bacteria (LF). Background consists of a spirochete-rich flora (S). Original magnification ×4,300. (*From Lisgarten MA. Structure of the microbial flora associated with periodontal health and disease in man. J Periodontol. 1976; 47:1–18.*)

With dietary sugars entering the bacterial cells in the dental plaque, anaerobic glycolysis results in acid production (acidogenesis) and accumulation of acid in the plaque. If no acid-consuming organisms (eg, *Veillonella*) occur in the environs to utilize the acids in their metabolism, the plaque pH drops rapidly from 7.0 to below pH 4.5. This drop is important because enamel begins to demineralize between pH 5.0 to 5.5. One possible outcome of the drop in pH may be the dissolution of the mineralized tooth surface adjacent to the plaque, resulting in cavitation of the tooth.[65] This destruction of host tissue may, however, also be considered an adaptation of a widespread *natural phenomenon*, whereby microorganisms come into contact with an organic coating on a mineral surface and produce extracellular acids that dissolve the mineral. This process provides the bacteria access to the inorganic elements (eg, calcium and phosphate) needed for their nutritional requirements. By adhering to the tooth surface via an organic layer of salivary origin, dental plaque bacteria obtain a supply of organic nutrients, which is also a widespread natural phenomenon.[87]

The same search for nutrients may explain the extension of bacteria from the supragingival plaque into the gingival sulcus.[88,89] Once the subgingival colonization begins, the host tissues defend against the bacterial challenge with antibacterial agents, such as antibodies in the gingival crevicular fluid and emigration of polymorphonuclear neutrophils from the adjacent connective tissue compartment into the gingival sulcus environment. The continued metabolic activity of the bacterial plaque in the subgingival environment is responsible for initiating the inflammatory response of the gingival tissues[90] and also may eventually cause progressive destruction of the attachment apparatus of the periodontium.

Until the extracellular matrix of the supragingival dental plaque mineralizes (ie, as dental calculus) and becomes firmly attached to the tooth, it can be removed by toothbrushing and flossing. Even so, as the plaque matures, it becomes more difficult to remove with a toothbrush. In one study, at 24, 48 and 72 hours after formation, 5.5, 7.8, and 14 g/cm² of pressure, respectively, was required to dislodge the plaque—almost three times as much pressure to remove on the third day as on the first.[91] Once dental calculus has formed on the tooth, professional intervention and instrumentation are *necessary* for its removal.

Question 3. Which of the following statements, if any, are correct?

A. Usually dental plaques exhibit uniform structures, composition, and properties.

B. The intercellular dental plaque matrix is probably some combination of host materials, such as salivary proteins, *and* bacterial metabolites.

C. The term "corn cob" designates one possible interconnection between different kinds of bacterial cells in the dental plaque matrix.

D. The acid dissolution of tooth mineral supplies calcium for both bacterial nutrition and calcium bonding.

E. Gingival inflammation is caused by the bacteria that reside in the dental plaque adjacent to the teeth.

DENTAL CALCULUS

A last stage in the maturation of some dental plaques is characterized by the appearance of mineralization in the deeper areas of the plaque to form dental calculus. The term *calculus* is derived from the Latin word meaning pebble or stone. The lay term *tartar* refers to an accumulated sediment or crust on the sides of a wine cask. Some people do not form calculus, others form only moderate amounts, and still others are heavy calculus formers.

Calculus is not in itself harmful. The major reason to prevent or remove calculus is because it is always covered by a layer of unmineralized, viable, metabolically active bacteria, which at a microscopic level is closely associated with the external calculus surface. Calculus *cannot* be removed by personal oral hygiene techniques, such as brushing or flossing. Often it is difficult to remove all the calculus, even professionally, without damaging the tooth, especially the softer root cementum. Calculus also needs to be removed because it makes routine oral hygiene more difficult or even impossible by forming calculus "spurs" (Figure 2–8), which may contribute to plaque accumulation and stagnation.

In addition to local factors contributing to calculus formation, behavioral and systemic conditions appear to hasten calculus formation. For example, smoking causes an accelerated formation of calculus.[92] Children afflicted with asthma or cystic fibrosis form calculus at approximately twice the

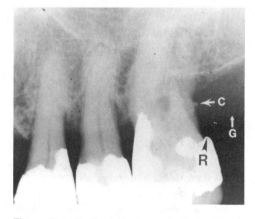

Figure 2–8. Radiograph demonstrating a "spur"-shaped deposit of calculus (C) on the distal side of the maxillary left first molar apical to the overhanging metallic restoration (R). The arrow (G) marks the coronal level of the gingival tissues indicating this is a subgingival deposit of calculus. (*Courtesy of Dr WK Grigsby, University of Iowa College of Dentistry.*)

rate as other children.[93] Similarly, non-ambulatory, mentally handicapped individuals who are tube-fed over long periods develop heavy calculus within 30 days, despite the fact that no food passes through the mouth.[94] Conversely, medications, such as beta-blockers, diuretics, and anticholinergics, can result in significantly reduced levels of calculus. The authors of the latter study[94] concluded that either the medications were excreted directly into the saliva affecting the rate of crystallization or they altered the composition of the saliva and thus indirectly affected calculus formation.[95]

Calculus results from the fact that saliva is saturated with respect to its concentrations of calcium and phosphate ions. These mineral elements in the saliva contribute to the formation of dental calculus, which is *mineralized dental plaque* that forms on a mineralized pellicle. The crystals in calculus include hydroxyapatite, brushite,

and whitlockite, all of which have different proportions of calcium and phosphate in combination with other ions, such as magnesium, zinc, fluoride, and carbonate.[96] *Supragingival calculus* forms on the tooth coronal to the margin of the gingival tissues and frequently develops opposite the duct orifices of the major salivary glands, such as on the facial surfaces of the maxillary molars. It is consistently found where saliva pools on the lingual surface of the mandibular incisors (Figure 2–9), and it can form in the fissures of teeth.[97] *Subgingival calculus* forms from calcium, phosphate, and organic materials derived from serum, which contributes to the mineralization of bacterial plaque within the gingival sulcus.[98]

One of the means by which the formation and growth of calculus is studied is by ligating a small strip of 0.001-in. thick plastic around the teeth and then removing the strips at periodic intervals.[99] In this way, the plaque that has accumulated on the plastic can be studied histologically and biochemically. It has been found that within 12 hours after the placement of the strips on teeth,

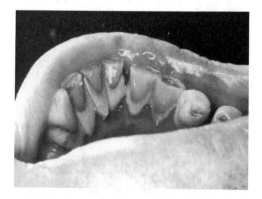

Figure 2–9. Deposits of supragingival calculus on the lingual surface of incisors and cuspids that could not be removed by brushing. (*Courtesy of Dr WK Grigsby, University of Iowa College of Dentistry.*)

x-ray diffraction studies demonstrate the positioning of mineral elements in the forming plaque. By the end of 3 to 4 days, the concentration of calcium and phosphate is significantly higher in the plaque of heavy calculus formers than in that of noncalculus formers.

Subgingival calculus is about 60% mineralized, whereas supragingival calculus is only about 30% mineralized.[100] Because of its greater hardness, being thinner and more closely interlinked to tooth surface imperfections, subgingival calculus can be more difficult to remove than supragingival calculus. The two types of calculus may differ in color. The supragingival calculus usually appears as a yellow-to-white mass, whereas the subgingival calculus appears gray to black. The dark coloration may be due to bacterial degradation of components of hemorrhagic exudate resulting from gingival inflammation. As a historical note, subgingival calculus was called *serumal calculus* by G.V. Black, who in 1882 postulated that its origin was from the blood serum.

It has been suggested that alkaline conditions in dental plaque may be an important predisposing factor in calculus formation.[101] On the other hand, calculus formation is not restricted to one bacterial species, or even to those growing at neutral or slightly acidic pH. This is evidenced by the caries-related streptococci, which may mineralize.[102] Not all bacterial plaques become mineralized, but a plaque that is destined to mineralize begins to do so within a few days of its initial formation, even though this early change is not detectable at a clinical level. Mineralization *begins in the intercellular plaque matrix* but eventually occurs within the bacterial cells. Bacterial phospholipids and other cell wall constituents may act as initiators of mineralization in dental plaque.[103]

Attachment of Calculus to the Teeth

At the tooth interface with the calculus, the enamel or root cementum are never perfectly smooth and invariably contain a variety of surface imperfections. The *normal* irregularities of the enamel and cementum such as the perikymata[d] and the point of origin of Sharpey's fibers[e] on the cementum appear to aid calculus attachment, as do defects in the enamel and cementum, such as areas of demineralization and cemental tears.[104] The attachment between the tooth and the calculus can be strong, indicating that the presence of calculus should *not* be regarded as only a surface precipitation. Scanning electron micrographs indicate a very close relationship between the matrix of the tooth surface and the matrix of the calculus; the crystalline structures of both are also very similar.[105]

Inhibiting Calculus Formation

Several agents are presently available to reduce calculus formation, including topical application using dentifrices that contain pyrophosphate ions or metal ions such as zinc.[106,107] One dentifrice contains two soluble phosphates, *tetrasodium pyrophosphate* and *disodium dihydrogen pyrophosphate*, in addition to fluoride.[107,108] The pyrophosphate ion not only serves as a structural analog of the orthophosphate ion, disrupting the formation of calcium phosphate crystals, but pyrophosphate also inhibits some strains of bacteria at concentrations significantly lower than the levels found in

---

[d] Perikymata are the numerous, small, transverse ridges on the exposed surface of the enamel of the permanent teeth.

[e] The tooth is anchored by connective tissue fibers that extend between the cementum and the bone; the ends embedded in the cementum are known as Sharpey's fibers.

dentifrices.[109,110] Thus, the daily combined mechanical action of toothbrushing and flossing and the chemical blocking effect on crystal formation by a dentifrice, can greatly reduce the frequency of need for professional calculus removal.

Question 4. Which of the following statements, if any, are correct?

    A. Intracellular polysaccharides are a source of energy that is available to the bacterial colony, but levans are available to only the synthesizing bacteria.

    B. An operational definition of calculus might be that it is "a mineralized dental plaque and pellicle that cannot be removed from the tooth by brushing or flossing."

    C. The flow of saliva over the tooth surfaces near the gland ducts keeps those teeth free of calculus deposits.

    D. Subgingival calculus is usually more densely mineralized that supragingival calculus.

    E. Pyrophosphate ion reduces the amount of calculus formation by preventing pellicle formation.

SUMMARY

Bacteria in dental plaque are the direct cause of the most widespread of all human diseases—dental caries and inflammatory periodontal diseases. These diseases, however, are not classical infections. They arise due to complex changes in plaque ecology and are affected by many factors in the host's protective responses. To understand the role of dental plaque in disease and how to prevent or control the plaque-associated diseases, it is essential to know the nature of dental plaque. Plaque forms initially on the preeruptive enamel cuticle as the tooth erupts into the oral cavity. Thereafter, salivary materials are deposited on the teeth, forming an acquired pellicle to which bacteria adhere. Adhesion is mediated by basic forces, including electrostatic interaction, hydrogen bonding, and hydrophobic interactions. The earliest of the primary bacterial colonizers are mainly Gram-positive cocci. They are then followed by a variety of Gram-positive and Gram-negative species, which are the secondary colonizers. Caries-related bacterial species have a greater ability than other bacterial species to adapt to excess sugars and their metabolites. With higher pH (ie, less acidity), some plaques mineralize to form dental calculus supragingivally and, in the event of periodontitis, subgingivally. The supragingival plaque is associated with caries and gingivitis, whereas the subgingival plaque is associated with gingivitis and periodontitis. As the plaque matures, mineralization begins in the extracellular matrix and eventually spreads to include the bacteria. Calculus is always covered by actively metabolizing bacteria, which can cause caries, gingivitis, and periodontitis. The acquired pellicle and the dental plaque can be removed by toothbrushing, flossing, and prophylaxis. Once dental plaque mineralizes to form calculus on the tooth, professional intervention and instrumentation are necessary for its removal. It is worth remembering that in spite of all the complexities of acquired pellicle, plaque, and calculus formation, and all the factors favoring retention or removal, growth or inhibition, if it were not for *stagnation* of pathogenic bacteria at risk sites, *neither dental caries nor inflammatory periodontal diseases would occur*. Later chapters deal with the wide range of nonsurgical methods, mechanical and chemical, increasingly used to control plaque and calculus formation. All of these methods have the aim of preventing, halting, or reversing the progression of dental caries and periodontal tissue inflammation.

ANSWERS AND EXPLANATIONS

1. B, C

   A—incorrect. The acquired pellicle is "acellular," indicating it is cell free.

   D—incorrect. The acquired pellicle begins to reform immediately and is reestablished within several hours.

   E—incorrect. Even though some binding sites are occupied by immunoglobulins, many more are for bacterial occupancy.

2. A, B, D, E

   C—incorrect. Like charges (ie, negative-to-negative or positive-to-positive) repel; unlike charges attract.

3. B, C, D, E

   A—incorrect. So many factors affect plaque formation that composition, structure, and properties are greatly varied.

4. B, D

   A—incorrect. It should be the reverse, with ICP available to the synthesizing bacteria, and levan to the surrounding bacteria having the enzyme, levanase.

   C—incorrect. The presence of high concentrations of calcium and phosphate ions at the duct opening results in more, not less calculus formation.

   E—incorrect. Pyrophosphate interferes with the formation of calcium phosphate crystals such as hydroxyapatite.

SELF-EVALUATION QUESTIONS

1. The stromatolites of the Precambrian era were quite similar to the dental _____.

2. The *acellular* salivary layer that covers the tooth prior to plaque formation is the _____.

3. Following prophylaxis, it requires about _____ hours for the acquired pellicle to completely reform.

4. Two of the host *defensive proteins* that compete with bacteria for receptor sites on the acquired pellicle are _____ and _____.

5. It takes approximately _____ hours for the initial plaque to form and about _____ days to double in mass; once formed, the growth is rapid for about _____ and finally stabilizes in mass around the _____.

6. (Water)(a toothbrush) or a (prophylaxis) is required to remove (1) materia alba, (2) plaque or (3) calculus.

7. Bacteria can attach to the acquired cuticle via _hydrophobic_ bonding, by calcium _bridging_, via attachment to the sticky _glucans_, and by surface proteins called _adhesins_.

8. The three places on the teeth where bacterial colonization is most abundant are _____, _____, and _____.

9. "Corn cob" figures are due to (cocci)(rods) radially attached to a central rod, whereas the _____ (figure) is due to rods radially attached to a central rod.

10. Between the cells of the plaque is the (ECP)(ICP) containing _____ and levans that serve as energy sources for the bacteria.

11. The "safe haven" where a bacterial colony can exist in the plaque environment is known as an _____.

12. Calculus is mainly made up of calcified _____.

13. One condition causing accelerated calculus formation is _____; reduced formation is seen after use of _____ (drugs).

14. Supragingival plaque derives its minerals from the _____, whereas the subgingival plaque derives them from the _____.

15. Two phosphates contained in dentifrices that inhibit calculus formation are _____ and _____.

REFERENCES

1. Keyes PH. The infectious and transmissible nature of experimental dental caries. Findings and implications. *Arch Oral Biol.* 1960; 1:304–320.
2. Listgarten MA. Structure of the microbial flora associated with periodontal health and disease in man. A light and electron microscopic study. *J Periodontol.* 1976; 47:1–17.
3. Schopf JW. The development and diversification of Precambrian life. *Orig Life.* 1974; 5:119–135.
4. Schopf JW. The age of microscopic life. *Endeavor.* 1975; 34:51–58.
5. Silverman G, Kleinberg I. Fractionation of human dental plaque and the characterization of its cellular and acellular components. *Arch Oral Biol.* 1967; 12:1387–1406.
6. Newman HN. Microbial films in nature. *Microbios.* 1974; 9:247–257.
7. Van der Velden U, Van Winkerhoff AJ, Abbas, de Graf J. The habitat of periodontopathic micro-organisms. *J Clin Periodontol.* 1986; 13:243–248.
8. Newman HN. The approximal apical border of plaque on children's teeth. I. Morphology, structure and cell content. *J Periodontol.* 1979; 50:561–567.
9. Meckel AH. The nature and importance of organic deposits on dental enamel. *Caries Res.* 1968; 2:104–114.
10. Ericson T. Adsorption to hydroxyapatite of proteins and conjugated proteins from human saliva. *Caries Res.* 1967; 1:52–58.
11. Meckel AH. The formation of biological films. *Swed Dent J.* 1965; 10:585–599.
12. Leach SA, Critchley P, Kolendo AB, et al. Salivary glycoproteins as components of the enamel integuments. *Caries Res.* 1967; 1:104–111.
13. Mayhall CW. Concerning the composition and source of the acquired enamel pellicle on human teeth. *Arch Oral Biol.* 1970; 15: 1327–1341.
14. Hardie JM, Bowden GH. The microbial flora of dental plaque: Bacterial succession and isolation considerations. In: Stiles HM, Loesche WJ, O'Brien TC, eds. *Proceedings Microbial Aspects of Dental Caries. Microbiol Abstr.* 1976; 1 (Spec Suppl): 63–87.
15. Lie T, Gusberti F. Replica study of plaque formation on human tooth surfaces. *Acta Odontol Scand.* 1979; 79:65–72
16. Baier RE. On the formation of biological films. *Swed Dent J.* 1977; 1:261–271.
17. Budtz-Jörgensen E, Theilade E, Theilade J, et al. Method for studying the development, structure and microflora of dental plaque. *Scand J Dent Res.* 1981; 89:149–156.
18. Tullberg A. An experimental study of the adhesion of bacterial layers to some restorative dental materials. *Scand J Dent Res.* 1986; 94:164–173.
19. Satou J, Fukunaga A, Satou N, et al. Streptococcal adherence on various restorative materials. *J Dent Res.* 1988; 67:588–591.
20. Leach SA, Critchley P. Bacterial degradation of glycoprotein sugars in human saliva. *Nature.* 1966; 209:506.
21. Hay DI, Oppenheim IG. The isolation from human parotid saliva of a further group of proline-rich proteins. *Arch Oral Biol.* 1974; 19:627–632.
22. Glenister DA, Salamon KE, Smith K, et al. Enhanced growth of complex communities of dental plaque bacteria in mucin-limited continuous culture. *Microbiol Ecol Hlth Dis.* 1988; 1:31–38.
23. Gibbons RJ, van Houte J. Bacterial adherence in oral microbial ecology. *Ann Rev Microbiol.* 1975; 29:19–44.
24. Williams RC, Gibbons RJ. Inhibition of streptococcal attachment to receptors on human buccal epithelial cells by antigenically similar salivary glycoproteins. *Infect Immun.* 1975; 11:711–718.

25. Kraus FW, Orstavik D, Hurst DC, et al. The acquired pellicle: Variability and subject dependence of specific proteins. *J Oral Pathol Med.* 1973; 2:165–173.

26. Orstavik D, Kraus FW. The acquired pellicle: Immunofluorescent demonstration of specific proteins. *J Oral Pathol Med.* 1973; 2:68–76.

27. Williams RC, Gibbons RJ. Inhibition of streptococcal attachment to receptors or human buccal epithelial cells by antigenically similar salivary glycoproteins. *Infect Immun.* 1975 11:711–718

28. Rogers AH, van der Hoeven JS, Mikx F. Inhibition of *Actinomyces viscosus* by bacteriocin producing strains of *Streptococcus mutans* in the dental plaque of gnotobiotic rats. *Arch Oral Biol.* 1978; 23:477–483.

29. Christersson LA, Grossi SG, Dunford RG, et al. Dental plaque and calculus: Risk indicators for their formation. *J Dent Res.* 1992; 71:1425–1430.

30. Baier RE, Glantz P-O. Characterization of oral in vivo film formed on different types of solid surfaces. *Acta Odontol Scand.* 1979; 36:289–301.

31. Liljemark WF, Schauer SV. Competitive binding among oral streptococci to hydroxyapatite. *J Dent Res.* 1977; 56:156–165.

32. Kuramitsu H, Ingersoll L. Molecular basis for the different sucrose-dependent adherence properties of *Streptococcus mutans* and *Streptococcus sanguis*. *Infect Immun.* 1977; 17:330–337.

33. Tanzer JM, Johnson MC. Gradients for growth within intact *Streptococcus mutans* plaque in vitro demonstrated by autoradiograph. *Arch Oral Biol.* 1976; 21:555–559.

34. Bjorn H, Carlsson J. Observations on a dental plaque morphogenesis. *Odontol Rev.* 1964; 15:23–28.

35. Furuichi Y, Linhe J, Ramberg P, et al. Patterns of de novo plaque formation in the human dentition. *J Clin Periodontol.* 1992; 19:423–33.

36. Howell, A Jr., Risso A, Paul F. Cultivable bacteria in developing and mature human dental calculus. *Arch Oral Biol.* 1965; 10: 307–313.

37. Listgarten MA, Mayo HE, Tremblay R. Development of dental plaque on epoxy resin crowns in man. A light and electron microscope study. *J Periodontol.* 1975; 46: 10–26.

38. Mehrotra KK, Kapoor KK, R Pradham BP, et al. Assessment of plaque tenacity on enamel surfaces. *J Periodont Res.* 1984; 18: 386–392.

39. Kolenbrander PE, London J. Ecological significance of coaggregation among oral bacteria. *Adv Microb Ecol.* 1992;12:183–217.

40. Newman HN. Diet, attrition, plaque and dental disease. *Br Dent J.* 1974; 136:491–497.

41. Leach SA. On the nature of interactions associated with aggregation phenomena in the mouth. *J Dent.* 1979; 7:149–160.

42. Rosenberg M, Judes H, Weiss E. Cell surface hydrophobicity of dental plaque microorganisms. *Infect Immun.* 1983; 42:831–834.

43. Doyle RJ, Rosenberg M, Drake D. Hydrophobicity of oral bacteria. In: Doyle RJ, Rosenberg M, eds. *Microbial Cell Surface Hydrophobicity.* Washington, D.C.: American Society for Microbiology; 1990:387–419.

44. Edgar WM. Studies of the role of calcium in plaque formation and cohesion. *J Dent.* 1979; 7:174–179.

45. Matsukubo T, Katow T, Takazoe I. Significance of Ca-binding activity of early plaque bacteria. *Bull Tokyo Dent Coll.* 1978; 19: 53–57.

46. Rose RK, Dibdin GH, Shellis RP. A quantitative study of calcium binding and aggregation in selected oral bacteria. *J Dent Res.* 1993; 72:78–84.

47. Newman HN, Britton AB. Dental plaque ultrastructure as revealed by freeze etching. *J Periodontol.* 1974; 45:478–488.

48. Germaine GR, Harlander SK, Leung W-LS, et al. *Streptococcus mutans* dextransucrase: Functioning of primer dextran and endogenous dextransucrase in water-soluble and water-insoluble glucan synthesis. *Infect Immun.* 1977; 16:637–648.

49. Gibbons RJ, van Houte J. Bacterial adher-

ence and the formation of dental plaque. Receptors and recognition. In: Beachey EH, ed. *Bacterial Adherence*. London: Chapman and Hall, Ltd; 1980; 6:63–104.

50. Ofek I, Perry A. Molecular basis of bacterial adherence to tissues. In: Mergenhagen SE, Rosan B, eds. *Molecular Basis of Oral Microbial Adhesion*. Washington, DC: American Society for Microbiology; 1985: 7–13.

51. Gibbons RJ. Adherent interactions which may affect microbial ecology in the mouth. *J Dent Res*. 1984; 63:378–385.

52. Weerkamp AH, van der Mei HC, Engelen DPPE, et al. Adhesion receptors (adhesins) of oral streptococci. In: ten Cate JM, Leach SA, Arends, J, eds. *Bacterial Adhesion and Preventive Dentistry*. Oxford: IRL Press; 1984:85–97.

53. Clark WB, Wheeler TT, Lane MD, et al. Actinomyces adsorption mediated by type-1 fimbriae. *J Dent Res*. 1986; 65: 1166–1168.

54. Irwin RT. Hydrophobicity of proteins and bacterial fimbriae. In: Doyle RJ, Rosenberg M, eds. *Microbial Cell Surface Hydrophobicity*. Washington, DC: American Society of Microbiology; 1990:137–177.

55. Cao CF, Aeppli DM, Liljemark WF, et al. Comparison of plaque microflora between Chinese and Caucasian population groups. *J Clin Periodontol*. 1990; 17:115–118.

56. Listgarten MA. Structure of the microbial flora associated with periodontal health and disease in man. A light and electron microscope study. *J Periodontol*. 1976; 47:139–147.

57. Tinanoff N, Gross A, Brady JM. Development of plaque on enamel. Parallel investigations. *J Periodont Res*. 1976; 11:197–209.

58. Lie T. Ultrastructural study of early plaque formation. *J Periodont Res*. 1978; 13:391–409.

59. Kolenbrander PE, London J. Adhere today, here tomorrow: Oral bacterial adherence. *J Bacteriol*. 1993; 175:3247–3252.

60. Theilade J, Fejerskov O, Hørsted M. A transmission electron microscopic study of 7-day old bacterial plaque in human tooth fissures. *Arch Oral Biol*. 1976; 21:587–598.

61. Newman HN. Retention of bacteria on oral surfaces. In: Bitton G, Marshall KC, eds. *Adsorption of Microorganisms to Surfaces*. New York: Wiley-Intersciences; 1980:207–251.

62. Hardie JM, Bowden GH. The normal microbial flora of the mouth. In: Skinner FA, Carr JG, eds. *The Normal Microbial Flora of Man*. London: Academic Press; 1974: 47–83.

63. Socransky SS. Microbiology of periodontal disease—present status and future considerations. *J Periodontol*. 1977; 48:497–504.

64. van Houte J, Gibbons RJ, Banghart SB. Adherence as a determinant of the presence of *Streptococcus salivarius* and *Streptococcus sanguis* on the human tooth surface. *Arch Oral Biol*. 1970; 15:1025–1034.

65. Donoghue HD, Newman HN. Effect of glucose and sucrose on survival in batch culture of *Streptococcus mutans* C67-1 and a non-cariogenic mutant, C67-25. *Infect Immun*. 1976; 13:16–21.

66. Kilian M, Rölla G. Initial colonization of teeth in monkeys as related to diet. *Infect Immun*. 1976; 14:1022–1027.

67. Weerkamp AH. Coaggregation of *Streptococcus salivarius* with Gram-negative oral bacteria: Mechanism and ecological significance. In: Mergenhagen SE, Rosan B, eds. *Molecular Basis of Oral Microbial Adhesion*. Washington, DC: American Society for Microbiology; 1985:177–183.

68. Ciardi JE, McCray GFA, Kolenbrander PE, et al. Cell-to-cell interaction of *Streptococcus sanguis* and *Propionibacterium acnes* on saliva-coated hydroxyapatite. *Infect Immun*. 1987; 55:1441–1446.

69. Lamont RJ, Rosan B. Adherence of mutans streptococci to other oral bacteria. *Infect Immun*. 1990; 58:1738–1743.

70. Shah HN, Gharbia SE. Microbial factors in the aetiology of chronic inflammatory periodontal disease. In: Newman HN, Williams DN, eds. *Inflammation and Immunology in Chronic Inflammatory Periodontal Disease*. Northwood, England: Science Reviews Limited; 1991:1–32.

71. Van der Hoeven JS, de Jong MH, Kolenbrander PD. In vivo studies of microbial adherence in dental plaque. In: Mergenhagen SE, Rosan B, eds. *Molecular Basis of Oral Microbial Adhesion.* Washington, DC: American Society for Microbiology; 1985:220–227.

72. Globerman DY, Kleinberg I. Intra-oral pO_2 and its relation to bacterial accumulation on the oral tissues. In: Kleinberg I, Ellison SA, Mandel ID, eds. *Proceedings: Saliva and Dental Caries.* (A special supplement for *Microbiol. Abst.*) New York: Information Retrieval; 1979:275–292.

73. Newman HN. The organic films on enamel surfaces. 2. The dental plaque. *Br Dent J.* 1973; 135:106–111.

74. Kolenbrander PE. Coaggregation: Adherence in the human oral microbial ecosystem. In: Dworkin M, ed. *Microbial Cell–Cell Interactions.* Washington, DC: American Society for Microbiology; 1991:316.

75. Newman HN, McKay GS. An unusual microbial configuration in human dental plaque. *Microbios.* 1973; 8:117–128.

76. Cisar JO, Brennan MJ, Sandberg AL. Lectin-specific interaction of *Actinomyces* fimbriae with oral streptococci. In: Mergenhagen SE, Rosan B, eds. *Molecular Basis of Oral Microbial Adhesion.* Washington, DC: American Society for Microbiology; 1985:159–163.

77. Kolenbrander PE, Andersen RN. Use of coaggregation-defective mutants to study the relationship of cell-to-cell interactions and oral microbial ecology. In: Mergenhagen SE, Rosan B, eds. *Molecular Basis of Oral Microbial Adhesion.* Washington, DC: American Society for Microbiology; 1985:164–166.

78. Gibbons RJ, van Houte J. Bacterial adherence in oral microbial ecology. *Ann Rev Microbiol.* 1975; 29:19–44.

79. Mattingly SJ, Daneo-Moor L, Shockman GD. Factors regulating cell wall thickening and intracellular iodophilic polysaccharide storage in *Streptococcus mutans. Infect Immun.* 1977; 16:967–973.

80. Critchley P, Wood JM, Saxton CA, et al. The polymerization of dietary sugars by dental plaque. *Caries Res.* 1967:112–129.

81. McDougall WF. Studies on the dental plaque. IV. Levans and the dental plaque. *Aust Dent J.* 1964; 9:1–5.

82. Da Costa T, Gibbons RJ. Hydrolysis of levan by human plaque streptococci. *Arch Oral Biol.* 1968; 13:609–617.

83. Manly RS, Richardson DT. Metabolism of levan by oral samples. *J Dent Res.* 1968; 47:1080–1086.

84. Edgar W, Jenkins G, Hillman D. Salivary precipitation and the development of plaque matrix. In: Leach SA, ed. *Dental Plaque and Surface Interactions in the Oral Cavity.* Eynsham, England: Information Printing, Ltd; 1980:197–210.

85. Bowen GH, Hardie JM, Fillery ED, et al. Microbial analyses related to caries susceptibility. In: Bibby BG, Shein RJ, eds. *Proceedings of Methods of Caries Prediction. Microbiol Abst.* 1978:83–87.

86. Conference report. Eleventh international conference on oral biology—Chemical control of plaque. *J Dent Res.* 1988; 67: 1535–1537.

87. Brock TD. *Principles of Microbial Ecology.* Englewood Cliffs, New Jersey: Prentice-Hall; 1966:72–75.

88. Newman HN. Structure of approximal human dental plaque as observed by scanning electron microscopy. *Arch Oral Biol.* 1972; 17:1445–1453.

89. Soames JV, Davies RM. The structure of subgingival plaque in a beagle dog. *J Periodont Res.* 1975; 9:333–341.

90. Löe H, Theilade E, Jensen SB. Experimental gingivitis in man. *J Periodontol.* 1965; 36:177–187.

91. Mehrotra KK, Kapoor KK, Pradhan BP, et al. Assessment of plaque tenacity on enamel surface. *J Periodont Res.* 1983; 18: 386–392.

92. Ennever J, Streckfuss JL, Riggan LJ, et al. Proteolipid and calculus matrix calcification in vitro. *J Dent Res.* 1977; 56:140–142.

93. Wotman S, Mercadante J, Mandel ID, et al. The occurrence of calculus in normal children, children with cystic fibrosis, and

children with asthma. *J Periodontol.* 1973; 44:278–280.

94. Klein FK, Dicks JL. Evaluation of accumulation of calculus in tube-fed mentally handicapped patients. *J Am Dent Assoc.* 1984; 108:352–354.

95. Turesky S, Breur M, Coffman G. The effect of certain systemic medications on oral calculus formation. *J Periodontol.* 1992; 63: 871–875.

96. Ellwood D, Melling J, Rutter P. The accumulation of organisms on the teeth. In: Society for General Microbiology. *Adhesion of Microorganisms to Surfaces.* New York: Academic Press; 1979:137–164.

97. McDougall WA. Analytical transmission electron microscopy of the distribution of elements in human supragingival dental calculus. *Arch Oral Biol.* 1985; 30:603–608.

98. Galil KA, Gwinnett AJ. Human tooth-fissure contents and their progressive mineralization. *Arch Oral Biol.* 1975; 2:559–562.

99. Turesky S, Renstrup G, Glickman I. Histologic and histochemical observations regarding early calculus formation in children and adults. *J Periodontol.* 1961; 32:7–14, 69–100.

100. Sundberg M, Friskopp J. Crystallograph of supragingival human dental calculus. *Scand J Dent Res.* 1985; 93:30–38.

101. Schroeder HE. *Formation and Inhibition of Dental Calculus.* Bern, Switzerland: Hans Huber Publishers; 1969; 559–562.

102. Newman HN. *Dental Plaque: The Ecology of the Flora on Human Teeth.* Springfield, Ill. Charles Thomas Publishers; 1980:49.

103. Streckfuss JL, Smith WN, Brown LR, et al. Calcification of selected strains of *Streptococcus mutans* and *Streptococcus sanguis.* *J Bacteriol.* 1974; 120:502–506.

104. Moskow BS. Calculus attachment in cemental separations. *J Periodontol.* 1969; 4: 125–130.

105. Selvig KA. Attachment of plaque and calculus to tooth surfaces. *J Periodont Res.* 1970; 5:8–18.

106. Feldman RS, Bravacos JS, Rose CL. Association between smoking different tobacco products and periodontal disease indexes. *J Periodontol.* 1983; 54:481–488.

107. ten Cate JM. *Recent Advances in the Study of Dental Calculus.* Oxford: IRL Press; 1988: 143, 259.

108. Zacherl WA, Pfeiffer HJ, Swancar JR. The effect of soluble pyrophosphates on dental calculus in adults. *J Am Dent Assoc.* 1985; 110:737–738.

109. Drake DR, Chung J, Grigsby W, et al. Synergistic effect of pyrophosphate and sodium dodecyl sulfate on periodontal pathogens. *J Periodontol.* 1992; 63:696–700.

110. Drake D, Grigsby W, Krotz-Dielemann D. Growth-inhibitory effect of pyrophosphate on oral bacteria. *Oral Microbiol Immunol.* 1994; 9:25–28.

Chapter 3

The Developing Carious Lesion

Michael W. J. Dodds
James S. Wefel

Objectives

At the end of this chapter, it will be possible to

1. Name the four general types of carious lesions that are found on a tooth.
2. Trace the possible paths of diffusion of a liquid from the dental plaque to the dentinoenamel junction.
3. Describe the visual and polarizing microscope appearance of an incipient lesion.
4. Name the two bacteria most often indicted in the caries process, and indicate when they are present in the greatest numbers during the caries process.
5. Describe the series of events in a cariogenic plaque and subsurface lesion from the time of exposure to sugar till the pH returns to a resting state.
6. Discuss the characteristics of root caries and explain the differences and similarities to coronal caries.
7. List preventive measures to be taken against root and coronal caries.
8. Explain why so much time is taken by the profession in treating secondary caries.

Introduction

The development of dental caries is a dynamic process of demineralization of the dental hard tissues by the products of bacterial metabolism, alternating with periods of remineralization. This pathologic process occurs on a continuum, in which any lesion may range from changes at the *molecular level* to gross tissue destruction and cavity formation.

Carious lesions occur in four general areas of the tooth: (1) *pit and fissure caries*, which is found mainly on the occlusal surfaces of posterior teeth as well as in lingual pits of the maxillary incisors; (2) *smooth-surface caries*, which arises on intact enamel surfaces other than at the location of the pits and fissures; (3) *root surface caries*, which might involve any surface of the root; and (4) *secondary, or recurrent, caries*, which occurs on the tooth surface adjacent to an existing restoration. Smooth surface caries can be further divided into *free smooth-surface caries* (ie, caries affecting the buccal and lingual tooth surfaces) and approximal caries, affecting the contact area(s) of adjoining tooth surfaces (ie, mesial or distal surfaces).

THEORIES OF CARIES

Many theories of caries have been propounded through the ages, but it was not until the 19th century that coherent notions based on scientific experimentation began to emerge. In 1890 W. D. Miller, an American dentist working in Germany, published his *chemicoparasitic* theory, which established the basis of our present knowledge.[1] As a result of his extensive experimentation, he believed that the extraction of the "lime salts" by bacterial acids was the first step in tooth decay. Miller's work, however, failed to identify dental plaque as the source of the bacteria; his assumption was that fermentation of impacted carbohydrate foodstuffs occurred in situ by salivary microorganisms. The chemicoparasitic theory became more cogent when taken in conjunction with the findings of other contemporary dental researchers, including G. V. Black and J. L. Williams, who both described a "gelatinous microbic plaque"[2] as the source of the acids. Indeed, as Williams stated, "My general conclusions are that all softening of enamel is due to the action of acids, and chiefly or wholly to the acids excreted by bacteria in situ."[3]

The presently accepted theory of caries is based on Miller's chemicoparasitic theory although a number of refinements and additions have been made to the theory over the years, some of which are described in more detail in this chapter and in Chapter 11. Dental caries is a multifactorial disease process, often represented by the three interlocking circles depicted in Chapter 1 (Figure 1–5). For caries to develop three factors must occur simultaneously: (1) a susceptible tooth and host; (2) cariogenic, tooth-associated microorganisms; and (3) cariogenic diet for a nondefined, but finite period of time. When exposed to a suitable substrate (usually sugar), cariogenic bacteria present in the plaque on the tooth produce acid. If this occurs for a sufficiently long period, caries develop and progress. Each of the three main factors (ie, bacteria, host and diet) includes a number of secondary factors and can be modified to either protect or further damage the tooth. For example, fluoride incorporated into dental enamel increases host resistance (Chapters 8 and 9). Conversely, a reduction in the saliva flow (xerostomia) greatly increases the caries risk.

ENAMEL STRUCTURE

To comprehend the nature of the caries process, it is important to understand the structure of the tooth's tissues. Although enamel is the most highly mineralized tissue in the body, being made of 95% to 96% inorganic matter, it is also porous, with the inorganic component representing only 87% of the total volume. This means that some 13% of the volume of enamel is composed of organic material (matrix). This organic, protein-rich matrix is mainly water (11% of the total volume). Essentially, enamel consists of innumerable microscopic crystals of the mineral *hydroxyapatite* arranged in larger structural units, or *rods*, also known as *prisms*. (In fact, the mineral composing the enamel is better termed a carbonated apatite, because the biologic apatites have many impurities not found in pure mineral apatites). The hydroxyapatite crystals are oriented by a protein network that makes up the enamel matrix. The proteins of this matrix are collectively called *enamelins.* On this network the initiation of apatite crystal formation, called *nucleation,* first occurs; nucleation is in turn followed by an enlargement of the crystal nucleus, called *crystal growth.* Thus each of the millions of rods making up the enamel is composed of columns of innumerable crystallites, much like a brick column, with the bricks comparable to crystallites and the mortar to the protein matrix. The matrix exists both between hydroxyapatite crystals (intraprismatic water) and in certain areas of the enamel that are richer in matrix than others; these include the *dentinoenamel junction, incremental lines,* and the *striae of Retzius.*

When the ameloblasts begin their secretory activity at the dentinoenamel junction, they lay down a thin layer of protein matrix, which does not mineralize to the same extent as the remainder of the rod. This layer of hypomineralized enamel is known as the *dentinoenamel membrane.* As the cell continues to lay down the matrix in its journey to the site of the future enamel surface, it does not form one continuous homogenous rod. Instead the ameloblast is subject to a circadian rhythm. After moving approximately *4 μm* in the course of a 24-hour period, it decreases activity for a while and then begins to move another 4 μm. The period in which the ameloblasts are resting is histologically marked by a greater portion of matrix and less mineralization. These periodic hypomineralized areas that occur every 4 μm are known as *incremental lines.* Finally, at intervals of *28 to 32 μm,* a still wider stratum of protein formation and hypomineralization occurs, known as the *stria of Retzius* (Figure 3–1). The overall protein network, consisting of the dentinoenamel membrane, incremental lines, and stria of Retzius, as well as the interconnecting protein around the crystallites and rods, facilitates the diffusion of fluids, ions, and small-sized molecules throughout the enamel.[4]

The enamel rods, when viewed in cross section with an electron microscope, appear as a group of keyhole-shaped structures, approximately 6 to 8 μm in diameter, with the enlarged portion of the keyhole called the *head* and the narrow portion the *tail.* With this configuration, each head fits between two tails. The tail is always positioned toward the apex. In the head of the rod the long axes of the crystals, called the *C axis,* are parallel to the enamel rod. However, as the periphery of the rod is approached, the crystals assume an angle to the more central crystals; in fact, in the tail this angulation may be around 30° (Figures 3–2 and 3–3 A and B).

At the junction of two adjacent rods, the crystals closely approximate each other.

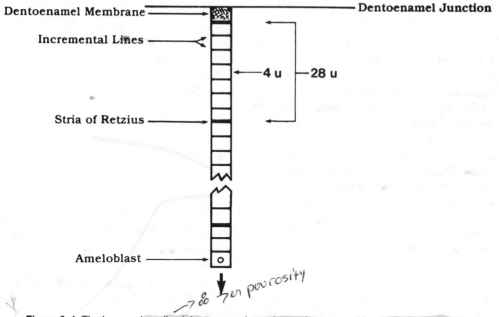

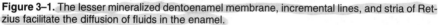

Figure 3–1. The lesser mineralized dentoenamel membrane, incremental lines, and stria of Retzius facilitate the diffusion of fluids in the enamel.

Yet a distinct delineation exists between the two due to a slight difference in orientation of the crystallites of each rod. In this interrod area submicroscopic spaces occur through which fluid can diffuse. Thus, between the availability of the hypomineralized areas along the protein network and the submicroscopic spaces between the crystals, *fluid diffusion can occur throughout the enamel.*[4]

At the time of eruption, many of the apatite crystals are not fully mineralized.[5] Once the tooth is exposed to saliva, however, considerable uptake of ions occurs in the crystals making up the outer 10- to 100-μm layer of the enamel rods. This physiologic mineralization process (*posteruptive maturation*) permits the mineral-deficient crystals to add calcium, phosphorus, fluoride, and other ions from the saliva, resulting in an enamel surface layer that is more mature and more resistant to dental caries. This may in part explain why newly erupted

teeth are more susceptible to caries than teeth that have been present in the mouth for some time.

PHYSICAL AND MICROSCOPIC FEATURES OF INCIPIENT CARIES

It usually takes a period of months or even years for a carious lesion to develop. Dental caries is not simply a continual, cumulative loss of mineral, but rather a dynamic process, characterized by alternating periods of *demineralization* and *remineralization.* Demineralization is the dissolution of the calcium and phosphate ions from the hydroxyapatite crystals, which are lost into the plaque and saliva. In remineralization, calcium, phosphate, and other ions in the saliva and plaque are redeposited in previously demineralized areas. It is possible to have demineralization and remineralization occurring without any loss of tooth mass. *A*

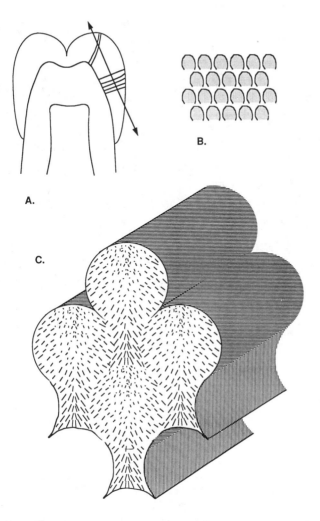

Figure 3–2. Enamel structure. **A.** The orientation of the enamel rods from the dentoenamel junction to the tooth surface. **B.** An arcade of rods seen at the section indicated by the line in **A. C.** The keyhole morphology of the rods. Shading differences represent different orientations of the crystals. (*Courtesy of MWJ Dodds, University of Texas Dental School at San Antonio.*)

lesion results when the cumulative, negative mineral balance exceeds the rate of remineralization over an extended period.

The development of a carious lesion occurs in two distinct stages. The earliest stage is the *incipient lesion*, which is accompanied by histologic changes of the enamel; this stage is followed by the *overt, or frank, lesion*, which is characterized by actual cavitation. If the time between the onset of the incipient lesion in one or more teeth and the development of cavitation is rapid and extensive, the condition is referred to as *rampant* dental caries. Usually rampant

caries occurs following either the excessively frequent intake of *sucrose* or the presence of a severe *xerostomia* (ie, dry mouth) or both. From a preventive dentistry standpoint, the early identification of the incipient lesion is extremely important, because it is during this stage that the carious process *can* be arrested or reversed. The overt lesion can only be treated by some form of operative intervention. Clinically, it is often difficult to recognize and diagnose the early lesion, and for this reason it is important to be familiar with its features from etiologic and histologic standpoints.[6]

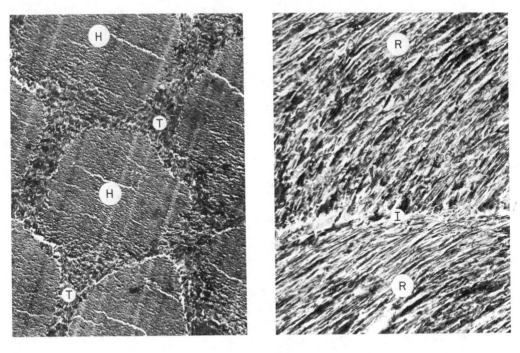

Figure 3–3. A. Electron micrograph of rod cut perpendicular to long axis, showing head (H) and tail (T) relationship. **B.** Electron micrograph of parallel to long axis showing two rods (R) and interrod area (I). Original magnification ×5000. (*From Meckel AH, Griebstein WJ, and Neal RJ. Structure of mature human dental enamel as observed by electron microscopy. Arch Oral Biol. 1965; 10:775–783.*)

The incipient lesion is macroscopically evidenced by the appearance of an area of opacity—the so-called *white spot lesion*. At this earliest clinically noticeable stage, the process at the microscopic level is well established with a number of recognizable zones. Probably the most important fact is that the surface of the enamel is relatively intact (although microscopically the surface is much more porous than sound enamel). The implication is that *the caries process can be retarded, arrested, or indeed reversed before any physical cavitation requiring clinical intervention has occurred.*

On the buccal and lingual surface of a tooth, the white spot may be localized, or it can extend along the entire gingiva, sometimes involving multiple teeth. Interproximally the incipient lesion usually starts as a small round spot immediately *gingival* to the contact point and then gradually expands to a small kidney shape, with the indentation of the kidney contour directed coronally.[7] In fissure caries the initial lesion comparable to the white spot usually occurs *bilaterally* on the two surfaces at the *orifice of the fissure* and eventually coalesces at the base[8] (Figure 3–4). Occasionally lesion formation begins along the wall of the fissure or at the base, either unilaterally or bilaterally.[9]

During the early stages the incipient lesion is not a surface lesion in which loss of

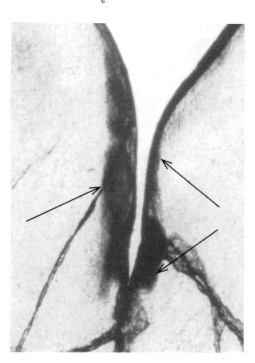

Figure 3–4. Incipient caries in an occlusal fissure. The bilaterality of the lesion is evident in the microradiograph. (*Courtesy of JS Wefel, University of Iowa College of Dentistry.*)

outer enamel has occurred. Instead the mature surface layer of 10 to 100 μm remains intact. If an explorer is used, the surface enamel feels hard and provides no indication of demineralization. However, microscopic pores extend through the mature surface layer to a point where subsurface demineralization occurs; the main body of the lesion is located at that point.[10]

The incipient lesion has been extensively studied and described by Silverstone.[7] Many of the observations of the incipient lesion have been based on the use of a polarizing microscope, which permits precise measurements of the amount of space—called *pore space*—that exists in enamel and enamel defects. Thus as demineralization progresses, more pore space occurs; conversely, as remineralization occurs, less pore space is present.

In the incipient lesion described by Silverstone, four zones are usually present. From the deepest zone of penetration to the mature layer, the four zones are the (1) *translucent zone*, (2) *dark zone*, (3) *body of the lesion*, and (4) *surface zone* (Figure 3–5).

Pore Spaces of the Different Zones

The translucent zone is seen in approximately 50% of the carious lesions examined.[11] In this zone, which is the advancing front of the lesion, slight demineralization occurs, with a *1%* pore space, compared with *0.1%* for intact enamel. In contrast, the dark zone occurs in approximately 95% of carious lesions and has a pore volume of *2% to 4%*. When teeth showing no dark zone are placed in a remineralizing solution, the dark zone becomes visible in its expected position between the translucent zone and the body of the lesion.[12] On the basis of this phenomenon, it is suggested that this zone is the site where remineralization can occur and that *a wider dark zone is indicative of a greater amount, or a longer period, of remineralization*.

Peripheral to the dark zone lies the main body of the lesion. In this zone pore volume ranges from approximately *5%* on the fringes of the lesion to about *25%* in the center.[13] Despite this considerable amount of demineralization, the crystals still maintain their basic orientation on the protein matrix.

The intact surface is slightly demineralized, with a pore volume of *1%*, the same as for the translucent zone. Despite the relatively intact status of the surface zone, some studies have indicated that bacteria may be present in the subsurface lesion. It is possible that the presence of bacteria sig-

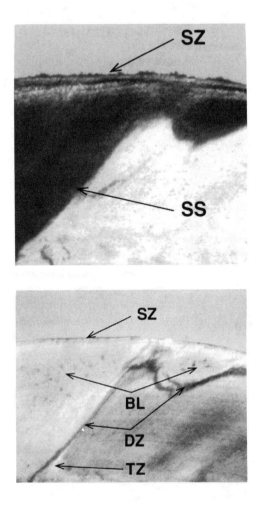

Figure 3–5. View of a natural incipient lesion seen in polarized light. **A.** The lesion immersed in water, with the dark subsurface (SS) body of the lesion and the surface zone (SZ) clearly visible. **B.** The same lesion imbibed in quinoline. The different zones of the incipient lesion are easily identifiable: (SZ) = surface zone; (BL) = body of the lesion (white); (DZ) = dark zone; and, (TZ) = translucent zone. (*Courtesy of JS Wefel, University of Iowa College of Dentistry.*)

nals the end of the incipient lesion and the beginning of the cavitation stage.

Question 1. Which of the following statements, if any, are correct?

A. *All* the following structures are involved in the passage of fluids in the enamel: subsurface cuticle, interrod space, intercrystalline matrix, dentoenamel membrane, incremental lines, striae of Retzius, and dentinoenamel membrane.

B. The head of the enamel rod is *always* oriented toward the incisal or occlusal surfaces of *both* the maxillary and mandibular teeth.

C. A rampant caries attack implies a previous rampant incipient lesion presence.

D. The incipient lesion usually starts incisal to the contact point in interproximal caries and at the base of the fissure in occlusal caries.

E. The dark and the translucent zones are centers of remineralization when "biologic repair" of the tooth is occurring.

THE CARIOGENIC BACTERIA

Following Miller's work, it was not until 1954 that fundamental experimental evidence proved that bacteria were the agents of acid production. F. J. Orland and colleagues[14] demonstrated that germ-free rats did not develop caries when fed a cariogenic diet. The *transmissible* nature of the disease in animals was demonstrated by the experiments of Keyes,[15] who showed that previously caries-inactive hamsters developed caries after contact with caries-active animals.

For caries to develop acidogenic (acid-producing) bacteria must be present, and a means must exist of containing the metabolic acids at the point where caries is to develop. Dental plaque fulfills both of these functions. Plaque can be defined as an adherent mass of bacterial deposits that covers tooth surfaces and that cannot be removed simply by rinsing the mouth. Chapter 2 describes the formation and development of dental plaque.

Of the 200 to 300 species of microorganisms inhabiting the plaque, the great majority are not directly involved in the caries process. Two bacterial genera are of special interest in cariogenesis[16,17]: (1) the *mutans streptococci* and (2) the *lactobacilli*.

Mutans Streptococci and Caries

The mutans streptococci (MS) are a group of bacterial species previously considered to be serotypes of the single species, *Streptococcus mutans*.[16] These bacteria are characterized by their ability to ferment mannitol and sorbitol, and to produce extracellular glucans from sucrose and by their cariogenicity in animal models. In the human population the two species of interest are *S mutans* and *S sobrinus*. *Streptococcus mutans* received its name in 1924 when J. K. Clarke in England isolated organisms from human carious lesions. He noted that they were more oval than round and assumed them to be a mutant form of a streptococcus.[18]

Mutans streptococci are now considered to be the *major* pathogenic bacterial species involved in the caries process. They have shown to be cariogenic when implanted into the mouths of animals, including rats, hamsters and monkeys. Several cross-sectional surveys have indicated an association between the presence of *S mutans* and dental caries.[19–21] This finding has been repeated to some extent in longitudinal studies of microbiology and caries incidence. Mutans streptococci are usually found in relatively large numbers in the plaque occurring immediately over developing smooth-surface lesions. In one longitudinal study, specific sites were periodically sampled for *S mutans* and the teeth

examined for caries. Teeth destined to become carious exhibited a significant increase in the proportions of *S mutans* from 6 to 24 months *before* the eventual diagnosis of caries.[22] Similarly, dental plaques isolated from sites overlying white spot lesions were characterized by a significantly higher proportion of MS than plaques sampled from sound enamel sites.[23] Increased numbers of MS in the saliva also parallel the development of the smooth-surface lesion. In another study *S mutans* counts from the saliva of 200 children indicated that 93% with detectable caries were positive for *S mutans*, whereas uninfected children were almost always caries-free.[24]

Certain physiological characteristics of the MS favor their position as a prime agent in caries. These traits include the ability to stick to tooth surfaces, production of abundant insoluble *extracellular polysaccharides* from sucrose, rapid production of *lactic acid* from a number of sugar substrates, *acid tolerance*, and the production of *intracellular polysaccharide* stores. These cariogenic features help the MS survive in an unfriendly environment under conditions called "feast or famine" due to the cycles of either very low concentrations of substrate (ie, between meals) through to periods of excessive concentrations of substrate (ie, during consumption of a sugary food). As a general rule, the cariogenic bacteria metabolize sugars to produce the energy required for their growth and reproduction. The by-products of this metabolism are acids, which are pumped out of the bacterial cells into the plaque fluid. The damage caused by *S mutans* is due mainly to lactic acid, although other acids, such as butyric and propionic, are present within the plaque.[25] In general *S mutans* is the most common of the human MS, and has the greatest evidence implicating it as the *most virulent odontopathogen*. Another of the MS, *S sobrinus*, differs from

S mutans in that it requires sucrose for attachment and growth in the plaque.

Lactobacilli and Caries

Lactobacilli (LB) are both *acidogenic* (acid-producing) and *aciduric* (acid-tolerant): their presence in the saliva of individuals with active, untreated caries and the subsequent reduction in their numbers following treatment of the caries[26] was thought to indicate a causal role for this organism. Indeed, from the early 1920s until the 1950s, lactobacilli were considered as the essential acidogenic bacteria causing caries. In 1954, Orland and coworkers demonstrated that when rodents living in a germ-free environment were infected with a lactic acid-producing enterococci (and no lactobacilli), they still developed caries.[14] This was the first time that it was known that lactobacilli were not requisite for caries development. However, the presence of an aciduric organism when acid conditions prevail does not prove cause and effect; in fact the numbers of lactobacillus species isolated from either saliva or plaque are so low as to be incapable of producing the range of pH values required for caries initiation.[27] Lactobacilli, specifically *L casei*, have been shown to colonize white spot lesions *prior* to cavitation, and associations have been demonstrated between the presence of lactobacilli and lesion development.[28] As a general rule, lactobacilli are found in greater numbers in the *more advanced*, smooth-surface lesions.[29] This is seen following irradiation for head and neck cancer, when extensive, multiple, carious lesions develop rapidly because of the destruction of the salivary glands. During the initial phases of the developing carious lesions, large numbers of *S mutans* appear, only to decrease later in number as the lactobacilli population increases.[30]

Based on some of the longitudinal studies of plaque microbiology and caries development, it appears that caries may be considered to be a *two-stage process*, with *S mutans* implicated in the *initiation* of the lesion and LB (specifically *L casei*) associated with its *progression*.[16,28] Other bacteria, particularly the actinomyces (*A odontolyticus*), have also been associated with lesion progression.[28]

ADHERENCE

Adherence to the solid tooth surface by *S mutans* is necessary both before and after colonization. The first bacteria must establish a foothold on the tooth surface and then maintain their positions while continuing to colonize in protected areas offered by the interproximal spaces along the gingiva or in the pits and fissures. Otherwise they would be swept away by the saliva.

Mutans streptococci are able to attach to the tooth surface by either of two mechanisms:[16,17,31] (1) sucrose-independent adsorption, in which the bacteria attach to the acquired pellicle through specific extracellular proteins (*adhesins*) located on the fimbriae (fuzzy coat) of these organisms; and (2) sucrose-dependent mechanisms, in which bacteria require the presence of sucrose to produce sticky extracellular polysaccharides, or *glucans*, which allow attachment and accumulation. *Streptococcus sobrinus* differs from *S mutans* in that it lacks the adhesin required for sucrose-independent attachment and therefore only accumulates on smooth surfaces in the presence of a sucrose-rich diet.[16] Thus the presence of the insoluble glucans is an important factor in establishing the presence and virulence of an organism. Sucrose is a disaccharide sugar, consisting of one glucose and one fructose unit (referred to as moieties) joined by a disaccharide bond. One of the key enzymes in the conversion of the glucose moiety of sucrose to glucan is *glucosyltransferase*. At times the enzyme may be altered, resulting in the production of a soluble glucan that does not support adherence or that at times can even function to inhibit adherence. These mutant strains that lack the insoluble glucan are usually noncariogenic.[32] Future advances in caries prevention may focus on displacing cariogenic strains of S mutans from their niches and substituting the non-cariogenic mutant strains.[33]

The effect of sucrose dependence for glucan production is seen in several clinical situations. Children who consume little or no sucrose because of sucrase or fructase enzyme deficiencies have a less cariogenic plaque. Similarly, individuals receiving long-term nourishment via stomach tube have less plaque and fewer S mutans.[34] Individuals restricting their sucrose intake have a decreased proportion of S mutans in their plaque, but the MS increases when sucrose is reintroduced into the diet.[35] Sugar restriction has also been shown to reduce the acidogenicity of dental plaque.[36,37]

ECOLOGY OF CARIES DEVELOPMENT

Several studies support the possibility that the initial colonizers can help to determine the eventual pathogenicity of the plaque.[38] Once a species of bacteria has established its ecologic niche, other bacteria introduced at a later date appear to have a more difficult task in colonizing. Once established, *a niche can be long-lasting*. For instance, children with the highest number of S mutans for deciduous teeth experienced a higher attack rate for the later permanent teeth.[39]

Streptococcus mutans requires a *solid surface* for successful colonization. During the first year of life, very few S mutans are found in the mouth.[40] These same bacteria, which are found only in minimal numbers prior to tooth eruption, rapidly colonize the plaque of newly erupting teeth, given the right conditions. It has been shown that an important route of infection of infants by S mutans is from their mothers by the mouth-to-mouth transmission, such as by sharing a spoon during feeding.[41] This observation, taken with the evidence that mothers with the highest S mutans counts had infants with similarly high S mutans counts,[42] and the fact that early infection by S mutans is associated with high decay rates,[43] suggests that an intriguing means of preventing caries in children would be to treat and prevent the disease in their mothers, possibly even *before* the child's birth.

Because no competition with other organisms occurs, these first bacterial populations probably have little difficulty in establishing their ecologic niches on the epithelial surfaces of the mouth and in the saliva. Once the teeth erupt, many of these oral reservoirs of bacteria participate in the formation of the plaque. Each firmly established niche can act as a "seeding" area for other areas of the mouth. This seeding can possibly be abetted by the use of *dental floss* or possibly with an *explorer* serving as the vehicle for the seeding.[44] *Streptococcus mutans* decrease in number as teeth are lost throughout life and practically disappear following full-mouth extraction.[45] After dentures are inserted, S mutans reappear, only to disappear again when the dentures are removed for an extended period.

The development of a cariogenic plaque depends on a number of factors. Frequent exposure of developing plaque to sugar, particularly in the form of sucrose, encourages a high concentration of acidogenic organisms. These organisms produce acid, thereby favoring growth of aciduric organisms, which are able to thrive in conditions both of excess sugar concentrations and at low pH. The cariogenic bacteria of the plaque also produce intracellular polysaccharide (ICP) stores, which allow them to survive between sugar exposures, and extracellular polysaccharides (ECP). The two main types of ECPs are the *glucans*, which are polymers of glucose, and the *fructans*, which are polymers of fructose. Fructans, which are produced by the enzyme, fructosyl transferase, are rapidly broken down for energy by the plaque bacteria. Glucans, produced by glucosyl transferase enzymes may be either soluble or insoluble; production of insoluble glucans (sometimes referred to as mutans) encourages growth of a thick plaque, which further aids bacterial attachment, as well as altering the diffusion characteristics of the plaque to encourage a low pH. Once a lesion develops, the stability of the immediate plaque population can change rapidly. The newly created aciduric environment often eliminates, or at least halts, the continuity of colonization of other organisms. *Streptococcus mutans* and *L casei* are metabolically active at pH 5.0, a pH at which many other plaque bacteria cannot survive. Certain bacteria may modulate the plaque pH by using some of the acids produced by other bacteria for their own metabolism. Species of *Veillonella*[46] and *Neisseria*[47] can both metabolize lactic acid, possibly modulating the overall acidogenic response of the plaque.

Question 2. Which of the following statements, if any, are correct?

A. *Streptococcus mutans* can be expected in increased numbers at an incipient lesion site in the early stages of demineralization.

B. Lactobacilli are usually found even earlier than mutans streptococci at the incipient lesion site.

C. Soluble glucans foster better bacterial adherence than insoluble glucans.

D. Mothers can be their child's worst dental friend.

E. Glucans provide energy for the bacteria producing it; fructans can supply an extracellular energy source for the surrounding bacteria.

CHEMICAL CHANGES IN THE PLAQUE

The incipient lesion is initiated by events that occur in the plaque. Almost immediately after exposure to a sugar (or acidogenic) challenge, the pH of the plaque begins to drop as the acidogenic plaque bacteria produce acids. A variety of acids are found in the plaque fluid (the fluid bathing the plaque bacteria and matrix). These include lactic acid, which is a strong acid, as well as weaker acids, such as acetic and propionic acids.[25] As the plaque pH drops in response to the production of these acids, a series of complex chemical and physical events start to occur. Plaque fluid is supersaturated with respect to calcium phosphate at normal, resting pH levels. However, as the pH falls, this level of saturation is not maintained, until at a pH of approximately 5.5 (the so-called *critical pH*), the plaque fluid is undersaturated with respect to calcium phosphate, and dissolution of the enamel may occur. The simplest explanation, therefore, for caries is that bacterial acid production following consumption of carbohydrate causes the pH of the tooth environment to fall; if it falls below the critical pH then the nonsaturation of the oral fluids with respect to calcium and inorganic phosphate allows the dissolution of enamel to take place. Thus physical degradation of enamel occurs. This concept does not, however, explain certain features of enamel caries such as the intact surface layer. The loss of mineral that occurs primarily in the body of the lesion may be explained by the fact that as the pH of the plaque falls, the proportion of undissociated acids in the plaque fluid increases. These acids, because they are uncharged, are able to diffuse through the porous matrix of the enamel down a concentration gradient. Once the acids penetrate to a certain depth, where the pH is higher, they dissociate, releasing protons, which attack the apatite lattice. Calcium and phosphate ions thus dissolved diffuse outwards into the plaque, or they may reprecipitate before escaping the enamel, thereby maintaining the surface zone. When the plaque pH returns to resting levels, calcium and phosphate may re-enter the enamel and repair some of the damaged crystallites in the process of remineralization (Figure 3–6). Fluoride acts as a *catalyst*, favoring remineralization and tending to inhibit demineralization.

The drop and recovery of plaque pH as a function of time following a glucose mouth rinse is often referred to as *Stephan's curve*, after Dr Robert Stephan, who originally reported on the phenomenon[48] (Figure 3–7). Plaque pH responses to simple sugar rinses have been shown to be differ-

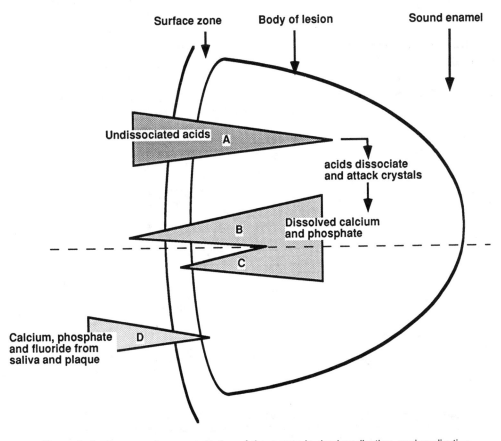

Surface zone   **Body of lesion**   **Sound enamel**

Undissociated acids A

acids dissociate and attack crystals

B

Dissolved calcium and phosphate

C

Calcium, phosphate and fluoride from saliva and plaque D

Figure 3–6. Diagrammatic representation of the events in demineralization–remineralization. Above the dotted line, demineralization is occurring, and below the line remineralization is occurring. The fall in plaque pH causes undissociated acids to diffuse through the surface layer into the subsurface layer, where they dissociate and attack the apatite crystals (A). Dissolved calcium and phosphate diffuse out and are either reprecipitated at the surface (B) or are lost into the plaque and saliva (C). When the pH is high, extrinsic calcium and phosphate may reenter the enamel, repairing the early damage (D). (*Courtesy of MWJ Dodds, University of Texas Dental School at San Antonio.*)

ent both in caries-free and caries-active individuals, as well as in different sites of the mouth. These differences point to an increased acidogenicity (ie, plaque pH falls lower) in plaque from either caries-active individuals or caries-prone sites of the dentition. As well as highlighting differences in caries susceptibility, plaque pH studies have been used to attempt to differentiate between different foods on the basis of their acidogenic potential, which could be useful in terms of diet advice in preventive dentistry.[49]

Ultrastructural Alterations in the Incipient Lesion

Demineralization of the surface enamel produces a ragged profile when seen with the electron microscope, with pores extending into the enamel structure[4] (Figure 3–8). Organic material, called the subsurface pellicle, immediately fills the microscopic voids. When conditions are optimum, this surface area is one of the first to remineralize.[50] The initial attack may be on the rod or between the rods or both.[51] The initial acid attack appears preferentially to dissolve the *core* of the crystals that make up the rods.

Small pores, or microchannels, have been observed by electron microscopy in the surface zone of incipient lesions, as well as a widening of the rod boundaries.[52] These initial enamel defects allow the ingress of acids to the subsurface region. The initial acid attack preferentially solubilizes the *magnesium* and *carbonate* ions and is followed by a removal of calcium, phosphorus,

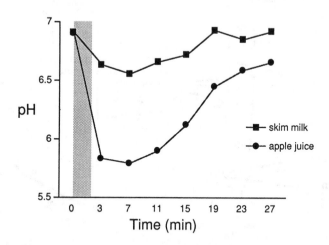

Figure 3–7. Stephan's curves. These curves show the typical plaque pH response to an oral rinse (indicated by the screened area). There is an immediate fall in the pH, followed by a gradual return to resting values after about 40 minutes. Each curve represents the mean of 12 subjects; the pH was measured by the sampling method (see Chapter 15) and therefore is an average value for the whole mouth plaque pH. In individual sites away from the salivary buffers, the pH values may fall close to 4.0. The upper curve was obtained from reconstituted powdered skim milk and the lower one from an apple-flavored drink, showing a large difference in the acidogenicity of these two drinks. (*Courtesy of MWJ Dodds, University of Texas Dental School at San Antonio.*)

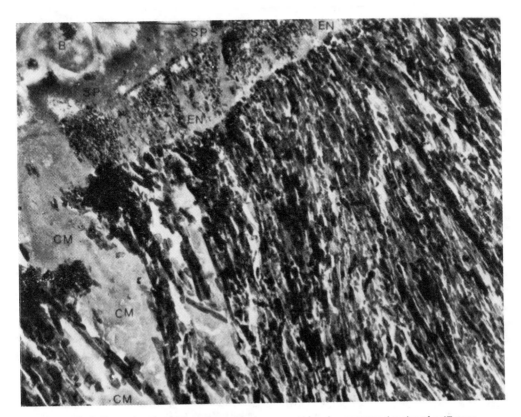

Figure 3–8. Enamel surface layer of a mesial brown spot in a lower second molar of a 47-year-old man. The carious attack has destroyed the enamel apatite crystals in external layer (EN) of about 0.8 µm wide. A small irregular defect filled with consolidated organic matrix (CM) extends into the depth of the lesion through the superficial enamel. Teaching comment: The break in the enamel with its consolidated matrix is a *pore* communicating with the subsurface lesion. Also, the consolidated matrix constitutes part of the *subsurface pellicle*. (*From Frank RM, Brendel A. Ultrastructure of the approximal dental plaque and the underlying normal and carious enamel. Arch Oral Biol. 1966, 11:909. Permission granted by Pergamon Press, Ltd., Oxford, England.*)

and other ions that are part of the crystal. If a cavity is to form eventually, the ions in the subsurface lesion must diffuse outward through the pores and pellicle and into the plaque. In the body of the lesion there appears to be a progressive demineralization that may occur preferentially along the striae of Retzius. Once the lesion reaches the dentinoenamel junction (DEJ), *lateral spread* also occurs along the DEJ (via the dentinoenamel membrane), which under-

mines the enamel. Eventually the mature surface layer begins to break down, with the process beginning on the surface and progressing inward. Concurrent with this change the more soluble protein is lost from the matrix. Once cavitation occurs, the zones of the incipient lesion become less clearly defined because of mineral loss and the presence of bacteria, bacterial end products, plaque, and residual substrate, which may support further lesion development.

ROOT CARIES

Although root caries as a disease entity separate from coronal caries was reported as early as 1884 by Darby,[53] it is only during the last 20 years that this topic has received attention. The prevalence of caries in children has declined during the past 15 or so years,[54] and a general demographic shift has occurred toward an increasing proportion of seniors within the population. Given that root caries occurs on the root surfaces, and that the prevalence of gingival recession increases with increasing age, the association between increasing age and root caries is obvious. Contributing to an expectation that root caries will become a greater oral health concern in the elderly population are three factors: more people are keeping their teeth longer, the population is aging, and more older people are taking medications known to reduce salivary flow. At present there is no standardized format for recording root caries, either clinically and epidemiologically. The development of such an instrument would permit a concerted, worldwide study and uniform reporting on the epidemiology of the disease, which could lead to its better control.

Katz and colleagues estimated that individuals going into their 30s have about 1 out of 100 surfaces with recession and root caries; when they leave their 50s, about 1 out of 5 exposed surfaces is involved.[55] By age 72, approximately 52% of these surfaces have been attacked.[56] The roots at greatest risk are the mandibular molars, and the mandibular incisors are at least risk.[55]

U.S. Department of Health and Human Services 1985–1986 *Survey of Oral Health in U.S. Adults* found that 63.5% of seniors had at least one decayed or filled root surface, with a mean of 3.1 surfaces per person. Buccal–lingual surfaces are more prone to root decay or fillings than proximal surfaces.[56] A Canadian study concluded that "the increase in the prevalence of root decay with age *may not be due to aging per se* but may be a product of the general deterioration in oral health which often accompanies growing old. Older adults with good oral health had low rates of tooth decay."[57] In a study of 5000 subjects in Finland, it was found that men had from 1.1 to 2.5 times more root caries than women. The greatest difference was in the group 60 to 69 years of age.[58]

A number of risk factors have been defined for root caries development, including age, gender, fluoride exposure, systemic illness, medications, oral hygiene, and diet.[59] In terms of the microbiology of root caries, despite early indications of a strong association between *Actinomyces* species and progressive root lesions,[60,61] more recent studies indicate that plaque and salivary concentrations of the mutans streptococci are correlated positively with the presence of root surface caries.[62,63]

Root caries differs from coronal caries in several aspects. A critical difference is that the tissues affected are fundamentally dissimilar. Enamel is much more highly mineralized than dentin or cementum. Because of the lower mineral content and higher organic content of the cementum–dentin complex, root caries may progress *both* by acid demineralization and by proteolytic breakdown of the organic component. These compositional differences therefore manifest in differences in the rate of lesion formation, histologic and visual appearance, and the potential for and rate of remineralization.[64] Clinically the lesion is initially noncavitated. It is soft and has a yellowish brown coloration. The lesion can eventually assume any outline and may involve multiple root surfaces (Figure 3–9). When cavitation does occur, lesions tend to spread laterally, have a depth of approximately 0.5 to 1 mm, and have a dark brown appearance.[65] Frequently lesions appear immediately below the cementoenamel junction, undermining but

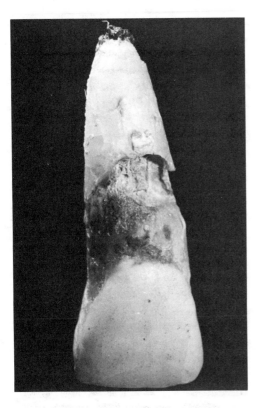

Figure 3–9. Root caries. The darker staining of the coronal half of the root indicates a considerable gingival recession, which is prerequisite to lesion development.

not involving the enamel. Root caries lesions may rarely occur subgingivally when loss of attachment has happened while the crest of the gingiva is coronal to or at the level of the cementoenamel junction.[59]

Histologic studies of the surface of normal exposed cementum indicate that it is hypermineralized in relation to unexposed cementum. The hypermineralization is probably due to calcium, phosphate, and other minerals derived from the saliva.[66] In the earliest stages of root caries, the surface hypermineralization can also result from the release of ions from the subsurface lesion, much as happens with coronal caries.[67] Also, like coronal caries, cemental caries is probably associated with periods of de-

mineralization and remineralization.[64] Root caries differs from coronal caries in that bacterial invasion of cementum and dentin occurs early on. At times the invasion features columns of organisms between spikes of relatively intact cementum. At other times a complete loss of cementum exposes the dentin.[61] Arrested caries that is dark and hard often demonstrates a layer of sclerotic dentin underlying the lesion. However, even in lesions clinically classified as arrested caries, areas of active caries may arise. Such lesions exhibit a mosaic pattern of active and arrested lesions.[68]

PREVENTION OF ROOT CARIES

The best prevention for root caries in old age is the prevention of periodontal disease in middle age or younger.[69] Frequent checkups, prophylaxes, professional applications of fluoride, plaque control measures, and the home use of fluoride dentifrices and mouth rinses are effective in preventing root caries.[65] All extensive periodontal surgery for pocket elimination should feature similar follow-up office and home care routines. Sugar restriction is especially important in reducing acidogenesis, as is good oral hygiene.[58,65] Fluoride plays a key role in root caries prevention. Water fluoridation is effective in reducing root caries,[70] and the use of topical fluorides to arrest or in reversing root lesions is often an alternative to restorations,[71,72] which is a desirable option in view of the difficulty in restoring root caries via operative procedures.

Secondary, or Recurrent, Caries

Lesions of secondary caries start in small imperfections or gaps between the tooth and the margins of a restoration. Bacteria are able to grow in these sites, sheltered from the protective effects of saliva, and eventually a so-called *wall lesion* develops. The diagnosis of these lesions is notoriously diffi-cult.[73] In one study, extracted teeth were cut so that the section included both a clinically sound amalgam margin and one defined as *ditched*. The prevalence of wall lesions in both sound and ditched sides was exactly the same at 54%, although it is unknown whether these lesions were recurrent or residual disease left during cavity prepara-tion.[74] The magnitude of the problem of sec-ondary decay is illustrated by studies in-dicating that the median survival time of restorations ranges from 5 to 10 years.[75] Replacement of restorations accounts for more operative dentistry time than the placement of first-time restorations.[76] Im-provements in this area are coming from the use of materials that bond directly to the tooth tissue, eliminating the gap between tooth and filling, and from restorative mate-rials that slowly release fluoride, such as glass ionomers and newer fluoride-releasing composites and amalgams.[77,78]

Question 3. Which of the following state-ments, if any, are correct?

A. The critical pH for enamel deminer-alization ranges between 6.0 to 5.5.
B. The initial caries attack on the enamel rod is along the C-axis.
C. Once the incipient lesions become overt, all the lesion zones disappear.
D. Root caries is *not* a part of the aging process but is usually a sign of previ-ous periodontal neglect.
E. A dentist usually inserts more res-torations as a result of secondary caries than for primary caries.

SUMMARY

Dental caries is a multifactorial disease of bacterial origin. The mutans streptococci, particularly *S mutans*, are associated with the beginning of smooth-surface lesions.

After the smooth-surface lesions are initi-ated by S mutans, lactobacilli are seen in increasing numbers. The first stage in the development of a cariogenic plaque is at-tachment to the tooth surface. The initial foothold is facilitated by the presence of spe-cific adhesins on the bacteria that bind stere-ochemically to complementary proteina-ceous receptors of the acquired pellicle. Once the foothold is established S mutans, lactobacilli, and other organisms produce a sticky glucan from dietary sucrose that pro-vides plaque bulk and allows more bacteria to become incorporated. The growth of aci-dogenic organisms in the plaque is sucrose-dependent. The end product of sucrose me-tabolism for S mutans is lactic acid. Acid production in the plaque following exposure to a fermentable carbohydrate substrate causes the pH of the plaque to fall, thus al-tering the chemistry of the enamel environ-ment so that demineralization can occur.

The first sign of caries is a white, frosty-appearing, incipient enamel lesion. The incipient lesion has four zones. Starting from the exterior, they are the surface zone, the body of the lesion, the dark zone, and the translucent zone. The surface and dark zones are associated with remineralization, the body of the lesion and the translucent zone with demineralization. During the life-time of a tooth, demineralization and re-mineralization occur continually. During the incipient caries phase the carious lesion can be arrested and reversed. It is only when demineralization exceeds remineral-ization over an extended period that cavita-tion occurs, signaling the beginning of the overt lesion.

ANSWERS AND EXPLANATIONS

1. A, B, C
    D—incorrect. The interproximal starting point is apical to the contact point; for

the pit-and-fissure lesion, it usually begins on the lateral walls of the fissure.
E—incorrect. The dark and the surface zones are the centers for remineralization; the body of the lesion and the *translucent* zones are centers for *demineralization*.

2. A, D, E
B—incorrect. The MS usually precede the lactobacilli.
C—incorrect. The bacteria producing glucans often are noncariogenic because of adherence problems; the insoluble glucans are usually produced by the cariogenic bacteria and facilitate adherence.

3. B, D, E
A—incorrect. The critical pH for enamel demineralization is from 5.5 to 5.0.
C—incorrect. The same zones are present but are less clearly defined due to the presence of bacteria, plaque, and debris.

SELF-EVALUATION QUESTIONS

1. In 1890, Miller proposed the _____ _____ theory for caries, which is still a basis for our present concept of the disease.
2. The two major stages of a carious lesion are the _____ lesion, which can be arrested or reversed by remineralization therapy, and the _____, which must be restored.
3. The four zones of an incipient lesion seen with the polarizing microscope (starting from the tooth surface) are the _____, _____, _____, and the _____ zones.
4. The zone of the incipient lesion that is the best indicator of *remineralization* is the _____ zone; the two most reliable indicator zones of *demineralization* are the _____ and the _____ zones.
5. The pore volume of the surface and translucent zones are approximately the same, that is _____ percent.
6. The critical pH for enamel demineralization is pH _____.
7. The plot of the drop and recovery of pH on a graph is often referred to as the _____ curve for the investigator who first published on the phenomenon.
8. Two possible sources of the calcium and phosphate accounting for the hypermineralized surface of root caries are _____ and _____.
9. The four major types (location) of caries are: _____, _____, _____, and _____.
10. Two causes for *rampant* caries are _____ (diet) and _____ (dry mouth).
11. The pore space in both the translucent and surface zones is 1%; dark zone approximately _____%, and the body of the lesion ranges up to _____%.
12. The two mutans streptococci most often associated with caries development are S _____ and S _____.
13. The surface of root caries is (hyper) (hypo) mineralized.
14. The species of lactobacilli most likely to cause caries is L _____.

REFERENCES

1. Miller WD. *The Microorganisms of the Human Mouth.* Philadelphia, SS White Dental Manufacturing Company; 1890. Reprinted Basel, Switzerland. Karger; 1973.
2. Black GV. Dr. Black's conclusions reviewed again. *Dental Cosmos.* 1898; 40:440–451.
3. Williams JL. On structural changes in human enamel; with special reference to clinical observations on hard and soft enamel. *Dental Cosmos.* 1898; 40:505–537.

4. Frank RM, Brendel A. Ultrastructure of the approximal dental plaque and the underlying normal and carious enamel. *Arch Oral Biol.* 1966; 11:883–912.

5. Crabb HSM. The porous outer enamel of unerupted human premolars. *Caries Res.* 1976; 10:1–7.

6. Dodds MWJ. Dilemmas in caries diagnosis—applications to current practice, and need for research. *J Dent Educ.* 1993; 57: 433–438.

7. Silverstone LM. The structure of carious enamel, including the early lesion. *Oral Sci Rev.* 1973; 3:100–160.

8. König KG. Dental morphology in relation to caries resistance with special reference to fissures as susceptible sites. *J Dent Res.* 1963; 42:461–476.

9. Juhl M. Localization of carious lesions in occlusal pits and fissure of human premolars. *Scand J Dent Res.* 1983; 91:251–255.

10. Zahradnik RT, Moreno EC. Progressive stages of subsurface demineralization of human tooth enamel. *Arch Oral Biol.* 1977; 22:585–591.

11. Silverstone LM. The primary translucent zone of enamel caries and of artificial caries-like lesions. *Br Dent J.* 1966; 120:461–471.

12. Silverstone LM. Remineralization phenomena. *Caries Res.* 1977; 11 (Suppl. 1):59–84.

13. Darling AI. Studies of the early lesion of enamel caries with transmitted light, polarized light, and microradiography. Its nature, mode of spread, points of entry and its relation to enamel structure. *Br Dent J.* 1958; 105:119–135.

14. Orland FJ, Blayney JR, Harrison RW, et al. Use of germ-free animal technique in the study of experimental dental caries. I. Basic observations on rats reared free of all microorganisms. *J Dent Res.* 1954; 33:147–174.

15. Keyes PH. The infections and transmissible nature of experimental dental caries—findings and implications. *Arch Oral Biol.* 1960; 1:304–320.

16. Loesche WJ. Role of *Streptococcus mutans* in human dental decay. *Microbiol Rev.* 1986; 50:353–380.

17. Tanzer JM. On changing the cariogenic chemistry of coronal plaque. *J Dent Res.* 1989; 68 (Special Issue):1576–1587.

18. Clarke JK. On the bacterial factor in the aetiology of dental caries. *Br J Exp Pathol.* 1924; 5:141–147.

19. Littleton NW, Kakehashi S, Fitzgerald RJ. Recovery of specific "caries-inducing" streptococci from carious lesions in the teeth of children. *Arch Oral Biol.* 1970; 15:461–463.

20. Keene HJ, Shklair IL. Relationship of *Streptococcus mutans* carrier status to the development of carious lesions in initially caries free recruits. *J Dent Res.* 1975; 53:1295.

21. Loesche WJ, Rowan J, Straffon LH, et al. Association of *Streptococcus mutans* with human dental decay. *Infect Immun.* 1975; 11:1252–1260.

22. Loesche WJ, Eklund S, Earnest R, et al. Longitudinal investigation of bacteriology of human fissure decay: Epidemiological studies in molars shortly after eruption. *Infect Immun.* 1984; 46:765–772.

23. van Houte J, Sansone C, Joshipura K, et al. In vitro acidogenic potential and mutans streptococci on human smooth-surface plaque associated with initial caries lesions and sound enamel. *J Dent Res.* 1991; 70: 1497–1502.

24. Edelstein B, Tinanoff N. Screening preschool children for dental caries using a microbial test. *Pediatr Dent.* 1989; 11:129–132.

25. Geddes DAM. Acids produced by human dental plaque metabolism in situ. *Caries Res.* 1975; 9:98–109.

26. Kesel RG, Shklair IL, Green GH, et al. Further studies on lactobacilli counts after elimination of carious lesions. *J Dent Res.* 1958; 37:1077–1087.

27. Gibbons RJ. Bacteriology of dental caries. *J Dent Res.* 1964; 43:1021–1028.

28. Boyar RM, Bowden GH. The microflora associated with the progression of incipient lesions in teeth of children living in a water-fluoridated area. *Caries Res.* 1985; 19:298–306.

29. Ikeda TH, Sandham HJ, Bradley EL Jr. Changes in *Streptococcus mutans* and lactobacilli in plaque in relation to the initiation

of dental caries in Negro children. *Arch Oral Biol*. 1973; 18:555–566.

30. Brown LR, Dreizen S, Handler S. Effects of elected caries regimens on microbial changes following radiation-induced xerostomia in cancer patients. In: Stiles HM, Loesche WJ, O'Brien TC, eds. *Proceedings: Microbial Aspects of Dental Caries*. 1976: 275–290, Washington, D.C., Information Retrieval.

31. Gibbons RJ. Bacterial adhesion to oral tissues: A model for infectious diseases. *J Dent Res*. 1989; 68:750–760.

32. Murchison H, Larrimore S, Curtiss R. In vitro inhibition of adherence of *Streptococcus mutans* strains by nonadherent mutants of *S mutans* 6715. *Infect Immun*. 1985; 50: 826–832.

33. Kuramitsu HK, Smorawinska M, Yamashita Y. Molecular biology of *Streptococcus mutans* virulence. In: Bowen WH, Tabak LA, eds. *Cariology for the Nineties*. Rochester, NY. University of Rochester Press; 1993: 300–307.

34. Littleton NW, McCabe RM, Carter CH. Studies of oral health in persons nourished by stomach tube. II. Acidogenic properties and selected bacterial components of plaque material. *Arch Oral Biol*. 1967; 12:601–609.

35. de Stoppelaar JD, van Houte JS, Backer-Dirks O. The effect of carbohydrate restriction on the presence of *Streptococcus mutans*, *Streptococcus sanguis* and iodophilic polysaccharide-producing bacteria in human dental plaque. *Caries Res*. 1970; 4:114–123.

36. Dodds MWJ, Edgar WM. Effects of dietary sucrose levels on pH fall and acid-anion profile in human dental plaque after a starch mouthrinse. *Arch Oral Biol*. 1986; 31:509–512.

37. Sgan-Cohen HD, Newbrun E, Huber R, et al. The effect of previous diet on plaque pH response to different foods. *J Dent Res*. 1988; 67:1434–1437.

38. Gibbons RJ, van Houte JH. Bacterial adherence and the formation of dental plaques. In: Beachey EH, eds. *Bacterial Adherence*. London, Chapman & Hall; 1980:61–104.

39. Zickert I, Emilson C-G, Krasse B. Effect of caries preventive measures in children highly infected with the bacterium *Streptococcus mutans*. *Arch Oral Biol*. 1982; 27: 861–868.

40. Carlsson J, Grahnen H, Jonsson G. Lactobacilli and streptococci in the mouth of children. *Caries Res*. 1975; 9:333–339.

41. Berkowitz RJ, Jones P. Mouth-to-mouth transmission of the bacterium *Streptococcus mutans* between mother and child. *Arch Oral Biol*. 1985; 30:377–379.

42. Köhler B, Bratthall D. Intrafamilial levels of *Streptococcus mutans* and some aspects of the bacterial transmission. *Scand J Dent Res*. 1978; 86:35–42.

43. Zickert I, Emilson C-G, Krasse B. Correlation of level and duration of *Streptococcus mutans* infection with incidence of dental caries. *Infect Immun*. 1983; 39:982–985.

44. Loesche WJ, Svanberg ML, Pape HR. Intra-oral transmission of *Streptococcus mutans* by a dental explorer. *J Dent Res*. 1979; 58: 1765–1770.

45. Carlsson J, Soderholm G, Almfedt I. Prevalence of *Streptococcus sanguis* and *Streptococcus mutans* in the mouth of persons wearing full-dentures. *Arch Oral Biol*. 1969; 14:243–249.

46. Ng SKC, Hamilton IR. Lactate metabolism by *Veillonella parvula*. *J Bacteriol*. 1971; 105:999–1005.

47. Hoshino E, Yamada T, Araya S. Lactate degradation by a strain of *Neisseria* isolated from human dental plaque. *Arch Oral Biol*. 1976; 21:677–683.

48. Stephan RM. Changes in hydrogen-ion concentration on tooth surfaces and in carious lesions. *J Am Dent Assoc*. 1940; 27:718–723.

49. Dodds MWJ, Edgar WM. The relationship between plaque pH, plaque acid anion profiles and oral carbohydrate retention after ingestion of several 'reference foods' by human subjects. *J Dent Res*. 1988; 67:861–865.

50. Tinanoff N, Glick PL, Weber DF. Ultrastructure of organic films on the enamel surface. *Caries Res*. 1976; 10:19–32.

51. Johnson NW. Some aspects of the ultrastructure of early human enamel caries seen with the electron microscope. *Arch Oral Biol.* 1967; 12:1505–1521.

52. Haikel Y, Frank RM, Voegel JC. Scanning electron microscopy of the human enamel surface layer of incipient enamel lesions. *Caries Res.* 1983; 17:1–13.

53. Darby ET. The etiology of caries at the gum margin and labial and buccal surfaces of the teeth. *Dental Cosmos.* 1884; 26:218–232.

54. Glass RL. The first international conference on the declining prevalence of dental caries. *J Dent Res.* 1982; 61 (special issue):1304–1383.

55. Katz RV, Hazen SP, Chilton NW, et al. Prevalence and intraoral distribution of root caries in an adult population. *Caries Res.* 1982; 16:265–271.

56. US Department of Health and Human Services. *Oral Health of United States Adults.* Bethesda, Maryland, NIH Publication 87-2868, 1987.

57. Locker D, Slade GD, Leake JL. Prevalence of and factors associated with root decay in older adults in Canada. *J Dent Res.* 1989; 68:768–772.

58. Vehkalahti MM, Paunio IK. Occurrence of root caries in relation to dental health behavior. *J Dent Res.* 1988; 67:911–914.

59. Banting DW. Epidemiology of root caries. *Gerodontology.* 1986; 5:5–11.

60. Jordan HV, Hammond BF. Filamentous bacteria isolated from human root surface caries. *Arch Oral Biol.* 1972; 17:1333–1342.

61. Sumney D, Jordan H. Characterization of bacteria isolated from human root surface carious lesions. *J Dent Res.* 1974; 53:343–351.

62. van Houte J, Jordan HV, Laraway R, et al. Association of the microbial flora of dental plaque and saliva with human root-surface caries. *J Dent Res.* 1990; 69:1463–1468.

63. Bowden GHW. Microbiology of root surface caries in humans. *J Dent Res.* 1990; 69:1205–1210.

64. Mellberg JR. Demineralization and remineralization of root surface caries. *Gerodontology.* 1986; 5:25–31.

65. Nyvad B, Fejerskov O. Active root surface caries converted into inactive caries as a response to oral hygiene. *Scand J Dent Res.* 1986; 94:281–284.

66. Selvig KA. Biological changes at the tooth–saliva interface in periodontal disease. *J Dent Res.* 1969; 48:846–855.

67. Hals E, Selvig KA. Correlated electron probe microanalysis and microradiography of carious and normal dental cementum. *Caries Res.* 1977; 11:62–75.

68. Schüpbach P, Guggenheim B, Lutz F. Histopathology of root surface caries. *J Dent Res.* 1990; 69:1195–1204.

69. Newbrun E. Prevention of root caries. *Gerodontology.* 1986; 5:33–41.

70. Burt BA, Ismail AI, Eklund SA. Root caries in an optimally fluoridated and a high-fluoride community. *J Dent Res.* 1986; 65:1154–1158.

71. Mellberg JR, Sanchez M. Remineralization by a monofluorophosphate dentifrice in vitro of root dentin softened by artificial caries. *J Dent Res.* 1986; 65:959–962.

72. Teranaka T, Koulourides T. Effect of a 100-ppm fluoride mouthrinse on experimental root caries in humans. *Caries Res.* 1987; 21:326–332.

73. Kidd EAM. Caries diagnosis within restored teeth. *Adv Dent Res.* 1990; 4:10–13.

74. Kidd EAM, O'Hara JW. The caries status of occlusal amalgam restorations with marginal defects. *J Dent Res.* 1990; 69:1275–1277.

75. Elderton RJ. Longitudinal study of dental treatment in the General Dental Service in Scotland. *Br Dent J.* 1983; 155:91–96.

76. Elderton RJ. Clinical studies concerning restoration of teeth. *Adv Dent Res.* 1990; 4:4–9.

77. Skartveit L, Wefel JS, Ekstrand J. Effect of fluoride amalgams on artificial recurrent enamel and root caries. *Scand J Dent Res.* 1991; 99:287–294.

78. Dijkman GEHM, de Vries J, Lodding A, et al. Long-term fluoride release of visible light-activated composites in vitro: A correlation with in situ demineralisation data. *Caries Res.* 1993; 27:117–123.

Chapter 4

The Role of Dental Plaque in the Etiology and Progress of Inflammatory Periodontal Disease

Donald E. Willmann
Eros S. Chaves

Objectives

At the end of this chapter it will be possible to

1. List each of the components of the periodontium and describe its function.
2. Discuss some of the key characteristics of the normal gingival sulcus and of the tooth and epithelium-related components of the subgingival plaque.
3. Differentiate between gingivitis and periodontitis.
4. Describe briefly the progress of periodontal disease from the time of bacterial invasion of the gingival sulcus until bone and connective tissue are involved.

Introduction

Inflammatory periodontal disease is a dental plaque-induced disease.[1-3] In its mildest form, periodontal disease is characterized by slight inflammatory changes of the surface tissues surrounding the teeth; in its severest form massive loss of tooth-support-ing structures and subsequent tooth loss occurs.[4] When periodontal disease is limited to the surface tissues (ie, the gingiva), it is referred to as *gingivitis*; gingivitis can usually be reversed with primary preventive measures. Periodontal disease that affects the deeper tooth-supporting structures is called *periodontitis*. Periodontitis is normally not reversible with primary preventive mea-

61

sures.[5] These same preventive measures, however, can play a critical role in *controlling* disease once periodontal health has been reestablished in a patient with periodontitis.[6]

Until approximately 1950, periodontal disease was accepted to be the result of the physiologic aging process, compounded by the lifetime presence of calculus and the absence of oral hygiene. From 1950 to 1970 it was considered to be a nonspecific disease in which the metabolic end products of many then-unknown oral bacteria contributed to the condition. However, since 1970 sufficient progress has been made in differential diagnosis to conclude that the term *periodontal disease* is an umbrella designation that includes *several* diseases of the periodontium that appear to be caused by different combinations of microbial agents. Taken as a group, the periodontal diseases are widespread. Gingivitis, an inflammation of the soft tissues, affects nearly everyone at some time. Periodontitis has been estimated to affect one fourth to one half of the adults in the United States,[7,8] with advanced disease affecting 8% of the overall population and 15% of seniors.[9] This latter statistic for seniors is somewhat misleading because it implies that periodontal disease is a result of the aging process. Instead, studies have shown that periodontal health is more closely related to personal oral hygiene habits than to age. Elderly individuals with good continuing oral hygiene habits *can* have good periodontal health.

Much debate exists about possible changes in the prevalence and severity of periodontal diseases in the future. The prevalence of inflammatory periodontal diseases may increase because (1) longer American life spans are increasing the *time* that teeth are at risk and (2) people are taking better care of their teeth, thus increasing the *number* of teeth at risk.[10] On the other hand, information about periodontal disease has exploded, including better techniques for diagnosis and treatment. Any additional progress in this direction should result in more effective disease control measures with the possibility that the prevalence and severity of periodontal disease will decline in the future, much as has occurred with caries. Based on the results of large-scale studies, it has been concluded that the severity of periodontal disease is indeed *decreasing*[11] and the need for treatment of periodontitis is less than previously estimated.[12]

Whatever future changes may occur in the prevalence and severity of periodontal disease, primary preventive measures, especially plaque control regimens, will continue to be an important factor in maintaining periodontal health in the United States.

THE PERIODONTIUM

Five anatomic structures function together to support the teeth in the jaws: (1) *alveolar bone*, (2) *cementum*, (3) the *periodontal ligament*, (4) the *dentogingival junction*, and (5) the *gingiva*. Collectively, these five structures are called the *periodontium* (Figs 4–1, 4–2). The five components of the periodontium can be functionally divided into three categories: (1) the bone, cementum, and periodontal ligament fibers, which serve to *anchor* the teeth in the bone sockets of the maxilla and mandible, (2) the dentogingival junction, which acts as a *seal* to isolate the anchoring components from the oral environment, and (3) the covering gingival tissues, which *protect* the dentogingival junction from excessive masticatory stresses.

The *principal fibers* of the periodontal ligament have different orientations and

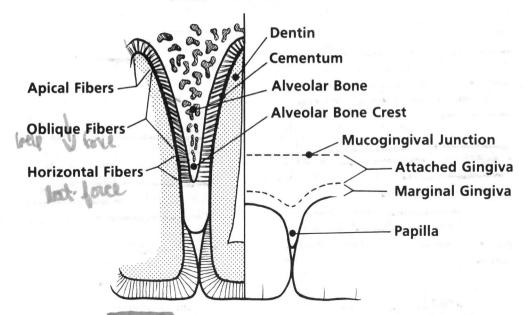

Figure 4–1. Periodontium: Apical, oblique, and horizontal fibers make up the *periodontal liga-ment,* which connects the cementum of the tooth to the alveolar bone. Marginal gingiva follows the contour of the tooth. Dentogingival junction is shown in Figure 4–2.

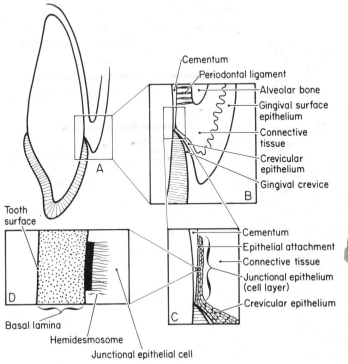

Figure 4–2. Dentogingival junction: The junction between the tooth and gingival soft tissues **A** and **B** occurs where a few layers of junctional epithelial cells **C** are joined to the tooth by an attachment mechanism that consists of hemidesmosomes located in each cell and a basal lamina between the cell body and the tooth **D**.

EP att. to enamel

Know

functions at various levels on the tooth root (Fig 4–1). The apical fibers are generally parallel to the long axis of the tooth; those at the midpoint on the root are oblique to the tooth surface, with the cemental origin apical to the bony insertion; and those of the cervical area are nearly horizontal. The *oblique fibers* act as a sling to help resist downward pressures, and the *horizontal fibers* resist lateral forces. In addition, a network of blood vessels within the fibers serves as a hydraulic cushion to protect the bone and periodontal fibers from occlusal forces. The complex arrangement of the fibers of the periodontal ligament is shown in Figure 4–3.

The dentogingival junction, which is the biologic seal interposed between the anchoring components of the periodontium and the oral environment, is made up of the following components:

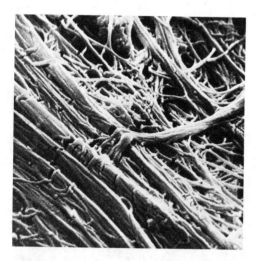

Figure 4–3. Electron scanning microscopic view of collagen bundles in the periodontal ligament space. Note narrow bundle crossing thick bundle at right angle. (*From Svejda J, Skach M. The periodontium of the human teeth in the scanning electron microscope (stereoscan). J Periodont. 1973;44:478–484.*)

1. A layer of epithelial cells that, following eruption, extend a short distance along the enamel surface near to but not over the cementoenamel junction. Because these cells are located at the base of the gingival sulcus[a] and are part of the dentogingival *junction,* they are termed *junctional epithelial cells (JE cells),* a designation that can be used interchangeably with *epithelial attachment* (Fig 4–2C)
2. The tooth surface
3. An ultrathin, 800 to 1200 Å (80–120 nm), *basal lamina* interposed between the tooth surface and the junctional epithelial cells (Fig 4–2D)

The junctional epithelial cells are attached to the tooth via *hemidesmosomes.* Hemidesmosomes are submicroscopic structures located on the inner side of a cell membrane that serve to attach the cell body to adjacent cells or tissues. Hemidesmosomes are also the mechanism of attaching the crevicular epithelium to connective tissue at the basement membrane.[13]

The junctional epithelium forms a strong and resistant seal between the oral environment and the periodontal ligament (Fig 4–2). If however, the dentogingival junction were to be exposed continuously to the direct forces of mastication, the epithelial cells might be torn from the tooth and the seal broken. This possibility is prevented by the protection afforded by the *free margin* of the gingiva. The free margin is a narrow, coronal extension of the *attached gingiva,* which in turn is attached by collagen fibers to the cementum and

---

[a] The terms *sulcus* and *crevice* will be used interchangeably throughout the book.

periosteum of the alveolar bone. The free margin encircles but is not attached to the cervical area of the tooth. Thus, a space potentially exists between the free margin of the gingiva and the tooth. This narrow crevice is called the *gingival sulcus (or crevice)*, and the epithelial lining of the sulcus is called *sulcular (or crevicular) epithelium*.

THE SUPRAGINGIVAL COLLAGEN FIBER APPARATUS

The marginal gingiva is held firmly against the tooth by a complex arrangement of collagen fibers. This close and firm contact of the marginal gingiva to the tooth is necessary to prevent food from forcefully entering the gingival sulcus during eating and causing damage to the epithelial attachment. These fibers, arranged into bundles and known as the supraalveolar fiber apparatus, are divided into groups according to their orientation and insertion into the tissues. Some fibers encircle the tooth and are called *circumferential fibers*. Others are in-

serted into cementum and extend into the crest and periosteum of the alveolar bone and are known as *dentoperiosteal fibers*. Another group of fibers extends into the gingival connective tissue from the cementum of the adjacent tooth and are called *transseptal fibers* (Figs 4–1, 4–2, and 4–4). Together all these fibers are responsible for maintaining the close contact of the free gingiva to the tooth.

THE GINGIVAL SULCUS

As previously discussed, the gingival sulcus is the space between the free margin of the gingiva and the tooth (Fig 4–2). The gingival sulcus, which is normally 2 to 3 mm in depth, is bounded on the outer side by a thin sulcular epithelium and on the inner side by the tooth; the orifice of this sulcus opens into the oral cavity, whereas the apical termination of the sulcus is the dentogingival attachment.

In a longitudinal section of the free gingiva, the tissues encountered in going

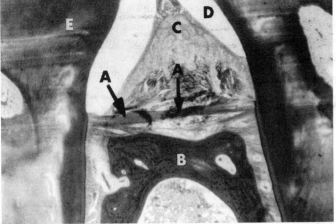

Figure 4–4. Cross-sectional view of interdental papillae showing **A.** transseptal fibers, **B.** alveolar crest, **C.** dental papillae, **D.** enamel space, and **E.** dentin. (*Courtesy of Dr. Don Willmann, University of Texas Dental School at San Antonio*).

from the sulcus to the oral vestibule[b] are (1) sulcular epithelium, (2) connective tissue, and (3) gingival surface epithelium. The sulcular and gingival surface epithelium merge at the crest of the free margin. In the interposed connective tissue there are plexi of blood vessels and nerves supplying both surfaces (Fig 4–2B).

When gingival inflammation is present, fluid flows *from* the depths of the gingival sulcus. This *gingival sulcular fluid* (GSF) is a transudate derived from blood vessels adjacent to the sulcus and is one of the first detectable signs of impending gingivitis. It is present prior to the development of the overt signs of inflammation,[14] and the flow rate is primarily dependent on the inflammation.[15] The flow rate of GSF can be increased by the muscular action of the cheeks or tongue or by mechanical stimulation such as brushing, which exerts pressure against the gingiva.

A flow of GSF of up to 20 μL/h has been measured, which amounts to replacing the normal volume in the sulcus (0.5 μL) 40 times per hour.[16] Gingival sulcular fluid serves several protective functions. It can help clear bacteria from the gingival sulcus and may also serve as the vehicle for leukocytes, antibodies to plaque bacteria, complement, and assorted enzymes of lysosomal origin. Sulcular fluid is believed to serve as one of the first lines of host defense against the bacteria causing periodontal disease. The presence of detectable amounts of gingival fluid has been related to the presence and severity of gingivitis but *not* to the severity of periodontitis.[17]

Immediately beneath the sulcular epithelium the entire resources of the host defense system are available in case antigens penetrate the lining epithelium.

---

[b] The oral vestibule is the space located between the teeth and alveolus and the lips and cheeks.

Question 1. Which of the following statements, if any, are correct?

A. The application of primary preventive procedures can usually *reverse* periodontitis.

B. The term *periodontal disease* includes several periodontal pathologies with separate specific manifestations.

C. *All* the principal fibers of the periodontal ligament are parallel to the long axis of the tooth.

D. The gingival sulcular fluid originates from *saliva* flowing *into* the sulcus.

E. A predictable increase in the flow of gingival sulcular fluid can be expected that parallels the severity of gingivitis but not the severity of periodontitis.

THE DEVELOPING GINGIVAL LESION

Because the free margin of the gingiva constitutes the first line of defense for the periodontium, this is usually the *initial site* of periodontal disease. If plaque is allowed to accumulate on a tooth surface adjacent to the gingiva, inflammation of the free margin results. In a healthy mouth following cessation of oral hygiene measures, it takes only 9 to 21 days before gingivitis can be observed clinically.

In most cases of gingivitis, the extent of the gingival involvement appears to parallel the extent of the plaque buildup. Early clinically evident gingival change includes alterations in color, contour, and consistency. The color changes are from pink to red, contour changes are from knife-edged to enlarged, and consistency changes are from firm to spongy. In addition, the sulcus often bleeds on gentle manipulation or probing of the free margin of the gingiva. At these early stages, the developing inflammatory process can be *completely reversed* by effective personal oral hygiene procedures.

PERIODONTAL MICROFLORA

Many investigators have attempted to characterize the microflora associated with gingivitis and periodontitis. Historically, two hypotheses have guided most thinking about periodontal microflora: the *nonspecific plaque hypothesis* and the *specific plaque hypothesis*. The nonspecific hypothesis simply relates disease progression to the overall amount of plaque present; the more plaque, the more disease. The specific plaque hypothesis attributes the various periodontal diseases to "specific" bacteria, similar to certain systemic diseases, such as streptococcal pharyngitis, which is caused by a specific microorganism.

Chronic gingivitis appears to behave as though it conforms more to the nonspecific hypothesis because many bacterial species can initiate gingival inflammation if the bacteria are present in high numbers because of inadequate oral hygiene.

Periodontitis appears to conform more to the specific hypothesis because certain bacterial species have been associated with most destructive periodontal diseases.[18] It must be pointed out that even at this time Koch's postulates have not been fulfilled for any periodontal microorganisms. However, much evidence incriminates certain microorganisms in periodontitis.[19,20] The microbial species that appear to be associated with the most common variety of periodontitis (adult periodontitis) are *Actinobacillus actinomycetemcomitans, Porphyromonas gingivalis, Prevotella intermedia, Bacteroides forsythus, Fusobacterium* species, *Peptostreptococcus micros, Campylobacter rectus,* and *Treponema denticola.* This list

may seem long, but keep in mind that 300 to 400 different species can inhabit the oral cavity.[21,22] Another rare type of periodontitis (localized juvenile periodontitis) appears to conform more closely to the specific hypothesis, because this disease is usually accompanied by infection with *Actinobacillus actinomycetemcomitans.*[23]

In general, as health status of the periodontium deteriorates, a proportional shift takes place in the plaque bacteria from aerobic, Gram-positive, nonmotile organisms, to anaerobic, Gram-negative, motile genera and species.

Periodontal Health. A healthy sulcus harbors few bacteria and these are characterized by Gram-positive *cocci and rods*,[24,25] which are predominantly aerobic. Direct microscopic examination reveals minimal numbers of both motile rods and spirochetes.[26]

Gingivitis. Plaque associated with chronic gingivitis is characterized by Gram-positive and facultative bacteria, but Gram-negative and anaerobic organisms are nearly as numerous. Direct microscopic examination reveals motile rods and spirochetes composing approximately 20% of the microorganisms.[27,28]

Periodontitis. Plaque taken from patients with periodontitis is characterized by Gram-negative anaerobic bacteria. Direct microscopic examination reveals few cocci, but large numbers of motile rods and spirochetes[24] are present.

Several currently accepted types of periodontitis exist, such as adult and juvenile, and the microflora of each of these diseases has been studied in some detail. Modern therapy for these destructive diseases often can target some of the specific microorganisms with antibacterial medications. However complex the therapy needed to treat patients with these diseases, primary preventive measures still play a critical role in maintaining disease control once periodontal health has been reestablished following therapeutic intervention.

FROM GINGIVITIS TO PERIODONTITIS

Note that the events leading to the conversion of gingivitis to periodontitis are not clear.[4] For instance, all periodontitis is preceded by a gingivitis, but not all untreated gingivitis progresses to periodontitis. At present a diagnosis of gingivitis or periodontitis is based primarily on clinical findings. A diagnosis of gingivitis or periodontitis implies that the actual level of soft tissue attached to the tooth root is at or near the cemento-enamel junction. A diagnosis of periodontitis implies that an apical migration of the epithelial attachment (JE cells) has taken place. This migration usually creates a deeper gingival sulcus between the tooth and the epithelium, called a periodontal *pocket*. The formation of the periodontal pocket with its relatively inaccessible subgingival plaque (to plaque control measures) creates the need for periodontal therapy. Also, as the pocket deepens with the migration of the epithelial attachment, a corresponding loss of the principal fibers occurs.

Question 2. Which of the following statements, if any, are correct?

A. Gingivitis is *completely* reversible by use of effective personal oral hygiene procedures.

B. Gingivitis is an example of a disease conforming to the specific plaque hypothesis, whereas periodontitis conforms to the nonspecific plaque hypothesis.

C. The bacteria found in the deep pockets of advanced periodontitis are usually motile, anaerobic, and Gram-negative.

D. The apical migration of the epithelial attachment and the subsequent increases in depth of the gingival sulcus eventually create the need for periodontal surgery.

E. The apical migration of the JE cells can occur without loss of principal fibers.

THE PLAQUE OF THE DEEPENING POCKET

As the pocket deepens, subgingival plaque acquires new characteristics that differentiate it from the supragingival plaque. In the supragingival plaque, the bacteria and the interbacterial matrix are well confined to the coronal areas by the adhesive glucans. In the subgingival plaque, this containment is much more limited. Instead, a two-compartment subgingival plaque system begins to evolve, that is made up of (1) the *tooth-associated plaque* and (2) the *epithelium-associated plaque.*[29]

The tooth-associated subgingival plaque is initially an apical extension of the supragingival plaque into the deepening crevicular area. The bacterial population consists mainly of *nonmotile Gram-positive* organisms. This plaque provides the basis for calculus formation. In turn, the presence of calculus offers a larger surface area on which additional plaque can accumulate. The mineralized mass also serves to shelter the plaque bacteria from routine plaque control measures, such as toothbrushing and flossing.

In the tooth-associated plaque, acidogenic organisms and extracellular polysaccharides occur that because of their proximity to the cementum *can initiate root caries.* Possibly a combination of diet and a prolonged food retention triggers the cariopathogenic potential of these organisms.

The epithelium-associated subgingival plaque is peripheral to the tooth-associated plaque and can be compared to a swarm of bees around a beehive, with the beehive in this case being the tooth-associated plaque. The organisms of the epithelium-associated plaque are highly *motile*, *Gram-negative* organisms that are immersed in crevicular fluid and tissue exudates. Bacteroides and spirochetes are consistent inhabitants of the periodontal pocket.[30] The halo of Gram-negative organisms extends much deeper into the pocket and is believed to be the plaque component *responsible for the damage to the dentogingival attachment.*

THE SUBGINGIVAL BACTERIA SEEN WITH PHASE-CONTRAST MICROSCOPY

When the phase microscope is used to view a sample of crevicular fluid and debris from a healthy sulcus, only a relatively few forms of bacteria can be seen. They include mainly nonmotile coccal forms, with the only action being confined to a few vibrios moving erratically in the field. In the diseased gingival sulcus, the flora is markedly different and has been described as follows:

> Static masses of bacteria apparently adhere to tooth surfaces as seaweeds cling to the surfaces of submerged rocks. Innumerable spirochetes and large gliding rods tend to migrate to the surfaces of the static, nonmotile masses of organisms where they affix one end of themselves to form configurations that resemble bristles on a brush. These microorganisms flex and beat together, often in synchronous ripples, setting up wave upon wave of

pulsating motion. Amoebae usually glide over the rapidly gyrating ends of the spirochetes and flexing rods, while blood cells, in numbers too numerous to count, assemble in spaces peripheral to the turbulent bacterial surfaces. The turbulent movements of the motile populations probably induce circulation of toxic bacterial agents throughout the circumradicular spaces.[31]

Because of the gross bacteriologic differences between health and disease, the phase, or dark-field, microscope may be used to assess the effectiveness of the patient's personal dental care. Although it is not possible to use these microscopes to quantitate objectively the numbers and types of bacteria present, the contrasting differences in microbial activity seen at the two ends of the spectrum of periodontal health and disease may permit subjective evaluations to be made (Fig 4–5).[32,33]

Controlled scientific research has not demonstrated that phase-contrast microscopic monitoring is a valid means of assessing disease activity. Some investigators have concluded that microscopic assessments are of limited value, because commonly used clinical parameters of periodontal disease activity, such as bleeding on probing, loss of attachment, and changes in probing depths, may provide a more time-effective and site-specific means of detecting disease activity and appropriate therapy.[30]

THE BACTERIAL CHALLENGE

Bacterial end products in the subgingival plaque are capable of destroying the cellular and intercellular components of the crevicular epithelium, the dentogingival junction, and the underlying connective tissue. The subgingival plaque contains enzymes, endotoxins, and exotoxins, as well as

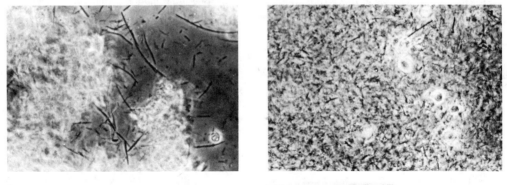

Figure 4–5. A. Few plaque organisms (dark figures) from a relatively healthy crevice as seen with a phase microscope. **B.** Great increase in number of organisms seen in moderate-to-severe marginal gingivitis.

a great number of antigens that have the potential for initiating antigen–antibody reactions. Examples of bacterial enzymes that degrade selected tissue components include collagenase, protease, keratinase, arylsulfatase, neuraminidase, fibronectin-degrading enzymes, and phospholipase A.[22] Once the crevicular epithelium is breached, both spirochetes and other bacteria are capable of directly invading the underlying connective tissue.[34,35] Even though bacteria can invade connective tissue in adult periodontitis, more damage appears to result from the penetration of bacterial end products and cell fragments that can directly damage the tissues or cause immune pathology.[22,36]

Question 3. Which of the following statements, if any, are correct?

A. The supragingival and the subgingival tooth-associated plaque are associated with calculus *and* caries formation.

B. The subgingival epithelium-associated plaque is *peripheral* to the subgingival tooth-associated plaque.

C. The phase microscope is used to quantitate the number and types of organisms seen in a specimen from the gingival sulcus.

D. Amoebae and spirochetes can usually be visualized by use of the phase-contrast microscope in specimens obtained from deep pockets.

E. The *intensity, duration*, and *kinds of bacteria metabolic end products usually* determine whether the crevicular epithelium is breached and invaded by bacteria.

HOST DEFENSES

If the free margin of the gingiva was healthy until the onset of gingivitis, the sulcular epithelium could probably act as a physical barrier for a limited time against the damaging metabolic products being generated in the plaque. Even if the toxic end products pass through the sulcular epithelium, tissue repair is possible, *provided that the insult from metabolic end products is minimal and of short duration.* When the gingiva and the crevicular epithelium are *chronically* exposed to the detrimental effects of the plaque bacteria, it triggers the body's humoral and cellular defense system and the initiation of the four cardinal signs of inflammation: *heat, redness, swelling,* and *pain.*

The heat and the change in color of the marginal gingiva towards red is a result of the increased blood flow to the area. The gingival swelling is due to the edema caused by leakage of fluids from the dilated capillaries. The fluid pressure of edema on nerve endings causes the pain. When the pain and swelling of gingivitis are sufficiently great, disuse and loss of function result, causing altered eating habits.

Accompanying the signs of inflammation are the histologic changes that occur with inflammation anywhere in the body. The noxious products from the dental plaque cause the release of substances within the connective tissue called *chemotactic* agents, which activate the cellular defense system. These defense cells arrive in a definite sequence. Initially, during the *acute* phase of inflammation, large numbers of *polymorphonuclear neutrophils* (PMNs) saturate the area. The acute phase may last from a few days to a few weeks. As the condition becomes more chronic, the *subacute* stage begins. The PMNs greatly decrease in number and are replaced by *lymphocytes*. This stage lasts for a few weeks to a few months. Finally, if healing still does not take place, the disease process is considered *chronic*, in which case the lymphocytes are mainly replaced by *plasma* and *mast* cells.

The same sequence of changes can be seen in the development of gingivitis. If plaque is allowed to accumulate in a previously clinically healthy mouth, free of inflammation, the same predictable histologic changes occur. Within 2 to 4 days of plaque accumulation, the microscopic picture is one of acute infection. Vasculitis is present in the area of the junctional epithelium. Extravascular PMNs begin to appear in large numbers in the area, with some migrating into the gingival sulcus. Edema is present, and perivascular collagen fibers are altered. From 4 to 7 days after the initial plaque buildup, further histologic changes occur.

The vasculitis is more apparent. Concentrations of PMNs in the connective tissue beneath the sulcular epithelium become greater, and lymphocytes increase in number. From 2 to 4 weeks following the initial accumulation, the histologic changes are those of chronic infection, with a notable increase in the number of plasma cells, lymphocytes, and macrophages.

Although the results of the cellular defenses in acute, subacute, and chronic disease are generally beneficial, detrimental side effects may occur. For instance, the cytoplasm of the PMNs contains many *lysosomes*, which are organelles that contain enzymes that normally aid in the phagocytosis of cellular debris. Because the PMNs are often destroyed by the bacterial toxins, their enzymes are released into the tissues and destroy host tissue in the vicinity. The release of these enzymes can also be triggered by the presence of endotoxins released by Gram-negative bacteria. The additional death and destruction of host tissues serve to intensify the inflammatory reaction, thus accentuating and perpetuating the chronicity of the periodontal lesion.

Though much investigation is still needed to understand the immunobiology of the periodontal diseases, it is clear that periodontal inflammatory responses are at least in part immunologic.[37–39] It is likely that antibodies play a major protective role in moderating infections caused by periodontal microorganisms and can interrupt the development of periodontal disease at a very early stage. In a recent publication[18] current knowledge about the immunobiology of the periodontal diseases was summarized as follows: (1) periodontopathic organisms can lead to host responses that result in tissue *destruction*; (2) the neutrophil–antibody–complement axis is critical for protection against microorganisms associated with periodontal disease, and any abnormalities of this axis can result in increased susceptibility to periodontal disease; and (3) regulators of inflammation play an important role in the resolution of inflammation and healing of the periodontal tissues.

TERMINAL EVENTS

To complete the story of the periodontal disease process, a few of the concluding events need to be mentioned. As the chronic inflammation continues, the dentogingival attachment slowly migrates apically. For each millimeter of apical migration, an equal loss occurs in periodontal fibers supporting the teeth. Eventually, this continuing loss of supporting fibers results in a loosening of the tooth. Also, with each millimeter of migration of the junctional epithelium, the depth of the gingival crevice increases where subgingival plaque can accumulate. Concurrent with the loss of soft tissue attachment is a loss of the supporting alveolar bone (Fig 4–6). This destruction of hard and soft tissues can continue until little or no support remains for the tooth. Extraction then becomes necessary, at which time all five components of the periodontium are lost forever.

PRIMARY PREVENTIVE DENTISTRY IMPLICATIONS

The most important strategy for the prevention of periodontal disease is *mechanical and chemical* plaque control. Mechanical plaque control begins at home with the correct *daily* use of a toothbrush and dental floss to remove plaque. This daily procedure is required to remove the plaque that accumulates along the free margin of the gingiva and in the gingival crevices. Antiplaque mouth rinses, which have been approved by the American Dental Association, can be used to supplement, *but not replace,* the

home mechanical plaque control programs. Finally, periodic primary prevention visits are necessary for dental office care. At this time, poorly contoured and overhanging restorations should be replaced or corrected. The dental hygienist is then responsible for completing a prophylaxis procedure to remove all plaque and any accumulated calculus, and to counsel the patient on oral hygiene procedures that will help achieve a more effective home care program. The importance of daily plaque removal is emphasized by the fact that *in the absence of plaque, no caries, gingivitis, or periodontitis can occur.*

The main challenge in preventing plaque is to increase public awareness that excellent oral health can be maintained by home care programs. An effective supragingival plaque control program that is established early minimizes the conditions leading to the establishment of the subgingival plaque. It was long believed that once the subgingival plaque was permanently organized, supragingival plaque control activities had no effect on this subgingival plaque. However, recent evidence has demonstrated that this is not so; meticulous supragingival plaque control measures *can* influence the initiation and composition of the subgingival plaque.[40–42]

Procedures for treating gingivitis are the *same* as those used to prevent it: mechanical and chemical plaque control procedures at home, and prophylaxis procedures in the dental office. If, however, the gingivitis converts to periodontitis, with accompanying destruction of the principle fibers of the periodontal ligament, it is not possible to return the periodontium to its original, disease-free state without additional professional intervention.

Question 4. Which of the following statements, if any, are correct?

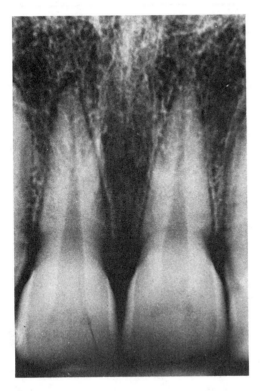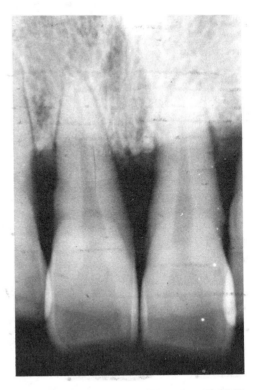

A   B

Figure 4–6. A. X-ray film of two central incisors showing only slight interproximal bone loss. **B.** A much greater bone loss is seen in advanced periodontal disease. (*Courtesy of Dr O Langland, University of Texas Dental School at San Antonio.*)

[handwritten: want teeth no bony socket exists, no cemendum, no principle fibers, no junctn epith, no gingiva]

A. Subgingival plaque has two distinct subcomponents: *tooth-associated plaque,* which is prominent in *root caries,* and *epithelium-associated plaque, which is associated with periodontitis.*

B. The invasion of *bacteria* into the tissues is *mainly* responsible for periodontal inflammation. *[handwritten: end prod. of Bact metabolism trigger inflam. Resp.]*

C. In periodontal inflammation the defensive cells arrive in the following sequence: first the plasma cells, then the lymphocytes, and finally the polymorphs.

D. Components of the periodontium still remain after all teeth are extracted.

E. Personal oral hygiene procedures that affect the bacteria in the supragingival plaque can result in changes in the subgingival plaque.

SUMMARY

Five anatomic structures function together to support the teeth in the jaws: (1) *alveolar bone,* (2) *cementum,* (3) the *periodontal lig-*

ament, (4) the *dentogingival junction*, and (5) the *gingiva*. Collectively, these five structures are called the *periodontium*.

Periodontal ligament principal fibers extend between the alveolar bone and the cementum to anchor the teeth; the epithelial attachment of the dentogingival junction acts as a seal to protect the anchoring components, and the gingiva protects the epithelial attachment from direct trauma from foods being forced into the gingival sulcus.

The inflammatory periodontal diseases are caused by bacteria and include two broad categories: gingivitis and periodontitis. Periodontitis is an inflammatory disease of the surface tissues.

Supragingival plaque is the initiating factor in gingivitis and caries. Subgingival plaque is composed of two components: the tooth-associated plaque, which is associated with root caries, and the epithelial-associated plaque, which is associated with periodontitis. The plaque bacteria present during oral health tend to be aerobic, Gram-positive, and nonmotile. In periodontitis, the organisms tend to be Gram-negative, motile, and anaerobic.

The bacterial etiology of gingivitis and periodontitis is well established, but it is not completely understood.

Primary preventive measures to prevent, arrest, or reverse gingivitis consist of daily use of mechanical and chemical plaque control measures, and of prophylaxes at appropriate intervals. These measures can be supplemented by antiplaque mouth rinses (ie, chemical plaque control agents). Gingivitis can usually be completely reversed by appropriate plaque control strategies, but periodontitis rarely can be reversed, although it can be maintained in an arrested state. With continued effective plaque control throughout life, the periodontal structures can be retained in a healthy state.

ANSWERS AND EXPLANATIONS

1. B, E
   A—incorrect. Reversal of gingivitis is possible; the reversibility of periodontitis is usually not possible.
   C—incorrect. Horizontal and oblique fibers are also not parallel.
   D—incorrect. The gingival sulcus fluid originates from the connective tissue beneath the sulcular epithelium.

2. A, C, D
   B—incorrect. Just the reverse. Gingivitis exemplifies the nonspecific hypothesis, whereas periodontitis can be better classified under the specific hypothesis.
   E—incorrect. For every one millimeter migration of the epithelial attachment, one millimeter of principal fiber support is lost.

3. A, B, D, E
   C—incorrect. The phase microscope provides a *qualitative* evaluation of the number and types of organisms as well as their motility.

4. A, E
   B—incorrect. It is probably due to the end products of bacterial metabolism that trigger the inflammatory response.
   C—incorrect. It is the reverse—first, the polymorphs, then the lymphocytes, and finally the plasma cells.
   D—incorrect. Without the teeth, no boney socket exists, there is no cementum, no principal fibers, no junctional epithelium and no gingiva—in summary, no periodontium.

SELF-EVALUATION QUESTIONS

1. The five components of the periodontium are the alveolar bone, Cementum, Perio ligament, dento gin junc, Gingiva, and Alveolar Bone

2. The components of the periodontium that *anchor* the teeth are the ___Bone___, ___cementum___, and ___perio ligament fibers___

3. The structure that acts as a *seal* between the gingival sulcus and the principal fibers is the ___dentogingival junct^n___

4. The structure that **prevents** food being forced down into the gingival sulcus to **damage** the JE junction is the ___Gingiva___ (anatomic structure).

5. The name given to the countercurrent of fluid arising from the depth of the gingival sulcus is ___Gin Sulcular fluid GSF___; its source is from the ___blood vessels adjacent to sulcus (connectives tissue)___

6. The supraalveolar collagen fiber apparatus is composed of the following fibers: _____; the dentoperiosteal fibers connecting the ___cementum___ and the ___periostium___; the transseptal group extending from ___ging connective tissue___ to ___adjacent tooth___; and the _____ group extending from the cementum into the marginal gingiva.

7. State the boundaries of the gingival sulcus: Lateral, ___Sulcular epithelium___; inner side, ___by tooth___; top, ___oral cavity___; and, bottom ___dentogingival junct^n___

8. The initial site of periodontal disease is the ___Free Marg. of the Ging___ (name of soft tissue structure) adjacent to the plaque buildup.

9. Bleeding caused by toothbrushing can be considered a manifestation of ___gingivitis___ (type of periodontal pathology).

10. It requires about ___9___ to ___21___ days without oral hygiene for gingivitis to develop; it takes about _____ to _____ days for it to resolve with appropriate personal oral hygiene measures.

11. *Initial* marginal gingivitis is usually attributed to pathogens in the (supra) (sub) gingival plaque.

12. The bacteria attached to calculus in the subgingival plaque is that of the (tooth-)(epithelium-) associated plaque.

13. The subgingival plaque can be subclassified into two components: the one related to *root caries* is the ___Tooth Ass SG plaque___ plaque, and the one related to periodontitis is the ___Epith Ass. S.G. plaque___

14. The *four cardinal signs* of inflammation are ___Edema___, ___Erythema___, ___Heat___, and ___Pain___.

15. In periodontitis, the eventual loosening of the tooth is due to an apical migration of the ___dento ging. junct^n___

REFERENCES

1. Periodontal therapy: A summary status report. 1987–1988. *J Periodontol.* 1988; 590: 306–310.

2. Socransky SS, Haffajee AD. The bacterial etiology of destructive periodontal disease. *J Periodontol.* 1992; 63:322–331.

3. Loesche WJ, Syed SA, Schmidt EF, et al. Bacterial profiles of subgingival plaques in periodontitis. *J Periodontol.* 1985; 56:447–456.

4. Williams RC. Periodontal disease. *N Engl J Med.* 1990; 322:373–376.

5. Greenstein G. Periodontal response to mechanical non-surgical therapy: A review. *J Periodontol.* 1992; 63:118–130.

6. McFall WT Jr. Tooth loss in 100 treated patients with periodontal disease: A long-term study. *J Periodontol.* 1982; 53:539–549.

7. Douglas CW, Gilling D, Sollecito W, et al. National trends in the prevalence and severity of the periodontal diseases. *J Am Dent Assoc.* 1983; 107:403–412.

8. Survey of Adult Dental Health. *J Am Dent Assoc.* 1987; 114:829–830.

9. Brown LJ, Oliver RC, Loe H. Periodontal diseases in the U.S. in 1981: Prevalence, severity, extent, and role in tooth mortality. *J Periodontol.* 1989; 60:363–370.

10. Douglas C, Gillings D, Sollecito W, et al. The potential for increase in the periodontal

diseases of the aged population. *J Periodontol*. 1983; 54:721–730.

11. Hunt RJ. Is it time to reassess the public health implications of periodontal diseases? A review of current concepts. *J Public Health Dent*. 1988; 48:241–244.

12. Oliver RC, Brown LJ, Loe H. An estimate of periodontal treatment needs in the U.S. based on epidemiological data. *J Periodontol*. 1989; 60:371–380.

13. Stern JB. Current concepts of the dentogingival junction. The epithelial and connective tissue attachments to the tooth. *J Periodontol*. 1981; 52:465–476.

14. Cimasoni G. Crevicular fluid updated. *Oral Sci*. 1983; 12:1–152.

15. Griffiths GS, Sterne JA, Wilton JM, et al. Associations between volume and flow rate of gingival crevicular fluid and clinical assessments of gingival inflammation in a population of British male adolescents. *J Clin Periodontol*. 1992; 19:464–470.

16. Conference Report: 11th International Conference on Oral Biology—Chemical Control of Plaque; Hong Kong. September 5–7, 1988.

17. Hancock EB, Cray RJ, O'Leary TJ. The relationship between gingival crevicular fluid and gingival inflammation. *J Periodontol*. 1979; 50:13–19.

18. Genco RJ. Host responses in periodontal diseases: Current concepts. *J Periodontol*. 1992; 63:338–355.

19. Socransky SS, Haffajee AD. Microbial risk factors for destructive periodontal diseases. In: Bader JD, ed. *Risk Assessment in Dentistry*. Chapel Hill NC: University of North Carolina Dental Ecology, 1991:79–90.

20. Slots J. Bacterial specificity in adult periodontitis. *J Clin Periodontol*. 1986; 13:912–917.

21. Moore WED. Microbiology of periodontal disease. *J Periodont Res*. 1987; 22:335–341.

22. Socransky SS, Haffajee AD. Microbial mechanisms in the pathogenesis of destructive periodontal diseases: A critical assessment. *J Periodontol Res*. 1991; 26:195–212.

23. Slots J, Rams TE. Microbiology of periodontal disease. In: Taubman MA, ed. *Contemporary Oral Microbiology and Immunology*. St. Louis, Mo. Mosby; 1992:425–443.

24. Friedman MT, Barber PM, Mardan NJ, et al. The "plaque-free zone" in health and disease: A scanning electron microscope study. *J Periodontol*. 1992; 63:890–896.

25. Slots J. Microflora in the healthy gingival sulcus in man. *Scan J Dent Res*. 1977; 85: 247–254.

26. Loe H, Theilade E, Borglum JS. Experimental gingivitis in man. *J Periodontol*. 1965; 36:177–187.

27. Slots, J, Moenbo D, Langeback J, et al. Microbiota of gingivitis in man. *Scan J Dent Res*. 1978; 86:174–181.

28. Tanner ACR, Haffner C, Bratthall GT, et al. A study of the bacteria associated with advancing periodontitis in man. *J Clin Periodontol*. 1979; 6:278–307.

29. Sanz M, Newman MG. Dental plaque and calculus. In: Newman MG, Nisengard R. *Oral Microbiology and Immunology*. Philadelphia, Pa. WB Saunders; 1988:367–380.

30. Armitage GC, Dickinson WR, Jendersick RS, et al. Relationship between the percentage of subgingival spirochetes and the severity of periodontal disease. *J Periodont*. 1982; 53:550–556.

31. Keyes PH. Personal communication. 1980.

32. Keyes PH, Wright WE, Howard SA. The use of phase-contrast microscopy and chemotherapy in the diagnosis and treatment of periodontal lesions—an initial report (I) *Quint Int*. 1. Rep. 1978; 1:51–56.

33. Keyes PH, Wright WE, Howard SA. The use of phase-contrast microscopy and chemotherapy in the diagnosis and treatment of periodontal lesions—an initial report (II). *Quint Int*. 1978; 2:69–76.

34. Manor A, Lebendiger M, Shiffer A, et al. Bacterial invasion of periodontal tissues in advanced periodontitis in humans. *J Periodontol*. 1984; 53:567–573.

35. Frank RM. Bacterial penetration in the apical pocket wall of advanced human periodontitis. *J Periodont Res*. 1980; 15:563–573.

36. Liakona H, Barber P, Newman HN. Bacterial penetration of pocket soft tissues in

chronic adult and juvenile periodontitis cases. *J Clin Periodontol*. 1987; 14:22–28.

37. Page R. The role of inflammatory mediators in the pathogenesis of periodontal disease. *J Periodont Res*. 1991; 26:230–242.

38. Ebersole JL. Host resistance and immune function. In: Newman MG, Nisengard R. *Oral Microbiology and Immunology*. Philadelphia, Pa. WB Saunders; 1988:11–53.

39. Taubman MA. Immunologic aspects of periodontal diseases. In: Slots J, Taubman MA. *Contemporary Oral Microbiology and Immunology*. St. Louis, Mo: Mosby; 1992: 542–554.

40. Dahlen G, Lindhe J, Sato K, et al. The effect of supragingival plaque control on the subgingival microbiota in subjects with periodontal disease. *J Clin Periodontol*. 1992; 19: 802–809.

41. Katsanoulas T, Renee I, Attstrom R. The effect of supragingival plaque control on the composition of the subgingival flora in periodontal pockets. *J Clin Periodontol*. 1992; 19:760–765.

42. Corbet EF, Davies WI. The role of supragingival plaque in the control of progressive periodontal disease: A review. *J Clin Periodontol*. 1993; 20:307–313.

Chapter 5

Toothbrushing and Toothbrushing Techniques

Samuel L. Yankell

Objectives

At the end of this chapter it will be possible to

1. Give a brief history of the toothbrush, describe its parts in detail, and explain why there is no one "ideal" brush for all situations.
2. Compare natural and nylon bristles for their uniformity of length, diameter, and durability.
3. Compare various toothbrush products for handle and head profile and shape.
4. Compare the manual with the powered toothbrush in effectiveness and motions used during brushing.
5. Name and explain the various methods that have been recommended for toothbrushing.
6. Explain why different amounts of time are needed by different individuals for toothbrushing, and discuss how the effectiveness and safety of toothbrushing can be evaluated.
7. Discuss modifications of toothbrushing techniques applicable to special patient care, patients using prostheses and those under orthodontic care.

Introduction

After teeth have been completely cleaned by the dental professional or by the individual, soft microbial dental plaque continually re-forms on the tooth surfaces. With time, plaque is the primary agent in the development of caries, periodontal disease, and calculus—the three conditions for which individuals most often seek professional services. If plaque, particularly at interproximal and gingival areas, is completely removed with home care procedures, these dental disease conditions can be prevented. Unfortunately, a great majority of the population is unable or unwilling or does not realize the need to spend the time to remove plaque adequately from all tooth surfaces.

Plaque deposits can be removed either mechanically or chemically. The focus of this chapter is the mechanical removal of plaque, using toothbrushes and toothbrushing techniques. The following two chapters emphasize the use of products and auxiliary aids with toothbrushes in removing plaque. The primary purpose of these materials is the maintenance of healthy teeth and gingival tissues.

HISTORY OF THE TOOTHBRUSH

The exact origin of mechanical devices for cleaning teeth is unknown.[1,2] Ancient peoples chewed twigs from plants with high aromatic properties. Chewing these twigs not only freshened the breath but also spread out fibers at the tips of the twig. These were then used for cleaning the tooth and gum surfaces. Published studies[3,4] proved that African chew sticks not only helped to clean teeth but also, because they contained antibacterial oils and tannins, helped prevent or remove plaque. Later, twigs were purposely chewed or hammered into fibers or bristles for cleaning the teeth. The Arabs before Islam used a piece of the root of the arak tree because its fibers stood out like bristles. This device was called a *siwak*. After several uses the bristle fibers became soft, and a new "brush" was created simply by stripping off the end and again making new bristle fibers. In the seventh century Mohammed gave rules for the proper use of the *siwak*. His requirements for oral hygiene became a religious obligation. It was recommended that the brush be used on the tongue, on buccal surfaces, and guided into interdental spaces. To this day the Arabs still use the *siwak*, which is composed from aromatic types of wood.

The Chinese are given credit for inventing the modern toothbrush during the Tang dynasty (618–907 AD). They used hog bristles similar to those in some contemporary models. In 1780, in England, William Addis manufactured what was termed "the first effective toothbrush."[5] This instrument had a bone handle and holes for placement of the natural hog bristles, which were held in place by wire. In 1789, Isaac Greenwood, the first native-born American practitioner of dentistry and the man whose son became George Washington's family dentist, advertised a double-ended toothbrush with a long brush at one end for general cleaning and a short one at the other end for specifically cleaning the lingual surfaces of the teeth.[1] By 1857, a brush was marketed in the United States by H. N. Wadsworth. In the early 1900s celluloid began to replace the bone handle, a changeover that was hastened by World War I when bone was in short supply. As a result of the blockade of high-quality natural hog bristles from China and Russia during World War II, nylon bristles were ushered in. Initially, nylon bristles were copies of natural bristles in length and thickness. They were stiffer than natural bristles of similar diameter, because they did not have the hollow stem of natural bristles and did not absorb water.

TOOTHBRUSH DESIGN

A manual toothbrush consists of a *head* with bristles and a *handle* (Fig 5–1). When the bristles are bunched together, they are known as *tufts*. A constriction, termed the *shank*, usually occurs between the handle and the head. The head is arbitrarily divided into the *toe*, which is at the extreme end of the head, and the *heel*, which is closest to the handle. Many toothbrushes are manufactured in different sizes—*large, medium,* and *small* (or *compact*)—to adapt better to the oral anatomy of different individuals.[6] Toothbrushes also differ in their defined hardness or stiffness, usually being classified as *hard, medium,* or *soft.* Descriptions and measurements of selected toothbrushes are shown in Table 5–1.

Toothbrushes vary in size, shape, texture, and design more than any other category of dental products.[7] Prior to 1960 many publications dealt with the advantages and disadvantages of the different characteristics of toothbrushes, but few

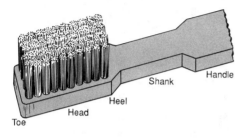

Figure 5–1. Parts of a toothbrush.

user-preference studies are reported. In a 1980 study,[8] 7-year-olds expressed a "preference" for larger—rather than smaller—headed brushes. In a 1993 publication,[9] both children and their parents responded similarly to a preference questionnaire on toothbrush handle designs. Much of the earlier data comparing the efficacy of various toothbrush designs is contradictory because of (1) the lack of quantitative methods used to measure cleaning (plaque removal), (2) the many sizes and shapes of toothbrushes used, and (3) the lack of standardized toothbrushing procedures used in the study. Recently, toothbrush heads have been altered to vary bristle lengths and placement in attempts to better reach interproximal areas.[10–12] Handles have also been ergonomically designed to accommodate better adults' or children's dexterity levels.[9,12] In clinical studies, new plaque evaluation methods have been introduced to detect differences between toothbrushes more accurately.[13,14]

Lateral Profile

When viewed from the side, tooth brushes have four basic lateral profiles: concave, convex, flat, and multileveled (rippled or scalloped). The concave shape can be useful for improved cleaning of facial surfaces, whereas convex shapes appear more useful for improved cleaning of lingual surfaces.[7] In a comparison of a convex-shaped brush with a conventional flat toothbrush,[15] the flat toothbrush appeared significantly more effective than the convex toothbrush based on planimetric plaque measurements. In short-term clinical plaque removal studies, toothbrushes with a multileveled lateral profile were more effective than flat toothbrushes.[16,17] Lateral profiles of selected toothbrushes commercially available in the United States are shown in Figure 5–2.

TABLE 5–1. DESCRIPTION AND MEASUREMENTS OF SELECTED TOOTHBRUSHES

Name	Manufacturer	Shape		Number of Tufts	Head Length (cm)	Head Width (cm)	Bristle Length (cm)	Handle Length (cm)
		Top	Bottom					
Advanced Design Reach	Johnson & Johnson Products Inc.	Oval	Oval	46	2.9	1.2*	1.1	15.9
Aquafresh	Smith Kline Beecham	Oval	Oval	43	3.1	1.1*	1.1	15.8
Colgate Plus	Colgate-Palmolive Co.	Oval	Oval	46	3.2	1.1*	1.2	15.1
Colgate Precision	Colgate-Palmolive Co.	Oval	Flat	57	2.7	1.5	1.1	16.2
Crest Complete	Procter & Gamble	Flat	Flat	38	2.9	1.1*	1.0	16.0
GUM 4.1	J.O.Butler Co.	Oval	Flat	42	3.0	1.1	1.1/0.9	16.4
Lactona M-39	Lactona Corp.	Oval	Flat	43	3.3	1.3	1.2	16.0
Oral B 35	Oral-B Laboratories	Flat	Flat	40	2.6	1.1	1.2	15.2
Oral B 40	Oral-B Laboratories	Flat	Flat	48	3.1	1.3	1.2	15.8
Oral B 60	Oral-B Laboratories	Flat	Flat	60	3.8	1.3	1.2	15.7
Pepsodent	Chesebrough-Ponds	Oval	Flat	50	3.6	1.1	1.1	16.0
Pepsodent Professional	Chesebrough-Ponds	Oval	Oval	34	2.5	0.9	1.0	19.2
Pycopay Softex	Block Drug Company, Inc.	Flat	Flat	51	3.3	1.2	1.1	16.4
Reach (compact head)	Johnson & Johnson Products, Inc.	Oval	Oval	34	2.3	1.4	1.1/1.0	18.0
Sensodyne Gentle	Block Drug Company, Inc.	Flat	Flat	51	3.0	0.9	1.1	16.5

*Maximum (for "diamond"-shaped toothbrushes).

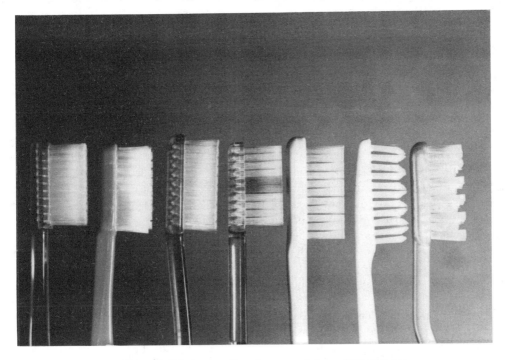

Figure 5–2. Lateral profiles of commercially available brushes.

Cross-Sectional Profile

In cross section, most commercially available toothbrushes in the United States have a flat profile, as exemplified by the Oral-B brush (C) in Figure 5–3. Three toothbrushes with shapes that are uniquely different are the Reach, which has a flat U shape, the Butler GUM, which is slightly convex, and the Colgate Precision with an angled outer row of bristles. From the working surface, the overhead appearance of most toothbrushes is an overall rectangle.

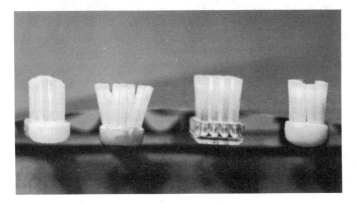

Figure 5–3. Cross-sectional profiles of four toothbrushes: **A.** Butler Gum; **B.** Colgate Precision; **C.** Oral-B; **D.** Reach.

The "diamond head" shape is available in several toothbrushes with flat or rippled lateral bristle configurations (Fig 5–4).

Bristle Shape

No standard criteria exist for labeling bristle configurations; bristle shapes are still subjectively classified by each manufacturer. With today's technology, nylon bristles have a uniform diameter and a wide range of predictable firmnesses. Firmness is defined as bristle resistance to pressure and is also referred to as texture, stiffness, and hardness. Originally, individual bristles were cut bluntly and often had sharp end configurations. In 1948, Bass reported that these bristle tips could damage the soft tissues and that rounded, tapered, or smooth bristle tips were less abrasive[18]—a concept that had its first origin in 1868 when the end-rounded tip was patented.[19] Although Bass' research was not performed according to strict research protocol, his findings have remained undisputed for more than 30 years. Indeed, advertisers still recommend end-rounded tips to promote toothbrush sales. When toothbrushes are examined under low magnification, most bristles labeled as "rounded" do in fact appear

smooth or end-rounded. However, at higher magnification, as shown in Figure 5–5, many of these "rounded" bristles take on different configurations.[7,20]

During use, the bristles in these brushes become smoother and more end-rounded. With continued use the bristles of the tuft expand and spread out.[21] No standard criteria exist for labeling bristle configurations; bristle shapes are still subjectively classified by each manufacturer. A 1988 scanning electron microscope study[20] compared end rounding of bristles from eight marketed types. Based on statistical analysis of 30 toothbrushes of each type, acceptability varied from 22% to 88%, indicating to these authors that some brushes are not sufficiently rounded and are likely to produce gingival damage. In addition, they have abrasive potential on dentin and cementum. A 1992 study[11] compared a ripple design with a flat profile brush using a stereoscopic microscope with fiberoptic lighting. Close to 90% of the bristles of the ripple brush were end-rounded, whereas the flat brush had an average of 52% rounded bristles. Apparently, the degree of end rounding depends on a manufacturer's specifications and not on toothbrush design. If bristles are

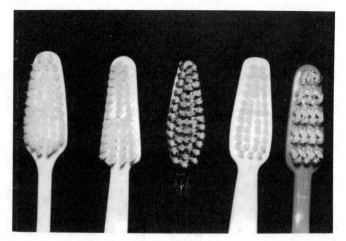

Figure 5–4. Overhead appearance of selected toothbrushes, from left to right: Advanced Design Reach; Aquafresh; Colgate Plus; Crest Complete; Jordan V.

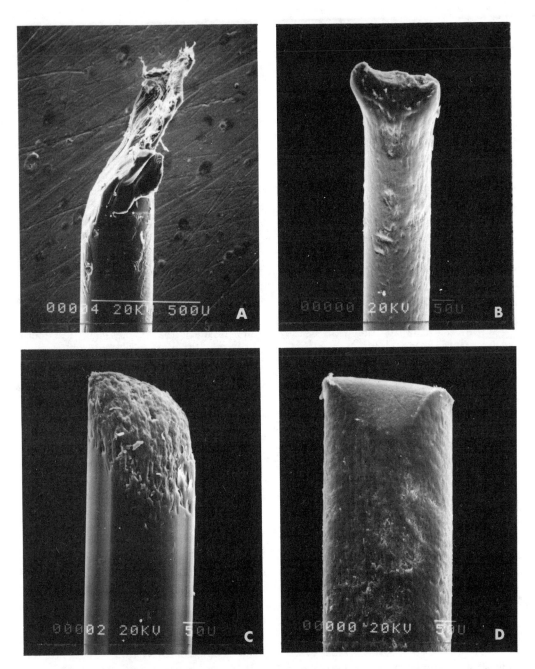

Figure 5–5. Toothbrush bristle ends as seen with the scanning electron microscope. **A.** A coarse-cut toothbrush bristle end, probably the result of an incomplete single-blade cut during the manufacturing process. These sharp projections can reduce the bristles' overall cleaning efficiency and damage oral tissues (SEM 85x). **B.** A slightly enlarged, bulbous nylon bristle end, resulting from a double-blade or scissor cut during the manufacturing process (SEM 170x). **C.** A tapered or round-end nylon bristle produced by heat or a mechanical polishing process (SEM 170x). **D.** The scrubbing, mechanical action of a toothbrush wear machine has nicely rounded off this bristle removed from a brush that was originally coarse cut. (SEM 170x). (*Courtesy of Park KK, Matis BA, and Christen AG. Indiana University Dental School.*)

cut sharply, are frayed, or are hollow, it is likely that they may also harbor bacteria or viruses. To examine this possibility, a study was conducted in which toothbrush bristles were purposely exposed to cultures of herpes simplex virus.[22] When the brushes were held in a moist environment, virus was recovered 7 days later. In another study[23] marketed brushes *currently in use* were cultured for bacteria and showed a wide range of organisms present, including species of enterobacteria and streptococci.

Bristle Firmness

The firmness or texture of a bristle is related to its (1) composition, (2) diameter, (3) length, and (4) number of individual bristles per tuft. In the manufacturing process, the diameter of nylon bristles can be well controlled. Because the majority of toothbrushes contain bristles 10 to 12-mm long, the diameter of the bristle becomes the critical determinant of texture. The usual range of diameters for adult toothbrush bristles is from 0.007 to 0.015 in. Those from 0.007 to 0.009 in. in diameter are generally considered *soft*. Those with a diameter of 0.010 to 0.012 in. are considered *medium*, and bristles with a diameter of 0.013 and 0.014 in. are considered *hard*. Those numbered 15 (0.015 in.) are *extra hard*. In children's brushes the bristles are shorter; therefore the diameter must be reduced to 0.005 in. to approximate the soft adult brush. Factors such as temperature, uptake of water (hydration), and toothbrush-use frequency affect firmness.

Firmness labeling is not standardized. Individual manufacturers label their brushes according to their testing criteria. Thus one manufacturer's "soft" grade may be stiffer than another manufacturer's "medium" grade. The International Organization for Standardization (ISO) has formulated testing procedures that permit manufacturers to label their brushes in a consistent manner.[24] The American Dental Association is a member of ISO.

Nylon Versus Natural Bristles

The nylon bristle is superior to the natural (hog) bristle in several aspects. Nylon bristles flex as many as 10 times more often than natural bristles before breaking; they do not split or abrade and are easier to clean. The configurations and hardness of nylon bristles can be standardized within specified and reproducible tolerances. As a result of the advantages of nylon, as well as its ease and economy of production, few natural bristle toothbrushes are sold. The only advantage that can be cited for the natural bristle is that it may cause less tooth abrasion, due to its extreme flexibility when wet. Bristle diameters vary greatly in any one tuft of natural bristles, ranging in diameter from 0.002 to 0.02 in.

Bristle Actions

Toothbrushing consists of one of four basic motions or combinations thereof: (1) horizontal reciprocating, (2) vertical sweeping, (3) rotary, and (4) vibratory. In any one of these motions the effectiveness of the brushing is due to bristle action. Bristles can exhibit *splay, lag, skip, slap, bunching, pulsing*, and *vibration* as the toothbrush head proceeds through the various motions. These actions are illustrated in Figure 5–6. Due to pressures on the toothbrush while brushing, one or all of these actions can be occurring with different bristles in different tufts as they encounter different contoured surfaces on the teeth and gingiva. Different methods of brushing and different pressures on the brush can emphasize one action over another. Each of the bristle actions can be detrimental to the cleaning process under some conditions and favorable under others.

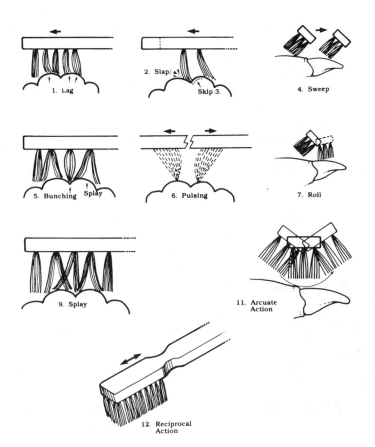

Definitions

1. Lag: Free end of bristle held in contact by friction while bristle shaft bends with handle movement.
2. Slap: As friction of lag is overcome, bristle springs against adjacent tooth surface.
3. Skip: Bristles miss proximal tooth surface areas in the course of a slap.
4. Sweep: A driving movement of bristles across surfaces by bodily movement of brush handle.
5. Bunching: Concentration of bristles in interproximal areas.
6. Pulse: Rhythmic bending of bristle shaft as hand moves back and forth.
7. Roll: Rotation of handle causing unidirectional arcuate movement of bristle ends.
8. Scour: Hard rubbing of bristles across surfaces for harsh frictional effect.
9. Splay: Bristles spread out under pressure.
10. Vibrate: Rapid to-and-fro movement over very short distance.
11. Arcuate action: Mechanical rotation of brush handle through a limited arch at right angle to its long axis.
12. Reciprocal action: Back-and-forth mechanical action in direction of long axis (limited).

Figure 5–6. Bristle action during brushing. (*Courtesy of Dr J. Kartman.*)

Bristle actions due to different brushing motions are illustrated in a 1992 publication[12] that measured and quantified three-dimensional individual movements during brushing. Data frames were filmed to create a computer-generated reanimation of brushing motions in order to design new toothbrush bristle conformations. These authors concluded that an individual's brushing techniques do not vary and are inadequate; therefore bristle configurations in newly designed toothbrushes should be adaptable to any brushing style.

Question 1. Which of the following statements, if any, are correct?

A. The toothbrush became commercially available in the United States just before the Civil War; the celluloid handle became popular during World War I; and nylon bristles appeared just before World War II.

B. A *hard* toothbrush has bristles with a diameter ranging from 0.007 to 0.009 in.; a *soft* bristle is approximately 0.014 in. in diameter.

C. The cross section of the average toothbrush in the United States has a flat head and a flat bristle profile.

D. Texture, stiffness, firmness, and hardness are synonyms that describe the resistance of a bristle or a toothbrush under pressure.

E. Lag, skip, and slap are a logical *sequence* of events for a tuft of bristles moving over, first, the contour of the crown, then over a groove onto another contour.

Handle Design

Many of the commercially available toothbrushes in the United States have a flat handle design. Modifications, such as triangular extrusions for better grasp, indentations along the sides, and various angle bends to permit better access to various parts of the mouth, have been introduced. The handle length is approximately 5 to 6 in. long for adults and 4 to 5 in. long for children. However, even shorter handled brushes are available for very young children.

Four basic types of toothbrush handle designs are shown in Figure 5–7. Several

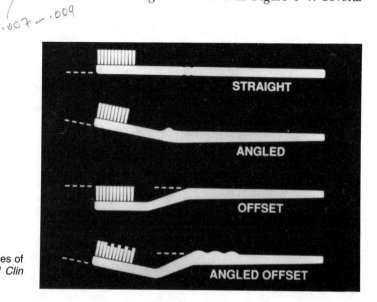

Figure 5–7. Four basic shapes of toothbrush handles. FSN (*J Clin Dent.*)

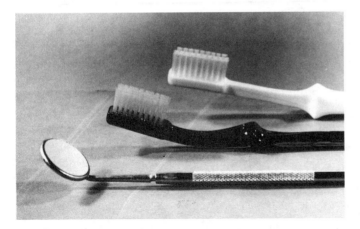

Figure 5–8. Similarity of angled toothbrushes and a dental mirror.

brushes have recently been marketed with an "angled" design, stated to be like a dental instrument. As shown in Figure 5–8, these toothbrushes are similar to a dental professional's mirror. Brushes are also available, as depicted in Figure 5–9, with a handle on the same plane as the bristle tips, as are dental instruments used for caries evaluations and prophylaxes. With both the offset and angled offset designs, points of bristle contact are in line with the longitudinal axis of the handle during brushing.

Although handle design does not have a major effect on clinical efficacy, it does affect comfort during use and brushing compliance.[12] This is particularly true of toothbrushes for children, whose dexterity may not be highly developed.[9]

TOOTHBRUSH CLEANING EFFICIENCY

Clinical advantages of various toothbrush head configurations for removing dental plaque and debris (cleaning efficacy) have been difficult to substantiate. This is attributed to the wide variations among individuals in toothbrushing times, brushing motions, brushing pressures, and shape and

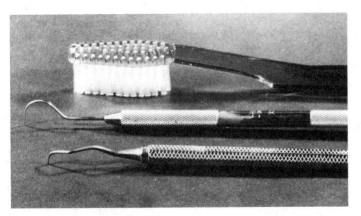

Figure 5–9. Similarity of two dental instruments and a toothbrush with the head on the same plane as the handle.

number of teeth present. A toothbrushing apparatus has been developed[25] that accurately standardizes all of the above factors, in addition to length and number of toothbrushing strokes over simulated anterior or posterior teeth (Fig 5–10).

Efficacy is determined by measuring the maximum width or interproximal access recorded on pressure-sensitive paper placed around the simulated teeth. In initial studies, interproximal access efficacy was directly related to increasing brushing weights and inversely correlated with bristle texture (the "softer" the texture, the higher the interproximal access efficacy).[25] More recently, laboratory access results[25–28] were predictive of clinical plaque removal when plaque assessments focusing on interproximal areas were used.[10,16,17,29]

The Council on Dental Materials, Instruments and Equipment of the American Dental Association (ADA) has established guidelines to enable manufacturers to obtain an acceptable rating and use the ADA Seal of Acceptance. These guidelines require only equivalency in plaque and gingivitis reduction compared with an already acceptable ADA toothbrush. The clinical protocol is summarized in Table 5–2.

The life expectancy of a toothbrush is determined more by the method of brushing than by the length of time of use.[30] The average life of a toothbrush has been stated to be 3 months. This estimate can vary greatly however, due to differences in brushing habits. For example, an evaluation of toothbrush age and wear in relation to plaque removal showed that in a group of 40 subjects, if new toothbrushes were supplied every 2 weeks rather than every 10 weeks, significantly more plaque was removed.[31] If brushes need to be replaced too often, the patient's brushing technique should be checked. Even if the brushing technique is acceptable or has been corrected, the toothbrush should still be replaced frequently. It is a good practice to have several toothbrushes and to stagger their use by always maintaining two or three in daily use while rotating a new brush into use for every toothbrush needing replacement because of splayed, bent, or broken bristles. Dental professionals should be familiar with various toothbrush products, primarily from their own use experience,

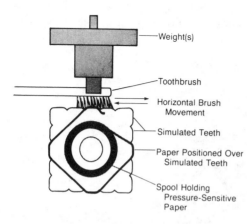

Figure 5–10. Essential components of a toothbrushing apparatus. The patterns of interproximal Horizontal brushing. *(From Yankell J Soc Cosmet Chem. 1983; 34:151–157.)*

Labels in figure:
- Weight(s)
- Toothbrush
- Horizontal Brush Movement
- Simulated Teeth
- Paper Positioned Over Simulated Teeth
- Spool Holding Pressure-Sensitive Paper

TABLE 5–2. SUMMARY OF THE AMERICAN DENTAL ASSOCIATION ACCEPTANCE PROGRAM CLINICAL STUDY GUIDELINES FOR TOOTHBRUSHES

1. Minimum of 28 healthy adult subjects assigned to
   a. A commercially available ADA-accepted toothbrush
   b. The test brush
2. Single-blind design (investigators not aware of product assignment)
3. Measurements at baseline, 15 days and 30 days
   a. Safety
   b. Plaque
   c. Gingivitis
4. Appropriate statistical analysis of data

and have examples of toothbrushes demonstrating various degrees of splaying or bending. These should be demonstrated when prevention methods are being discussed with the patient.

POWERED TOOTHBRUSHES

The heads of most powered or mechanical toothbrushes are smaller than manual toothbrushes and are usually removable to allow for replacements (Fig 5–11). The head follows three basic patterns when the motor is started: (1) reciprocating, a back-and-forth movement; (2) arcuate, an up-and-down movement; and (3) elliptical, a combination of the reciprocating and arcuate motions. Research to date has not indicated clearly significant advantages of one motion over another.[32–34] In studies ranging from one time use through 30 days, powered toothbrushes are consistently superior to manual toothbrushes in plaque removal.[32,35,36]

Motivation to improve oral hygiene appears to be a key factor for patients to purchase powered toothbrushes.[37,38] Often this motivation disappears after the novelty

has worn off. In a survey by the ADA, of the 139 respondents who owned powered toothbrushes, 21.6% used them regularly, and 25.2% used them occasionally.[37] This survey does not indicate the toothbrushing frequency of the remaining 53%. A published study on the use of powered toothbrushes found that when consumers first purchased the electric brush they increased their frequency of use. Unfortunately, after approximately a 3-month period, the use of electric toothbrushes decreased considerably until it was below the original frequency measurement. In the control group using hand toothbrushes, toothbrushing frequency and regularity remained essentially the same throughout the study.[38] More recently,[39] a survey conducted 6 months after subjects completed a clinical efficacy study indicated that most subjects were not using their powered device twice a day.

The ADA regards the electric toothbrush as an acceptable device and has developed criteria for acceptance based on both safety and efficacy. (1) Laboratory evidence of electric safety, that is, no electric shock hazard; (2) clinical evidence of both hard and soft tissue safety under unsupervised conditions; (3) clinical evidence of efficient cleaning when used according to the manufacturer's directions; and (4) evidence of proper labeling and advertising claims that may mention plaque reduction but not improvement of any existing oral disease. A listing of powered oral hygiene devices considered acceptable has been published by the ADA.[40] The required statement for labeling and commercial claims on powered toothbrushes authorized by the American Dental Association is as follows: Acceptable as an effective cleansing device for use as part of a program for good oral hygiene to supplement the regular professional care required for oral health.[11]

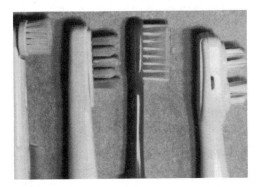

Figure 5–11. Toothbrush heads from powered toothbrushes. From left to right: Braun; Interplak; Panasonic; Plak Trac; Rota-dent; Sonicare.

Powered Special Uses

Powered toothbrushes can be particularly beneficial for parental brushing of children's teeth; for patients who are physically handicapped, mentally retarded, aged, arthritic, or otherwise with poor dexterity; and for those patients who are poorly motivated. These brushes are especially recommended for patients who require a larger handle, because powered models are easier to grasp.

Question 2. Which of the following statements, if any, are correct?

A. By the use of existing laboratory and clinical tests, the relative effectiveness of different toothbrushes can be compared and *specific brushes* identified as outstanding for removal of plaque.

B. Interproximal access *decreases* as the textures of the bristles *increases*.

C. Interproximal access is better with vertical brushing procedures, compared with a horizontal motion of the brush head.

D. All other factors being equal, a manual (hand) brush can remove plaque as effectively as an electric toothbrush with rotating tufts.

E. The interproximal plaque index is used to measure interproximal toothbrush cleaning efficiency.

TOOTHBRUSHING METHODS

Many toothbrushing methods have been developed, and most are identified by an individual's name, such as Bass, Stillman, Charters, or by a term indicating a primary action to be followed, such as roll or scrub. The objectives of toothbrushing are to (1) remove and disturb plaque formation; (2) clean teeth of food, debris and stain; (3) stimulate the gingival tissue; and (4) apply fluoride dentifrice. The toothbrushing methods most emphasized are horizontal scrub, Fones', Leonard's, Stillman's, Charters', Bass', rolling stroke (press roll), and Smith-Bell. All of these techniques are applicable to the cleaning of the facial, lingual, and occlusal surfaces; all are relatively ineffective in cleaning interproximal areas; and, only the Bass technique is effective in cleaning the sulcus. The brush motions used in each of these techniques are summarized in Table 5–3.

Natural Methods of Brushing

The most natural brushing methods used by patients uneducated in toothbrushing are a reciprocating *horizontal scrub technique*, a *rotary motion* (Fones' technique),[41] or a simple *up-and-down* motion over the maxillary and mandibular teeth (Leonard's technique).[42] Patients managing effective toothbrushing with these methods without causing traumatic problems or disease should not alter their brushing methods just for the sake of change.[43–45]

TABLE 5–3. BRUSH MOTIONS USED IN TOOTHBRUSHING METHODS

I. Horizontal reciprocating scrub
II. Vibratory
  Bass (sulcular technique)
  Stillman's
  Charters'
III. Vertical sweeping
  Rolling stroke (press roll)
  Modified Stillman's
  Modified Charters'
  Modified Bass
  Leonard's
  Smith-Bell (physiologic technique)
IV. Rotary
  Fones'

Horizontal. The horizontal scrub technique is probably the most used method. The toothbrush bristles are positioned perpendicular to the tooth crown. The brush is moved back and forth in short horizontal strokes. The bell-shaped anatomy of children's primary teeth is most effectively cleansed by the scrub technique.[46] Over prolonged periods excessive pressure and abrasive dentifrices, however, can result in gingival recession and tooth damage at the cementoenamel junction.

Fones. The Fones' technique is similar to the horizontal scrub method except that rotary strokes are used. Fones cautioned about possible gingival damage but encouraged stimulating the gingiva with rotary strokes. In addition, Fones advocated mouth brushing, which included teeth, gingivae, and tongue.

Leonard. In Leonard's method, an up-and-down brushing motion is used over the facial surfaces of the clenched posterior teeth to provide both tooth cleaning and gingival stimulation.[42]

Often all three natural motions are used by the same individual during brushing, and it is impossible to determine a dominant motion in removing debris and stains from the smooth tooth surfaces; all stimulate and sometimes harm the gingiva.

Stillman. Stillman's method was originally developed to provide gingival stimulation.[47] The toothbrush is positioned with the bristles inclined at a 45° angle to the apex of the tooth, with part of the brush resting on the gingiva and the other part on the tooth (Fig 5–12). A vibratory motion is used with a slight pressure to stimulate the gingiva. In this technique, the bristles are mainly pulsed. The brush is lifted and then re-

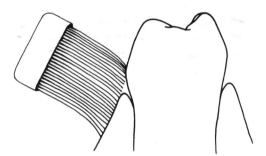

Figure 5–12. Stillman's technique seen diagrammatically.

placed in the same area, and pulsing is repeated.

Charters. Charters advocated a pressure–vibratory technique to clean interproximal areas.[48] Charters' original intent was to reduce the incidence of interproximal caries. The toothbrush should be placed at a 90° angle to the long axis of the teeth so that the bristles are gently forced between the teeth but do not rest on the gums. The brush is moved in several small rotary motions so that the sides of the bristles are in contact with the gum margin. After two or three such motions the brush is removed and replaced in the same area and the motions repeated. According to Charters these movements crowd the sides of the bristles into the V-shaped spaces between the teeth so that the gingivae are massaged. This method is useful in cleaning the abutting surfaces or fixed bridges, around fixed orthodontic appliances, and when interproximal tissues are missing. When normal papillae are present, other methods are easier to use and are equally effective in cleaning interproximal areas.

Bass. It is important to note that the Bass technique was the first to focus on the removal of plaque and debris from the gingival sulcus by the combined use of a soft toothbrush and unwaxed dental floss. Bass, a physician and former dean at the Tulane Medical School, published his initial paper in the *Journal of the Louisiana State Medical Society*[49]—not in a dental journal. The method is effective for removing plaque adjacent to and directly beneath the gingival margins as part of the self-care regimen for controlling periodontal disease and caries.

Bass advocated specific qualities for the toothbrush used in sulcular brushing (Fig 5–13). Some key requisites are that the toothbrush be

- An individualized size
- Easily and effectively manipulated
- Readily cleaned and aerated
- Impervious to moisture
- Durable
- Inexpensive

In the Bass technique the toothbrush is positioned in the gingival sulcus at a 45° angle to the tooth apex.[49] The bristles are then gently pressed to enter the sulcus. A vibratory action, described as a back-and-forth horizontal jiggle, causes a pulsing of the bristles to clean the sulci[50] (Fig 5–13). Ten strokes are advised for each area.

The Rolling Stroke. The rolling stroke (press roll) method involves the general cleaning of the gingiva and the teeth without emphasis on the sulcus.[45] It offers preparatory instruction for the modified Stillman's, modified Charters', and modified Bass, techniques. The toothbrush bristles are positioned parallel to and against the attached gingiva, with the toothbrush head level with the occlusal plane. The wrist is then turned to flex the toothbrush bristles first against the gingiva and then the facial surface. An arcuate sweeping motion is continued until the occlusal or incisal surface is reached (Fig 5–14). The toothbrush bristles are at right angles to the tooth surface as the brush passes over the crown. The press roll action is repeated at least five times before proceeding to the next site. Overlapping the tooth areas ensures a more thorough cleaning. With the rolling stroke method patients may miss the gingival third of the teeth if rotation begins with the brush on the crown instead of on the attached gingiva. If the

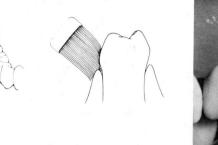

A

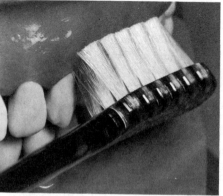

B

Figure 5–13. Bass technique: **A.** graphically; **B.** pictorially.

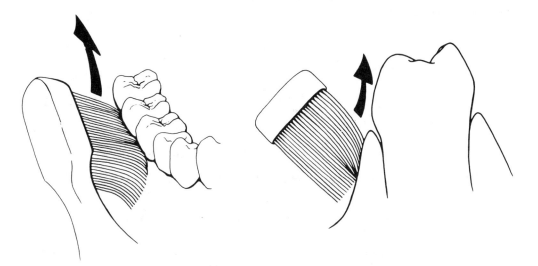

Figure 5–14. Rolling stroke technique.

toothbrush is positioned too deep in the buccal vestibule, the mucrogingival junction and alveolar mucosa can be traumatized.

Modified Brushing Methods

In attempts to enhance brushing of the entire facial and lingual tooth surfaces, the original techniques of Stillman, Charters, and Bass have been modified to include the rolling stroke method.

In the modified Stillman's and Charters' methods, the toothbrush bristles are placed in approximately the same position as advocated in the original method, and a pulsing action is started. Then the toothbrush is slowly press-rolled coronally. A continued vibratory motion is used during this rolling stroke.

In the modified Bass technique, sulcular brushing is done either before or after the use of the rolling method. The Bass sulcular brushing and the rolling stroke should not be combined into one continuous movement, because this may result in an inadequate amount of pulsing or the brush not being positioned correctly in the sulci. Lingual surfaces are cleaned in the same manner by using small, circular, vibratory motions.

The "physiologic" method of Smith-Bell is mentioned for historic interest.[51] The toothbrush bristles are positioned at the incisal or occlusal surfaces and are swept toward the gingiva. The direction of the brushing motion from the occlusal to the gingiva was an attempt to duplicate what was believed to be nature's self-cleansing mechanism, where the downward flow of food over the smooth surfaces of the buccal and lingual surfaces would remove plaque.

Table 5–4 summarizes the various toothbrushing techniques and their claimed benefits.

Question 3. Which of the following statements, if any, are correct?

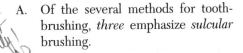

A. Of the several methods for toothbrushing, *three* emphasize *sulcular* brushing.

TABLE 5–4. TOOTHBRUSHING METHODS SUMMARIZED

Technique	Bristles Positioning	Brushing Motion	Effect Claimed
Horizontal scrub	90° to tooth	Horizontal strokes	Supragingival cleansing, gingival stimulation
Fones	90° to tooth	Large circles over teeth and gingiva	Supragingival cleansing, gingival stimulation
Leonard	90° to tooth	Vertical strokes	Supragingival cleansing, gingival stimulation
Smith-Bell (physiologic)	at occlusal surface	Sweep gingivally	Supragingival cleansing
Rolling stroke (press roll)	apically against attached gingiva	Sweep in arc occlusally	Supragingival cleansing, gingival stimulation
Stillman	45° to apex; part on gingival margin, part on cervix of tooth	Vibratory pulsing	Gingival stimulation
Modified (above plus)		Sweep occlusally	Supragingival cleansing
Charters	90° to tooth	Circular vibratory	Gingival stimulation, interproximal cleansing
Modified (above plus)		Sweep occlusally	Supragingival cleansing
Bass	45° apex; in sulcus	Vibratory horizontal jiggle	Subgingival cleansing, gingival stimulation
Modified (above plus)		Sweep occlusally	Supragingival cleansing

B. Stillman's method emphasizes bristle action in the interproximal areas, whereas the method of Charters provides better stimulation of the gingiva.

C. The interproximal access of bristles is probably greater using the press roll stroke or Leonard's technique than Fones' or the horizontal scrub technique.

D. The Bass technique is the *only* technique of those mentioned that results in a mechanically cleansed sulcus.

E. All the modified methods of brushing involve the original method plus the addition of the press roll stroke.

The following considerations are important when teaching patients a particular toothbrushing technique: (1) the patient's oral health status, including number of teeth, their alignment, patient's mouth size, presence of removable prostheses, orthodontic appliances, periodontal pockets, and gingival condition; (2) the patient's systemic health status, including muscular and joint diseases, and mental retardation; (3) the patient's age; (4) the patient's interest and motivation; (5) the patient's manual dexterity; and (6) the ease and effectiveness with which the professional can explain and demonstrate proper toothbrushing procedures.

TOOTHBRUSHING TIME AND FREQUENCY

For many years the dental professional advised patients to brush their teeth after every meal. The ADA has modified this position by use of the statement that patients should brush "regularly." Research has indicated that if plaque is *completely* removed every other day, there will be no deleterious effects in the oral cavity.[52] On the other hand, because few individuals *completely* remove plaque, daily brushing is still extremely important to maximize sulcular cleaning as a periodontal disease control measure as well as to afford an opportunity to use fluoride dentifrices more often in caries control. Where periodontal pockets exist, even more frequent oral hygiene procedures are indicated.

Studies have been done in which patients were asked to brush exactly as they did at home and then covertly monitored to determine the length of time of brushing. The average brushing time was approximately 1 minute, even though these individuals claimed that they usually brushed for 2 or 3 minutes.[53,54] These results demonstrate that people either grossly overestimate their efforts or else are telling their professionals what they would like them to believe.

Thorough toothbrushing requires a different amount of time for each individual, depending on such factors as the innate tendency of a person to accumulate plaque and debris; the psychomotor skills of the individual; and the adequacy of clearance of foods, bacteria and debris by the saliva. Only after patients have repeatedly brushed their teeth under the supervision of a dental professional can the adequacy of cleaning in a given time be determined. Often a compromise is made by suggesting 5 to 10 strokes in each area or by advocating the use of a 3-minute egg timer. This amount of time, which might be adequate for the average person, may not be sufficient for patients in most need of maximum plaque control programs. To ensure continued commitment to a personal oral hygiene program, the benefits of proper oral care must be well explained and demonstrated to patients.

TOOTHBRUSHING PROCEDURE

The occlusal surfaces may be cleaned by either (1) short vibratory strokes, with pressure being maintained to accomplish as deep a penetration of the pits and fissures as possible; or (2) a rapid up-and-down vibrating motion to force the bristles into the pits and fissures, followed by a sweeping motion to expel the dislodged debris. Long, sweeping, horizontal strokes are contraindicated, because the toothbrush bristles have minimum contact in the deeper and more critical fissures (Fig 5–15). The orifices of the pits and fissures are too narrow for bristle penetration and, whatever the technique, are inaccessible for adequate cleaning. This helps explain why more than 66% of all carious lesions in the mouth are found on the occlusal surface, even though most individuals attempt to brush this surface.

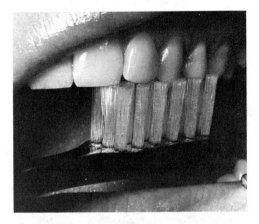

Figure 5–15. Occlusal brushing dislodges debris in the pits and fissures of posterior teeth (commonest site of caries) as well as in interproximal incisal areas.

The Anterior Lingual Areas

In all methods access to the lingual surfaces of the mandible and maxilla is difficult. Brushing in these areas can be facilitated by cutting off all tufts on a brush, except the first four or five rows in the toe. This modified brush has unimpeded access to the gingival sulci and lingual fossae areas (Fig 5–16). In the lower arch the heel of the brush can be used for the same purpose.

Brushing Sequence

A routine brushing pattern should be established to avoid exclusion of any area. One systematic pattern is to teach patients to begin on the occlusal surfaces at one molar end of the maxillary arch. Patients are taught to begin with the distal surface of the most posterior tooth and to continue brushing the occlusal and incisal surfaces around the arch until the last molar on the other side of the arch has been reached. The lower arch is then brushed in a similar manner.

Patients tend to apportion more time and effort on the facial areas of the anterior teeth.[55] Often right-handed people do not brush the right side of the arch as well as the left side; left-handed people similarly neglect the left side over the right side.

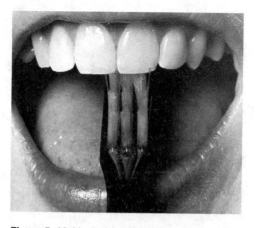

Figure 5–16. Vertical position of the toothbrush for the often-constricted lingual area.

CLINICAL ASSESSMENTS OF TOOTHBRUSHING

Whatever techniques are recommended, the main purpose of toothbrushing is to remove dental plaque from the teeth, including any in the gingival crevice, with the minimum amount of damage to the teeth and surrounding structures.[56] Disclosing agents provide the means of evaluating the thoroughness of cleaning the teeth[16,43,56] Hartzell first proposed use of disclosing agents in a 1930 issue of the *Journal of the American Dental Association.*[57] Staining agents have included iodine, mercurochrome, food coloring, bismarck brown, basic fuchsin and erythrosin. The latter two compounds are now regarded as carcinogenic. The most widely marketed red disclosing agent products contain FD&C Red #28.

Disclosing agents may be in either a liquid or tablet form. The chewed-up tablet or the liquid disclosant should be swished around the mouth for 15 to 30 seconds and then expectorated. Home use of disclosants by the patient should be encouraged to permit self-evaluation of the effectiveness of plaque control programs. Clinical assessments should be made for evidence of improper toothbrushing. Minor damage that may be noted includes abrasion to the soft tissues (scuffing, bruising, and punctate lesions) or damage to the tooth surface.

"Pink toothbrush" indicates gingival bleeding or is a sign of improper or infrequent brushing and flossing. Other damage includes gingival recession (exposure of the root surface) and tooth abrasion. Gingival recession occurs from excessive pressure or trauma from hard bristles, frayed and broken bristles, and bristles positioned beyond the attached gingiva. The areas generally affected are the gingivae, facial surfaces, especially around the cuspids, or teeth that prematurely contact the brush due to malalignment.

Toothbrush abrasion, or the wearing away of tooth substances, occurs from the use of highly abrasive dentifrices, too hard a brush, incorrect brushing methods, and excessive pressure during brushing. Common abrasion locations are on the surfaces of the teeth displaced facially and on the cervical areas of exposed root surfaces. Because enamel is harder than cementum, tooth damage usually occurs as a V-shaped, horizontal notch immediately apical to the cementoenamel junction. Further progress of the abrasion can be minimized by use of soft-bristle brushes, changes in brush angulation, pulsing instead of stroking, and the use of less abrasive dentifrices.

SUPPLEMENTAL BRUSHING

Tongue Brushing

The brushing of the tongue and palate helps to reduce the debris, plaque and number of oral microorganisms. The papillae on the tongue provide an area especially conducive to bacterial and debris retention. Tongue cleansing is accomplished by placing the side of the toothbrush near the middle of the tongue, with the bristles pointed toward the throat. The brush is swept forward, and this motion is repeated six to eight times in each area.[59] The palate should also be cleansed with a sweeping motion. A dentifrice should be used with this brushing of soft tissues to improve cleansing action.

SOME SPECIAL NEEDS

Abutment Teeth

The *abutment teeth* of a fixed bridge must be kept clean of all dental plaque near and below the gingival margin. A vibratory technique, or combination of techniques used with interdental aids, can maintain the meticulous hygiene needed. The gingival (tissue) surface of a dental bridge, beneath pontics and correctors, can often be cleansed of plaque by using Charters'[48] technique along with auxiliary aids such as floss threaders.

Orthodontic Appliances

Fixed orthodontic appliances require special emphasis on sulcular brushing to prevent gingivitis and thorough cleansing between the appliances and gingiva to prevent dental caries. A preteen or teen-aged patient is normally prone to dental caries; therefore a rigid, preventive program is required. A soft brush, an orthodontic brush, and auxiliary aids are used in combination with a vibratory technique and short horizontal strokes. The Bass technique for the facial sulci, Charters' technique[48] for the facial appliances, and a modified Stillman's technique[47] on the lingual surfaces can provide the means of cleaning the teeth and gingiva and stimulating the gingiva of the patient with full banding.

Denture patients with *full dentures* can meet their oral hygiene needs with a soft nylon brush for the oral tissues and a denture brush that cleans all areas of the denture. The denture brush that carries a nonabrasive cleaner should reach into the recessed alveolar ridge area of the denture to ensure maximum cleansing. The oral tissues should be brushed at least once a day with a gentle vibration and long straight strokes from the posterior to anterior mouth regions.[60]

Patients with *removable partial dentures* and *removable orthodontic appliances* need at least two toothbrushes, one for the natural teeth and another for the appliance. Brushing clasps, wires, and other metal parts can wear out a regular toothbrush. A clasp brush—2 or 3 in. long, narrow, and tapered—can be obtained as a third brush. Special care is needed to carefully clean the clasps of all plaque as a preventive measure for the supporting teeth.

Handicapped Patients

Handicapped patients like to brush their own teeth and can often do so with support and encouragement from dental personnel and the use of special brushes. A manual brush with an enlarged handle, elastic cuff, or small strap attached to the brush or a long-handled holder for patients who cannot raise their arms or do not have hands permits the patient to brush.[61] The elastic cuff is fitted around the hand and holds the toothbrush in the patient's palm. Patients who are unable to reach their mouths for brushing can at times attach the brush in a stationary upright position by using a clamp.[62] The patients bend over to position the brush in the mouth. The National Foundation of Dentistry for the Handicapped is developing a preventive program to encourage toothbrushing to the beat of music. Mentally retarded patients can often brush using a soft toothbrush with the plastic handle bent for better grasping. A horizontal scrub is often the best that these patients can manage.

Question 4. Which of the following statements, if any, are correct?

A. For the *average* person striving for plaque control, a meticulous, once-every-other-day program is probably more pragmatic and effective than daily morning and evening brushings.

B. The high incidence of caries that occurs on the occlusal surface is usually traceable to inadequate brushing.

C. Charters' method is probably more practical for an individual with orthodontic appliances than is the Smith-Bell technique.

D. For a person with a partial denture, the toothbrush used for the natural teeth is not adequate for cleaning the clasps.

E. It is necessary for handicapped persons to have others aid in brushing their teeth.

SUMMARY

Toothbrushing alone cleans buccal and lingual tooth surfaces. Toothbrushing used in conjunction with a dentifrice results in better cleaning, probably because of increased brushing time. No single toothbrushing technique adequately cleans occlusal pits and fissures. No toothbrushing procedure removes all interproximal and subgingival plaque, especially around malposed teeth and fixed prostheses. Interproximal cleaning aids are necessary to complete the tooth cleaning process. No one toothbrush design has been demonstrated to be *most* effective for *all* patients in long-term studies. Although manufacturers are advertising variations in bristle shape, bristle size, and number of filaments, *no* accepted criteria exist for product labeling. The American Dental Association does not yet consider one toothbrush design superior to another but is developing guidelines, associated with gingivitis reduction. Thoroughness and frequency of brushing is probably more important than a specific toothbrushing method and toothbrushing products. Any method that is taught should be effective, not damaging to the hard or soft tissues, and routinely used. In initiating effective toothbrushing, it is necessary to (1) select the appropriate toothbrush(es) suitable for the patient; (2) instill in individuals the goals of toothbrushing and the need for good oral physiotherapy; (3) teach a technique or combination of brushing methods needed to meet special needs; and (4) assess the ability of persons to accomplish thorough and effective toothbrushing as a part of the total oral hygiene program.

ANSWERS AND EXPLANATIONS

1. A, C, D, E

   B—incorrect. It should be the reverse. The higher the number, the firmer the bristle.

2. B, C, E

   A—incorrect. Laboratory and clinical testing has not yet attained the precision to permit meaningful comparisons of commercial toothbrushes.

   D—incorrect. The manual (hand) brush is not as effective as the powered toothbrush with rotating tufts.

3. C, D, E

   A—incorrect. Only the Bass technique includes sulcular brushing.

   B—incorrect. The reverse is true. Stillman's method emphasizes gingival stimulation, whereas Charters' emphasizes interproximal brushing.

4. C, D

   A—incorrect. It is true that one good cleaning would do the job, but so few people do a good job, that several cleanings might be equal to one good try.

   B—incorrect. No matter how well the occlusal surface is brushed, the deep pits and fissures cannot be adequately cleaned with a brush.

   E—incorrect. Handicapped persons can often manage brushing with slightly modified oral hygiene aids or with specially developed brushing devices.

SELF-EVALUATION QUESTIONS

1. The three *general* reasons that people do not spend adequate time for personal oral health care are _unwilling_, _ignorance_, and _____.

2. Wadsworth introduced the toothbrush into the United States just before the _Civil War_ war.

3. The constricted part of the toothbrush between the handle and the head is the _shank_. The end of the head is arbitrarily termed the _Toe_, the part closest to the handle is called the _Heel_.

4. Four lateral profiles of brushes sold in the United States are _Concave_, _convex_, _flat_, and _multileveled (rippled)_.

5. The American Dental Association Council on _____, (name) continually accomplishes scientific evaluations of devices used in dentistry. To support standardization of professional devices, the ADA is a member of the International _organizat⁼ for stnd⁼_, which has as its objective the establishment of consistency of labeling.

6. Three synonyms for hardness of bristles and toothbrushes are _texture_, _stiffness_, and _hardness_. Firmness of bristles is due to three general characteristics of bristles; they are _composit^n_, _diameter_, _length_, and _#indv. bristles_. A medium hard bristle has a diameter of approximately _____ in.

7. Five different bristle actions in addition to splay are _lag_, _skip_, _slap_, _bunching_, and _vibrat^n_. The ability of a bristle to enter the interproximal space is indicated by the _Interprox Plaq Index_ index.

8. Three basic motions of electric toothbrushes with heads are _back & forth_, _up & down_, and _elliptical_.

9. Three groups of people who can especially benefit from use of electric toothbrushes are _children_, _handicapped_, and _arthritic_, _aged ment. ret_

10. Four objectives of toothbrushing are _Remove & Disrupt plaq_ _Clean teeth/food/stain_, and _to apply fl. cont_. The three *natu-* _stimulate ging. tissue_

OSC

ral methods of tooth brushing are _horizontal scrub_, _fones_, and, _venord_. The motion of the brush in blank no. 1 is _reciprocating_ in blank no. 2 is _rotary_; and in blank no. 3 is _up & down_.

11. The toothbrushing method originally developed to protect gingival health was _Stillman's_ method; to reduce caries, _Charters_ method; and to accomplish sulcular cleaning, _Bass_ method. The modified methods all include the use of the _Rolling stroke_ method.

12. From a research point of view, the *least* number of meticulous plaque removals that can be accomplished, consistent with continuing good oral health is _every other day_ (frequency); however, from a practical viewpoint, it is more desirable to have the patient develop the habit of brushing _daily_ (frequency). The amount of time a patient should brush is _dep. on_. (Explain your answer). _psychomotor innate skag_

13. The sign of tooth damage due to abrasion is _among left part_; the sign of soft tissue damage is _recession_. Three disclosants that have been used in the past are _food col_, _iodine_, and _Bismarck Brown_.

14. The cleaning of the tissue under a pontic can be accomplished by _Charters_ (method); the best way to maintain cleanliness of orthodontic appliances is _____; full dentures should be brushed _____ (frequency); and partial dentures require at least _____ (number) brushes to clean teeth and clasps.

REFERENCES

1. Hirschfeld I. *The Toothbrush: Its Use and Abuse*. Brooklyn, NY. Dental Items of Interest Publishing Co; 1939.

2. Taylor GC. *A History of Dentistry*. Philadelphia, Pa. Lea & Febiger; 1922.

3. Akpata ES, Kinrinisi A. Antibacterial activity of extracts from some African chewing sticks. *Oral Surg.* 1977; 44:717–722.

4. Wolinsky LE, Soto EO. Isolation of natural plaque-inhibiting substances from Nigerian chewing sticks. *Caries Res.* 1984; 18:216–225.

5. Addis R. The history of the toothbrush. *Br Dent J.* 1939; 66:532–533.

6. Smith TS. Anatomic and physiologic conditions governing the use of the toothbrush. *J Am Dent Assoc.* 1940; 27:874–878.

7. Yankell SL, Emling RC. Understanding dental products: What you should know and what your patient should know. *U Pa Cont Dent Educ.* 1978; 1:1–43.

8. Updyke JR, Terrell ME. Toothbrush selection of a young child. *Pedodontics.* 1980; 4:295–298.

9. Benson BJ, Henyon G, Grossman E. Plaque removal efficacy of two children's toothbrushes: A one-month study. *J Clin Dent.* 1993; 4:6–9.

10. Benson BJ, Henyon G, Grossman E. Clinical plaque removal efficacy of three toothbrushes. *J Clin Dent.* 1993; 4:21–25.

11. Mulry CA, Dellerman PA, Ludwa RJ, et al. A comparison of the end-rounding of nylon bristles in commercial toothbrushes: Crest Complete and Oral-B. *J Clin Dent.* 1992; 3:47–50.

12. Mintel TE, Crawford J. The search for a superior toothbrush design technology. *J Clin Dent.* 1992; 3C:1–4

13. Rustogi KN, Curtis JP, Volpe AR, et al. Refinement of the modified navy plaque index to increase plaque scoring efficiency in gumline and interproximal tooth areas. *J Clin Dent.* 1992; 3C:9–12.

14. Benson BJ, Henyon G, Grossman E, et al. Development and verification of the proximal/marginal plaque index. *J Clin Dent.* 1993; 4:14–20.

15. Thevissen E, Quirynen M, van Steenberghe D. Plaque removing effect of a convex-shaped brush compared with a conventional flat brush. *J Periodontal.* 1987; 58:861–867.

16. Yankell SL, Green PA, Greco PM, et al. Test procedures and scoring criteria to evaluate toothbrush effectiveness. *Clin Prev Dent.* 1984; 6:3–8.

17. Volpe AR, Emling RC, Yankell SL. The toothbrush—A new dimension in design, engineering, and clinical evaluation. *J Clin Dent.* 1992; 3C:29–33.

18. Bass CC. The optimum characteristics of toothbrushes for personal oral hygiene. *Dent Items Int.* 1948; 70:697–718.

19. Maury TF. Improved toothbrush, U.S. Patent 74, 560. 1868.

20. Silverstone LM, Featherstone MJ. A scanning electron microscope study of the end rounding of bristles in eight toothbrush types. *Quintessence Int.* 1988; 19:87–107.

21. Nygaard-Ostby P, Yankell SL. Evaluation of the end-roundedness of toothbrushes filaments in laboratory and clinical studies. *J Dent Res.* 1981; 60:394.

22. Glass RT, Jensen HG. More on the contaminated toothbrush: The viral story. *Quintessence Int.* 1988; 19:713–716.

23. Glass RT, Lare MM. Toothbrush contamination: A potential health risk. *Quintessence Int.* 1986; 17:39–42.

24. International Organization for Standardization. *Dentistry—Stiffness of the Tufted Area of Toothbrushes.* References ISO 8627: 1987.

25. Nygaard-Ostby P, Edvardsen S, Spydevold B. Access to interproximal tooth surfaces by different bristle designs and stiffnesses of toothbrushes. *Scand J Dent Res.* 1979; 87: 424–430.

26. Emling RC, Shi X, Benson BJ, et al. Laboratory interproximal testing of three toothbrushes. *J Dent Res.* 1993; 72:414.

27. Yankell SL, Shi X, Emling RC. Comparative laboratory evaluation of three toothbrushes regarding interproximal access efficacy. *J Clin Dent.* 1992; 3C:5–8.

28. Yankell SL, Shi X, Emling RC. Comparative laboratory evaluation of two new toothbrushes regarding interproximal access efficacy. *J Clin Dent.* 1993; 4D:1–4.

29. Singh SM, Deasy MJ. Clinical plaque removal performance of two manual toothbrushes. *J Clin Dent.* 1993; 4D:13–16.

30. Craig TT, Montague JL. Family oral health survey. *J Am Dent Assoc.* 1976; 92:326–332.

31. Glaze PM, Wade AB. Toothbrush age and wear as it relates to plaque control. *J Clin Periodontol.* 1986; 13:52–56.

32. Emling RC, Raidl A, Greco MR, et al. Clinical evaluations of the Plac Trac toothbrush. *J Clin Dent.* 1991; 2:57–62.

33. Breuer MM, Cosgrove R, Hardy D, et al. A comparison of the plaque-removal efficacies of two electric toothbrushes. *Quintessence Int.* 1989; 20:501–504.

34. Ciancio SC, Mather ML. A clinical comparison of two electric toothbrushes with different mechanical actions. *Clin Prev Dent.* 1990; 12:5–7.

35. Mueller LJ, Darby ML, Allen DS, et al. Rotary electric toothbrushing. Clinical effects on the presence of gingivitis and supragingival dental plaque. *Dent Hygiene.* 1978; 52:546–550.

36. McKinney J, Burns S, Killoy W. A comparison between the counter-rotational toothbrush and multi-action toothbrush. *J Clin Dent.* 1990; 2:39–42.

37. American Dental Association. *Dentists' Desk Reference: Materials, Instruments and Equipment. Aids to Oral Hygiene and Oral Health: Powered Toothbrushes,* 2nd ed. Chicago; 1983.

38. Muhler JC. Comparative frequency of use of the electric toothbrush and hand toothbrush. *J Periodontol.* 1969; 40:268–270.

39. Baab DA, Johnson RH. The effect of a new electric toothbrush on supragingival plaque and gingivitis. *J Periodontol.* 1989; 60:336–341.

40. American Dental Association. *Clinical Products in Dentistry: A Desktop Reference.* Chicago; 1992.

41. Home care of the mouth. In: Fones AC, ed. *Mouth Hygiene,* 4th ed. Philadelphia, Lea & Febiger; 1934:294–315.

42. Leonard HJ. Conservative treatment of periodontoclasia. *J Am Dent Assoc.* 1939; 26:1308–1318.

43. Arnim SS. The use of disclosing agents for measuring tooth cleanliness. *J Periodontol.* 1963; 34:227–245.

44. Carranza FA, ed. *Glickman's Clinical Periodontology*, 7th ed. Philadelphia. W B Saunders; 1990.

45. Jones SC. Toothbrushes and toothbrushing technique. In: Harris NO, Christen AG, eds. *Primary Preventive Dentistry*, Reston, Va. Reston Publishing Company; 1982:76–99.

46. Tsamtsouris A, White CE, Clark ER. The effect of instruction and supervised toothbrushing on the reduction of dental plaque in kindergarten children. *J Dent Child.* 1979; 465:204–209.

47. Stillman PR. A philosophy of the treatment of periodontal disease. *Dent Dig.* 1932; 38: 315–319.

48. Charters WJ. Home care of the mouth I. Proper home care of the mouth. *J Periodontol.* 1948; 19:136–137.

49. Bass CC. An effective method of personal oral hygiene, Part II. *J Louisiana State Med Soc.* 1954; 106:100–112.

50. Gibson JA, Wade AB. Plaque removal by the Bass and roll brushing techniques. *J Periodontol.* 1977; 48:456–459.

51. Bell DG. Home care of the mouth, III. Teaching home care to the patient. *J Periodontol.* 1948; 19:140–143.

52. Lang KP, Cumming BR, Löe H. Toothbrushing frequency as it relates to plaque development and gingival health. *J Periodontol.* 1973; 44:396–405.

53. Emling RC, Flickinger KC, Cohen DW, et al. A comparison of estimated versus actual brushing time. *Pharm Therap Dent.* 1981; 6:93–98.

54. Saxer UP, Emling R, Yankell SL. Actual vs. estimated toothbrushing time and toothbrush used. *Caries Res.* 1983; 17:179–180.

55. Tsamtsouris A. Effectiveness of toothbrushing. *J Pedodontics.* 1978; 2:296–303.

56. Woodall IR, Dafoe BR, Young NS, et al. *Comprehensive Dental Hygiene Care,* 3rd ed. St. Louis, Mosby; 1989.

57. Hartzell TB. Clinical experiments on the efficiency of ultraviolet light in the treatment of dental disease. *J Am Dent Assoc.* 1930; 17:138–141.

58. Yankell SL, Emling RC. A study of gingival irritation and plaque removal following a three-minute toothbrushing. *J Clin Dent.* 1994; 5:1–4.

59. Christen AG, Swanson BZ Jr. Oral hygiene: A history of tongue scraping and brushing. *J Am Dent Assoc.* 1978; 96:215–219.

60. Wilkins EM. *Clinical Practice of the Dental Hygienist,* 6th ed. Philadelphia, Lea & Febiger; 1989.

61. Fuller L, Dunn MJ. An occupational therapist's role in oral hygiene for the handicapped. *Am J Occup Ther.* 1966; 20:35–36.

62. Birch RH, Mumford JM. Electric toothbrushing. *Dent Prac.* 1963; 13:182–186.

Chapter 6

Dentifrices, Mouth Rinses, and Tooth Whiteners

Stuart L. Fischman
Samuel Yankell

OBJECTIVES

At the end of this chapter, it will be possible to

1. Differentiate between a cosmetic and a therapeutic dentifrice or mouth rinse.
2. Explain the three phases of research necessary when applying to investigate a new drug (IND)—the process that precedes receiving a new drug application (NDA), which is necessary to market a new product.
3. Discuss how approval or nonapproval of a new product by the Food and Drug Administration (FDA) differs from an acceptance or rejection by the American Dental Association (ADA).
4. Explain the various reasons that the same abrasive material in a toothpaste can cause differing levels of abrasion on tooth structure.
5. Name the usual dentifrice ingredients and their percentages in a dentifrice.
6. Name the agents used in dentifrices to produce anticaries, anticalculus, and antihypersensitivity effects.
7. Name two antiplaque, antigingivitis mouth rinses: one sold over the counter, the other as a prescription item.

Introduction

Dentifrices and mouth rinses are the major products for routinely administering effective cosmetic and therapeutic agents in the mouth. These products are the most widely used by consumers, generating the largest sales of all dental products.

Dentifrices and mouth rinses differ considerably. Dentifrices are complex and difficult to formulate. Tremendous innovations have occurred in the past 20 years in the appearance and packaging of dentifrices. The contemporary consumer is faced with many alternatives in appearance (pastes, clear gels, stripes, sprinkles), and forms and packaging (conventional tubes, stand-up tubes, pumps) as well as in products marketed specifically for children. In addition, numerous claims are made for dentifrices. They are said to prevent tartar and caries, to whiten teeth and to eliminate hypersensitivity.

Because they are routinely used by the public, usually 1 to 3 times per day, dentifrices are the most beneficial dental products. Some of this benefit is lost if a person rinses immediately after brushing because rinsing decreases the concentration or reservoir of the active agent(s) in the oral cavity.

Mouth rinses are available in liquid form, the traditional method for stabilizing and delivering many pharmaceutically active agents. Mouth rinses are considered by consumers to have primarily cosmetic benefits (ie, breath fresheners) and are therefore not used as frequently or routinely as dentifrices in the daily oral hygiene regimen. Two mouth rinses, Listerine and chlorhexidine (Peridex), have been recognized by the American Dental Association (ADA) as effective against plaque and gingivitis. The Food and Drug Administration (FDA),

however, has recognized *only* chlorhexidine, and only as a *prescription* product. The two agencies differ in their acceptance criteria, which places the responsibility for selecting an effective product on the dental professional.

MONITORING THE SAFETY AND EFFECTIVENESS OF THERAPEUTIC DENTAL PRODUCTS

Caution is needed before introducing a new therapeutic product to the market. Some of the concerns surrounding new products are: Will the active agent disrupt the "normal" bacterial balance of the mouth? Should the search for an ideal bacteriocidal or bacteriostatic agent focus on depressing or eliminating specific disease-related organisms or a broad spectrum of organisms? Should a product be used to preserve a disease-free state while risking the possibility of developing a drug resistance? Regardless of the apparent effectiveness of any new product in the laboratory, *public safety is paramount.*

The process by which oral care agents are evaluated and regulated in the United States has recently been reviewed by Trummel.[1] Safety and efficacy standards apply not only to prescription medications but also to over-the-counter (OTC) drugs. There are three levels of regulation of oral chemotherapeutic agents. The *governmental level* includes the *Food and Drug Administration (FDA)* and the United States Pharmacopoeial Convention. The professional, or *voluntary*, level includes the Council on Dental Therapeutics of the *American Dental Association.* The third level of review includes *consumer advocacy organizations*, advertising standards review panels, and the Federal Trade Commission.

In addition, each of the major television networks has their own in-house review committee.

An ongoing review of all OTC products is conducted by the Food and Drug Administration. One aim of regulation is to protect the patient–consumer from useless or harmful products. All approval or disapproval decisions by the FDA have the *force of law*.

The stages of FDA approval include *preclinical research* and development (animal testing and toxicity) followed by *clinical research* and development, which is conducted with an approved investigational new drug application (IND). The IND usually includes *three phases*. In phase 1, the study is limited in scope and uses a *few subjects* to determine the safe dose for humans. For dental products, this usually involves ingestion or exaggerated (three or four times per day) topical applications or both. Phase 2 involves *more subjects* to demonstrate the clinical efficacy of the drug and define the dose range. Phase 3 generally includes *double-blind*, controlled trials to demonstrate long-term safety and efficacy. After the company receives an approved new drug application (NDA), marketing may begin, but *post-marketing surveillance* of the product is mandatory.

Over the years the commissioner of the FDA has requested manufacturers of OTC products to submit a listing of the *active and inactive* ingredients in their products as a basis for helping to codify regulations governing OTC sales. Among the many recommendations of the FDA advisory panel[2] that provide for better control of OTC oral therapeutic products is the stipulation that all inactive ingredients be listed on the label in descending order by quantity. Active ingredients, as well as inactive agents, should be in *no higher concentrations than necessary for the intended purpose*. The panel also recommended that the indicated objective of the active agent must be on the label and that the inclusion of the name of an active agent without stating its proposed benefits is considered misleading. Proof must exist to substantiate any claim for a specific therapeutic benefit. For instance, dentifrices that have not been subjected to laboratory or clinical trials but that list the inclusion of "decay-fighting fluorides" in their products cannot claim that the dentifrice is anticariogenic, only that it contains fluoride. It is possible that the fluoride in the untested dentifrice might not be compatible with other dentifrice ingredients, or the fluoride may not be released in active ionic form and therefore be totally ineffective.

Recommendations also apply to *packaging* and *labeling*, as well as to guidelines regulating advertising. For example, the recommendations suggest that all containers for OTC therapeutic dentifrices, rinses, and gels containing fluoride have a label to identify the product, for example, "anticaries dentifrice"; its use, for example, "aids in the prevention of dental caries"; a warning, such as "Do not swallow. Developing teeth of children under 6 years of age may become permanently discolored if excessive amounts of fluoride are repeatedly swallowed"; and directions for use, such as: "Adults and children 6 years of age or older should brush teeth thoroughly at least twice daily, or as directed by a dentist or physician."

After years of ignoring claims of *antigingivitis efficacy* for various OTC dentifrices and rinses, in 1988 the FDA advised manufacturers of such products they must either cease making such claims or substantiate them. In the 1990 published summary of its call for data the FDA announced

The Food and Drug Administration is announcing a call for data for ingredients containing products bearing anti-plaque and antiplaque related claims, such as "for the reduction or prevention of plaque, tartar, calculus, film, sticky deposits, bacterial buildup and gingivitis." The agency will review the submitted data to determine whether these products are generally regarded as safe and effective and not mis-branded for the label uses. This notice also describes the Attorney General's enforcement of policy governing the marketing of over-the-counter (OTC) drug products bearing antiplaque and antiplaque related claims during the pendency of this review. This request is part of the ongoing review of OTC drug products conducted by the FDA.[3]

In addition to the FDA's regulation of OTC products, the American Dental Association's Council on Dental Therapeutics (CDT) continually reviews dental products. The council is directed to study, evaluate and disseminate information with regard to dental therapeutic agents, their adjuncts and dental cosmetic agents that are offered to the public or to the profession.[1] The most important activity of the CDT in meeting this charge is its acceptance program. Unlike the IND process, submission by a manufacturer to the ADA program is voluntary. If the product is safe and effective, the Seal of Acceptance is granted and can be used by the manufacturer in marketing the product. The seal provides assurance to dental professionals and to the public.

The council recognized that plaque control might best be demonstrated by clinically significant reduction of gingivitis. In 1986, the council issued "Guidelines for Acceptance of Chemotherapeutic Products for the Control of Supragingival Dental Plaque and Gingivitis."[4] The guidelines for acceptance are presented in Table 6–1.

The purpose of the separate and independent actions of the FDA and the ADA is to ensure the *effectiveness and safety* of OTC products and to *prevent mislabeling* and thus misleading information.

Question 1. Which of the following statements, if any, are correct?

A. The Food and Drug Administration (FDA) and the American Dental Association (ADA) have *both* recognized Listerine and chlorhexidine as antiplaque agents.

B. The decisions of *both* the Food and Drug Administration and of the American Dental Association to approve a product have the force of law.

C. To receive the ADA's seal of acceptance an antiplaque agent must pre-

TABLE 6–1. AMERICAN DENTAL ASSOCIATION GUIDELINES FOR ACCEPTANCE OF CHEMOTHERAPEUTIC PRODUCTS FOR THE CONTROL OF SUPRAGINGIVAL DENTAL PLAQUE AND GINGIVITIS

The 1986 American Dental Association Council on Dental Therapeutics Guidelines require the following clinical study efficacy criteria:

- Two independent studies should be conducted.
- The study populations should represent typical product users.
- The test product should be used in a normal regimen and compared to a placebo.
- The study design should be either parallel or crossover.
- Each study should be at least six months in duration.
- The plaque and gingivitis scoring procedure should be conducted at baseline, after six months and at an intermediate period of time.
- Microbiological profile should demonstrate that pathogenic or opportunistic microorganisms do not develop over the course of the study.

vent or reduce the severity of some disease caused by the plaque.

D. The sales of *both* therapeutic and over-the-counter dental products are regulated by the FDA.

E. A manufacturer must secure the ADA's seal of acceptance before marketing a dental product.

DENTIFRICES

According to *Webster's*, the term *dentifrice* is derived from *dens* (tooth) and *fricare* (to rub). A simple, contemporary definition of a dentifrice is a mixture used on the tooth in conjunction with a toothbrush. The historic aspects of dentifrice use was reviewed by Fischman.[5]

Dentifrices are marketed as toothpowders, toothpastes, and gels. All are sold as either *cosmetic* or *therapeutic products*. If the purpose of a dentifrice is therapeutic, it must reduce some disease process in the mouth. Usually the actual or alleged therapeutic effect is to reduce caries incidence, gingivitis, calculus formation, or tooth sensitivity. The sales appeal of a product, however, is strongly linked to its flavor and foaming action.

In 1970, the dentifrice market amounted to an estimated $355 million; by 1988 it had increased to $1 billion; and the 1992 market is estimated at $1.4 billion.

Packaging

The development of the toothbrush in 1857 provided the stimulus to market commercial dentifrices. Toothpowders were popular because boxes and cans from which they could be dispensed already existed. The formulas consisted of little more than water, soap, and flavor.

Toothpastes began to appear on the market following the development of *lead*

tubes for packaging. When it was realized that some of the lead was combining with the dentifrice ingredients, the tube lining was coated with wax. Later tubes were made more malleable by alloying the lead with tin. During World War II, the shortage of lead and tin spurred the development of plastic tubes. This revolutionary change to plastic packaging simultaneously (1) eliminated the possibility of the user ingesting lead, (2) reduced the possibility of incompatibility of the tube and paste components, (3) aided the expelling of the paste by squeezing, (4) permitted an easier and more economic production of tubes, and (5) provided a good surface for the printing of decorative designs and information.

In 1984, Colgate introduced the pump dispenser to the market. Procter and Gamble began marketing Crest in 1991 in an upside-down tube that rests on its cap (Neat Squeeze). Colgate followed with their Stand Up product. In 1992, Chesebrough-Ponds introduced a dual-chamber pump dispenser to keep the peroxide and baking soda components of their dentifrice, Mentadent, separate until delivered together on the toothbrush. Examples of these packages are shown in Figure 6–1.

Dentifrice Ingredients

Dentifrices were originally used for cosmetic effect. They are effective in removing *extrinsic* stains, those that occur on the *surface* of the tooth. These stains, which are often the end products of bacterial metabolism, range in color from green to yellow to black. They also may be stains from foods, coffee, and tea. Dentifrices do not remove *intrinsic* stains, which are a result of altered amelogenesis, such as the white-to-brown color changes seen in fluorosis or the grayish-blue appearance of enamel following administration of tetracycline. Dentifrices are also ineffective in altering the yellowing

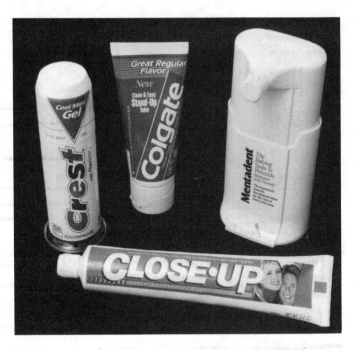

Figure 6-1. Examples of contemporary dentifrice containers; packaging pump (Crest), stand-up tube (Colgate), dual-chamber pump (Mentadent), and traditional tube (Close-Up).

color of teeth seen with physiologic aging and in correcting the hues of tooth color produced by the differing shades of dentin.

Most toothpastes contain several or all of the ingredients listed in Table 6–2. More recently gel dentifrices have appeared in the marketplace that contain the same components as the toothpastes, with the exception that the gels have a higher proportion of the thickening agents. Both toothgels and toothpastes are equally effective in plaque removal and in delivering active ingredients.

Abrasives

Early dentifrices were manufactured with the prime objective of cleaning teeth. Abrasiveness was emphasized, with little concern about possible damage to tooth structure. Dr Lyon's toothpowder was an example. In 1934, the American Dental Association (ADA) began its publication of Accepted Dental Remedies, and classified dentifrices as acceptable or nonacceptable on the basis of effectiveness and reasonableness of claims for the product. In 1940, after 70 years of sales, Dr Lyon's toothpowder was listed as unacceptable because of its excessive abrasiveness. In 1947, the ADA dropped the policy of evaluating dentifrices for any characteristic other than proven therapeutic value.

The degree of dentifrice abrasiveness depends on the (1) inherent *hardness* of the

TABLE 6–2. **TOOTHPASTE CONSTITUENTS**

Ingredient	Percentage
Abrasives	20–40
Water	20–40
Humectants	20–40
Foaming agent (soap or detergent)	1–2
Binding agent, up to	2
Flavoring agent, up to	2
Sweetening agent, up to	2
Therapeutic agent, up to	5
Coloring or preservative, less than	1

abrasive, (2) *size* of the abrasive particle, and (3) *shape* of the particle. Several other variables can affect the abrasive potential of the dentifrice: the brushing technique, the pressure on the brush, the hardness of the bristles, the direction of the strokes, and the number of strokes can all contribute to the cumulative effect of the abrasive. Also, the abrasive tested alone can differ from the same abrasive tested as part of a dentifrice formula. The salivary characteristics of individuals may also affect dentifrice abrasiveness.

Calcium carbonate and calcium phosphates were previously the most common abrasives used. These agents often reacted adversely with fluorides. Now silicon oxides, aluminum oxides, and bicarbonate and chalk are used.

Abrasiveness Testing. The Council on Dental Materials and Devices of the American Dental Association periodically publishes data on the relative abrasiveness of dentifrices. Independent studies are also carried out (Table 6–3). The majority of the data originates from laboratory tests and cannot be directly extrapolated to in vivo expectations.

Standard laboratory testing uses a machine with several brushes. The length of the reciprocating stroke, number of strokes, and pressure of the brush can be adjusted. Depending on the experimental objectives, enamel, dentin, or cementum is then brushed, and the amount of calcium or phosphorus in the resultant slurry is analyzed. A more accurate method has been developed in which the extracted teeth are placed in a nuclear reactor to activate some of the tooth phosphorus to radioactive phosphorus. After brushing root surfaces of sound canines and molars, the amount of radioactive phosphorus removed is more accurately assessed than with classical

TABLE 6–3. LABORATORY DENTINAL ABRASIVITY VALUES FOR SELECTED U.S. DENTIFRICES

Brand Name	RDA*
Colgate	44.7
Viadent	52.0
Pepsodent	61.8
Peak	71.0
Aim	73.0
Toms of Maine	80.0
Ultra-Brite	81.0
Gleem	86.0
Sensodyne	87.0
Colgate Tartar Control	94.0
Crest Tartar Control	121.0

*RDA = Percentage of the abrasivity value of $CaCO_3$ adjusted to 100%. (*Adapted from Cornell J. In vitro abrasion of dentifrices. J Clin Dent. 1988; 1: A9–A10.*)

chemical analyses. Results are referenced against the amount of tooth substance removed by the use of the control abrasive, calcium pyrophosphate.[6]

Abrasives usually do not damage enamel, but may dull the tooth luster. To compensate for this, *polishing agents* are added to the dentifrice formulation. These polishing agents are usually small-sized particles of aluminum, calcium, tin, magnesium, or zirconium compounds. Usually the manufacturer blends the abrasives and the polishing agents to form an *abrasive system.* Agents, such as chalk or silica, may have both polishing and abrasive effects. Smaller particles (1 μm) have a polishing action, and larger particles (20 μm) have an abrasive action.[7] In selecting a dentifrice, the abrasiveness and polishing characteristics should meet individual needs. For instance, up to 20% of the population does not accumulate visible stain when engaged in their own style of personal oral hygiene.[8] For these individuals, a dentifrice with high polishing and low abrasion should be recommended. For the average individual, an additional amount of abrasive is needed to control accumulating stain. The stains on neglected teeth may be green, orange, or black chromogenic stains of bacterial origin or yellow and brown stains from smoking. As the abrasive level increases, greater care must be taken to perfect brushing techniques that do not cause self-inflicted injury to the teeth or soft tissues. Such injuries can result from excessive pressure, hard bristles, and prolonged brushing. When toothbrushing is done without toothpaste, there is little possibility of abrasion. When damage does occur, it usually manifests as a V-shaped notch in the *cementum* immediately below the cementoenamel junction (Fig 6–2). This area is vulnerable, because enamel is about 20 times harder than dentin or cementum. More serious defects usually occur in older individuals who maintain a very high level of oral hygiene.

Problems of Liquid–Powder Formulations

Toothpaste consisting only of a toothpowder and water resulted in a product with several undesirable properties. In time the solids in

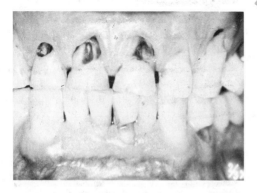

Figure 6-2. V-Shaped notches in central incisors resulting from use of a dentifrice with a harsh abrasive system. *(Courtesy of Dr B Baker, University of Texas Dental School at San Antonio.)*

the paste tended to settle out of solution and the water to evaporate. This resulted in a caking of the remaining dentifrice. Until the 1930s, most toothpastes had a short shelf life because of this problem. Once the tube was opened, the first expelled paste was too liquid, but the last paste in the tube was either impossible to expel or too hard to use. To solve this problem, *humectants* were added to maintain the moisture. Commonly used humectants are sorbitol, mannitol, and propylene glycol. These humectants are nontoxic, and mold or bacterial growth can occur in their presence. For this reason, *preservatives* such as sodium benzoate are added.

Humectants help to maintain the consistency of toothpaste; but despite their presence, the solids tend to settle out of the paste. To counteract this, *thickening* or *binding* agents are added to the formula. Gums, such as gum tragacanth, were first used. These were followed by colloids derived from seaweed, such as carrageenan, which in turn were replaced by synthetic celluloses. These celluloses in low concentration are also often used as humectants; in higher concentrations they function as gelling agents in the formulation of gel dentifrices. At high concentrations (>40%), humectants also act as preservatives.

Soap and Detergents

Because toothpastes were originally manufactured to keep the teeth clean, soap was the logical cleansing agent. As the toothbrush bristles displace the plaque, the *foaming* or *sudsing* action of the soap aids in the removal of the loosened debris. Soap has several disadvantages, however: (1) it can be irritating to the mucous membrane; (2) its flavor is difficult to mask and often causes nausea; and (3) many times soap is incompatible with other ingredients, such as calcium.

When the detergents appeared on the market, soaps largely disappeared from dentifrices. Sodium lauryl sulfate (SLS) is the most used detergent. It is stable, possesses some antibacterial properties, and has a low surface tension, which facilitates the flow of the dentifrice over the teeth. SLS is active at a neutral pH, has a flavor that is easy to mask, and is compatible with the current dentifrice ingredients. Barkvoll[9] has suggested that patients who suffer from various oral mucosal diseases should avoid the use of dentifrices containing sodium lauryl sulfate.

Question 2. Which of the following statements, if any, are correct?

A. Gel dentifrices are the same as regular dentifrices, except that they contain a greater proportion of thickening agent.

B. The abrasiveness of an abrasive agent depends on (1) inherent *hardness* of an abrasive, (2) *size* of the abrasive particles, and (3) *shape* of the abrasive particle.

C. The V-shaped damage to the tooth from using an excessively abrasive dentifrice occurs *coronal* to the cementoenamel junction.

D. Synthetic celluloses are now used as thickening agents for toothpastes and gels.

E. If sodium lauryl sulfate is added to the dentifrice formula, foaming can be expected when brushing.

Flavoring and Sweetening Agents

Flavoring Agents. Flavor, along with smell, color, and consistency of a product, is an important characteristic that leads to public acceptance of a dentifrice. If dentifrices did not possess these characteristics, they would probably be poorly accepted. For taste acceptance the flavor must (1) be pleasant, (2) provide an immediate taste sensation, and (3) be relatively long-lasting. Usually essential oils and synthetic flavors are blended to provide the desired taste. Spearmint, peppermint, wintergreen, cinnamon, and other flavors give toothpaste a pleasant taste and refreshing aftertaste. It is difficult to formulate a flavor that is universally acceptable, because people have different color and taste preferences.

Sweetening Agents. In early toothpaste formulations, sugar and honey were used as sweeteners. Now saccharin, cyclamate, sorbitol, and mannitol serve as primary noncariogenic sweetening agents; the latter two also serve a dual role as sweetening agents and humectants. Glycerine, which also serves as a humectant, adds to the sweet taste. A new sweetener in dentifrices is xylitol. In laboratory studies, it is not metabolized by bacteria to produce acid. In human studies, where it was placed in chewing gums and food, xylitol was noncariogenic. In addition, it demonstrated an anticaries capability by facilitating the remineralization of incipient carious lesions.

Other Tooth Cleaning Products

Some toothpastes and cleaning agents have been developed for special circumstances or for specific cleaning devices. For example, an ingestible dentifrice was developed for use by astronauts on space missions. The ingestion of the dentifrice following brushing obviates the need to carry the small but highly critical, additional weight of water needed for rising. This dentifrice has a low calcium content and contains glycerine, carboxylmethylcellulose (a thickening agent), saccharin, and water, with no oils or detergents. The same dentifrice can be prescribed for patients who have difficulty in rinsing and spitting following brushing.

Baking Soda Dentifrices

Baking soda (sodium bicarbonate) has a long history of use as an oral hygiene aid. Arm and Hammer, manufacturer of one of the original baking soda toothpastes, states that "two out of three dentists and hygienists recommend brushing with baking soda for healthier teeth and gums." Three major baking soda dentifrices are on the U.S. market. They are manufactured by Arm & Hammer, Procter & Gamble, and Colgate. In addition, Chesebrough-Pond's recently introduced Mentadent, a product containing baking soda and hydrogen peroxide. *All contain fluoride*, but only the last three have been awarded the ADA's Seal of Acceptance for caries protection. These products obtained the seal because they also contain hydrated silica as an abrasive ingredient. Hydrated silica is contained in most ADA-approved products and has been demonstrated to be compatible with fluoride and effective in laboratory, animal, and clinical studies. The currently marketed baking soda dentifrices are presented in Appendix 6–1.

Baking Soda and Hydrogen Peroxide.

Hydrogen peroxide and baking soda have been used as part of a daily oral hygiene regimen since the turn of the century. The mixture has been prescribed as an alternative to the use of commercial dentifrices by some dentists. Allegorically, many patients attribute benefit to routine use of the product. Hydrogen peroxide is used routinely or semiroutinely by approximately 14% of the population in conjunction with baking soda. The recently marketed Mentadent delivers a combination of 0.75% stable peroxide gel in conjunction with baking soda and 1100 ppm sodium fluoride. This material is packaged in a two-chamber pump to permit the baking soda and peroxide components to be mixed at the time of delivery (see Fig 6–1). The product has been demonstrated to be safe,[10] and the low level of hydrogen peroxide does not present problems alleged to result from higher levels of peroxide in early animal studies.[11] The product has been widely accepted by consumers,[12] reaching a 12% market share following introduction in the Northeast.

Therapeutic Dentifrices

The most commonly used therapeutic agent added to dentifrices is fluoride, which aids in the control of caries. In 1960, the Council on Dental Therapeutics of the American Dental Association classified Crest toothpaste as a caries prophylactic dentifrice based on several studies that indicated its effectiveness. For the first time, a therapeutic dentifrice was awarded the seal of *provisional* acceptance. In 1964, on the basis of further new and favorable data,[13] the classification was upgraded to full acceptance.

The level of fluoride in OTC dentifrices and gels is restricted to no more than *120 mg* of fluoride, and the package must include a *safety closure*. Therapeutic toothpastes may contain up to 260 mg of fluoride. The following fluorides are generally recognized as effective and safe for OTC sales: 0.22% *sodium fluoride* (NaF), 0.76% *sodium monofluorophosphate (MFP)*, and *0.4% stannous fluoride* (SnF_2). Recently, levels were increased for the "extra-strength" products of Crest (sodium fluoride) and Aim (sodium monofluorophosphate).

Multiple clinical studies of fluoride dentifrices containing NaF, MFP, or SnF_2 in the presence of compatible abrasives and stable formulations have been submitted to and been accepted by the ADA; the association, therefore, accepts fluoride dentifrices based on laboratory data if they comply with previously submitted data.[14]

The fluoride dentifrices currently accepted by the Council on Dental Therapeutics of the American Dental Association are presented in Appendix 9–1. Not all fluoride-containing dentifrices have demonstrated anticaries activity, however. The level of active fluoride must be adequate and must be maintained over the shelf life of the dentifrice. The seal of acceptance of the American Dental Association is one assurance of an active product. Fluoride dentifrices are discussed more extensively in Chapter 9.

Most intriguing is the concept of chemical plaque control, in which chemical compounds are used to supplement the usual brushing, flossing, and use of auxiliary aids employed in mechanical plaque control. Antiplaque agents can act directly on the plaque bacteria or can disrupt different components of plaque to permit easier and more complete removal during toothbrushing and flossing. This opportunity to use chemistry to enhance oral hygiene procedures is important, especially because manual plaque control methods are difficult to teach and monitor, tedious to perform, time-consuming, impossible to accomplish by some physically and mentally handicapped persons, and not used by nonmotivated individuals.

The present plaque control agents should not be considered a panacea because they have *not* been proven to be a total substitute for routine oral hygiene measures. Excessive emphasis on chemical control may encourage some patients to deemphasize proven oral hygiene methods.

At the present time, an agent (or agents) analogous to fluoride is being sought to control gingivitis and prevent periodontitis. The properties of an ideal form of such an agent are listed in Table 6–4.

TABLE 6–4. PROPERTIES OF AN IDEAL AGENT TO CONTROL GINGIVITIS

High immediate and intrinsic antimicrobial activity
Broad-spectrum efficacy against bacteria and yeasts
Chemical stability in formulations and in the oral cavity
Substantivity (ability to stick) to oral tissues, and be released over time in an active form
Toxicologic and ecologic safety
  No topical adverse reactions (staining, burning)
  No taste or aftertaste problems
  No inhibition of taste perception
  No systemic toxicity
    No change in oral or GI flora
    Neither carcinogenic nor teratogenic
No adverse reactions
Compatibility with dentifrice or mouthwash formulations

Stannous Salts. Stannous fluoride has been reported to be active against gingivitis.[15] Clinically, the stannous ion has been shown to have both antiplaque and antigingivitis effects.[16]

Numerous clinical trials have demonstrated the ability of an optimally formulated dentifrice containing stannous pyrophosphate and zinc citrate to maintain gum health. The efficacy of this dentifrice in reducing the development of gingival bleeding, measured by the probe method, was noted in two experimental gingivitis studies.[15,17] In a six-month double-blind trial,[15] a significant reduction in plaque, numbers of bleeding sites, and calculus formation was attributed to a stannous fluoride–stannous pyrophosphate dentifrice.

Triclosan. Triclosan is a broad-spectrum antibacterial agent marketed for use in European oral products under the trade name Irgacare. It is effective against a wide variety of bacteria and is widely used as an antibacterial agent in OTC consumer products in the United States including deodorant soaps and antibacterial skin scrubs (Clearasil soap). It has also been shown to be a useful antibacterial agent in oral products. A review of the available pharmacologic and toxicologic information concluded that "Triclosan can be considered safe for use in dentifrice and mouthrinse products."[18]

At least two products containing triclosan have been subjected to clinical evaluation. Many dentifrices containing triclosan are marketed in Europe, but at present, they are not available in the United States. Approval by the FDA is pending. A Colgate product contains triclosan and polyvinylmethyl ether maleic acid (PVA/MA) copolymer. Volpe and colleagues[19] reviewed several long-term clinical efficacy studies and concluded that this product provides clinically and statistically "meaningful benefits with regard to supragingival plaque, gingivitis and supragingival calculus efficacy, compared to a placebo dentifrice." A Unilever product containing zinc citrate and triclosan has also received considerable attention. Clinical evaluation has shown this to be effective in reducing plaque formation and in preventing gingivitis. Six-month clinical trials indicated that subjects who brushed with the zinc citrate–triclosan formula had 75% less plaque and developed 70% less gingival bleeding than those who brushed with a normal fluoride toothpaste.[20,21] A summary of the zinc citrate–triclosan studies was recently published in the *International Dental Journal*.[22]

Antitartar Dentifrices

In the late 1970s, anticalculus dentifrices began to appear on the market without any evidence of effectiveness.[23] In 1985, Procter & Gamble supplemented their existent Crest anticariogenic toothpaste with a similar anticaries formula that also contained a combination of tetrasodium phosphate and disodium dihydrogen pyrophosphate. The soluble pyrophosphates are crystalgrowth inhibitors, which retard the formation of cal-

culus.[24] This combination has been demonstrated in clinical studies to reduce significantly the amount of calculus formed compared with a control dentifrice. The dentifrice is marketed as Crest Tartar Control. The formula received the ADA Seal of Acceptance but only as a caries control product and only because of its fluoride content. Other similar anticalculus products are now on the market; all contain NaF. Zinc citrate trihydrate is used to inhibit calculus formation in the tartar control versions of both Aim and Close-Up. Clinical studies[25] have shown that zinc citrate does not affect the caries inhibition of fluoride. Rolla and Saxegaard[26] have noted, however, the possibility of "crystal poisons," such as pyrophosphates and phosphonates, inhibiting remineralization. Such inhibition might adversely affect the anticaries effect of the fluoride in this type of tartar control dentifrice.

Despite favorable anticalculus data, the ADA seal has not been awarded to anticalculus products, because the ADA considers calculus inhibition as a cosmetic, *not* a therapeutic effect. Two simultaneous beneficial effects—caries control and calculus inhibition—are available with one brushing operation. The major currently marketed tartar control products are presented in Appendix 6–2.

Question 3. Which of the following statements, if any, are true?

A. Baking soda, peroxide, and *fluoride* are incompatible in a dentifrice.

B. The present consensus is that chemical plaque control is only a *supplement* to mechanical plaque control.

C. Stannous fluoride is both an anticaries and an antigingivitis agent.

D. Triclosan is an effective antibacterial agent.

E. Crest Tartar Control toothpaste has received the ADA's Seal of Acceptance as an anticalculus product.

ANTIHYPERSENSITIVITY PRODUCTS

Many people experience pain when exposed areas of the root, especially at the cementoenamel junction, are subjected to heat or cold. To address this issue the ADA has formed the Ad Hoc Committee on Dentinal Sensitivity. Several OTC dentifrices have been accepted—Denquel, Sensodyne, and Protect—with the active agents being *potassium nitrate*, *strontium chloride*, and *sodium citrate*, respectively.[27] Potassium citrate has also been accepted by the British Department of Health.

The ADA's Council on Dental Therapeutics has approved a dentifrice—Sensodyne F—with a combination of active ingredients, which has demonstrated *both* antihypersensitivity and caries-preventive benefits. This was the *first* therapeutic dentifrice on the market directed at solving two problems, caries and hypersensitivity, with the *same* brushing operation.

Appendix 6–3 presents the desensitizing dentifrices accepted by the American Dental Association as of January, 1993.[27]

TOOTHPOLISHES AND WHITENERS

Considerable controversy surrounds the use of stain removers and tooth whiteners. Products are being marketed for professional use or for use by the patient at home. Many claims for efficacy and safety are under review by agencies and government panels.

These dentifrices have been divided into two categories: with or without peroxide. Representative products without peroxide are shown in Appendix 6–4. Although the public perceives these as more abrasive than ordinary toothpastes, their abrasiveness is usually intermediate among the products tested.

The second category of products (with peroxide) usually are marketed as tooth whiteners (Appendix 6–5). They are available as a dentifrice or gel or are used in a two- or three-step treatment "process." These products usually contain *hydrogen peroxide* or *carbamide peroxide* as their bleaching or whitening ingredient. Carbamide peroxide breaks down to form urea and hydrogen peroxide. Hydrogen peroxide in turn forms a free radical containing oxygen, which is the active bleaching molecule. Home bleaching products may contain other chemicals to aid in the delivery of the bleaching agent. Glycerine or propylene glycol are commonly added to thicken the solution and prolong contact with the tooth surface. In the two- or three-step products, agents can be delivered to teeth via a custom-made tray or by toothbrushing.

There is concern that regular use of the peroxides or their breakdown products may enable overgrowth of undesirable organisms, including yeasts, possibly leading to "black hairy tongue." In addition, peroxides may damage the pulp or the soft tissues of the mouth. Delayed wound healing is also a concern, as is the possible mutagenic effect of strong oxygenating agents. The Food and Drug Administration has sent a regulatory letter to producers of those commercial tooth whitening agents containing peroxides to inform them that these products are *classified as drugs*. The letter asked for information about possible side effects, such as delayed wound healing, periodontal harm, and mutagenic potential. The ADA's Council on Dental Therapeutics has stated that "These products may be safe and effective, but the Council has not been provided with supporting data by the distributors." *None* of the commercially available polishing or whitening products is currently recommended by the Council on Dental Therapeutics.[28]

MOUTH RINSES

Freshening bad breath has been the traditional purpose of mouth rinses. The 1992 market for such products is estimated at $635 million, with 3% anticipated annual growth. In addition to the traditional cosmetic use, therapeutic mouth rinses are now available.

The active ingredients of most mouth rinses include quaternary ammonium compounds, boric and benzoic acids, and phenolic compounds. As with dentifrices, commercial sales of a rinse are closely related to taste, color, smell, and the pleasant sensation that follows use. The pleasant sensation is often enhanced by the addition of *astringents*. Commonly used astringents are alum, zinc stearate, zinc citrate, and acetic or citric acids. Zinc sulfate has been added to mouth rinses as an antiplaque ingredient.

Alcohol in the mouth rinse is used as a solvent, a taste enhancer, and an agent providing an aftertaste. The alcohol content of commercial rinses, ranging from zero to 27%, constitutes a *danger for children*, especially those from 2 to 3 years of age. According to the National Poison Center Network, 5 to 10 oz of a mouth rinse containing alcohol can be lethal for a child weighing 26 lb. Between 1987 and 1991, the nation's poison control centers logged more than 10,000 reports of children younger than 6 years old drinking mouth rinses containing alcohol; 3 died and another 40 children had life-threatening conditions or suffered permanent injuries.[29] The American Academy of Pediatrics has recommended that OTC liquid preparations be limited to 5% ethanol, that safety closures be required, and that the packaged volume be kept to a "reasonable minimum to prevent the potential for lethal ingestion."[30]

The Council on Dental Therapeutics of the ADA *requires* child-resistant caps on all alcohol-containing mouth rinses that bear the ADA Seal of Acceptance.[29] The council also requires manufacturers of ADA-accepted mouth rinses that contain more than 5% alcohol to include the following statement on the label: "Warning: Keep out of reach of children. Do not swallow. Contains alcohol. Use only as directed." The attorneys general of 29 states have petitioned the U.S. Consumer Products Safety Commission to require child safety caps on bottles of mouth wash that contain more than 5% alcohol.

Research from the National Cancer Institute has linked alcohol and mouth wash to *mouth and throat cancers*.[31] After taking into account participants' smoking and drinking habits, it was found that cancer patients were more likely than the control group to have rinsed regularly with a high-alcohol (25% or more) mouth wash. The researchers concluded that alcohol may or may not cause cancer in and of itself but may promote the disease by dissolving and dispersing other cancer-causing substances within the mouth and throat. In response to these and other studies, several *alcohol-free* mouth rinses (eg, Choice) have been introduced on the market.

For the dental professional, it may be important for patients to use a mouth rinse prior to aerosol-generating procedures. Unless an effective dry-field technique is used, the bacterial aerosol generated by a high-speed turbine in a 30-second period is roughly *equivalent* to the patient sneezing in the dentist's face.[32] A study by Wyler and coworkers[33] found that even a preliminary water rinse temporarily reduced the bacterial aerosol population by 61%, brushing alone by 85%, and an antibacterial mouth rinse by 97%. Recently, Fine[34] and coworkers, using a simulated office visit model, showed that preprocedural use of an antimicrobial mouth rinse (Listerine) resulted in a 93.6% reduction in the number of viable bacteria in a dental aerosol produced by ultrasonic scaling. The effect of this reduction on actual disease transmission has not been determined.[35]

Cosmetic Mouth Rinses

Alcohol All 3

Halitosis. Oral malodor has been a neglected research area. Indeed, the first scientific symposium on halitosis research was not held until 1991. Further research and education is needed in this important area because many practicing dental professionals still believe that bad breath usually comes from the stomach. Identifying the cause of halitosis and developing an appropriate treatment plan can be difficult.[36] Published studies by Spouge[37] and by Tonzetich[38] have demonstrated that oral malodor usually derives from the mouth itself and may be reduced following oral hygiene.[38] To motivate improvement in oral hygiene, dental professionals should advise patients that bad breath may result from microbial putrefaction within the mouth. Rosenberg[39] notes, "bad breath is a cause of concern, embarrassment, and frustration on the part of the general public. Oral malodor, whether real or perceived, can lead to social isolation, divorce proceedings, and even 'contemplation of suicide'." A body of science currently exists to permit the quantitative assessment of bad breath, which should be able to verify product claims for treating this important sign of disease.

Chlorhexidine

One prescription plaque control rinse, Peridex, has been approved by the FDA and the ADA as effective for the control of dental plaque and gingivitis. It is manufactured by the Procter and Gamble Company and contains 0.12% chlorhexidine. Directions call for a twice daily, 30-second rinse with 1 oz of the solution. A second chlorhexidine product, Perio Guard, has recently

been marketed by Colgate but has not yet received the ADA seal.

Chlorhexidine has proved one of the most effective antiplaque agents to date.[40] Chlorhexidine is a cationic compound that binds to the hydroxyapatite of tooth enamel, to the pellicle, to plaque bacteria, to the extracellular polysaccharide of the plaque,[41] and especially to the mucous membrane.[42] The chlorhexidine adsorbed to the hydroxyapatite is believed to inhibit bacterial colonization.[43] After binding, the agent is slowly released in active form over *12 to 24 hours*.[44] This ability of the oral tissues to adsorb an active agent and to permit its slow release in active form over a prolonged period is known as *substantivity*. As the substantivity of an antiplaque agent decreases, the frequency of use needs to be increased.

Chlorhexidine has not proved beneficial as the sole method of treating periodontitis with deep pockets. Following root planning, prophylaxis, or periodontal surgery, chlorhexidine may be effective in helping to control inflammation and subgingival plaque.[45]

In some countries, such as the United States, chlorhexidine products are available only by prescription. In others, such as the United Kingdom, it is available over the counter. Although chlorhexidine is quite effective, it is not active against all relevant anaerobes. A high minimal concentration is necessary for efficacy. Some side effects are associated with its use, of which *stain* is the most common. Occasionally altered taste sensation is reported.[46,47] Increased calculus formation,[48] superficial desquamation of tissue, and hypersensitivity have also been noted.[49,50] Chlorhexidine is inactivated by most dentifrice surfactants and, therefore, *should not be used immediately before or after regular tooth brushing*. For this reason, it is not included in dentifrices.

Although chlorhexidine is more effective than any other current antiplaque agent and has a definite role in preventive and control dental procedures, it is *not* a "magic bullet." Its side effects and inadequate activity range somewhat limit its use.

Listerine

Listerine antiseptic is the first OTC antiplaque and antigingivitis mouth rinse to be approved by the ADA.[51] Patients are recommended to rinse twice daily with 20 mL of Listerine for 30 seconds, in addition to their usual oral hygiene regimen. Listerine has been used as a mouth rinse for more than 110 years. The active ingredients are thymol, menthol, eucalyptol, and methyl salicylate. The original formula contained 26.9% alcohol. A flavor variation of the product, Cool Mint Listerine Antiseptic, which also has received the ADA seal, contains 21.6% alcohol. Microorganisms *do not develop a resistance* to the antibacterial effects of essential oils, such as clove oil (eugenol) and thyme oil (thymol).[52] Two generic versions of original Listerine have also been granted the ADA seal and are marketed under numerous trade names.[27]

In long-term clinical trials, Listerine has been shown to reduce both plaque accumulation and severity of gingivitis by up to 34%.[53] Microbial sampling of plaque in these trials has demonstrated no undesirable shifts in the composition of the microbial flora. As with chlorhexidine, rinsing with Listerine per se is unlikely to be effective in treating periodontitis because the solution does not reach the depths of the periodontal pockets. Irrigation studies, using irrigator tips designed to deliver solutions subgingivally, suggest that Listerine and Peridex may have some value as adjuncts to mechanical therapy.

Xerostomia Mouth Rinses

Many people experience dry mouth (*xerostomia*) traceable to several possible causes, such as damage to the salivary glands following radiation therapy for head and neck cancer; Sjögren's syndrome; and use of tranquilizing drugs, especially the tricyclic antidepressants. In such cases the mucous membrane is continually dry and uncomfortable. To ameliorate the dryness, artificial salivas have been developed, which are used ad libitum by the patient to moisten the mucous membrane.

Because xerostomia is correlated with an *increased caries incidence*, the rinses usually contain *fluoride* as well as chemical compounds in concentrations that closely parallel those of saliva. The rinses that contain fluoride may, in reality, be remineralizing solutions. Several artificial salivas have been accepted by the ADA, among which are Glandosane, Moi-Stir, Salivart, and Xero-Lube.[27]

Question 4. Which of the following statements, if any, are correct?

A. Sensodyne F was the first dentifrice approved by the ADA as containing active agents that could help relieve *two* dental problems with one brushing.

B. The ADA has awarded its Seal of Acceptance to a whitener containing carbamide peroxide.

C. The agent in cosmetic mouth rinses that poses the greatest danger to 2-to-4-year-old children is *alcohol*.

D. Chlorhexidine mouth rinses are most effective when used immediately after brushing.

E. Tricyclic antidepressants often cause a xerostomia, which in turn is a factor in cariogenesis.

SUMMARY

Both dentifrices and mouth rinses can be categorized as either *cosmetic* or *therapeutic*. Cosmetic products have traditionally been used to remove debris, provide a pleasant "mouth feel" and temporarily reduce halitosis. To improve on their marketability, flavors and colors have been added to dentifrices and mouth rinses. Recently, other ingredients have also been added to depress temporarily the oral bacterial population or to prevent or moderate some disease process in the mouth. In 1960, Crest toothpaste with stannous fluoride as an active anticaries ingredient was introduced, and the term *therapeutic dentifrice* became a part of the dental lexicon. At about the same time mouth rinses with added fluoride ushered in the *therapeutic mouth rinse* era. Soon, the widespread use of therapeutic fluoride dentifrices and mouth rinses were helping to reduce the worldwide prevalence of dental decay. Other agents are now being used to target other oral health problems. Toothpastes containing potassium nitrate, strontium chloride, and sodium citrate have antihypersensitivity properties; other toothpastes with tetrasodium phosphate and disodium dihydrogen pyrophosphate retard the formation of calculus. Chlorhexidine is a highly effective antiplaque, antigingivitis agent. Listerine, which has been popular for over a century, has demonstrated the same properties. Thus, the self-use of dentifrices and mouth rinses is proving to be an important preventive dentistry measure.

Although these new items have great potential for improving oral health because they are so extensively available, there is also the possible danger of exposing vast populations to known and as yet unknown carcinogens, teratogens, or mutagens. This concern prompted the government, through the Food and Drug Administration, to develop rigid guidelines for testing the safety and efficacy of products *prior* to their introduction on the market. Part of the function of the regulatory process, is to differentiate between products whose potential risks are sufficiently low as to be sold over the counter and those whose possible hazards justify restriction to prescription use.

ANSWERS AND EXPLANATIONS

1. C, D
   A—incorrect. The ADA has recognized both mouth rinses; the FDA has recognized only chlorhexidine.
   B—incorrect. Only the FDA decisions have the force of law.
   E—incorrect. The award of the Seal of Acceptance is a *voluntary* relationship between the manufacturer and the ADA after ensuring safety and efficacy of a product.
2. A, B, D, E
   C—incorrect. The V-shaped notch is just below the CE junction and in the softer cementum.
3. B, C, D
   A—incorrect. They are compatible.
   E—incorrect. The toothpaste does have the Seal of Acceptance, but it was bestowed for the toothpaste's anticaries action, not for its anticalculus properties; tartar accumulation is considered a cosmetic problem, not a disease.
4. A, C, E
   B—incorrect. The ADA has *not* approved *any* whitening preparations.
   D—incorrect. The use of the two should be separated in time.

SELF-EVALUATION QUESTIONS

1. The key government organization regulating the marketing of new dental products is the ___FDA___ (name of agency).
2. For an approved over-the-counter (OTC) product found safe and effective by the ADA, a Seal of ___Approval___ is granted.

3. Up to _____ 5 % _____ % of a toothpaste is composed of the therapeutic agent.

4. The detergent that replaced soap in dentifrices is _Sod. Laural Sulphate (SLS)_.

5. The abrasive often used in baking soda dentifrices is _hydrated silica_.

6. For safety purposes, an OTC dentifrice can contain no more than _120_ mg of fluoride.

7. Both Listerine and chlorhexidine have _Substantivity_, meaning that they can be adsorbed onto the target tissues, and gradually release the active therapeutic agent in active form.

8. Triclosan is an (anticaries) (antigingivitis) agent.

9. The toothpaste _Sensodyne-F_ has ingredients that provide antihypersensitivity and anticaries benefits at the same brushing.

10. The agent in tooth whiteners that causes the whitening is _Oxygen_ Hydrogen peroxide (Carbamid)

11. The alcohol in mouth washes has been linked to an increased risk of cancer of the _mouth_ and _throat_ (sites).

12. Foul-smelling breath is termed _Halitosis_.

13. The ingredients in Listerine that provide the antibacterial effects are the _essential_ oils. (clove(eugenol) thyme (thymol))

14. Two (of several) conditions that cause xerostomia are _H & N Rad'n therapy_ and _Antidepress. Drugs_.

REFERENCES

1. Trummel C. Regulation of oral chemotherapeutics in the United States. *J Dent Res* 1994; 73:704–708.

2. Department of Health, Education, and Welfare, Food and Drug Administration. Establishment of a monograph on anticaries drug product for over-the-counter human use; proposed rulemaking. *Federal Register*. March 28, 1980. Part IV.

3. Over-the-counter dental and oral health care drug products for antiplaque use; safety and efficacy review. *Federal Register*. September 9, 1990; 55:38560–38562.

4. American Dental Association, Council on Dental Therapeutics. Guidelines for acceptance of chemotherapeutic products for the control of supragingival dental plaque and gingivitis. *J Am Dent Assoc*. 1986; 112:529–532.

5. Fischman S. Hare's teeth to fluorides, historical aspects of dentifrice use. In Embery G, Rolla G, eds. *Clinical and Biological Aspects of Dentifrices*. Oxford, Oxford Univ Press; 1992; 1–7.

6. Hefferren J J. A laboratory method for the laboratory assessment of dentifrice abrasivity. *J Dent Res*. 1976; 55:563–573.

7. Adams D, Addy M, Absi E. Abrasive and chemical effects of dentifrices. In Embery G, Rolla G, eds. *Clinical and Biological Aspects of Dentifrices*. Oxford, Oxford Univ Press; 1992:345–355.

8. Kitchen PC, Robinson HBG. How abrasive need a dentifrice be? *J Dent Res*. 1948; 27:501–506.

9. Barkvoll P. Considerations concerning the sodium lauryl sulphate content of dentifrices. In Embery G, Rolla G, eds. *Clinical and Biological Aspects of Dentifrices*. Oxford, Oxford Univ Press; 1992: 171–180.

10. Fischman S, Truelove R, Hart R, et al. The laboratory and clinical safety evaluation of a dentifrice containing hydrogen peroxide and baking soda. *J Clin Dent*. 1992; 3:104–110.

11. Marshall M, Kuhn J, Fischman S, et al. Carcinogenicity bioassay of a H_2O_2 containing dentifrice. *J Dent Res*. 1992; 71:195.

12. Fischman S, Kugel G, Truelove R, et al. The motivational benefits of a dentifrice containing baking soda and hydrogen peroxide. *J Clin Dent*. 1992; 3:88–92.

13. American Dental Association. Council on Dental Therapeutics. American dental reclassification of Crest toothpaste. *J Am Dent Assoc*. 1964; 69:195–196.

14. American Dental Association. Clinical uses

of fluorides: a state-of-the-art conference on the uses of fluorides in clinical dentistry. *J Am Dent Assoc.* 1984; 109:472–474.

15. Svatun B. The effect of toothbrushing with a stannous fluoride/stannous pyrophosphate dentifrice on dental plaque and gingivitis-six months results. *J Dent Res.* 1983; 62:686. Abstract.

16. Bay I, Rolla G. Plaque inhibition and improved gingival condition by use of a stannous fluoride toothpaste. *Scand J Dent Res.* 1980; 88:313–315.

17. Tinanoff N, Manwell M, Zameek R, et al. Clinical and microbiological effects of daily brushing with either NaF or SnF$_2$ gels in subjects with fixed or removable prostheses. *J Clin Periodontol.* 1989; 16:284–290.

18. DeSalva S, King B, and Lin Y. Triclosan: A safety profile. *Am J Dent.* 1989; 2:185–196.

19. Volpe A, Petrone M, DeVizio W, et al. A review of plaque, gingivitis, calculus, and caries clinical efficacy studies with a dentifrice containing Triclosan and PVM/MA copolymer. *J Clin Dent.* 1993; 4:31–41.

20. Stephen K, Saxton C, Jones C-L, et al. Control of gingivitis and calculus by a dentifrice containing a zinc salt and Triclosan. *J Periodontol.* 1990; 61:674–679.

21. Svatun B, Saxton C, Rolla G. Six month study of a dentifrice containing zinc citrate and Triclosan on plaque, gingival health and calculus. *Scand J Dent Res.* 1990; 98:301–304.

22. Fischman S. Self-care: Practical periodontal care in today's practice. *Int Dent J.* 1993; 43:179–183.

23. American Dental Association. Council on Dental Therapeutics. *Accepted Dental Therapeutics.* 38th ed. Chicago, Ill: American Dental Association; 1979: 345–346.

24. Zacherl WA, Pfeiffer HJ, Swancar JR. The effect of soluble pyrophosphates on dental calculus in adults. *J Am Dent Assoc.* 1985; 110:737–738.

25. Stephen K, Creanor S, Russell J, et al. A three-year oral health dose-response study of sodium monofluorophosphate dentifrices with and without zinc citrate: Anti-caries

results. *Community Dent Oral Epidemiol.* 1988; 16:321–325.

26. Rolla B, Saxegaard E. Critical evaluation of the composition and use of topical fluorides, with emphasis on the role of calcium fluoride. *J Dent Res.* 1990; 60:780–785.

27. American Dental Association. Council on Dental Therapeutics. *Clinical Products in Dentistry—A Desktop Reference.* Chicago, Ill. 1993.

28. Berry J. What About whiteners? *J Am Dent Assoc.* 1990; 121:223–225.

29. American Dental Association. CDT acts on mouthrinses. *J Am Dent Assoc.* 1993; 124:26.

30. American Academy of Pediatrics, Committee on Drugs. Ethanol in liquid preparations intended for children. *Pediatrics.* 1984; 73:405.

31. Winn D, Blot W, McLaughlin J, et al. Mouthwash use and oral conditions in the risk of oral and pharyngeal cancer. *Cancer Res.* 1991; 51:3044–3047.

32. Miller RL, Micik RE. Air pollution and its control in the dental office. *Dent Clin North Am.* 1978; 22:453–476.

33. Wyler D, Miller R, Micik R. Efficacy of self-administered preoperative oral hygiene procedures in reducing the concentration of bacteria in aerosols generated during dental procedures. *J Dent Res.* 1990; 50:509.

34. Fine D, Yip J, Furgang D, et al. Reducing bacteria in dental aerosols: Pre-procedural use of an antiseptic mouthrinse. *J Am Dent Assoc.* 1993; 124:56–58.

35. Molinari J, Molinari G. Is mouthrinsing before dental procedures worthwhile? *J Am Dent Assoc.* 1992; 123:75–80.

36. McDowell J, Kassebaum D. Diagnosing and treating halitosis. *J Am Dent Assoc.* 1993; 124:55–64.

37. Spouge J. Halitosis. A review of its causes and treatment. *Dent Pract Dent Rec.* 1964; 14:307–317.

38. Tonzetich J. Production and origin of oral malodor, a review of mechanisms and methods of analysis. *J Periodontol.* 1977; 48:13–20.

39. Rosenberg M. Halitosis—The need for further research and education. *J Dent Res.* 1992; 71:424.

40. Addy M. Chlorhexidine compared with other locally delivered antimicrobials. A short review. *J Clin Periodontol.* 1986; 13:957–964.

41. Turesky S, Warner V, Lin PS, et al. Prolongation of antibacterial activity of chlorhexidine adsorbed to teeth. *J Periodontol.* 1977; 48:646–649.

42. Rolla G, Löe H, Schiott CR. The affinity of chlorhexidine for hydroxyapatite and salivary mucins. *J Periodont Res.* 1970; 5:90–95.

43. Yankell S, Moreno OM, Saffir AJ, et al. Effects of chlorhexidine and four antimicrobial compounds on plaque gingivitis and staining in beagle dogs. *J Dent Res.* 1982; 61:1089–1093.

44. Axelsson P, Lindhe J. Efficacy of mouthrinses in inhibiting dental plaque and gingivitis in man. *J Clin Periodontol.* 1987; 14: 205–212.

45. Wieder SG, Newman HN, Strahan JD. Stannous fluoride and subgingival chlorhexidine irrigation in the control of plaque and chronic periodontitis. *J Clin Periodont.* 1983; 10:172–181.

46. Eriksen H, Gjermo P. Incidence of stained tooth surfaces in students using chlorhexidine-containing dentifrices. *Scand J Dent Res.* 1973; 81:533–537.

47. Flotra L, Gjermo G, Rølla G, et al. Side effects of chlorhexidine mouth washes. *Scand J Dent Res.* 1971; 79:119–125.

48. Löe H, Mandell M, Derry A, et al. The effect of mouthrinses and topical application of chlorhexidine on calculus formation in man. *J Periodontol Res.* 1971; 6:312–314.

49. Moghadam B, Drisko C, Gier R. Chlorhexidine mouthwash-induced fixed drug eruption. *Oral Surg.* 1991; 71:431–434.

50. Skoglund L, Holst E. Desquamative mucosal reactions due to chlorhexidine gluconate. *Int J Oral Surg.* 1982; 11:380–382.

51. American Dental Association. Council on Dental Therapeutics accepts Listerine. *J Am Dent Assoc.* 1988; 117:515–517.

52. Meeker HG, Linke HAB. The antibacterial action of eugenol, thyme oil, and related essential oils used in dentistry. *Comp Cont Educ Dent.* 1988; 9:32–40.

53. Menaker L, Weatherford TW, Pitts G, et al. The effects of Listerine antiseptic on dental plaque. *Ala J Med Sci.* 1979; 16:71–77.

APPENDICES OF CURRENTLY AVAILABLE DENTIFRICES AND WHITENERS

APPENDIX 6–1. BAKING SODA DENTIFRICE PRODUCTS

Product	Supplier	Ingredients	
		Fluoride	Abrasive
Aim (with baking soda)	Chesebrough-Pond's	MFP	Hydrated silica
Arm & Hammer paste	Arm & Hammer	NaF	Sodium bicarbonate
Arm & Hammer gel	Arm & Hammer	NaF	Sodium bicarbonate
Close Up with baking soda	Chesebrough-Pond's	NaF	Hydrated silica
Colgate baking soda	Colgate-Palmolive	NaF	Hydrated silica
Crest baking soda	Procter & Gamble	NaF	Hydrated silica
Mentadent	Chesebrough-Pond's	NaF	Hydrated silica
Pepsodent baking soda	Chesebrough-Pond's	NaF	Hydrated silica

APPENDIX 6–2. TARTAR CONTROL DENTIFRICE PRODUCTS

Product	Supplier	Fluoride	Abrasive	Active Agent
Aim	Chesebrough–Pond's	MFP	Hydrated silica	Zinc citrate trihydrate
Aquafresh	SmithKline Beechman	NaF	Hydrated silica	Tetrapotassium pyrophosphate; tetrasodium pyrophosphate
Arm & Hammer	Arm & Hammer	NaF	Sodium bicarbonate	Sodium pyrophosphate
Arm & Hammer gel	Arm & Hammer	NaF	Sodium bicarbonate and hydrated silica	Sodium pyrophosphate
Colgate tartar control gel	Colgate–Palmolive	NaF	Hydrated silica	Tetrasodium pyrophosphate and PVM/MA copolymer
Close-Up antitartar	Chesebrough–Pond's	MFP	Hydrated silica	Zinc citrate trihydrate
Crest paste & gel	Procter & Gamble	NaF	Hydrated silica	Tetrapotassium pyrophosphate; bisodium pyrophosphate tetrasodium pyrophosphate

APPENDIX 6–3. ANTIHYPERSENSITIVITY DENTIFRICES*

Product	Supplier	Active Agent (s)
Denquel	Procter & Gamble	Potassium nitrate
Protect gel	John Butler	Sodium citrate pluorionic gel
Sensodyne-SC	Block Drug	Strontium chloride hexahydrate
Sensodyne with fluoride	Block Drug	MFP, potassium nitrate

*With ADA seal (Accepted Therapeutic Products, January, 1993).

APPENDIX 6–4. STAIN REMOVAL–WHITENER PRODUCTS*

Product	Supplier	Active Agent(s)
Caffree	Block Drug	MFP; diatomaceous earth; aluminum silicate
Pearl Drops	Carter Wallace	MFP; hydrated silica; calcium pyrophosphate; dicalcium pyrophosphate
Plus White	CCA Industries	MFP; polishers; hydrated silica
Rembrandt	Den-Mat	MFP; dicalcium phosphate dihydrate; alumina; Papain; sodium citrate
Topol Smokers	Topol	MFP; hydrated silica; zirconium silicate
Ultrabrite	Colgate-Palmolive	MFP; hydrated silica

* Without peroxide.

APPENDIX 6–5. TOOTH WHITENER PRODUCTS*

Product	Supplier	Active Agent(s)
Dazzle	US Buyers Network	Citric acid; hydrogen peroxide; hydrated silica
Doctor's Tooth Whitener	Dental Concepts	Citric acid; hydrogen peroxide; hydrated silica
Instant White	Howe Chemical Labs	Citric acid; hydrogen peroxide; hydrated silica
Plus + White (one step action)	CCA Industries	Hydrogen peroxide
Plus + White	CCA Industries	Citric acid; hydrogen peroxide; hydrated silica
Stay-white	Dental Concepts	Hydrogen peroxide

* With peroxide.

Chapter 7

Personal Oral Hygiene: Auxiliary Measures to Complement Toothbrushing

Maureen C. Rounds
Terri S. I. Tilliss

Objectives

At the end of this chapter it will be possible to

1. State the reasons that supplemental oral hygiene care is needed to complement toothbrushing.
2. Identify factors, in addition to oral conditions, that influence selection of supplemental oral hygiene devices and techniques.
3. List the objectives for the use of supplemental oral hygiene devices.
4. State the purposes, indications, contraindications, techniques, advantages, and limitations of the following oral hygiene devices:
   a. Dental floss
   b. Dental floss holder
   c. Dental floss threader
   d. Knitting yarn
   e. Pipe cleaner
   f. Gauze strip
   g. Interdental tip stimulator
   h. Wedge stimulator
   i. Toothpick
   j. Toothpick holder
   k. Interdental brush
   l. Tongue cleaner
5. Describe the purpose and technique for the use of mouth rinses and oral irrigators.
6. Describe proper oral hygiene care for dental implants.
7. Describe proper oral hygiene care for partial and full dentures.

Introduction

Auxiliary plaque control measures are necessary to *complement* toothbrushing. Appropriately performed thorough toothbrushing removes plaque accumulations on the facial and lingual aspects of the clinical crowns and exposed roots of the teeth. Toothbrushing is effective in removing plaque from shallow, well-coalesced, occlusal pits and fissures and is marginally effective when deep, narrow, occlusal pits and fissures are present. By adhering to specific sulcular toothbrushing techniques, plaque can be effectively removed from the gingival sulcus. Additionally, the tongue, palate, and buccal mucosa can be gently brushed to remove plaque. The least accessible sites for toothbrush removal of plaque accumulations are the *interproximal tooth surfaces*, which are protected by the interdental papillae, and deep *gingival sulcus,* or *pocket, areas*. The inflammatory and caries processes may begin or continue in these protected areas unless additional oral hygiene measures are performed.

Therefore, for optimal plaque control, even in an apparently healthy oral environment, toothbrushing should be supplemented with additional means of interdental cleaning to prevent disease.[1] When the dentition or periodontal conditions are altered, different supplemental oral hygiene devices may be warranted. The oral hygiene measures required depend on various criteria, such as the size of the interdental spaces, tooth position and morphology, periodontal conditions, and presence of dental prostheses.

A wide variety of devices may be used to accomplish supplemental oral hygiene care. Dental floss and tape are the most commonly used interproximal cleaning aids. Others include yarn, wood wedges, toothpicks, plastic and rubber stimulator tips, floss holders, tongue cleaners, and various types of interproximal brushes. Use of all oral hygiene devices should be accomplished in a *systematic fashion and follow prescribed techniques*.

SUPPLEMENTAL ORAL HYGIENE CARE

The primary purpose of oral hygiene practice is to prevent dental disease by *reducing plaque accumulation* and by *promoting soft tissue circulation*. To determine which supplemental oral hygiene practices are needed, assessment data from the dental and periodontal examinations must be considered.

Appropriate supplemental oral hygiene devices are then selected according to the dictates of the patient's oral condition. Adequate instruction in the use of supplemental devices must be provided to the patient. Additionally, supervised practice sessions are important. After such instruction, success in plaque control ultimately rests with the *patient*. Principles of learning and motivation should be applied to encourage patient compliance.

DENTAL FLOSS

Effective use of dental floss accomplishes several objectives: It

1. Removes plaque and debris that adhere to the teeth; restorations; orthodontic appliances,[2] fixed prostheses and pontics;[3] gingiva in the interproximal embrasures;[4] and around implants[5–7]
2. Polishes the surfaces as it removes the debris

3. Massages the interdental papillae[8]
4. Aids in identifying the presence of subgingival calculus deposits, overhanging restorations, or interproximal carious lesions
5. Reduces gingival bleeding[9]
6. May be used as a vehicle for the application of polishing or chemotherapeutic agents to interproximal and subgingival areas.[10,11]

Dental floss can also promote the feeling of cleanliness sought by most patients. For plaque and debris removal, dental floss is most effective when the interdental papilla *fills* the embrasure space. When this is not the case, other oral hygiene devices may be more effective.

Although dental floss is thought to be a contemporary advancement in preventive dentistry, it was actually used for cleansing the interproximal surfaces in the early 1800s. Parmly, in 1819, recommended waxed silken thread for flossing the teeth. He wrote that "silken thread which, though simple, is the most important. It is to be passed through interstices of the teeth, between their necks and the arches of the gums, to dislodge that irritating matter which no brush can remove and which is the real source of disease."[12]

Prior to the advent of nylon, dental flosses were made from silk. During World War II, silk became unavailable, and synthetic materials were tried. In 1948, Bass was responsible for the research and development of the type of unwaxed floss currently in vogue.[13] He established the specifications for the type of floss and suggested that it should be a thin, nylon yarn strand made up of approximately 35 filaments loosely twisted along their long axis to form a stronger strand.

Not all interproximal contact areas, either anatomically or restoratively, are the same. Consequently, several types of floss, from thin, unwaxed varieties to thicker waxed tapes are available. Previous hypotheses about the superior effectiveness of unwaxed floss in removing plaque and concern for wax residue deposited on the tooth surface by waxed floss have been *rejected*. Clinical trials have shown no significant differences in cleansing ability between waxed and unwaxed floss.[1,14] Moreover, deposits have not been found on saliva-coated tooth surfaces cleaned with waxed floss.[15]

Unwaxed floss is frequently recommended because it is thinner and slips more easily through tight contact areas. Unwaxed floss may fray and tear, however, when crowded teeth, heavy calculus deposits, or defective and overhanging restorations are present. Floss breakage may frustrate the patient and discourage continued use. For these conditions, waxed or lightly waxed floss should be recommended. Another type of floss made of polytetrafluoroethylene (PTFE, also known as Goretex) is easy to insert and resists fraying.[16]

Waxed dental tape, unlike the round dental floss, is broad and flat, and may be effective in an interdental space without tight contact points. Some brands of dental floss and tape are colored and flavored. In addition to increased patient appeal, color provides a visual contrast to plaque and oral debris, thus enabling a patient to see what is being removed by flossing. Being able to see that flossing is removing debris can increase motivation to floss. One recent study indicated that patients preferred waxed over unwaxed floss and mint-flavored waxed floss over plain waxed floss.[17]

A floss variation, called Super Floss (Figs 7–1B, 7–2A), combines a stiff end with a section of unwaxed floss and an area of thicker, cylindrical, nylon meshwork. The stiff end of the Super Floss allows for threading under fixed bridges,[3,4] between

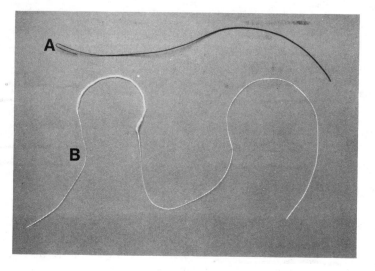

Figure 7–1. Floss variations. **A.** Nylon Postcare with stiff, hooked end. **B.** Super Floss with stiff straight end, cylindrical nylon meshwork, and unwaxed floss section.

orthodontic bands and wires, beneath tight contact areas, and through exposed furcations (Fig 7–3). Super Floss may be recommended for use in cleaning implant abutments[5,7] and areas with open contacts, wide embrasures, or where recession and bone loss permit access to furcations. Comparisons of the cleansing ability of Super Floss and other types of floss have yielded conflicting results.[18–21]

When recommending a type of floss, consider not only the specific oral conditions present, but also patient preference and ability.

Dental Flossing Methods

Two frequently used flossing methods are (1) the *spool* method and (2) the *circle, or loop,* method. Both facilitate control of the floss and ease of handling.

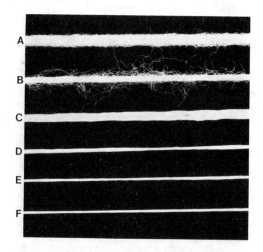

Figure 7–2. Variation of strands. **A.** Super Floss. **B.** Nylon yarn. **C.** Dental tape. **D.** Waxed floss. **E.** Bonded unwaxed floss. **F.** Unwaxed floss.

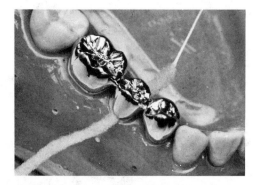

Figure 7–3. Super Floss. The stiffened section is used to thread between the teeth, under fixed bridgework and orthodontic appliances. The yarn-type section is used for cleaning under a bridge or an area where space permits. The unwaxed floss section (not shown) is used in the conventional manner.

The spool method is particularly suited for teenagers and adults who have acquired the level of neuromuscular coordination and mental maturity required to use floss correctly. The loop method is suited for children as well as adults with less nimble hands or physical limitations caused by conditions such as poor muscular coordination or arthritis. Until children develop adequate dexterity, flossing should be performed by an adult.

When using the spool method, a piece of floss approximately 18 in. long is taken from the dispenser. The bulk of the floss is lightly wound around the middle finger. Space should be left between wraps to avoid impairing circulation to the fingers (Fig 7–4A). The rest of the floss is similarly wound around the same finger of the opposite hand. This finger can wind, or "take up," the floss as it becomes soiled or frayed to permit access to an unused portion. The last three fingers are clenched and the hands are moved apart, pulling the floss taut, thus leaving the thumb and index finger of each hand free (Fig 7–4B). The floss is then secured with the index finger and thumb of each hand by grasping a section 3/4 to 1 in. long between the hands (Fig 7–4C).

When using the loop method, a piece of floss approximately 18 in. long is made into a circle and tied securely (Fig 7–5A). All fingers except the thumbs are placed within the loop (Fig 7–5B) so that the finger or thumb tips used to place the floss between the teeth are 3/4 to 1 in. apart. The floss is guided with the two index fingers for the mandibular teeth (Fig 7–5C) and with two thumbs or one thumb and one index finger for the maxillary teeth (Fig 7–5D). As teeth are flossed, the loop is rotated so that each proximal area receives an unused floss portion.

Whether using the spool or the loop method of flossing, the same basic proce-

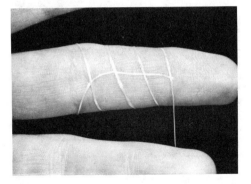

A

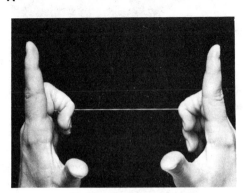

B

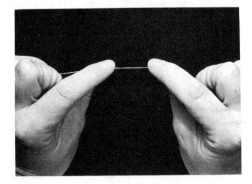

C

Figure 7–4. Spool method for dental flossing. **A.** Floss is lightly wound and spaced around the middle finger of each hand. **B.** The last three fingers are clenched, pulling the floss taut and leaving the index finger and thumb of each hand free. **C.** The floss is held with the index finger and thumb of each hand by grasping a section 3/4 to 1 in. long between the hands.

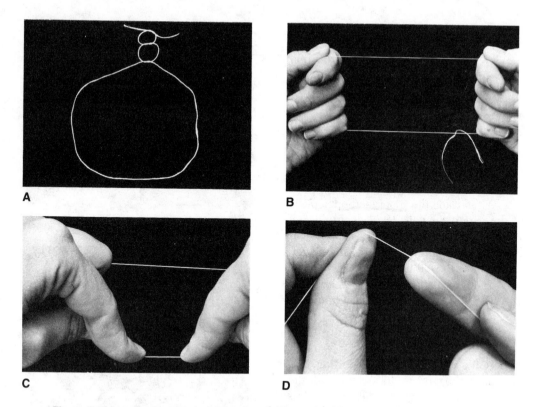

Figure 7–5. Loop method for dental flossing. **A.** The ends of floss are tied securely to form a loop. **B.** All fingers except the thumbs are placed within the loop for easy maneuverability. **C.** For the mandibular teeth, the floss is guided with the two index fingers. **D.** For the maxillary teeth, the floss is guided with two thumbs or one thumb and one index finger.

dures are followed. The thumb and index finger of each hand are used in various combinations to guide the floss between the teeth. To insert, the floss is *gently eased between the teeth* while sawing it back and forth at the contact point. This seesaw motion flattens the floss, making it possible to ease it through the contact point (Fig 7–6). The floss is seesawed gently to prevent snapping it through the contact point, thus avoiding trauma to the sulcular gingiva. Once past the contact point, the floss is adapted in turn to each interproximal surface by creating a C-shape. The floss is then directed apically into the sulcus and back to the contact area several times or until the

tooth surface is clean. The procedure is repeated on the adjacent tooth in the proximal area, again using care to prevent damage to the papilla while readapting to the adjacent tooth. A clean, unused portion should be used for *each* proximal area.

In general, flossing is best performed by adhering to the procedures in a progressive fashion, cleaning each tooth *in succession*, including the distal surface of the last tooth in each quadrant. The patient should be assisted with problem areas and encouraged to experiment with each method to achieve proficiency. Criteria for evaluation are based on the success of plaque removal and the safety of the patient's method.

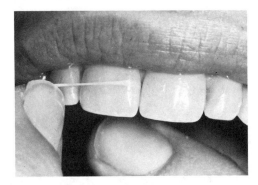

Figure 7–6. Note the flattening and widening action of unwaxed filaments as dental floss is eased past the contact point.

Plaque removal is easily evaluated using a disclosing solution to stain any remaining soft deposits. Evaluation of the safety of the patient's flossing method is a more complicated procedure. The clinician may observe the patient's flossing technique during a scheduled appointment but not during daily routine home care. Often an incorrect flossing technique can be detected through clinical observations of the gingiva. Signs that suggest a patient is not using dental floss correctly include cuts occurring primarily in the papilla and gingiva, and cervical wear on proximal root surfaces. If any of the preceding conditions occur, further instruction should be given until the patient has become adept at performing the technique. With instruction and practice, most motivated adult patients can master either the spool or loop method of flossing. In certain circumstances, the use of a floss holder, floss threader, or Super Floss may be more effective.

Dental Floss Holder

The floss holder is a device that eliminates the need for placing fingers in the mouth. It is recommended for individuals (1) with physical disabilities, (2) lacking manual dexterity, (3) with large hands or a limited opening to the mouth, (4) with a strong gag reflex, or (5) lacking motivation to floss. The floss holder may also be helpful when one person is assisting another in flossing.

The limited scientific data available comparing finger-manipulated flossing to the use of floss holders show *no differences* in effectiveness. Studies have found that when compared, a significant majority of individuals preferred the floss holder over finger-manipulated flossing.[22,23] It has been emphasized that effective initial education and reinforcement are necessary for proper use of the floss holder. The findings of these studies indicate that use of a floss holder aids in developing a flossing habit.

Floss holders usually consist of a yoke-like device with a 3/4 to 1 in. space between the two prongs of the yoke. The floss is secured *tightly* between the two prongs (Fig 7–7). The patient grasps the handle of the device to guide it during use. The width and length of the handle are important considerations when recommending the use of a floss holder to patients with limited gripping abilities.[24] Most floss holders require that floss be strung around various parts of the holder prior to each use. This assembly mechanism allows for quick rethreading of the floss whenever its working portion becomes soiled or begins to fray. Patients with limited manual agility may require a floss holder that contains a supply of floss in the handle. The floss is advanced by turning a knob, thus eliminating the need for constant rethreading (Fig 7–A, E, H). Strict attention should be given to achieving the desired floss tension when assembling the floss holder. To ensure *tautness*, the prongs can be forced together while securing the floss. The most persistent problems with the yokelike devices are the difficulties in maintaining tautness of the floss between the prongs and decreased ability to adapt the

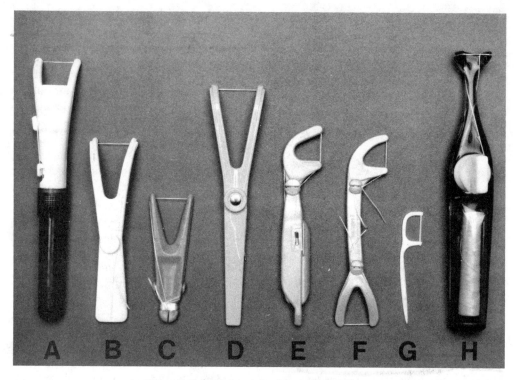

Figure 7–7. A–H. A variety of dental floss holders.

floss into a C shape around the proximal surface. No device should be recommended that does not allow for ease of threading, maintenance of proper tautness, or ease in manipulation by the user.

When using a holder, the floss is inserted interproximally, using the same technique used for finger-manipulated flossing. Once through the contact point, the floss and holder must be pushed distally to clean the mesial surface of a tooth or pulled mesially to clean the distal surface (Fig 7–8). This pulling or pushing motion creates a conformity to the tooth convexities, thus allowing the floss to slide apically into the sulcus. The floss is then activated in the same manner as with finger-manipulated flossing.

Dental Floss Threader

A floss threader is a needlelike device with an opening at one end through which the dental floss is threaded. The floss threader is used to carry the limp floss under an appliance, through an interdental embrasure, or between teeth whenever it cannot be inserted at the incisal edge and through the contact points. It is used to carry floss (1) through embrasure areas under defective contact points that are too tight for floss insertion, (2) between the proximal surface and gingiva of abutment teeth of fixed prostheses, (3) under pontics, (4) around orthodontic appliances, and (5) under splinting.

Different types of floss threaders are made from (1) a soft, thin, plastic loop (Fig 7–9A); (2) twisted wire (Fig 7–9B); and (3)

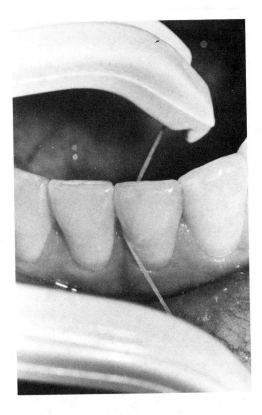

Figure 7–8. Dental floss holder. Insertion of dental floss between the mandibular anterior teeth while pushing the floss holder distally to clean the mesial surface.

plastic with a closed eye (Fig 7–9C). Selection of a floss threader should be determined by the patient's oral condition. The patient should be able to assemble and use it easily, with emphasis on effective plaque removal. A portion of an *18-in.* piece of floss is inserted through the eye of the floss threader, which is then inserted under the contact point or pontic if space permits (Fig 7–10A). Care should be taken not to cause trauma by forcing the point of the floss threader into the gingival tissues. For cleaning under a fixed bridge, the floss threader is pulled through completely from the facial to the lingual aspect until only the floss is against the abutment or pontic. The floss

may then be disengaged from the threader. The floss is adapted to one abutment tooth surface in the area of the embrasure (Fig 7–10B) and moved up and down to remove plaque from the proximal surface. The floss is then slid through the space between the pontic and the gingiva (Fig 7–10C) to the contact area of the opposite proximal surface (Fig 7–10D). Removal of the floss from between the abutment and pontic is accomplished by pulling it out from the facial aspect. For flossing a closed contact area, the threader is inserted under the contact and disengaged from the floss. The floss is removed by pulling it out from the facial aspect.

OTHER MATERIALS FOR INTERDENTAL CLEANING

Knitting Yarn

In areas where the interdental papillae have receded and the interdental embrasure is *wide open*, knitting yarn is often used for proximal cleaning. Several types have been suggested for dental use: (1) four-ply cotton, (2) two- or three-ply nylon, (3) three-ply rayon. Wool knitting yarn is not recommended because the wool fibers tend to burn and irritate the gingival tissues. White yarn is preferable to colored yarn, which contains dyes. A piece of yarn about 8 in. long is folded so that the yarn's width is doubled. It should be *moistened* before use. When access to the embrasure is limited, dental floss or a floss threader with a large threading eye may be used to insert the yarn into the embrasure. The floss threader is used as previously described. When dental floss is used to insert the yarn into the embrasure, about 8 in. of floss should be looped through and doubled. The double strand of floss is inserted through the contact point (Fig 7–11A); then the yarn is

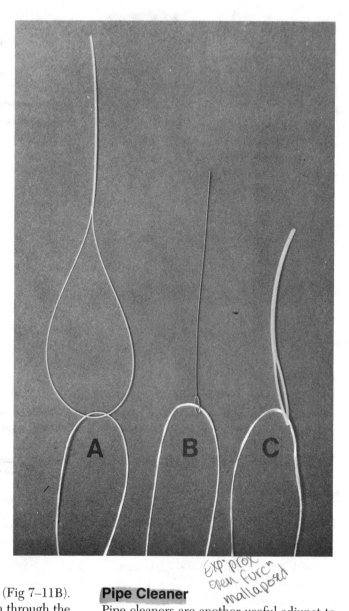

Figure 7–9. A–C. A variety of dental floss threaders.

drawn through the embrasure (Fig 7–11B). Once the yarn has been drawn through the embrasure, the technique is the same as for using regular dental floss. The double yarn is excellent for cleaning not only wide embrasure areas but also mesial and distal abutments, isolated teeth, teeth adjacent to edentulous areas, teeth separated by a diastema, and implant abutments.

Pipe Cleaner

Pipe cleaners are another useful adjunct to dental flossing for the removal of plaque and debris from (1) exposed proximal surfaces, (2) open furcation areas, and (3) malposed or separated teeth. A pipe cleaner is not recommended unless severe loss of tissue and bone has occurred. A pipe cleaner for oral use should have a soft covering with

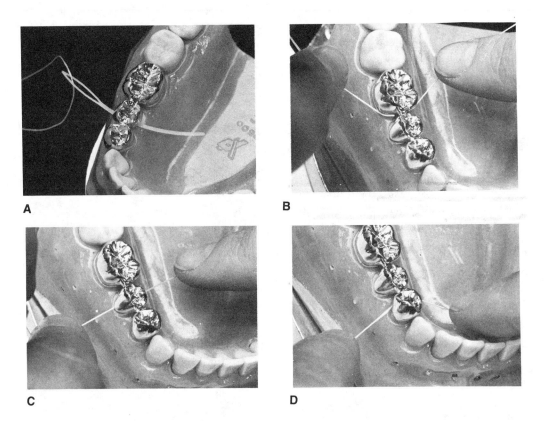

Figure 7–10. Use of a dental floss threader. **A.** Floss threader inserted under pontic. **B.** Floss adaption to mesial of abutment. **C.** Floss slid underneath pontic. **D.** Floss adaption to distal of abutment.

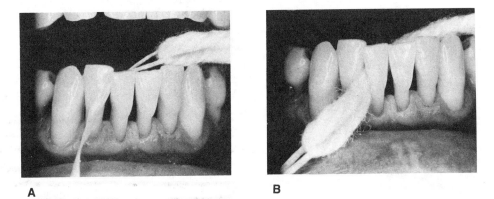

Figure 7–11. Use of knitting yarn in wide open embrasure. **A.** Yarn is looped through dental floss and inserted through the contact point. **B.** Yarn is drawn through the embrasure.

a minimum of exposed wire. Caution is advised because the sharp wire center can *scratch* the cementum or *traumatize* the gingival tissue. Once inserted, the pipe cleaner is moved in a buccolingual direction to clean proximal surfaces (Fig 7–12).

Gauze Strip

A gauze strip is an effective device for cleaning the proximal surfaces of teeth adjacent to edentulous areas, teeth that are widely spaced, and implant abutments. To prepare the strip, a 1-in. wide gauze bandage is cut into a 6-in. length and folded in half. The lengthwise edge of the gauze is positioned with the fold *toward the gingiva* (Fig 7–13). It is necessary to fold any loose ends inward to avoid gingival irritation. The gauze is adapted by wrapping it around the exposed proximal surface to the facial and lingual line angles of the tooth. A buccolingual "shoeshine" stroke is used to loosen and remove plaque and debris.

Question 1. Which of the following statements, if any, are correct?

A. Waxed dental floss is better for removing *interproximal* dental plaque than is unwaxed.

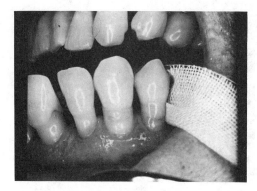

Figure 7–13. A 6-in. length of 1-in. gauze bandage folded in half with the folded edge adjacent to the gingiva for subsequent adaptation.

B. A major problem encountered with the dental floss holder is maintaining *tautness* of the floss.

C. The spool method of using interdental floss is the preferable technique for introducing children to flossing.

D. Flossing with a floss holder is easier *but not as effective* as flossing with the spool or loop methods.

E. In using a gauze strip for cleaning, the fold should be towards the gingival surface.

ADDITIONAL INTERDENTAL DEVICES

Interdental Tip Stimulator

The interdental stimulator consists of a conical, flexible rubber or plastic tip attached to a handle or to the end of a toothbrush (Fig 7–14). It can be used to remove plaque and debris from exposed furcation areas, open embrasures, and along the gingival margin. The tip is placed at a 90° angle to the long axis of the tooth and traced with moderate pressure along the gingival margin (Fig 7–15). In an open embrasure area the tip is moved in and out in a buccolingual direc-

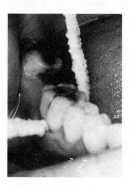

Figure 7–12. Use of pipe cleaner in area between roots where the furcation has been exposed.

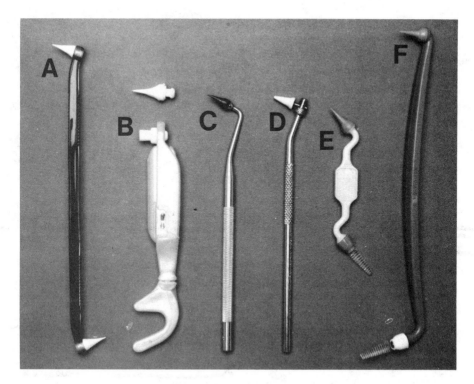

Figure 7–14. A–F. A variety of interdental tip stimulators.

tion. The use of a tip attached to an angled shank rather than a toothbrush handle may allow for greater ease of access and adaptation. To prevent damage to the soft tissues, patients should be *cautioned* against insertion of the tip subgingivally.

It has been suggested that the rubber tip may stimulate the tissue when used to massage the gingiva. The rubber tip is also recommended by some practitioners following surgery. No clinical data supports either practice.

Wedge Stimulator

Wedge stimulators are made of wood (usually balsa or birch) or plastic and are triangular in cross section (Fig 7–16). The wedge stimulator may be used for cleaning interdental areas where tooth surfaces are ex-

posed and interdental gingiva is missing. It is also used to massage the underlying interdental gingiva. The triangular design is meant to slide easily between teeth. The wedge is inserted interproximally from the buccal aspect with the flat surface of the base of the triangle resting on the gingiva. The tip of the wedge is angled coronally (Fig 7–17) and is moved in a buccolingual direction. If a wooden wedge is used, the pointed end can be softened in the mouth by moistening it with saliva. The wedge should be discarded if the wood becomes splayed. Splayed wood could force splinters into the gingiva. Plastic wedges can be thoroughly washed and reused.

Wedge stimulators do *not* completely remove plaque from the proximal surface of teeth, but they may reduce the amount of

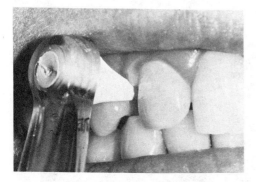

Figure 7–15. Use of interdental tip stimulator to remove plaque. The tip is placed at a 90° angle to the long axis of the tooth and traced along the gingival margin or moved in a buccolingual direction in an open embrasure area.

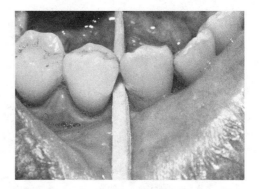

Figure 7–17. Wood wedge interdental stimulator. The base of the triangular wedge is inserted coronally into the embrasure to follow the contour of the interdental papilla. Without disengaging the wedge, it is moved in and out while applying a burnishing stroke to each side of the embrasure.

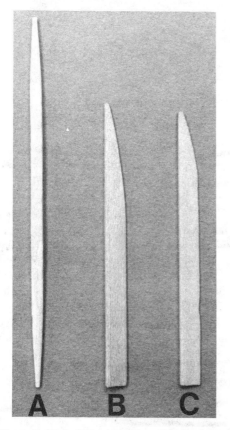

Figure 7–16. A–C. A variety of wedge stimulators.

accumulated plaque on these surfaces. In studies of oral hygiene and bleeding interdental gingiva, it was found that plaque removal with wooden interdental (wedge) cleaners was effective in reducing inflammation more in the coronal regions of the interdental pocket than in the apical regions.[25] Numerous studies have compared the effectiveness of various wood and plastic wedge stimulators.

Toothpicks

The toothpick may date back to the days of the caveman, who probably used sticks to pick out food from between the teeth.[26] Over the ages, the nobility and the affluent have used elaborate toothpick kits of metal, ivory, and carved wood; the less affluent have whittled sticks for the same purpose.

With the advent of the toothbrush, the toothpick began to lose its appeal as the prime means for oral hygiene. There is little research to indicate a definite role for the toothpick. Many people use a toothpick because it is available and because of peer acceptability. The toothpick can help to remove plaque left behind by toothbrushing.

Plaque removal is achieved by tracing the gingival margin around each tooth and in each interproximal area with moderate pressure. Interproximally, the toothpick is inserted and reinserted in a buccolingual direction to remove plaque and stimulate tissue.

Toothpick Holder

The toothpick holder is an instrument designed to increase effective application of the traditional toothpick by holding it securely at the proper angle. A variety of toothpick holders are available commercially (Fig 7–18). The toothpick is inserted into an adjustable, plastic, contraangled handle, with the excess wood end broken off by snapping the toothpick off in a downward direction. This leaves a stem to prevent the tip from falling out of the holder. The handle is angled acutely on one end to access lingual surfaces and obtusely on the other end to adapt to buccal surfaces. The use of a toothpick holder is indicated for (1) plaque removal along the gingival margin and within gingival sulci or periodontal pockets, (2) interdental cleaning of concave proximal surfaces (Fig 7–19), (3) cleaning of accessible furcation areas, (4) cleaning around orthodontic appliances and fixed prostheses, and (5) application of chemotherapeutic agents.

The toothpick may be moistened with saliva prior to use to soften the wood. It is applied at the gingival margin by placing the blunt tip perpendicular to the long axis of

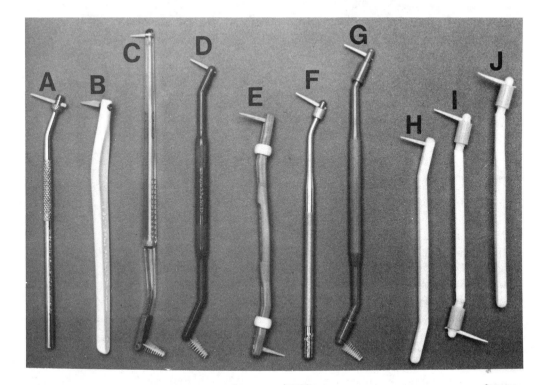

Figure 7–18. A–J. A variety of toothpick holders.

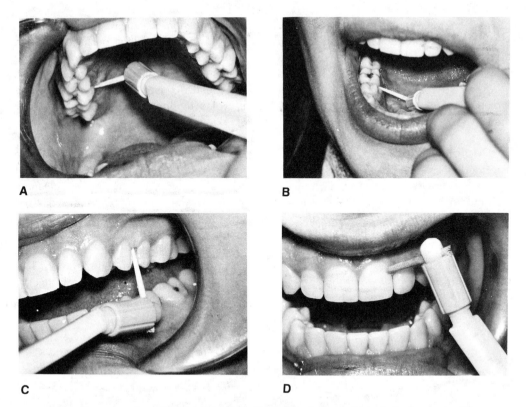

Figure 7–19. Use of a toothpick holder. **A, B**. Tip is placed perpendicular to the long axis of the tooth to clean along gingival margins. **C**. Tip is placed at less than a 45° angle on the tooth to clean along marginal gingiva. **D**. Frayed tip is used to burnish or brush the tooth surface. (*Courtesy of Marquis Dental Manufacturing Company, 15370 H. Smith Road, Aurora, CO, 80011.*)

the teeth. Care should be taken to *avoid* subgingival insertion or vigorous interproximal use because the gingiva or teeth could be damaged.

Interdental and End-Tuft Brushes

An interdental brush is a small, spiral, bristle brush (Fig 7–20) used (1) to clean spaces between teeth and around furcations (Fig 7–21B), orthodontic bands, and fixed prosthetic appliances with spaces that are large enough to easily receive the device; (2) to provide some stimulation to the gingival tissues, and (3) to apply chemotherapeutic agents. Interdental brushes may be preferable to dental floss in cleaning interdental

areas where the papilla is missing. The brushes are tapered or cylindrical in shape and are available in soft, medium, and hard textures. The core of the brush that holds the bristles is made of plastic, wire, or nylon-coated wire.

When determining the appropriate size of interdental brush, the diameter of the bristles should be slightly larger than the space to be cleaned. The brush is moistened, then inserted into the area at an angle approximating the normal gingival contour (Fig 7–22). An in-and-out motion is used to remove plaque and debris. Caution should be exercised to prevent damage to the tooth or soft tissue from the firm wire or plastic

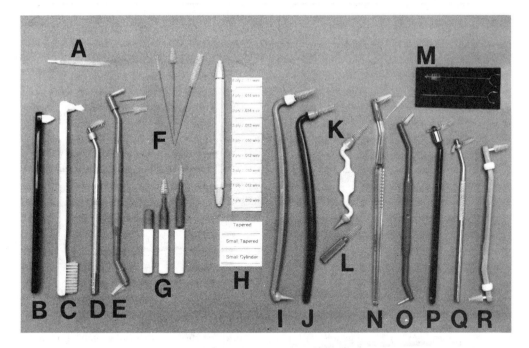

Figure 7–20. A variety of interdental brushes.

core. When used to clean implant abutments, extreme caution should be exercised to prevent scratching of the titanium surface.[27]

The end-tuft brush is most efficient for cleaning (1) mesial and distal surfaces of teeth adjacent to edentulous spaces, (2) furcations and fluted root surfaces (mesial of maxillary first premolars and mandibular first molars) that have been exposed due to gingival recession or periodontal surgery, (3) wide-open embrasures where papillae

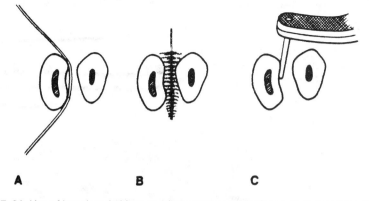

Figure 7–21. Use of interdental aids to reach concave tooth surfaces. **A.** Dental floss does not reach bottom of concavity. **B.** Interdental brush reaches both the concave and convex surfaces. **C.** A toothpick contacts the tooth surface at bottom of concavity.

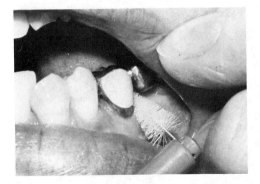

Figure 7–22. Interdental brush. Proxabrush used to remove plaque from around a fixed bridge by inserting the brush between the abutment tooth and pontic at an angle approximating the normal gingival contour.

have been lost and (4) around dental appliances, including implants. The end of the tuft is directed into the interproximal area by combining a rotating motion with intermittent pressure. The end-tuft brush has also been suggested for application of chemotherapeutic agents.

TONGUE CLEANER

Tongue cleaning and scraping have been practiced since antiquity.[28] Studies on tongue scraping have renewed interest in this auxiliary measure to complement toothbrushing.[29] The papillary structure of the tongue dorsum affords a large surface area favoring the accumulation of oral microorganisms and oral debris. The fungiform papillae do not extend as high as filiform papillae and therefore create elevations and depressions that may entrap debris and microorganisms. The tongue is therefore an excellent substratum for bacterial growth. The availability of oral debris from these sites *contributes to plaque formation* in other areas of the mouth. Reduction of this debris by mechanical tongue debridement can retard the initial rate of plaque formation, total plaque accumulation, and oral malodor. Currently available tongue cleaners are strips of flexible plastic or stainless steel that can be bent into an arc (Fig 7–23). A soft-bristled toothbrush can also be used, stroking in a posterior-to-anterior direction. The tongue cleaner is placed on the dorsal surface of the tongue as close to the base as possible and pulled forward, pressing lightly against the surface of the tongue (Fig 7–24). The tongue cleaner is particularly indicated for those who smoke or have tongues that are coated, deeply fissured, or have elongated papillae (hairy tongue).

RINSING

The use of a toothbrush and supplemental oral hygiene devices disperses and loosens food debris and plaque. The removal of food debris may be aided by vigorous rinsing of the mouth.

For maximum effectiveness, a technique should be adopted whereby fluid is forced through the interdental areas of the *clenched* teeth with as much pressure as possible, in order to loosen debris. Lip,

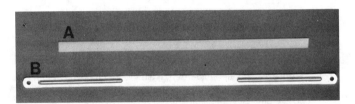

Figure 7–23. A and **B**. Tongue cleaners.

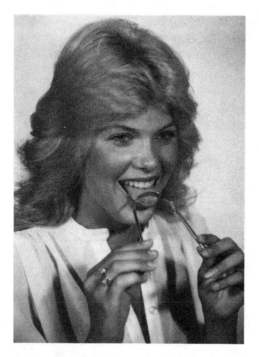

Figure 7–24. Stainless steel Lila tongue cleaner strip bent into an arc. (*Courtesy of Venk Enterprises, Inc, 6 Castle Creek Place, Shawnee, OK 74801.*)

tongue, and cheek action aids in forcing the fluid back and forth between the teeth prior to expectoration. Rinsing is also recommended after meals and snacks when toothbrushing and supplemental oral hygiene care may not be possible. Although rinsing does not remove attached plaque, it may *help* return the mouth to a neutral pH following the acid production that results from ingesting fermentable carbohydrates.

IRRIGATION DEVICES

Rinsing is a means of flushing the entire mouth; irrigation devices are a means of irrigating *specific* areas of the mouth. An irrigation device for home use provides a steady or pulsating stream of fluid (Fig 7–25). The pressure of the fluid flow can be regulated to a safe, yet effective level. In at least three situations use of an irrigating device is desirable: (1) to help remove accumulated debris from interdental areas where access is difficult; (2) to aid in the personal oral hygiene of individuals with orthodontic devices, complex restorations, crowns, and fixed bridges; and (3) where indicated, to help irrigate deeper gingival sulci.

Some disadvantages to the use of irrigating devices are (1) the motor-powered units are expensive, (2) patients who use an irrigating device often overestimate its effectiveness and reduce the time used for the more effective toothbrushing and flossing, (3) even more important, if an excessive water pressure is used, the irrigation fluid and air may be forced into the underlying tissues and thereby into the blood stream.[30,31] This possibility of a *bacteremia* is especially hazardous to those prediposed to *bacterial endocarditis*. Included in this high-risk group are patients with a history of endocarditis and those with rheumatic and congenital heart disease. Also at considerable risk are those who have had bone marrow transplants or surgery for placement of cardiac pacemakers, cardiovascular prostheses, prosthetic joint implants, and vascular grafts. Irrigation devices are also contraindicated for patients with acute necrotizing ulcerative gingivitis or a periodontal abscess.

The ADA Council on Dental Materials, Instruments and Equipment recommends that an oral irrigating device be used as an *adjunct* to toothbrushing and interdental plaque removal, that it be used at the lowest effective setting, and that the tip be in motion during use.[32] During irrigation procedures, the nozzle of the irrigator should be at a *right angle* to the long axis of the tooth. This provides circulation in the pockets,

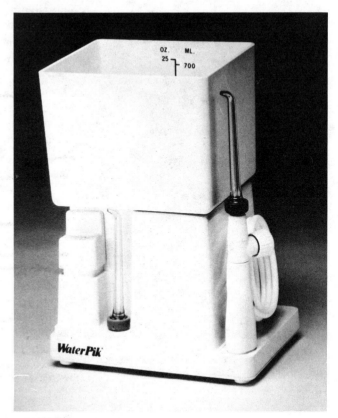

Figure 7–25. An irrigation device with detachable nozzles for individual family members. The detachable reservoir can be filled with either therapeutic or nontherapeutic irrigating solutions.

which both displaces and disrupts the bacteria of the unattached plaque yet does not force the bacteria into the surrounding tissues. In view of the mounting interest in irrigators, the ADA has developed guidelines for acceptance of these devices.[33]

Presently many irrigation devices are being used with active agents, such as chlorhexidine[34–36] sanguinarine,[37,38] and Listerine.[39] Water has also been shown to be effective.[40] For any agent to be useful, the irrigation fluids must be able to reach the target areas. In one study it appeared that their effectiveness was greatest in crevices from 0 to 2 mm, still obvious at 2 to 4 mm, and less effective in deeper pockets.[41] In another study in which pockets exceeded 7mm, deep, 100% penetration occurred only 3% to 6% of the time.[42] Yet another study, however,

showed that patients could irrigate to 80% of the depth of 6.9 to 7.8 mm pockets.[43] Use of a cannula-type tip rather than a standard tip also adds to the depth of penetration.[44]

IMPLANT HOME CARE

Meticulous home care is essential in maintaining dental implants. Plaque and calculus *adhere to implant abutments* in the same way as they adhere to the natural dentition.[45,46] Because bacterial inflammation can contribute to implant failure, effective plaque removal is necessary.[47] Plaque has been correlated with gingivitis[48] and bone loss around implants.[49,50]

The loss of natural teeth that necessitates the use of implants is often due to past poor oral hygiene resulting in dental disease. An understanding of the importance of adequate, daily home care is essential for implant patients. Cleaning the abutment posts and bars, as well as the implant suprastructure, presents a challenge to the patient. This can be even more demanding than cleaning natural teeth. Ideally, the complexity and cost of the procedure serve as motivating factors toward diligent plaque control. As with natural teeth, a combination of devices is usually needed to remove plaque from all surfaces. The goal is for the patient to remove soft deposits *without altering the surface of the implants*. Damage to titanium implants can increase corrosion and affect the molecular interaction between the implant surface and host tissue.[49] Such damage may lead to increased plaque accumulation due to scratching.[50]

An effective brushing technique should be the first component of the implant home regimen. A soft, manual toothbrush can be used; however, the Rota-dent electric toothbrush is frequently recommended.[51] This rotary type electric brush does not damage the polished implant surface[52] and can be effective in areas where access is difficult.[51] Whatever brush is used, patients should be shown how to adapt the brush to the facial and lingual sides of abutment posts and replaced teeth. The dentifrice should meet ADA standards to ensure that it is not excessively abrasive. To aid in plaque removal from abutment posts a cone or cylindrically shaped interproximal brush or an end-tuft brush is recommended (Fig 7–26). These are used with an in-and-out motion to clean the abutment posts. The interdental brush must have a nylon-coated core wire rather than the standard metal wire to *prevent scratching* the implant with the tip of the interdental brush. To help control bacteria the rotary or the interproximal brush may be dipped into an antimicrobial solution before use. Chlorhexidine digluconate (0.12%) is usually recommended for this purpose. Alternatively, a cotton swab can be used to apply the agent. Rinsing with chlorhexidine is not considered to be the delivery mode of choice due to concerns about staining the prosthesis.

Some type of floss, yarn, or tape should be used for *circumferential plaque removal* around abutment posts. In some cases traditional floss can be used with a floss threader, or Super Floss or gauze can be used with an up-and-down, shoeshine motion after placing it in a 360° loop around the abutment post. Alternatively, floss products designed specifically for use with implants can be used. These include flossing yarn and ribbon, which are wide, woven, sometimes braided, gauzelike versions of floss. One product has a hook on the end of the floss ribbon to allow for wrapping the floss around an entire post by inserting from the facial aspect only, thus eliminating insertion from both facial and lingual surfaces. Placing a small amount of toothpaste on the floss or ribbon can help to polish the posts.

Oral irrigators can be helpful for cleaning around abutments.[53-55] The water spray should be used on the lowest setting and should not be directed subgingivally.

As with standard oral hygiene, only the minimal number of cleaning devices needed for plaque accumulation should be recommended. With proper instruction, the motivated patient can maintain implants successfully.

DENTURE MAINTENANCE

Patients who wear full or partial dentures should be instructed in the proper care and cleaning of both the dentures and the underlying tissues. According to one survey, *only 40% of dentures worn by the elderly are adequately cleaned.*[56]

Routine care of the soft tissues on which a denture rests includes removing the

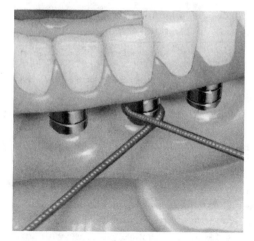

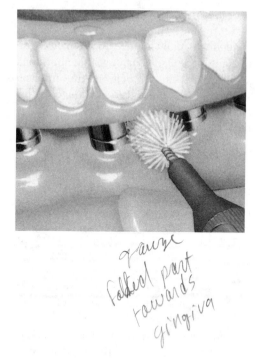

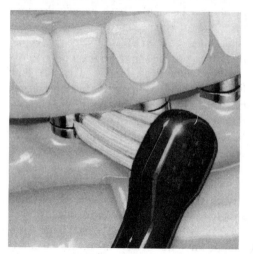

Figure 7–26. Cleaning implants: (Top left) Circumferential placement of Postcare braided nylon cord. (Top right) Interproximal brush. (Bottom) End-tuft brush. *(Courtesy of John O. Butler Co., 4635 W. Foster Ave., Chicago, IL 60630.)*

denture overnight or for a substantial time each day, cleaning and massaging the tissues under the denture daily,[57,58] and performing regular oral self-examinations to observe and report any irritation or chronic changes in appearance of the tissues. Failure to remove the denture may result in excessive alveolar ridge resorption.

Cleaning and massaging of the soft tissues can be performed simultaneously by brushing with a soft-bristled toothbrush or by massaging with the thumb or forefinger wrapped in a clean face cloth.

Deposits that form on dentures include pellicle, plaque, calculus, oral debris (eg, desquamated epithelial cells), and food debris.

Routine, effective cleaning of dentures not only serves to enhance a patient's sense of oral cleanliness, but more importantly, to prevent denture stomatitis or other tissue irritation. Denture stomatitis is common, occurring in 60% to 70% of denture wearers.[59] Cleaning methods commonly practiced by denture wearers are immersion or brushing or a combination of both.

Immersion Cleaners

Immersion cleaners, also known as chemical soaks, employ a liquid cleaning agent in which the denture is soaked. An advantage of this type of cleaner is that it reaches all parts of a denture, whereas with brushing, areas of the denture may be missed.

When selecting an immersion cleaner, denture materials must be taken into consideration. Alcohol or essential oils found in commercial mouthwashes are not compatible with denture acrylic, which may become dry or lose color due to prolonged contact with these substances.

Hypochlorite solutions (which contain bleach) are used to dissolve organic substances in the denture plaque matrix upon which stains and calculus form.[60] Hypochlorite solutions also act as antifungal and antibacterial agents.[61] Soaking a denture overnight in a mixture of 1 tsp household bleach, 2 tsp water softener and 8 oz of water, loosens debris, which can then be removed by brushing and rinsing under running water.[58] Hypochlorite solutions *may corrode metal alloys*, however, and patients should be cautioned about the use of these cleaners for metallic appliances.[60]

Alkaline peroxide cleaners typically contain sodium perborate, sodium percarbonate, monopersulfates or troclosene potassium, plus alkaline detergents and are available commercially as powders or tablets. They aid in the removal of lightly adhering plaque and stain and have an antibacterial effect.[60] When dissolved in water, these agents decompose and release oxygen bubbles, which mechanically loosen debris on the denture surface. The alkaline substances and detergent enhance the mechanical effect of the oxygen bubbles. Enzymes have been incorporated into some brands of alkaline peroxide cleaners to increase their antifungal effect.[62] Regular use of these types of cleaners, in combination with brushing, (Fig 7–27) can keep a denture reasonably clean and prevent the buildup of tenacious deposits.

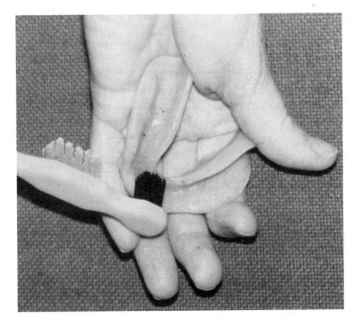

Figure 7–27. Brushing the alveolar surface of a full denture with a denture brush. Note the firm hold to prevent the denture slipping out of the hand.

Other Denture Cleaners

Dilute hydrochloric acid is sometimes used by patients to remove calculus from a denture. This practice is *not* advisable because the acid is not only caustic, but can also corrode metallic parts of a denture.[62]

Brushing alone, brushing in conjunction with an abrasive agent, or brushing a denture before and after it has soaked in an immersion cleaner, can aid in the removal of deposits. A brush with medium or soft, end-rounded bristles, if used properly, should not abrade denture materials. A denture brush provides access to all surfaces of a denture. Poor manual dexterity, however, may result in incomplete removal of deposits,[63,64] which the dental professional should take into account when instructing a patient in denture home care.

Nonabrasive agents, such as soap or baking soda, may be safely used in conjunction with a brush. However, other agents sometimes used by patients may be harmful to denture materials.

Daily cleaning of dentures by immersion in an alkaline peroxide cleanser, in conjunction with brushing and rinsing may be sufficient to keep dentures clean. Patients should be instructed to seek the help of the dental professional if deposits cannot be removed by this means.

Ultrasonic or *sonic devices* are available for home denture cleaning. They utilize a cleaning solution in conjunction with agitation produced by ultrasonic (inaudible, high-frequency) or sonic (audible) sound waves to remove debris and stains. Supplemental brushing can promote more thorough cleaning.[60] Use of one of these devices may be particularly helpful for individuals with limited manual dexterity or for the personal care staff of long-term care facilities.

Whichever method is used, the denture should be thoroughly rinsed under running, tepid water before reinsertion into the mouth in order to remove any substances that could irritate soft tissue.

Instruction of the patient in the recommended method of home care of a denture and of the tissues upon which it rests is critical to successful denture maintenance. It is the responsibility of the dental professional to be certain that the patient understands both the "why" and "how" of denture maintenance and the potential consequences of poor home care. This can often best be accomplished by explaining the procedure, demonstrating the correct method, and then asking the patient to demonstrate his or her comprehension and ability.

PATIENT FACTORS IN SUPPLEMENTAL AID SELECTION

In addition to oral conditions, several patient factors affect the appropriate selection and use of supplemental oral hygiene devices. The patient's dexterity in performing oral hygiene procedures, motivation to practice home care, and preferences for specific devices should be assessed when recommending supplemental oral hygiene devices and techniques. When a device is introduced to the patient, it is essential to ensure that the patient can demonstrate its proper use in all areas of the mouth and that he or she understands the potential for damage if used improperly.

Despite adequate dexterity and ability, attainment of optimal oral health requires motivation and daily compliance in performing oral care. To enhance compliance and skill development, the number of recommended oral hygiene devices *should be limited*. Studies examining patient compliance and effectiveness indicated that patients develop proper skills and are more willing to use supplemental oral hygiene devices on a regular basis when the number of devices is limited. It has been suggested that patients be instructed in the use of no more than *two* devices to supplement toothbrushing.[65,66]

The patient's preferences for particular oral hygiene devices should also be considered. Although a specific device may be preferred by the clinician, it will be ineffective if the patient does not use it. If a patient has already shown a preference for a particular device, its use should be encouraged. For example, if the patient is a toothpick user and oral hygiene appears inadequate, the clinician should consider (1) instruction to enhance the patient's effectiveness with the toothpick, (2) introduction of a toothpick holder to facilitate access and manipulation of the toothpick, or (3) use of the interdental wedge device because of its similarity to the toothpick.

Patient factors, such as level of understanding, dexterity, motivation, and preference, should be given serious consideration when determining appropriate supplemental oral hygiene devices and techniques.

Question 2. Which of the following statements, if any, are correct?

A. Implants accumulate dental plaque and thus can contribute to the development of periodontal disease.

B. Plaque removal from an implant can be best accomplished with a pipe cleaner.

C. The stream of solution from an irrigating device should be directed apically to clean the sulcus.

D. Immersion cleaning of dentures is usually more effective than brushing, because immersion ensures that the cleaning agent reaches all areas of the denture.

E. After providing instructions on auxiliary methods of oral hygiene, the patient should be given the devices

for the *four or five options* recommended.

SUMMARY

To achieve optimal oral health, toothbrushing must be supplemented with the use of specific interdental cleansing devices. A detailed evaluation of the periodontium and dentition is necessary to identify which oral conditions require which type of supplemental oral hygiene care. The comparative merits of the various oral hygiene devices and the techniques, abilities, and motivation of each patient should be carefully considered when recommending specific oral hygiene measures to meet the needs of each individual.

ANSWERS AND EXPLANATIONS

1. B, E

   A—incorrect. There is no evidence to indicate that one is better than the other.

   C—incorrect. The circle (or loop) method is best for children who do not yet have the dexterity needed for the spool method.

   D—incorrect. The floss holder might be easier to use for some, but certainly not more effective than the spool or loop method, if properly accomplished.

2. A, D

   B—incorrect. Circumferential plaque removal from an implant is best accomplished with a soft material that can be wrapped around its circumference: floss, tape, or wool.

   C—incorrect. It should be at right angles to the long axis of the tooth; otherwise bacteria can be forced into the blood supply to the area.

E—incorrect. It is best to restrict the recommendations to one or two options; otherwise compliance becomes a problem.

SELF-EVALUATION QUESTIONS

1. The tooth surface least accessible to the toothbrush is the (occlusal) (interproximal) (buccolingual).

2. Nylon floss contains approximately _35_ (number) of fine filaments twisted along the long axis. The (waxed) (unwaxed) floss frays and breaks more frequently on contact with calculus and restoration overhangs. The spool method of flossing requires (more) (less) psychomotor coordination than is required for the circle method. When using floss, approximately _18_ inch(es) is needed, of which only about _3/4 - 1"_ inch(es) is/are held between the fingers to insert the floss between the teeth. A new segment of floss (is)(is not) used to clean each interdental space. If floss is forced too deeply into the sulcus, it can cause _cuts_ in the gingiva, whereas if it is whipsawed buccolingually with too much force, it causes _cervical wear_ of the cementum. If a periodontal condition exists, there is/are usually (one best) (several satisfactory) device(s) for plaque removal from areas with difficult access.

3. Four indications for the use of a dental floss holder in lieu of regular finger flossing are _dexterity lack_, _phys. disab._, _____, and _____.

4. Three indications for the use of a floss threader are _lg hands_, _strong gag_, and _lack motivat_.

5. Research (has)(has not) proved the value of the toothpick in maintaining oral health.

6. Irrigation devices should be used with extreme caution, *or not at all*, by patients with a history of _Endocarditis_, _Cong. H diseas_, _Reumatic Hdis_, and _Prosth Jt, Bone Marrow tran, pacemaker_.

7. Scratching the titanium implant while removing plaque can cause a more rapid buildup of _plaque_ and hence pose a greater risk of gingivitis and periodontitis.

8. The wrapping of floss around an implant post for cleaning is termed _circumfrential_ plaque removal.

9. One study indicates that as few as _40_ % of the dentures worn by the elderly are adequately cleaned. Failure to maintain clean dentures can result in denture _stomatitis_ (name of inflammation), a condition which is seen in 60%–70% of denture wearers.

10. The two most frequently used methods of cleaning dentures are brushing and _immersion cleaners_.

11. When providing oral home care instruction to a patient who wears dentures, the practitioner should instruct the patient to care for both the denture itself and the _alveolar ridge soft tissue_.

12. Four objectives that may be accomplished by proper use of dental floss are: _interprox plag. rem._, _polished_, _massage int. pap._, and _gin bleed_.

13. Two auxiliary cleaning aids that can be used to safely and effectively clean under a fixed bridge are _floss threaders_ and _irrigation devices_.

REFERENCES

1. Graves RC, Disney JA, Stamm JW. Comparative effectiveness of flossing and brushing in reducing interproximal bleeding. *J Periodontol.* 1989: 60:243–247.

2. Saloum FS, Sondhi A. Preventing enamel decalcification after orthodontic treatment. *J Am Dent Assoc.* 1987; 115:257–261.

3. Tolboe H, Isidor F, Budtz-Jorgensen E, et al. Influence of oral hygiene on the mucosal conditions beneath bridge pontics. *Scand J Dent Res*. 1987; 95:475–482.

4. Schwab C. Flossing compliance. *Dent Hy News*. 1989; 2:5.

5. Brough Muzzin KM, Johnson R, Carr P, et al. The dental hygienist's role in the maintenance of osseointegrated dental implants. *J Dent Hyg*. 1988; 62:448–453.

6. Stefani LA. The care and maintenance of the dental implant patient. 1988; *J Dent Hyg*. 62:447, 464–466.

7. Jensen RL, Jensen JH. Peri-implant maintenance. *Northwest Dent*. 1991; 70:14–23.

8. Bonfil JJ, Fourel J, Falabregues R. The influence of gingival stimulation on recovery from human experimental gingivitis. *J Clin Periodontol*. 1985; 12:828–836.

9. Walsh MM, Heckman BL. Interproximal subgingival cleaning by dental floss and the toothpick. *Dent Hygiene*. 1985; 59:464–467.

10. Smith BA, Shanbour GS, Caffesse RG, et al. In vitro polishing effectiveness of interdental aids on root surfaces. *J Clin Periodontol*. 1986; 13:597–603.

11. Newman HN. Modes of application of antiplaque chemicals. *J Clin Periodontol*. 1986; 13:965–974.

12. Parmly LS. *A Practical Guide to the Management of the Teeth*. Philadelphia, PA: Collins & Croft; 1819.

13. Bass CC. The optimum characteristics of dental floss for personal oral hygiene. *Dent Items Int*. 1948:70:921–934.

14. Lamberts DM, Wunderlich RC, Caffesse RG. The effect of waxed and unwaxed dental floss on gingival health. Part 1. Plaque removal and gingival response. *J Periodontol*. 1982; 53:393–400.

15. Perry DA, Pattison G. An investigation of wax residue on tooth surfaces after the use of waxed dental floss. *Dent Hygiene*. 1986; 60:16–19.

16. Ciancio SG, Shilby O, Farber GA. Clinical evaluation of the effect of two types of dental floss on plaque and gingival health. *Clin Prevent Dent*. 1992; 14:14–18.

17. Beaumont RH. Patient preference for waxed or unwaxed floss. *J Periodontol*. 1990; 61:123–125.

18. Ong G. The effectiveness of three types of dental floss for interdental plaque removal. *J Clin Periodontol*. 1990; 17:463–466.

19. Smith BA, Collier CM, Caffesse RG. In vitro effectiveness of dental floss in plaque removal. *J Clin Periodontol*. 1986; 13:211–216.

20. Spidel L, Person P. Floss design and effectiveness of interproximal plaque removal. *Clin Prevent Dent*. 1987; 9:3–6.

21. Wong CH, Wade AB. A comparative study of effectiveness in plaque removal by Super Floss and waxed dental floss. *J Clin Periodontol*. 1985; 12:788–795.

22. Kresch CH. Finger-manipulated and floss-holder flossing: A comparison of the habit formation. *Gen Dent*. 1976: 24:35–36.

23. Kleber CJ, Putt MS. Evaluation of a floss-holding device compared to hand-held floss for interproximal plaque, gingivitis, and patient acceptance. *Clin Prevent Dent*. 1988: 10:6–14.

24. Mulligan R, Wilson S. Design characteristics of floss-holding devices for persons with upper extremity disabilities. *Spec Care Dent*. 1984; 4:168–172.

25. Caton J, Bouwsma O, Polson A, et al. Effects of personal oral hygiene and subgingival scaling on bleeding interdental gingiva. *J Periodontol*. 1989; 60:84–90.

26. Bahn PG. Early teething troubles. *Nature*. 1989; 337:693.

27. Steele DL, Orton GS. Dental implants: Clinical procedures and homecare considerations. *Pract Hyg*. 1992; 1:9–12.

28. Gillette WA, Van House RL. Ill effects of improper oral hygiene procedures. *J Am Dent Assoc*. 1980; 101:476–480.

29. Ralph WJ. Oral hygiene—why neglect the tongue? *Aust Dent J*. 1988; 33:224–225.

30. Romans AR, App GR. Bacteremia, a result from oral irrigation in subjects with gingivitis. *J Periodontol* 1971; 42:752.

31. Felix JE, Rosen S, App GR. Detection of bacteremia after use of an oral irrigation device in subjects with periodontitis. *J Periodontol*. 1971; 42:785.

32. American Dental Association. *Dentist's Desk Reference Materials, Instruments and Equipment*, 2nd ed. Chicago; American Dental Association; 1983.

33. Naylor WP, Stewart DM. The end tuft toothbrush for the partially edentulous patient. *J Prosthet Dent.* 1984; 52:311.

34. Walsh TF, Glenwright HD, Hull PS. Clinical effects of pulsed oral irrigation with 0.2% chlorhexidine digluconate in patients with adult periodontitis. *J Clin Periodontol.* 1992; 19:245–248.

35. Itic J, Serfaty R. Clinical effectiveness of subgingival irrigation with a pulsed jet irrigator versus syringe. *J Periodontol.* 1992; 63: 174–181.

36. Jolkousky DL, Waki MY, Newman MG, et al. Clinical and microbiological effects of subgingival and gingival marginal irrigation with chlorhexidine gluconate. *J Periodontol.* 1990; 61:663–669.

37. Parsons LG, Thomas LG, Southard GL, et al. Effect of sanguinaria extract on established plaque and gingivitis when delivered as a manual rinse or under pressure in an oral irrigator. *J Clin Periodontol.* 1987; 14: 381.

38. Southard GL. Effect of sanguinaria extract on development of plaque and gingivitis when subgingivally delivered as a manual rinse or under pressure in an oral irrigator. *J Clin Periodontol.* 1987; 14:377.

39. Ciancio SG, Mather ML, Zambon JJ, et al. Effect of a chemotherapeutic agent delivered by an oral irrigation device on plaque, gingivitis, and subgingival microflora. *J Periodontol.* 1989; 60:310–315.

40. Flemming T, Newman MG, Doherty FM, et al. Supragingival irrigation with 0.06% chlorhexidine in naturally occurring gingivitis I. Six month clinical observations. *J Periodontol.* 1990; 61:112–117.

41. Bossi J. Experiments with a toothbrush. (Interspace Toothbrush). *Dent Health.* 1965; 4:59–62.

42. Toon S. Rubbing out the bad guys. *R D H.* 1987; 7:10,11,15.

43. Braun RE. Periodontal pocket depth of delivery with a subgingival irrigating tip. *J Dent Res.* 1990; 69(Special Issue):248.

44. Boyd RL, Hollander BN, Eakle WS. Comparison of a subgingivally placed cannula oral irrigator tip with a supragingivally placed standard irrigator tip. *J Clin Periodontol.* 1992; 19:340–344.

45. Duckworth J. Microbial morphology of subgingival plaque surrounding single-tooth ceramic alumina implants. *J Dent Res.* 1986; 65(Special Issue):260.

46. Rams TE, Roberts TW, Tatum H Jr, et al. The subgingival flora associated with human dental implants. *J Prosthet Dent.* 1984; 11: 93–100.

47. Lundquist S, Carlsson GE. Maxillary fixed prostheses on osseointegrated dental implants. *J Prosthet Dent.* 1983; 50:262–270.

48. Zarb GA, Symington JM. Osseointegrated dental implants: Preliminary report on a replication study. *J Prosthet Dent.* 1983; 50: 271.

49. Schroeder A, van der Zypen E, Stich H, et al. The reaction on bone, connective tissue, and epithelium to endosteal implants with titanium-sprayed surfaces. *J Maxillofac Surg.* 1981; 9:15–25.

50. Klawitter J, Weinstein A, Cooke F, et al. An evaluation of porous alumina ceramic dental implants. *J Dent Res.* 1977; 6:768–776.

51. Meffert RM. The soft tissue interface in dental implantology. *J Dent Educ.* 1988; 52: 810–811.

52. Thomson-Neal D, Evans G, Meffert RM, et al. A SEM evaluation of various prophylactic modalities on different implants. *Int J Periodont Restor Dent.* 1989; 9:301–311.

53. Balshi TJ, Mingledorff EB. Maintenance procedures for patients after complete fixed prosthodontics. *J Prosthet Dent.* 1977; 37: 420–431.

54. Bodine R, Mohammed C. Implant denture histology: Gross and microscopic studies of a human mandible with a 12-year subperiosteal implant denture. *Dent Clin North Am.* 1970; 14:145–159.

55. Rams T, Link C. Microbiology of failing implants in humans: Electron microscope observations. *J Oral Implantol.* 1973; 11:93–100.

56. Hoad-Reddick G, Grant AA, Griffith CS. Investigation into the cleanliness of dentures in an elderly population. *J Prosthet Dent.* 1990; 64:48–52.

57. Tautin FS. The beneficial effects of tissue massage for the edentulous patient. *J Prosthet Dent*. 1982; 48:653–656.

58. Zarb GA, Bolender CL, Hickey JC, et al. *Boucher's Prosthetic Treatment for Edentulous Patients*, 10th ed. St. Louis. Mosby; 1990.

59. Budtz-Jorgensen E, Knudsen AM. Chlorhexidine gel and steradent employed in cleaning dentures. *Acta Odontol Scand*. 1978; 36:83–87.

60. American Dental Association, Council on Dental Materials, Instruments and Equipment. Denture cleaners. *J Am Dent Assoc*. 1983; 106:77–79.

61. Budtz-Jorgensen E. Materials and methods for cleaning dentures. *J Prosthet Dent*. 1979; 42:619–623.

62. Minagi S, Tsunada T, Yoshida K, et al. Objective testing of the efficiency of denture-cleaning agents. *J Prosthetic Dent*. 1987; 58: 595–598.

63. Dills SS, Olshan AM, Goldner S, et al. Comparison of the anti-microbial capacity of an abrasive paste and chemical-soak denture cleaner. *J Prosthet Dent*. 1988; 60:467–470.

64. Palenik CJ, Miller CH. In vitro testing of three denture cleaning systems. *J Prosthet Dent*. 1984; 51:751–754.

65. Heasman PA, Jacobs DJ, Chapple IL. An evaluation of the effectiveness and patient compliance with plaque control methods in the prevention of periodontal disease. *Clin Prevent Dent*. 1989; 11:24–28.

66. Johansson LA, Oster B, Hamp SE. Evaluation of cause-related periodontal therapy and compliance with maintenance care recommendations. *J Clin Periodontol*. 1984; 15: 689–699.

Chapter 8

Water Fluoridation

Norman O. Harris
D. Christopher Clark

Objectives

1. Recall the historic highlights leading to the discovery of the benefits of fluoride.
2. Explain the cause, characteristics, and treatment of dental fluorosis.
3. State the optimal amount of fluoride in parts per million needed to give near maximum caries reduction and near minimum fluorosis.
4. Outline the normal metabolism of the fluoride ion in humans.
5. Explain the principal of the probable toxic dose (PTD) for fluoride, and discuss the emergency treatment for fluoride poisoning.
6. Briefly describe the equipment, chemicals, and techniques used to fluoridate and defluoridate communal drinking water.
7. Outline alternative methods of fluoride administration that are used in lieu of water fluoridation.
8. Discuss political objections to water fluoridation, and elaborate on means to overcome these objections.

Introduction

Based on nearly 50 years of experience, controlled water fluoridation continues to be the *safest* and most *economic* method to prevent dental decay for *all socioeconomic groups*. The widespread availability of, first, water fluoridation and later, of fluoride from several dental and food products has been the reason attributed to the continued decrease of caries in the Western world.[1]

Despite these impressive results, the practice of fluoridating community water supplies continues to generate controversy on an unprecedented scale. Opposition still surfaces in some communities when a decision is made to add fluoride to the water supply. Court battles are still waged over this issue. Bearing in mind the political contentiousness surrounding fluoridation, let us look at some of the facts about the dental benefits of fluorides and the "great fluoride controversy."[2]

HISTORIC

At the turn of the 20th century, two reports appeared in the literature, the importance and relationship of which were not to be appreciated until many decades later. In 1901, Eager, a U.S. Public Health Service physician, reported on the prevalence of mottled teeth in Italy.[3] The cause of the mottling was unknown. At the same time, a fluoride preparation—known as Fluoridens—was widely sold in Europe as being a "remedy for decay of the teeth." Unfortunately, for unknown reasons, this over-the-counter item disappeared from the market at the turn of the century.[4]

In 1907, Dr. Fredrick McKay of Colorado Springs, without knowledge of the aforementioned events, began a classic epidemiology study to find the cause of the mottled enamel[a] that was endemic in the Rocky Mountain area. By 1916, with the aid of Dr. G. V. Black, an outstanding teacher and researcher, McKay had alerted the dental profession of the widespread prevalence of the condition. In the approximately 25-year course of his studies, McKay observed (but did not pursue his casual observation) that *teeth with the stain (mottling) appeared to have fewer caries.* It was not until the

early 1930s that Churchill, a chemist with the Aluminum Company of America, *associated* an excess of fluoride with mottled teeth. This finding was immediately followed by a report by Smith and Smith of the University of Arizona, conclusively demonstrating that fluoride did *cause* mottling.[2] For the first time, the mottling could be correctly called *dental fluorosis*.

In 1938, Trendley Dean of the U.S. Public Health Service completed a series of studies in which he measured the number of carious lesions in a community, the number of teeth with fluorosis, and the amount of fluoride in the water.[5] He found that (1) the number of carious teeth and the amount of fluorosis were *inversely* related; and (2) the amount of fluoride in the water and the amount of fluorosis were *directly* related. Furthermore, a concentration ranging from about 0.6 to 1.2 ppm appeared to be the optimal range to result in both minimal caries and minimal dental fluorosis (Fig 8–1).

The next major step was to determine whether the *addition* of 1 ppm of fluoride to a communal water supply deficient in fluoride would prevent dental decay. In January 1945, the fluoride content of the water supply of Grand Rapids, Michigan, was adjusted to 1 ppm. This was the first city in the world to artificially fluoridate its water supply. The eventual reduction in decayed, missing, and filled teeth (DMFT)[b] for children 12 to 14 years of age was 55%. Similar studies in Evanston and Oak Park, Illinois, Newburgh and Kingston, New York, and Brantford and Sarnia, Michigan, showed similar reductions ranging from 48% to 70%, or from four to nine fewer DMFT.[6] By 1989, approximately 126,000,000 people in the United States

---

[a] Often referred to at the time as the Colorado, or Texas, brown stain.

[b] DMFT = Decayed, missing, filled permanent teeth.
   dmft = Decayed, missing, filled primary teeth.
   DMFS = Decayed, missing, filled permanent surfaces.
   dmfs = Decayed, missing, filled primary surfaces.

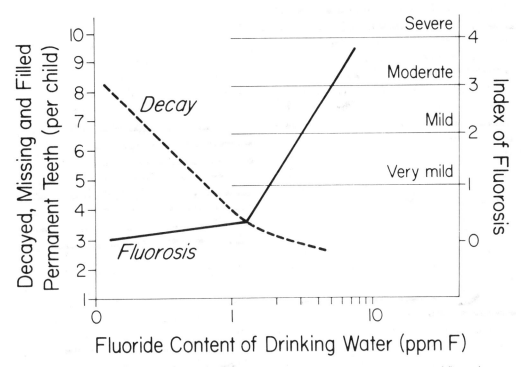

Figure 8–1. As the fluoride content of water increases beyond 1 ppm, the index of fluorosis escalates more rapidly than the DMF decreases. (*From Horowitz HS.* An Update for Dental Practice. *New York. American Academy of Pedodontics, MedCom, Inc; 1976.*)

were consuming water with *added* fluoride, and an additional 9,000,000 were receiving *naturally* fluoridated water—a total of approximately 65% of the U.S. population.[7,8] Among the many metropolitan centers in North America receiving adjusted fluoridated water are New York, Baltimore, Chicago, Philadelphia, and Toronto.

THE "HALO EFFECT" OF FLUORIDE

The outstanding success of the early studies created in the public's mind a belief that the benefits of water fluoridation would endure through time. This was not to be the case. By the 1990s the 50% to 60% reductions seen in earlier studies had dropped to about

20% to 40%.[9] It was apparent that in looking forward to the year 2000, the benefits from an optimally fluoridated water supply *alone* would not be as great as previously thought.

In retrospect, the dental benefits resulting from the use of fluorides can be arbitrarily viewed as occurring in two periods: (1) an *earlier era* from 1945 to 1960 when the reduction in dental caries and saved teeth could be attributed primarily to the ingestion of fluoride contained in the water and to a lesser extent from food; and (2) a *later era* when fluoride was being ingested by entire populations from *multiple* commercial sources. Important sources of fluoride include those contained in many soft drinks along with infant and adult foods that are prepared with water containing varying amounts of fluoride. Other significant sources are fluoride drops, lozenges, vitamins with fluoride, fluoride tablets for children; professionally applied liquid and gel topical applications in dental offices; mouth rinses available in schools; and over-the-counter products. Probably the most ubiquitous source of all is from fluoride dentifrices.[10] For instance, in 1964, Crest toothpaste was the only dentifrice fully accredited by the American Dental Association (ADA) as an anticariogenic toothpaste; by 1980, the percentage of fluoride-containing dentifrices had climbed to 98%.[11]

As dental researchers developed new technologies to increase the number of methods used to protect the teeth against dental caries, two major phenomena occurred. First, a *worldwide decline* began in caries *prevalence*. This decline has been documented by Kaminsky and coworkers, who listed 14 countries where even in *nonfluoridated* areas, the prevalence of caries had declined.[12] The decline is also well illustrated in the classic longitudinal study involving 63,000 examinations of Tansworth, NSW school children in Australia over a period of 24 years (Table 8–1).

Second, the percentage differences in caries *prevalence* between newly fluoridated communities and their nonfluoridated control cities, also began to *decrease*. Yet, despite the decrease, the overall relationship of oral health is contingent on the amount of fluoride in the water supply, as indicated in a recent study in England (Table 8–2).

It was now becoming more difficult to separate the effects of ingesting solely water-borne fluoride from the effects of swallowing fluoride contained in widely distributed beverages, food, and dental products.[13] Thus, as the apparent effectiveness of water fluoridation *alone* decreased as a dental public health measure, the difference was being compensated for by the increased ingestion of fluoride contained in the total gamut of commercial fluoride products. Most important is the fact that between the two, the total caries problem is diminishing. Research has shown that the increased fluoride ingestion from processed beverages and foods is extremely variable and depends on the source of water used during processing. In some nonfluoridated areas the ingestion of fluorides from these sources can be significant. Some have termed the benefits of this secondary exposure to imported fluoridated water in processed foods and beverages, as a *"halo effect."*

It should be noted that when access to commercial fluoride-containing products is minimal, as with many of the poor and elderly, water fluoridation still provides the *single most important* source of fluoride. For the more prosperous, the fluoride that is ingested directly from public water supplies constitutes but one of several sources.[14,15] It has been estimated that water fluoridation may result in a 40% benefit for the poor,

TABLE 8–1. ORAL HEALTH OF TANSWORTH SCHOOLCHILDREN IN NSW, AUSTRALIA, 24 YEARS AFTER INITIATING WATER FLUORIDATION

DMFT Values for	1963	1967	1970	1973	1979	1988
At 6 years of age	1.3	0.9	0.5	0.4	0.1	0.1
9	4.0	3.2	2.9	2.0	1.1	0.3
12	8.4	7.0	5.6	4.3	2.4	0.9
15	12.5	11.2	10.2	7.7	4.6	1.5

Note: The decline in DMFT of permanent teeth over the period of 1963–1988 is well demonstrated and occurred for all ages. (*From Sivaneswaran S. J Dent Res. 1990; 69:934. Abstract 9.*)

TABLE 8–2. A PATTERN OF DECREASING CARIES EXPERIENCE WITH INCREASING FLUORIDE WATER CONTENT AS SEEN IN 15-YEAR-OLD CHILDREN IN NORTH OF ENGLAND

Town	Number	Fluoride Content (ppm)	Mean DMFT (SE mean)	Mean DMFS (SE mean)	Percentage Caries-Free
Hartlepool	254	1.0–1.3	1.7 (0.13)	2.9 (0.26)	40
Newcastle	227	1.0	2.5 (0.16)	3.5 (0.27)	30
West Cumbria	145	1.0	2.7 (0.21)	4.6 (0.44)	24
South Shields	407	0.3	2.8 (0.13)	5.0 (0.30)	22
Sunderland	390	0.3–0.5	2.9 (0.14)	5.2 (0.33)	26
Middlesbrough	259	0.2	3.3 (0.26)	6.1 (0.46)	24
East Cumbria	180	0.1	4.2 (0.28)	8.8 (0.72)	18

Note: As fluoride water concentration (third column) *decreases* (from top-to-bottom) a parallel *decrease* occurs in caries-free teeth, and expected *increase* occurs in the mean DMFT and DMFS.
(*From Murray JJ, Nunn JH. J Dent Res. 1992; 71 (special issue): 726. Abstract 726.*)

whereas the affluent with ready and frequent access to commercial dental products and professional services may realize only a 1% to 20% reduction in caries from water fluoridation.[16] This socioeconomic difference was aptly demonstrated in a study in England, in which children from nonfluoridated and fluoridated areas were categorized into economic classes, ranging from high, (children of professionals) to low, (children of laborers or unemployed). In each area, the children from the highest economic groups in both communities had fewer caries, with the children in each group from the fluoridated community having the better oral status of the two.[17]

BENEFITS OF WATER FLUORIDATION

The decline of caries in the United States and the tremendous effect of fluoride on dental health are seen in the data resulting from a National Institute of Dental Research (NIDR) National Survey of Dental Health.[18] In this study, 39,000 U.S. children, 5 to 17 years of age were examined in 1986 and 1987 and compared with children from a similar study in 1979 and 1980 (Fig 8–2).

Approximately 50% of *all* American children younger than 17 have never had a cavity or a filling in their permanent teeth.[18] Another illustration of the effectiveness of fluoride is that about six times as many school-aged children living in a fluoridated area are free from any detectable dental decay, compared with children living in a nonfluoridated area.[18] Overall caries prevalence has declined by more than 75%, and that of interproximal tooth surfaces, by more than 90%.[19] Toothlessness has been drastically reduced. Other important benefits are freedom from pain, less time lost from school and work, and the retention of the chewing potential of the teeth.

Children residing continuously in fluoridated areas had 18% lower DMFS scores than did those from the nonfluoridated areas, even though fluoride-containing dental products were widely available in the nonfluoridated control areas.[18] An even more recent study in Canada demonstrated a 34% reduction, or a saving of approximately one surface per child.[20]

Fluoride Benefits All Ages

Recently, Newbrun has estimated that fluoridation now prevents 30% to 39% of the dental caries in the *primary* dentition; 11%

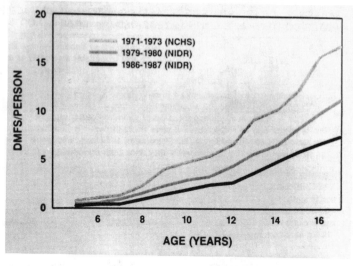

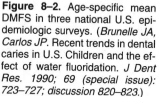

Figure 8–2. Age-specific mean DMFS in three national U.S. epidemiologic surveys. (*Brunelle JA, Carlos JP*. Recent trends in dental caries in U.S. Children and the effect of water fluoridation. *J Dent Res. 1990; 69 (special issue): 723–727; discussion 820–823.*)

to 38% of the *mixed* dentition; and 13% to 35% of the *permanent* dentition. Estimated reductions for adults, aged 20 to 44, range from 20% to 30% for *coronal* caries and 20% to 40% for *root* caries. Thus, the *maximum* attainable caries benefit for coronal and root caries derived from water fluoridation *alone* now appears to be a reduction of about 40%.[21]

The great majority of the early literature on water fluoridation focused solely on the benefits derived by children. With adults now retaining their teeth longer, the effect of fluoride on the adult dentition is being reassessed. These observations are overdue because root caries begin to occur with significant frequency in the 35 to 44 age group, doubles in the 45 to 54 age group, and redoubles in the 55 to 66 age group.[15]

Fluoride levels in cementum and root dentin increase with longer exposure to fluoridated water.[22] Stamm and colleagues compared the dental status of 502 lifelong residents in a naturally fluoridated community (Stratford, Ontario, 1.6 ppm) to 465 residents in a low fluoride community (Woodstock, 0.2 ppm). The mean DMFT for coronal caries was 11 for Stratford and 15 for Woodstock. The percentage of subjects with root caries experience was 21% for Stratford and 35% for Woodstock. It was also found that the reduction in the prevalence of root caries for adults was approximately the same percentage as for coronal caries for children.[15] Stamm's findings immediately highlight the following suggestion by Horowitz, which if implemented, could greatly extend the benefits of fluoride, "The current recommendation to discontinue dietary fluoride supplementation sometime in the teen years is incongruent with our present knowledge that *fluoride continues to benefit dentate persons throughout their lives.*"[23]

Cost of Water Fluoridation

Water fluoridation is economical. The annual cost of fluoridating the water supply of a city of over 200,000 is approximately 12 to 21 cents per person, and for cities with populations from 10,000 to 200,000, the cost is from 18 to 76 cents per capita. The national weighted average is 51 cents (Table 8–3).[24]

The economy of water fluoridation is further dramatized by comparing the 51-cent national average with the national aver-

TABLE 8–3. ESTIMATED ANNUAL COST OF FLUORIDE REGIMENS PER PERSON SERVED IN PUBLIC HEALTH PROGRAMS

Method	Cost ($)
Community water fluoridation	
>200,000 persons	0.12–0.21
10,000–200,000 persons	0.18–0.75
National weighted average	0.51
School water fluoridation	3.55–4.73
Fluoride supplements	0.81–5.40
Fluoride mouth rinse in schools	0.52–1.78

Note: No fluoride supplementation is as economical as water fluoridation. The use of mouth rinses, fluoride supplements, and school fluoridation are all more expensive. (*From Review of Fluoride. Benefits and Risks. Department of Health and Human Services Report of the ad hoc Subcommittee on Fluoride. Public Health Service. February, 1991.*)

age cost of one restoration, which is $51. Thus, the saving of only one restoration would defray the cost of a *lifetime* of fluoridation for one person.[25] This 100-fold savings is equally magnified by the realization that for every carious lesion initially prevented, the need is reduced for repeatedly restoring defective restorations and *recurrent* carious lesions several times over a lifetime.[26] This savings is important considering that the replacement rates for amalgam restorations because of secondary caries varies between 38% and 50% depending on the study.[27,28]

Another way to demonstrate the effectiveness of water fluoridation is to look at what happens when a community decides to cease water fluoridation. One community—Antigo, Wisconsin—initiated fluoridation in 1949. After 11 years, fluoridation was discontinued. In a survey taken 4½ years later, the incidence of caries greatly increased, with 92%, 183%, and 41% increases in DMF for kindergarten, second, and fourth grades, respectively. A year after the survey, Antigo reinstated fluoridation.[29] More re-

cently, the same result occurred in Wick, Scotland, where after 5 years of defluoridation, the DMFS increased by 40%, going from a low of 2.63 DMFS in 1979 to 3.9 in 1984.[30]

Question 1. Which of the following statements, if any, are correct?

A. Trendley Dean of the U.S. Public Health Service discovered the *cause* of dental fluorosis.

B. From the *1940s* to the *1960s* water fluoridation resulted in an approximate *50%* to *60%* caries reduction.

C. The poor, the uneducated, minorities, and the elderly *benefit the most* from water fluoridation.

D. Water fluoridation prevents *root caries* as well as coronal caries.

E. Antigo, Wisconsin, provided an example of how *rapidly* the prevalence of caries can increase following defluoridation.

METABOLISM OF FLUORIDE

The metabolism of fluoride is relatively uncomplicated. Fluoride can be absorbed from the stomach as well as from the intestine. About 86% to 97% of ingested fluoride is absorbed. Starvation increases the rate of absorption, whereas the presence of calcium, aluminum, and magnesium, which bind fluoride in the intestine, decreases absorption. Blood plasma fluoride levels begin to rise about 10 minutes after ingestion and reach maximal levels *within 60 minutes.* The plasma blood levels return to preingestion levels after 11 to 15 hours.[31] In experimental animals with little previous exposure to fluorides, the amount of fluoride absorbed can double in 10 to 90 minutes after intake—with approximately 50% of the dosage being deposited in bones.

More than 99% of the fluoride in the body is found in the calcified tissues.[32] As bone saturation is approached, excretion of fluoride increases. In geographic areas with lower than optimum water fluoride levels, bone fluoride content increased from approximately 200 ppm at 10 years of age to about 1200 ppm at 80. In areas with 9 ppm, the maximum bone accumulation in old age can approach 10,000 ppm.[33]

The fluoride can be deposited in the (1) *adsorbed layer* of the bone, (2) the *crystal structure*, and (3) the *bone matrix*.[34,35] The fluoride in the adsorbed layer is in equilibrium with the blood and can be rapidly raised or lowered, depending on ingestion patterns and the efficiency of kidney function. In crystal formation, the fluoride ion is probably involved in an ionic exchange with the hydroxyl moiety (see Fig 11–1). Once fluoride is incorporated into the crystals of the bone, it is more slowly removed, probably through the osteoclastic action seen in remodeling. In Bartlett, Texas, following defluoridation, the half-life[c] of loss was 120 weeks for adults and 75 weeks for children. In the initial weeks of loss following defluoridation, the fluoride loss was rapid. After the third month it increasingly slowed due partially to the fact that, following osteoclastic action, some of the released fluoride was redeposited in other newly forming bone before it could be eliminated by the kidneys.

The amount of fluoride that is not stored in bone is *rapidly* excreted through the kidneys. If 1 to 1.5 mg of fluoride is ingested (a fluoride tablet contains 1 mg), 20% to 25% of the dose is excreted in about 4 hours. The excretion rate rises rapidly for the first hour, then begins to fall for the next 3 hours, after which there is a low, continuous plateau. With a more continuous intake of fluoride as occurs through drinking fluoridated water, the excretion rate is more constant.

Up to 50% of the fluoride can be eliminated by extensive sweating. Feces can account for up to 25% of the fluoride eliminated, the amount depending on the presence of such dietary elements as calcium, magnesium, aluminum, and other binding agents. Little, if any, fluoride is excreted via the bile. In human milk, the concentration is approximately the same as in the blood (ie, 0.1 ppm). The blood plasma can vary widely from 2.4 and 0.7 ppm.

The concentration of fluoride in the saliva usually is within a range of 0.01 to 0.04 ppm, which is less than the blood plasma. The saliva concentration parallels that of the plasma, with the peak output of fluoride occurring approximately 1 to 1.5 hours after intake. The concentration in the plaque is usually 50 to 100 times higher than in the whole saliva.[35]

TOXICOLOGY OF FLUORIDE

The handling of fluorides is carefully regulated in industry by occupational safety health legislation and in the marketplace by the Food and Drug Administration. Commercial dental fluoride products and professional practices *can be toxic and even lethal* when used inappropriately. The lethal dose for an adult is somewhere between 2.5 and 10 g, with the *average lethal dose* being 4 to 5 g. The use of the "average lethal dose" is a very imprecise designation that makes it difficult to predict the outcome of an accidental swallowing of an excess of fluoride. To correct this problem, a *body-weight based, the probable toxic dose (PTD) standard*, has been recommended as a more practical ap-

---

[c] Half-life means that if in 120 weeks, half of the original fluoride stored in the body is lost; in the next 120 weeks, another half will be lost; in the third 120 weeks, another half of the still remaining fluoride is lost, and so on.

proach to making treatment decisions. With it, the urgency for first aid and more definitive emergency treatment can be determined rapidly. The PTD approach, first reported by Bayless and Tinanoff, bases the level and urgency of treatment on the number of multiples of 5 *mg/kg* of fluoride ingested (Table 8–4).[36]

If the amount ingested is less than 5 mg/kg, the office use of available calcium, aluminum, or magnesium products as first aid antidotes should suffice. If the amount is over 5 mg/kg, first aid measures should be expeditiously applied, followed by hospital observation for possible further care. Finally, if the amount of fluoride ingested approaches or exceeds 15 mg/kg, the immediate first aid treatment should be followed by a *most urgent* action to move the patient

swiftly into a hospital emergency room where cardiac monitoring, electrolyte evaluation, and shock support is available. Ingestion of 15 mg/kg fluoride can be lethal. Methods for quickly calculating the amount of fluoride ingested from dental products and use of professional practices are contained in Appendix 8–1.

Fluoride Toxicity

Fluoride acts in four general ways: (1) when a concentrated fluoride salt contacts moist skin or mucous membrane, hydrofluoric acid forms, causing a chemical burn; (2) it is a general protoplasmic poison that acts to inhibit enzyme systems; (3) it binds calcium needed for nerve action; and (4) hyperkalemia occurs, contributing to cardiotoxicity.

TABLE 8–4. EMERGENCY TREATMENT FOR FLUORIDE OVERDOSE

Milligram Fluoride Ion per Kilogram Body Weight*	Treatment
Less than 5.0 mg/kg	1. Give calcium orally (milk) to relieve GI symptoms. Observe for a few hours. 2. Induced vomiting not necessary.
More than 5 mg/kg	1. Empty stomach by inducing vomiting with emetic. For patients with depressed gag reflex caused by age (<6 months old), Down's syndrome, or severe mental retardation, induced vomiting is contraindicated and endotracheal intubation should be performed before gastric lavage. 2. Give orally soluble calcium in any form (for example, milk, 5% calcium gluconate, or calcium lactate solution). 3. Admit to hospital, and observe for a few hours.
More than 15 mg/kg	1. Admit to hospital immediately. 2. Induce vomiting. 3. Begin cardiac monitoring and be prepared for cardiac arrythmias. Observe for peaking T waves and prolonged QT intervals. 4. Slowly administer intravenously 10 mL of 10% calcium gluconate solution. Additional doses may be given if clinical signs of tetany or QT interval prolongation develops. Electrolytes, especially calcium and potassium, should be monitored and corrected as necessary. 5. Adequate urine output should be maintained using diuretics if necessary. 6. General supportive measures for shock.

*Average weight per age: 1–2 years = 10 kg; 2–4 years = 15 kg; 4–6 years = 20 kg; 6–8 years = 23 kg.
(*From Bayless JM and Tinanoff N. Diagnosis and treatment of acute fluoride toxicity. J Am Dent Assoc. 1985, 110:209–211.*)

When dry fluoride powder contacts the mucous membrane or the moist skin, a reddened lesion occurs, and later the area becomes swollen and pale; still later ulceration and necrosis may occur. In past years, skin burns of this type were common for many water engineers who emptied drums of fluoride agents into the hoppers feeding water supplies. Federal and state occupational safety acts have greatly reduced this danger.

Following *excessive ingestion* of fluoride, nausea and vomiting can occur. The vomiting is usually caused by the formation of hydrofluoric acid in the acid environment of the stomach, causing damage to the lining cells of the stomach wall. Local or general signs of muscle tetany ensue due to the drop in blood calcium. This can be accompanied by abdominal cramping and pain. Finally, as the hypocalcemia and hyperkalemia intensify, the severity of the condition becomes ominous with the onset of the three C's that can portend death— *coma, convulsions*, and *cardiac arrhythmias*. Generally, death from ingestion of excessive fluoride occurs within 4 hours; if the individual survives for 4 hours, the prognosis is guarded to good.

EMERGENCY TREATMENT

Four actions are salient in treating fluoride poisoning: (1) *immediate treatment*, (2) *induced vomiting*, (3) protection of the stomach by *binding fluoride* with orally administered calcium or aluminum preparations, and (4) *maintenance of blood calcium levels* with intravenous calcium. Urgent and decisive treatment is mandatory once the PTD of 15 mg/kg has been approached or exceeded. The speed of initiating proper treatment can be critical to a person's chance for survival.[37] The blood level reaches its maximum from 0.5 to 1 hour

after the fluoride is ingested. *By that time it can be too late.*

If an excessive amount of sodium fluoride is ingested, first aid treatment can be initiated. Milk, or better yet, milk and eggs should be given, for two reasons: (1) As demulcents, they help protect the mucous membrane of the upper GI tract from chemical burns; (2) they provide the calcium that acts as a binder for the fluoride. Lime water, (calcium hydroxide) or Maalox (an aluminum preparation), can be drunk to accomplish the same purpose. Plenty of fluid, preferably milk[d] should be ingested to help dilute the fluoride compound in the stomach. Vomiting is beneficial and often occurs spontaneously; it also can be induced by digital stimulus to the base of the tongue or with syrup of ipecac, if available. When vomiting does occur, the majority of the ingested fluoride is often expelled. Preferably, the patient should be taken directly to the emergency room of a hospital. Otherwise the closest emergency medical service unit or physician capable of dealing with fluoride toxicity is the alternative.[e] Once in a well-equipped medical facility, several options are possible, such as gastric lavage, blood dialysis, or oral or intravenous calcium gluconate to maintain the blood calcium levels. Every effort should be made to rid the body rapidly of the fluoride or to negate its toxicity before a refractory hyperkalemia and cardiac fibrillation become a greater problem than the fluoride intoxication.[38]

Chronic Fluoride Exposure

At high levels of industrial fluoride exposure, as experienced by cryolite and bauxite

---

[d] A can of condensed milk can be kept indefinitely for emergency use.

[e] The phone numbers of emergency services should be readily available in an office manual or conspicuously displayed in the office.

workers prior to the era of occupational safety regulations, the combined intake of fluoride through inhalation, ingestion, and water consumption often resulted in a daily dose of over 20 mg. This exceedingly high level of continual intake for 10 to 20 years resulted in a severe *skeletal fluorosis* characterized by osteosclerosis, calcification of the tendons, and the appearance of multiple exostoses. This same crippling bone fluorosis can also occur from long-term consumption of naturally fluoridated waters found in some parts of the world, which contain 14 ppm or more of fluoride. Other factors that increase the severity of the bone fluorosis are high temperatures with a concomitant increase in drinking episodes, an elevated intake of fluoride in food, nutritional diseases, and low-calcium diets. *No* cases of skeletal fluorosis have been reported in the United States where water fluoridation concentrations were under 3.9 ppm.[24]

HOME SECURITY OF FLUORIDE PRODUCTS

The lack of home storage security of over-the-counter (OTC) and prescription fluoride products poses hazards to consumers. As presently packaged, the fluoride content of OTC fluoride products can exceed the PTD for children.[39] For instance, the swallowing of 50 fluoride tablets, or 1.7 oz of a 1000-ppm dentifrice can be lethal to a 2- or 3-year-old child (See Table 8–4).[36] That the danger at home is real is attested by two deaths of children after swallowing fluoride tablets: one in Austria, and the other in Australia.[21] In one year (1986–1987), 13 cases of fluoride poisoning were reported to the North Carolina Poison Center. It was noted by the poison center that *no health care providers who contacted the center were familiar with the treatment of the GI symptoms*

induced by fluoride poisoning.[40] Clearly, *parents* need to be educated about the hazards of fluoride-containing dental products. Dentifrices, mouth rinses, and fluoride supplements need to be *securely stored*. Equally, *health professionals* need to be educated about the emergency treatment protocol following excessive intake of fluoride.

In a larger study, the American Association of Poison Control Centers reported that the number of fluoride-related calls had increased from 3856 cases in 1984 to 7794 in 1989. Of these, the number seeking clinical treatment was 366 in 1984 and 668 in 1989. In each of these years, young children were involved in 90% of the calls.[41]

DENTAL FLUOROSIS

Enamel opacities (mottling) may be classified into three categories: (1) *dental fluorosis* due to an above-optimal intake of fluoride; (2) *nonfluoride-induced mottling*, such as caused by other specific known agents, such as strontium and tetracycline; and (3) *idiopathic mottling*, in which the cause is unknown.[42] Microscopically, dental fluorosis demonstrates a subsurface porosity of enamel, the extent of which depends on the concentration of fluoride in the environment at the time of tooth development.[43,44] The exact cause of the hypoplastic enamel is not clear, but has been attributed by various investigators to altered metabolism in any or all of the phases of the enamel formation: altered ameloblastic activity, interference with crystal nucleation or growth, or even with several possible faulty enzymatic or cofactor interrelationships.[45]

The hypomineralization of dental fluorosis occurs beneath a well-mineralized enamel surface. The lesions are symmetric.[42] Clinically, the mildest changes are characterized by a white parchment-like color that first involves the incisal edges, or cusps of posterior teeth ("snowcapping"). The configuration of the white areas can range from a few white *flecks* to occasional *white spots*. In some instances, thin, irregular white opaque streaks, or *veining*, are noted, especially in the maxillary incisors. The next level of involvement is the presence of wisps of tan-to-dark brown staining included with any of the various combinations of previous parchment-like white coloration. Finally, in moderate to severe cases, *discrete pits* may occur that are 1 to 2 mm in diameter, or several pits may be merged into a *confluent* configuration. In the severest form, the surface contour of the enamel is altered by fractures of the brittle enamel, presenting a *corroded appearance*. The stains in the severest forms are widespread and range in color from *chocolate brown to almost black*.

According to Cutress and Suckling, the teeth are *not discolored at the time of eruption*; discoloration is caused by the uptake of exogenous stains from the diet.[42] There is no evidence to suggest that any systemic or topical applications of fluorides *after* enamel maturation causes dental fluorosis. Dental fluorosis per se is not a health hazard, in fact the increased resistance to dental caries might be considered an asset if esthetics were not a consideration. There is *no* indication that the *mild* forms represent any problem or concern to the public. Only the more moderate to severe forms of dental fluorosis, which are still quite rare, are considered to be a cosmetic problem.[46]

The assessment of the prevalence and severity of dental fluorosis continues to be the *primary* scientific means of *retrospectively* estimating fluoride ingestion. By the 1970s, a logical concern had arisen that the increased ingestion of fluoride, coupled with the worldwide decrease in caries, might signal an increase in fluorosis.[47] Ac-

cordingly, several studies were initiated to determine if this hypothesis was correct.

The detection of temporal changes in the prevalence of dental fluorosis is complicated by several factors. The first problem is that different indices have been used for the assessment of dental fluorosis in different areas by different investigators. Five principal indices have been introduced, and three are used commonly today. Historically, Dean's index, or the community fluorosis index (CFI), was the only index available for many years and was used extensively.[48] More recently, the Thylstrup and Fejerskov index (TF index),[49] the tooth surface index of fluorosis (Table 8–5),[50] the fluorosis risk index (FRI),[51] and the epidemiological index of developmental defects of dental enamel (DDE)[52] have introduced new systems for the measurement of dental fluorosis.

A second problem with dental fluorosis, especially in its mildest forms, is that it is difficult to diagnose.[43,53] Therefore, when different examiners use different indices to survey dental fluorosis in different areas, caution is warranted in comparing data of one survey with another. It is ironic that none of these indices was designed specifically to quantify esthetic problems or appearance of teeth, which is often the main (and sometimes the only) concern voiced by the public when water fluoridation is proposed.[54] Therefore, none of the cited studies relate to any specific public health problem, just to the prevalence and severity of the condition. An increase in dental fluorosis by itself is not as much a dental public health concern, as it is an indication that the total fluoride exposure may be more than necessary to prevent tooth decay. Prudent public health practice generally dictates using no more of a substance than the amount necessary to achieve the desired effect.[14]

A U.S. Public Health Service (USPHS) report[14] reported on investigations to deter-

TABLE 8–5. DESCRIPTIVE CRITERIA AND SCORING SYSTEM FOR THE TOOTH SURFACE INDEX OF FLUOROSIS (TSIF)

Numerical Score	Descriptive Criteria
0	Enamel shows no evidence of fluorosis.
1	Enamel shows definite evidence of fluorosis, namely areas with parchment-white color that total less than one third of the visible enamel surface. This category includes fluorosis confined only to incisal edges of anterior teeth and cusp tips of posterior teeth ("snowcapping").
2	Parchment-white fluorosis totals at least one third of the visible surface, but less than two-thirds.
3	Parchment-white fluorosis totals at least two thirds of the visible surface.
4	Enamel shows staining in conjunction with any of the preceding levels of fluorosis. Staining is defined as an area of definite discoloration that may range from light to very dark brown.
5	Discrete pitting of the enamel exists, unaccompanied by evidence of staining of intact enamel. A pit is defined as a definite physical defect in the enamel surface with a rough floor that is surrounded by a wall of intact enamel. The pitted area is usually stained or differs in color from the surrounding enamel.
6	Both discrete pitting and staining of the intact enamel exist.
7	Confluent pitting of the enamel surface exists. Large areas of enamel may be missing and the anatomy of the tooth may be altered. Dark brown stain is usually present.

(*From Horowitz HS, Driscoll WS, Meyers RJ et al. A new method for assessing the prevalence of dental fluorosis—the tooth surface index of fluorosis. J Am Dent Assoc. 1984; 109:37–41.*)

mine if the prevalence of dental fluorosis had increased. Three types of comparisons were used.

1. Comparison of dental fluorosis in the same cities, using the same index and the same examiners every 5 years
2. Comparison of dental fluorosis in the same cities as Dean's original surveys 30 or 40 years ago, using the same index, but different examiners
3. Comparison of dental fluorosis from the 1940s to the 1980s and 1990s in different cities, but with similar water fluoride concentrations, using the same index and different examiners

Given the possibility of examiner variation and other potential errors, the USPHS report of these studies[14] estimated that the prevalence of dental fluorosis in nonfluori-

dated and fluoridated areas, respectively, has increased by 5% (from about 1% to 6%) and 9% (from about 13% to 22%) over the last 30 to 40 years. The results confirmed that the great majority of the increase in dental fluorosis had occurred primarily in the milder or lower categories, and that the prevalence of moderate to severe cases remained essentially unchanged. In contrast to the foregoing USPHS findings, Pendrys and Stamm,[55] in a subsequent review of the topic, estimated that in areas with negligible to 0.3 ppm fluoride the prevalence of dental fluorosis increased from 1% in the 1940s to 10% during the 1980s, with a corresponding increase in optimally fluoridated areas from 13% to 23%. More recent reviews suggest even higher prevalences for nonfluoridated and fluoridated areas, in the range of 20% to 35% and 30% to 45%, respectively.[56,57]

In response to an increase of fluorosis in Hong Kong, the level of fluoride in the water was reduced from 1.0 ppm to 0.7 ppm in 1978. A further reduction to 0.4 to 0.5 ppm was made in 1988.[58] Using the level of fluorosis seen on the incisal edge of the upper right central incisor, it was found that following the downward adjustment of fluoride level, the prevalence of dental fluorosis decreased from 64% to 47%. Despite this change, the prevalence of caries continued to decline.[59]

Question 2. Which of the following statements, if any, are correct?

A. Following absorption, it takes approximately *10 hours* for the blood plasma to reach its maximum fluoride level.

B. The ingestion of 20 mg/kg for a 20-year-old adult is considered *below* the probable toxic dose.

C. The first aid treatment for fluoride toxicity is well known by *health professionals*.

D. The staining seen in dental fluorosis occurs *posteruption*.

E. Dental fluorosis prevalence has continued to *increase* despite the fact that water fluoride concentrations have remained *constant*.

Fluoride Ingestion and Fluorosis

The historic standard of 1 ppm as the optimum amount of fluoride necessary to reduce caries to a minimum without increasing the prevalence of fluorosis is a complex issue today because of the multiple sources of fluoride available. More important is the variability of ingestion that occurs from these sources. Although the cause for dental fluorosis is known; the ability to control the varying levels of fluoride ingestion by children is not easily managed.

Studies of fluoride intake show that there are three prime sources of ingested fluoride: fluoridated water, soft drinks, den-

tifrices (and to a lesser extent, fluoride supplements).[60,61]

In one study, the range of daily fluoride intake of a 2-year-old child with *1 ppm fluoridated water*, food, and dentifrice was estimated to range from 0.5 to 2.6 mg/day. In a nonfluoridated area with its minimal intake of water fluoride, a child receiving a *fluoride supplement* in addition to the food and a dentifrice, has an intake range from 0.7 to 2.8 mg/day.[55] Thus, in *both* cases, the risk of fluorosis increases as the intake exceeds 1.0 mg/day.[f] In another study involving 6-year-old children,[62] the average dietary fluoride intake was 0.86 mg/day in a *non*fluoridated area—an amount considered nearly optimal.[61] Beverages and drinking water contributed 75% of this total.

The amount of fluoridated water ingested from the tap varies considerably from area to area; the amount of fluoride in the water used for cooking can be concentrated by evaporation; and by the amount of fluoride in the water supply used by commercial food processors in preparing their products. When taken together, Armstrong and coworkers showed that children under the age of 3 consumed an average of 0.6 L of water per day, ranging between 0.1 and 0.9 L.[63] If these liquids are fluoridated at 1 ppm, then the mean daily intake of fluoride from tap water and tap-water-based beverages ranges from 0.1 to 0.9 mg for 3-year-olds. For children 3 to 5, the intake ranges from 0.4 to 1.5 mg.

In both fluoridated and nonfluoridated areas, the daily intake of fluoride depends strongly on the concentrations of fluoride in available commercial products, which as Levy points out, not only vary within the same product over time but oftentimes is unreported on the labels. The pattern of

---

[f] The World Health Organization has established a threshold of 1.5 mg/L, above which the risk of fluorosis increases rapidly.

soft drink consumption also varies widely.[60] These findings suggest that the use of fluoridated water in the processing of soft drinks and reconstituted juices is largely responsible for the "halo effect" seen in nonfluoridated communities.

The ingestion of fluoride toothpaste following toothbrushing is significant for children under age 6, especially considering the fact that this is during the period of tooth formation. Children under 6 years of age often brush in an unsupervised manner, and an excess of fluoride is swallowed, especially when using dentifrices containing 1000 and 1500 ppm.[64] Children can swallow from 35% to 50% of the fluoride from dentifrices while brushing.[65] For children between the ages of 3 and 6 years, the mean daily ingestion of fluoride from dentifrice ranges from 0.1 to 0.4 mg per brushing. At this level of intake, twice daily brushing would account for almost all of the optimal daily requirement of fluoride.[11,60] In one study, those children who brushed their teeth with fluoride dentifrices before 25 months of age, had 11 times the risk for fluorosis compared with those beginning brushing at a later date.[66]

Research on fluoride ingestion points out the difficulty in determining a child's intake accurately, primarily because of the multiple sources with varying concentrations of fluoride available in commercial and dental products. In considering the data on the range of fluoride ingested daily, Levy suggests that a significant number of children exceed their optimal daily fluoride requirements from the use of fluoride dentifrices alone.[60] Other sources of fluoride are supplemental fluoride drops and tablets, which will be discussed later.

Treatment of Dental Fluorosis

Most teeth with dental fluorosis are so mild in appearance that they are apparently acceptable esthetically. In more severe cases, two general methods have been used to improve the appearance of fluorosed teeth. The first is to attempt to *remove* the mottling and stain, and the second is to esthetically *cover* them. Both methods are being used either individually or in combination. The *removal* method requires that the stain and organic debris be removed from the micropores that make up the surface porosity. To accomplish this, a 35% hydrogen peroxide solution is applied to remove the stain from micropores extending into a thin layer of surface enamel. In some cases, this method is satisfactory. In others, the openings of the micropores are clogged by posteruptive mineral deposits from the saliva. As a result, many clinicians opt for the use of various concentrations of hydrochloric acid to uncover the micropores and to gain entry to the stained areas that are often within 0.1 mm from the enamel surface.

The next refinement was to combine the acid and bleaching techniques, using hydrochloric acid, Superoxal,[g] and ether to daub on the teeth.[67] Refinements include adding pumice to the solution to make a paste, which is slowly brushed on the teeth, or to use a 12-fluted finishing bur or stone to abrade off the acid-moistened superficial layer of enamel.[68] In the end, the acid-etched area is neutralized by the application of sodium bicarbonate or sodium hypochlorite, followed by flushing with water. For all procedures, a rubber dam is used. Each acid treatment of a tooth lasts for only a few minutes. The number of treatments needed depends on the desired end point, realizing that improvement, rather than total esthetic perfection, is often the expected objective.

Since the introduction of enamel adhesives as part of the repertoire of esthetic dentistry, impetus has grown for covering the enamel defect. Again, there are two approaches. In one, after acid-etching the sur-

[g] Superoxal = 35% hydrogen peroxide.

face of the tooth, a thin layer of an appropriate shade of the enamel adhesive is applied
with a brush.[69] At times, an initial coat of a
masking adhesive is needed to conceal very
marked enamel defects. A variation on the
brushed-on enamel adhesive is the veneer,[h]
which is placed over the entire labial surface of a tooth that is moderately to severely
mottled. For severely fluorosed teeth involving all surfaces, a tooth-colored crown
may be necessary. This assortment of options permits all fluorosed teeth—from the
mildest to the severest categories—to be
successfully and esthetically restored.

CONTINUING FLUORIDE RESEARCH

Basic and clinical research continues to improve understanding of the mechanisms of
fluoride action on bone and teeth, as well as
to identify any additional perceived risks
and benefits. For example, one of the current concerns is the relationship of fluoride
ingestion and the risk of bone fractures seen
in osteoporosis.

Interest in the connection between
bone and fluoride metabolism stems from
the following facts: (1) the number of osteoblasts increases in the presence of fluoride, (2) the rate of bone formation increases, and (3) the serum activity of
skeletal alkaline phosphatase rises.[70] Despite these cellular-level effects, the relationship between the lifelong ingestion of
fluoride and bone fractures is unclear. For a
time, the use of a high daily dosage of fluoride was advocated as a treatment for osteoporosis. Well-controlled studies, however,
have changed this opinion, and the current
consensus is that *high daily doses* of fluoride

have not demonstrated any beneficial effect
in either preventing or reversing osteoporosis.[71]

At least three investigations have examined the possible effect of consuming fluoridated drinking water on the incidence of hip
fractures: in the one in Finland[72] fewer hip
fractures occurred; in the two in the United
States more occurred. In the two U.S. studies, the fluoride water levels in one of the investigations was 4 ppm, which is above
drinking water standards.[73] In the second
U.S. study, the geographic relationship between the number of fractures seen in the
northern and southern United States was
much more significant than the relationship
of fluoride levels to hip fractures. This
prompted the authors of the study to conclude that no presently recognized factor or
factors could adequately explain the observed geographic differences in fracture incidence.[74] Because of the importance of the
subject, the National Institutes of Health
convened a conference to evaluate all of the
studies relating fluoride to bone health. In a
report published in 1992, the conference
participants concluded that "there was not
an adequate basis for making firm conclusions relating fluoride levels in drinking
water to hip fracture and bone health."[75] Future research was encouraged, however.

In 1987, the National Resources Defense Council (NRDC), a civilian activist organization, won a federal court decision
against the Environmental Protection
Agency (EPA). In this judgment, the EPA
was challenged on the adequacy of existing
research, claiming that naturally fluoridated
water with 2 to 4 ppm and above of fluoride could be carcinogenic. This litigation
prompted two federal studies: one by the
National Toxicology Program (NTP) of the
U.S. Public Health Service,[76] and the second by the Committee of Toxicology of the
National Research Council.

---

[h] A veneer is a thin, color-matched overlay that is permanently bonded to the facial surface of a tooth,
much like an artificial fingernail.

The NTP program involved rat and mice feeding studies routinely used to identify potential hazards of any chemical at various dosage levels. At the conclusion of the study, the peer review panel concluded that the evidence of carcinogenic activity from sodium fluoride was equivocal, based on the occurrence of a very small number of osteosarcomas in dosed rodents.

The second study was a major review by the National Research Council to determine whether the EPA's *maximum contaminant level (MCL)* of 4 mg of fluoride per liter of drinking water was appropriate. The study included the following areas: fluorosis; risk of bone fracture; reproductive effects; effect on renal, gastrointestinal, and immune systems; genotoxicity; and carcinogenicity of fluoride. The subcommittee concluded that the EPA's current MCL of 4 mg/L for fluoride in drinking water is appropriate as an interim standard.[77]

Even more important for direct applicability to humans, Hoover and coworkers at the National Cancer Institute expanded and extended an earlier major study of *all counties* in the United States to determine the relationship of cancer mortality to the fluoridation status of the drinking water.[78] Data were collected from cancer registries, originating as far back as 1973 and including 25 million individual entries for evaluation. The conclusion was "If fluoride presents any risks to the public at the levels to which the vast majority of us are exposed, those risks are so small that they have been impossible to detect in the epidemiological studies to date . . . In contrast, the benefits [of fluoride] are great and easy to detect."[79]

FLUORIDATION OF WATER

Previously we mentioned that 1 ppm of fluoride in the water supply provides maxi-

mum caries protection and minimum dental fluorosis. In the 1990s, this statement needs to be revised. First, it has been recognized that individuals living in colder climates drink less fluid than those residing in hotter areas. If the average daily consumption of water is more than a liter, then the 1 ppm fluoride concentration must be reduced proportionately; if less than 1 ppm, more must be added. Therefore, the optimum concentration of fluoride in community water supplies is dependent on the average daily fluid intake of the population, which in turn is dependent on the *annual average of maximum daily air temperatures* in a specific community and possible ingestion from other sources.[80] The relationship of temperature to fluoride augmentation is well recognized and is shown in Table 8–6. The increased ingestion of fluoride from all sources, however, has prompted experts worldwide to reexamine these recommendations. In fact, several countries have adjusted the recommended level of water fluoride downward.

The addition of 1 ppm of fluoride to the water involves no engineering problems beyond those already encountered and solved in dealing with chlorine and other

TABLE 8–6. RECOMMENDED OPTIMAL FLUORIDE LEVEL

Annual Average of Maximum Daily Air Temperatures (°F)*	Optimal Fluoride
40.0–53.7	1.2
53.8–58.3	1.1
58.4–63.8	1.0
63.9–70.6	0.9
70.7–79.2	0.8
79.3–90.5	0.7

*Based on temperature data obtained from a minimum of 5 years.
(*From Centers for Disease Control, National Center for Prevention Services, Dental Disease Prevention Activity.*)

water treatment processes. Fluoride does not affect the taste, odor, color, or turbidity of the water at the levels used for water fluoridation. The fluoride content can be maintained within a narrow range of concentration. In over 3000 checks of water fluoride content in Grand Rapids, Michigan, over a 10-year period, 99% of the tests showed a concentration between 0.8 and 1.2 ppm. In general, larger municipalities with full-time water engineers maintain a more constant fluoride concentration.

Occasionally, the problem encountered is that a community is not sufficiently prepared to fluoridate public water supplies. Inadequate training of operators, poor storage facilities, malfunctioning fluoride feed equipment, and lack of proper water analysis equipment have been noted. In the majority of cases this resulted in fluoride levels being consistently under the programmed level of 1 ppm.[81] To combat this problem of insufficient maintenance of waterworks, the Centers for Disease Control and Prevention maintains an ongoing program for consultation and guidance.[82]

The fluoridation of water may be accomplished using either dry compounds, such as fluorspar, sodium fluoride, and sodium silicofluoride, or solutions of hydrofluorosilicic acid. No single chemical is best for all conditions and for all sizes of water plants. Selection depends on the (1) size of the plant; (2) number of points at which fluoride is introduced into the water; (3) delivered cost of the fluoride agent; (4) use of an existing plant, with modifications, or a new plant; and (5) the plant manager's personal preference. The equipment for employing *dry* material consists of a hopper into which the fluoride compound is placed—usually from 100-lb bags or drums.

The hopper has a motorized unit at the bottom to ensure positive movement of the powder into a dissolving tank. Following so-lution of the salts in the dissolving tank, the saturated supernatant fluid is injected into the water line, using a *metering pump*. This pump is constructed to feed a given amount of fluoride solution continually into a proportionate amount of water being pumped (see Fig 8–3). Liquid fluoride feeders require only a metering pump between the container of the hydrofluorosilicic acid and the point of injection.[82]

The point of injection of fluoride into the water usually follows the steps in which alum coagulation and water filtration occur, because these processes tend to remove some of the fluoride. The possibility of excessive amounts of fluoride entering the

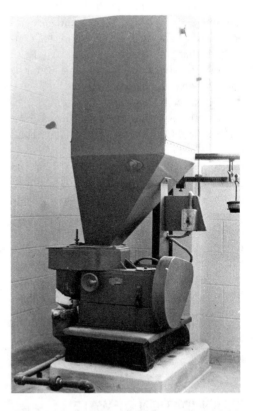

Figure 8–3. A volumetric roll-type dry feeder feeds sodium silicofluoride to a population of 10,000 people in Winchester, Tenn. (*Courtesy of Dr D.R. Collier, Tennessee Department of Health.*)

water supply is controlled by (1) the limited amount of fluoride maintained in the hoppers, (2) the positive controls on feeding fluoride from the hoppers into the dissolving tanks, and (3) the proven safety of a metering pump that is electrically connected to the water pump, so that if one fails, both stop operation.

In the period between the pioneer water fluoridation studies and 1993, five fatalities have occurred. The first occurred in Annapolis, Maryland, to an individual attached to a kidney dialysis unit at the same time a spill occurred at the water plant. Contrary to USPHS recommendations that mineral-free water be used for dialysis, tap water was used in this case.[83] Also contributing to this death was the fact that the individual did not seek medical care at the time of initial illness.

The second death, in 1992, occurred at Hooper Bay, a small village in northern Alaska. Several factors are believed to have contributed to this death: improper equipment, incorrect installation, and inadequate operator monitoring.[84]

The final three deaths occurred in 1993 in a Chicago kidney dialysis facility. This time the water fluoride level was not increased. Instead, the problem was a failure in the deionization unit intended to remove even low levels of fluoride and other ions. The preliminary findings indicate an unexplained release of a high concentration of fluoride from the deionizer.[85]

Question 3. Which of the following statements, if any, are correct?

A. In nonfluoridated areas, the risk of dental fluorosis is increased by the *"halo effect"* of water fluoridation.

B. The stain of dental fluorosis can be either removed by a bleach or covered over with a tooth-colored material.

C. A high daily dosage of fluoride is *beneficial* in the treatment of osteoporosis.

D. The amount of fluoride added to the water varies *inversely* with the average annual temperature of an area.

E. The *metering pump* should be electrically connected to the water pump in such a way that if the water pump stops, both stop.

DEFLUORIDATION OF WATER

The need to fluoridate water supplies to reduce dental caries is balanced by a similar obligation to remove excessive amounts of fluorides (defluoridate) from naturally over fluoridated waters. This obligation was made into law by the *1986 Congressional Safe Drinking Water Act*. Under this act, the EPA established 4.00 ppm as the maximum concentration of fluoride allowed in drinking waters in the United States. *Natural* water sources exceeding this level *must* be defluoridated.[86] At the same time, a secondary standard of 2 ppm for a *natural* source was also established as the *recommended* (but not federally enforceable) maximum. Under this secondary standard, when the water exceeds 2 ppm, community residents are informed of the greater risk for dental fluorosis.[86] Note that this regulation applies to natural water supplies. At the same time, it does not permit *adding* fluoride to a level higher than the 1 ppm optimum for a given temperature (See Table 8–6).

The ideal method for defluoridating a community's water supply is to blend the water from a well containing a low level of fluoride. Unfortunately, adjacent sources of water, one with a high and the other with a lower fluoride content, are not often encountered. Therefore, other chemical methods must be used to defluoridate natural water supplies that contain an excess of fluoride.

Defluoridation is carried out by adding chemicals to precipitate the fluoride or to absorb fluoride on other precipitated compounds. Chemicals usually used include *calcium* oxide (lime), *magnesium* compounds (dolomite), and *aluminum* sulfate (alum). Following the addition of these chemicals, mixing basins, flocculating units, settling basins, and filtering beds are needed to allow the precipitates and particulate matter to settle. These beds need to be cleaned constantly of the accumulating *sludges*.

Following defluoridation in Bartlett, Texas, dental fluorosis dropped from 80% to 18%, and the severity of the cases dropped from the originally severe and moderately severe to acceptably normal, questionable, or mild.

About 1100 water systems in the United States exceed the established maximum allowable fluoride concentration. Many municipalities have still not defluoridated despite the congressional mandate. Reasons for this slow response are varied: (1) defluoridation is approximately 10 times as expensive as water fluoridation, and compulsory defluoridation could bankrupt many municipalities, (2) little protest arises about mottling from individuals who have grown up in areas where dental fluorosis is endemic, and (3) the EPA must consider the availability of alternative water supplies for those municipalities in the event that the decision is made to close existent waterworks.

ALTERNATIVES TO WATER FLUORIDATION

Approximately 113,000,000 U.S. citizens do not receive the benefit of water fluoridation because they (1) are located in remote areas with no central water supplies, (2) reside in municipalities that do not have the money to fluoridate, (3) live in a community that refuses to institute fluoridation for a variety of reasons, or (4) consume bottled water deficient in fluoride. To overcome these obstacles, fluoride supplements were developed to provide systemic fluoride to children and adolescents without access to an optimally fluoridated water supply. Supplements come either in the form of drops, tablets, or lozenges. Generally, the drops are used by infants who can't chew a tablet or suck on a lozenge. Drops are usually administered with a dropper, from which 10 drops equals 1 mg of fluoride. Ten drops placed in 1 L of water containing no fluoride produces a concentration of 1 ppm of fluoride (1 mg/mL). Thus, if the local water supply contains only 0.3 ppm and there is a need, for say, 0.7 ppm as the optimum, 4 drops are added to a liter of water. If the entire liter of water is used during the day in place of regular tap water, the child receives the recommended amount of systemic fluoride for that day. Unfortunately, the daily preparation of water in this manner is time-consuming for parents and is often abandoned. To help improve compliance, current recommendations suggest that the drops be added directly to a glass of water or to juice for immediate consumption. This latter method provides a once-a-day peak fluoride level that is not as desirable as the more stable lower level that accompanies the more frequent drinking of fluoridated water.

Probably the most common method of supplementation is the use of tablets that contain 1 mg of fluoride. Like the drops, tablets and lozenges are dispensed by *prescription* in the United States. This is not the case in Canada and other parts of the world, where they are available over the counter. To improve safety, the American Dental Association recommends that no more than 264 sodium fluoride tablets be dispensed at any one time to minimize the possibility of reaching lethal accumulations in the medicine cabinet. As an additional safety measure, the tablets are usually scored (grooved) to permit using one half or even one quarter of a tablet to permit a more precise dosage. Some tablets are flavored to improve child acceptance, a practice which also adds to the danger of overdose. At times, the fluoride tablets may contain vitamins, especially vitamin C. This vitamin supplement neither augments nor detracts from the effectiveness of the tablet as a caries control measure; it only adds to the expense.

Tablets and lozenges have the advantage of being ready to use and requiring little time or effort to dispense. Yet, like fluoride drops, when tablet programs are conducted in the home, they are generally unsuccessful because of parent noncompliance. Tablets and lozenges also have disadvantages, probably the greatest being that they are overprescribed in both fluoridated and nonfluoridated communities. This is seen in a report by Kuthy and McTigue, who stated that errors are frequently made in prescribed dosages because recommended dosage schedules are not followed or because practitioners fail to estimate the child's daily fluoride intake from drinking water and from other sources.[87] To remedy overprescription requires an intensive educational program of all undergraduate and graduate health professionals involved in the prescribing chain, especially physicians, dentists and pharmacists. Recently, Dr. James Mason, Assistant Secretary for Health, provided an advisory in the *Journal of the American Medical Association* to explain to physicians the relationship of fluoride tablet dosage and dental fluorosis.[88]

Once a child is old enough to swish fluid around the mouth, it is suggested that the tablets be chewed and the fluoride-saturated saliva swished between the teeth for a minute before swallowing. In this way both a topical and a systemic dosage of fluoride is achieved.

TIMING OF FLUORIDE SUPPLEMENTS

The anticaries activity of fluoride is due to the (1) preeruptive effects on the morphology and mineralization of the developing teeth,[89] (2) sufficient concentrations of fluoride in the saliva to act as a plaque antibacterial agent,[90] and probably the most important, (3) its property of reducing demineralization and facilitating remineralization.[91]

There is still uncertainty about the role of preeruptive fluoride supplements. Presently, the tendency is to discount the belief that preeruptive incorporation of fluoride into the enamel is the *principal* mechanism for protection of the later erupting teeth.[92] The possibility of some important preeruptive benefits cannot be ruled out, however.[91] For example, it has been noted that in fluoridated areas, the cusps are rounder, the fossae shallower, and the fissure approximations tighter, all of which help to reduce the risk of occlusal pit-and-fissure caries.[93,94]

It is recommended that the timing of the fluoride administration should involve all stages of tooth development, although the most effective time seems to be during the pre- and posteruptive *maturation* periods.[13,95] Thylstrup believes that the most critical period for fluoride administration is immediately after the teeth erupt into the oral cavity.[96] To specifically identify whether the benefits of fluoride could be attributed to events before or after eruption, Groeneveld and associates reviewed the pre- and posteruptive effects of longitudinal data from the Culemborg (nonfluoridated) and Tiel (fluoridated) water study in the Netherlands. They stated that 66% of the reduction in pit-and-fissure caries came from preeruptive fluoride; on the smooth surfaces, however, this effect was reduced to 25%. For interproximal surfaces, the reduction was due half to pre- and half to posteruptive fluoride, although the total reduction in surfaces was greater for smooth surfaces compared with pit and fissures.[97]

Question 4. Which of the following statements, if any, are correct?

A. A *natural* water supply with over 4 ppm *must* be defluoridated; a supply between 2 and 4 pmm is *not* required by law to be defluoridated.

B. Home administration of fluoride drops and tablets in caries preventive programs have an *excellent* record of *parental compliance*.

C. The iatrogenic outcome of overprescription of fluoride supplements is dental fluorosis.

D. The *principal* protective effect of ingested fluoride occurs *preeruptively*.

E. It is believed that the greatest preeruptive effect of fluoride on teeth is to curtail the number of *pit-and-fissure* lesions.

Hargreaves showed that fluoride levels in primary enamel paralleled the fluoride levels in the drinking water up to 2.2 mg/L.[98] The need for early fluoride protection of the primary teeth of high-risk children is demonstrated in one study in which 20% of the children had carious lesions by age 2 and by age 3 over 50% were affected. Between the ages of 2 and 3, the permanent maxillary incisors are also developing, with the most critical times for the development of dental fluorosis of the incisal edge being

from 22 to 26 months.[99] Herein lies a dilemma.

In attempting to protect some teeth with fluoride supplements during the posteruptive maturation period, the risk of eventual fluorosis to other developing teeth in the preeruptive stage is increased. When water and food were the only sources of fluoride, the 1 ppm that balanced the reduction of caries against the extent of fluorosis was an acceptable working formula. Now, with the multiple sources of fluoride, this balance is tipping towards an increasing prevalence of dental fluorosis. Several partial solutions have been proposed.

1. Market toothpastes with lower concentrations of fluoride for children. This should be possible because the FDA requires that the concentration of fluoride in a dentifrice must be over 650 ppm to make caries prevention claims, a concentration considerably below that in several preparations now on the market with 1000 ppm or higher.[86]

2. Place a warning label on the tubes of all fluoride dentifrices indicating the concentration, and the fact that the paste should not be used by children under 6 without parental supervision.

3. Parents should supervise children up to the age of 6 to ensure that only a pea-sized amount of dentifrice is applied to the brush, and that the child thoroughly rinses and spits following each brushing. These precautions should be even more stringent if the child brushes more than once a day. The need for such precautions underlines the need for toothpastes with lower than conventional fluoride concentrations for pre school-aged children.[100]

4. Develop dentifrice dispensers with

a smaller orifice to limit the amount of dentifrice expelled. One study by Faller and colleagues indicated, however, that education was more important to limiting the amount of dentifrice dispensed than was a reduction of 25% in the size of the tube orifice.[101]

5. Label bottled water showing the fluoride concentration in parts per million.

Some of the discussions of separate scientific groups in Canada and Europe seeking to limit the ingestion of fluoride for children 0 to 3 years of age are of interest. Recommendations have been made to commence supplements at age 3 instead of at birth.[102,103] In view of past emphasis on the need for supplements, such a change to withhold fluoride tablets until a child reaches 3 would require a strong publicity campaign involving dentists, physicians, and the public. In Canada, where this change is already being implemented, both public and professional groups seem to have accepted this alternative without great difficulty.[104]

The recommendation's rationale is that the key *primary* preventive effect from fluoride is *remineralization*, which is a posteruptive phenomenon. With this in mind, the use of supplements starting at age 3 still afford significant preventive effects for the permanent teeth. The discussion that perhaps influenced many experts centered on the question: "For the small group of children who receive supplements before the age of 3, will they benefit and are they at risk for dental fluorosis?" Studies confirm that although few parents of children actually do comply with the use of supplements over the long term, for those that do, their children will probably have dental fluorosis. Data from numerous studies support this conclusion.[105–108]

The question then is, if the child needs the protection that supplements can offer, can the risk of dental fluorosis be reduced? The work of Evans and Stamm suggests that the developing permanent maxillary incisors are most susceptible to dental fluorosis between the ages of 18 and 30 months.[109] Therefore, if supplements are given at age 3, full posteruptive benefits will be realized while avoiding the risk of developing fluorosis of the permanent anterior dentition.

Further support for eliminating supplements before the age of 3 comes from the likelihood that the parents who give their children supplements, also brush their children's teeth with a fluoride-containing dentifrice, coincidentally contributing to additional intake of fluoride.[11] *This action alone prevents dental caries for most children*.

Discussions are now in progress to determine if dosage levels should be modified. One of the best literature reviews supporting this need is by Riordan who urges that the maximum fluoride ion content of a tablet be 0.5 mg and that there be no upper age level for supplementation because caries has no age limit.[110] Looking at the other end of the age spectrum, the possibility of adult supplementation needs to be addressed in nonfluoridated areas when the risk to either root or coronal caries is high. This need is especially apropos considering the key role fluoride plays in root caries prevention by concentrating it in the more permeable cementum.[111] Also, supplementation takes full advantage of the remineralization potential for both root and coronal caries.

SALT FLUORIDATION

In the 1940s in Switzerland, Wespi was studying the effects on the thyroids of newborns of different amounts of iodine in salt.

At that time he learned of Dean's work with fluoride in the United States.[112] By 1946, he had produced a table salt with both iodine and fluoride. By 1955, salt was available in Switzerland with 5 mg of potassium iodide and 90 mg of sodium fluoride. The amounts of iodide and fluoride were later increased in steps, until by 1981 the supplements had reached 10 mg of iodide and 250 ppm of sodium fluoride, a level that is still maintained. One-kilogram packages of salt with or without iodide or fluoride or without both are available in stores at no difference in cost. Fluoridated salt is not sold in Basel, which is the one Swiss city that has had water fluoridation since 1962.

The successful Swiss use of fluoridated salt was followed by programs in Colombia, Hungary, Finland, and Spain. The Pan American Health Organization is supporting such programs for developing countries of the western hemisphere.[113] In 1981, Mexico issued regulations for the iodinization and fluoridation of salt to be used for human consumption. As in Switzerland, provisions were made to provide a fluoride-free salt in areas where water fluoride levels are at an optimal level. Salt fluoridation appears to be the most effective method for delivering fluoride to a target population where water fluoridation is not possible or, as is the case in parts of Europe, of achieving a high level of caries control while avoiding the firestorm of antifluoridationist opposition.

Salt fluoridation has both advantages and disadvantages. Fluoridated salt is safe. A toxic level of the sodium chloride is reached long before toxic levels of fluoride can be ingested. No supervised waterworks nor water distribution systems are necessary, making it a practical method for many countries. The possibility of fluorosis is minimized by the fact that children use very little salt. There is freedom of choice, which

blunts a major rallying point for the fluorophobes. One of the most attractive features of salt fluoridation is the low cost. In Switzerland, as in Finland, an additional approximate \$0.012/kg of salt is required for the fluoride, manpower, and marketing. The disadvantages are few. Control of individual consumption is not as precise as is possible with water fluoridation, because salt intake varies greatly among people. Because children don't consume much salt, their ingestion of fluoride is less when they need it most. Another objection is that the international effort to reduce sodium intake to help control hypertension consequently reduces fluoride intake.

THE POLITICS OF FLUORIDATION

In 1954, Puerto Rico was the first political unit under the U.S. flag to legislate commonwealth fluoridation. Connecticut was the *first state* to mandate statewide fluoridation, followed by Illinois, Minnesota, Michigan, Georgia, Nebraska, Ohio, South Dakota, and others. Delaware, Maine, and Nevada require a referendum prior to municipal fluoridation; New Hampshire and Utah have "option out" laws whereby a municipality may indicate within a set time that it does not wish to fluoridate. In Massachusetts, the board of health may order fluoridation, but the public may vote to be exempted. In Tennessee, where there is no mandatory state law, 95% of its public water supplies have been fluoridated as a result of statewide education programs. In Maryland, the state supreme court has ruled that the state health department has the power to enforce fluoridation by withholding state formula funds.

Court challenges that fluoridation is unconstitutional on the basis of civil liberties and religion have been rejected.[114] One court case in Alton, Illinois, remained in litigation from 1967 to 1984, before being ruled constitutional by the Illinois supreme court. Many of the water fluoridation cases have been appealed to the U.S. Supreme Court, which has *never* accepted any such cases for review. In general, most public health laws survive legal challenges if they are shown to be reasonable attempts to protect and promote the public health and safety in a manner plausibly designed to accomplish such a goal.[115]

As a final note, state laws work well only if provisions for financial support are included in the law mandating fluoridation.

Proponents of Fluoridation

The safety and effectiveness of fluoridation of water have probably been the most extensively researched of all public health measures now in use. The American Medical Association has long endorsed water fluoridation, indicating that there is no evidence that any pathology results from the daily ingestion of water containing 2 ppm of fluoride. In this endorsement, it specifically pointed out that there is no evidence of adverse altered physiology or morphology of the kidneys, endocrine glands, soft tissues, liver, growth patterns, congenital anomalies, enzymes, placental transfer, milk, deafness, allergy, cancer, Down syndrome, or toxicities. This endorsement supporting the safety of water fluoridation is echoed by the USPHS, ADA, American Public Health Association, World Health Organization, National Cancer Institute, National Academy of Sciences, and other domestic and foreign health organizations.

Antifluoridation Strategies

As previously indicated, the opposition to water fluoridation started with its introduction in 1945 and has continued unabated to this day. Although the resistance to fluorida-tion has remained strong for a half a century, the issues and the nature of this opposition has changed little through time. Today, the *alleged* single most important issue is a moral one involving personal rights.[116]

Whenever a community initiates activity to fluoridate its water supply, letters to the editor begin to appear in the local newspaper providing misinformation about adverse effects of the ingestion of fluorides. The phone lines of local radio talk shows are clogged with antifluoridationists often voicing bizarre claims that confuse the public. According to Hastreiter,[117] antifluoridationist rhetoric in the United States has three basic themes: (1) fluoridation is not effective in reducing dental disease, (2) fluoridation is basically harmful to the human system, and (3) when fluoridation is applied as a public health measure, it deprives individuals of free choice by forcing them to accept medication against their will. The apparent strength of their arguments rests on three main factors. (1) The arguments are simple and easy to follow, and their weaknesses difficult for laypeople to grasp. (2) Their arguments are based on widely held cultural mores—individual rights, fear of the unknown, fear of poison, and fear of bodily harm. (3) There is a tendency to perceive the world as menacing.

In many respects the appeal to the populace by the antifluoridationists is similar to that seen in psychologic warfare: if the "big lie" is repeated often enough it becomes the "big truth." Little attention is paid to the scientific literature that rebuts these allegations.[118] Similarly, the fact that 10-year postfluoridation pediatric examinations in Newburgh and Kingston showed no differences in physical status, goes unheeded.[119]

Scientific refutation around the time of a referendum vote is usually ignored or misunderstood; reason and logic are subverted by politics and emotion. The confusion that is generated can then be followed by a very logical suggestion by the antifluoridationists to postpone the vote until a later date to allow time to study a particular issue further. Such a suggestion would be quite plausible were it not for the fact that the specific issue has probably been studied many times before. However, to the cautious politician, such a suggestion provides an expedient means of avoiding a decision that might cost votes. The methods of the antifluoridationists are becoming more sophisticated.[120] When fluoridation referendums are initiated, petitions are circulated among organizations with similar self-protection objectives—some environmentalists, individuals who desire publicity, and chronic dissident groups—in an attempt to secure sufficient signatures to negate the original referendum. The courts are being used increasingly to challenge either the outcome of a referendum or to seek injunctions against a city planning to fluoridate a water supply.

Now, instead of concentrating their activities only in those communities contemplating fluoridation, efforts are being made to influence lawmakers to rescind previous legislation, or at least to downgrade it to local option voting. In some instances, the opposition against fluoridation has gone beyond its customary stance by opposing other community preventive programs that incorporate fluoride procedures.

Securing Acceptance to Fluoridation

At least three approaches are recommended for implementing the fluoridation of water supplies. The first approach is for health professionals to determine the need, safety, and cost benefits of the program, after which health legislation is proposed, much as for the legal basis for chlorination of water. This method has been successfully used in several states. The second approach involves a long continuing-education program to acquaint the public with the advantages of fluoridation. This is the approach used in Tennessee. A third approach has emerged, with the federal government making preventive service block grants to the states. This procedure allows state health departments to establish their own spending priorities for public health programs. In many states this funding change has resulted in a net loss of financial support for water fluoridation.

Debates between antifluoridationists and profluoridationists have been found to be counterproductive. It is difficult to rebut successfully a barrage of often intentional untruths, partial truths, and disinformation. Essentially the profluoridationist is expected to adhere to scientific truths, but the antifluoridationist is not so shackled. A skilled fluorophobic speaker can often convince the uninformed that fluoridation is in the same category as uncontrolled radiation, toxic chemical waste, and acid rain.[121] Even the value of a debate as a means of changing opinion is questionable. For instance, at the end of one community debate, the moderator asked the audience how many had been persuaded to change their vote in the coming referendum. Not one hand was raised.[122]

A major problem is to make scientific facts understandable to the layperson. This challenge is formidable when it is considered that in a 1990 national health interview survey (NHIS), 41,104 U.S. adults were asked, "As you understand it, what is the purpose of adding fluoride to the public drinking water?" The responses were coded to fit one of the following categories: "prevent tooth decay," "protect teeth," "purify the water," "other or don't know." One third of the the answers indicated that adults of voting age could not correctly identify the purpose of fluoridation.[123]

The most effective means of winning a fluoridation campaign is to develop a dedicated committee that represents all the people of the area—unions, businesses, racial and ethnic groups, news media, churches, school officials, parent–teacher groups, and health professionals. Sufficient money is necessary for publicity, speakers, and education programs. One exception was in Phoenix, Arizona, where the direct costs for the 16-month campaign to win the support of a population of over a million totalled only $1,958.79.[124] Fluoride initiatives must be conducted as political campaigns, not as health issues. The ADA has established a Directorate of Fluoridation Activities to aid program planning, and the USPHS Centers for Disease Control provides technical expertise on installation of, as well as aid in developing strategies for, fluoridation campaigns.

Community apathy must be overcome to ensure continuous pressure on the political councils responsible for the decision to fluoridate. Many of the referendums are won or lost by a few percentage points. For example, in 1985 after a 2-year long acrimonious public debate complete with talk shows, water fluoridation was defeated in San Antonio, Texas, by 4% of the votes. Unfortunately it was the poor, the minorities, and the old—the people in the most need—who made up the negative swing vote.[125] One recent example of how to elicit community support was demonstrated in Squamish, British Columbia. Two days before the referendum, dental students along with dental hygiene and dental assisting students, helped local health professionals canvas 1800 homes in the city.[122] This campaign provided the information and publicity that contributed greatly to the success of the referendum.

Question 5. Which of the following statements, if any, are correct?

A. A child in a nonfluoride area receiving fluoride tablets and using a fluoride dentifrice is at *high* risk of developing dental fluorosis.

B. Fluoride tablets used to reduce root decay for adults could *cause* fluorosis.

C. Fluorosis of the anterior permanent maxillary teeth would not be a problem if tablet supplements were started *after* 3 years of age.

D. Public debates provide an *ideal* forum for public education of the benefits of water fluoridation.

E. The old, the poor, the uneducated, and the minorities are prone to vote *against* water fluoridation.

SUMMARY

Originally, the introduction of 1 ppm of fluoride into a water supply reduced caries by 50% to 60%. This protective effect has now been reduced to 20% to 40%. This reduction in perceived effectiveness of water fluoridation is related to the increased benefits due to the "halo effect." The decline in caries as being experienced throughout the western world is attributable *both* to the ingestion of fluoridated water and fluoride from other multiple sources. The present benefits of water fluoridation are highly skewed towards aiding the poor, dentally uneducated, handicapped, and the aged—many of whom do not have access to dental care, nor the money to purchase the commercial fluoride dental products needed for self-care. From a technical standpoint, fluoridation can be accomplished without the water engineer experiencing any major problems. In those parts of the world where adequate water distribution systems and supervised waterworks do not exist, salt fluoridation promises to be an economical and effective method of providing a near-optimal level of fluoride to large populations. The increasing ingestion of fluorides from multiple sources has led to an increase in mild dental fluorosis. This has prompted a search for means of reducing the daily intake of fluoride, especially by young children. One considered option has been a possible downward revision of the concentration of fluoride considered optimal for a water supply. Other suggested actions have included: to (1) advise health professionals strongly against prescribing supplements in areas already served by fluoridated water, or if supplements are prescribed in fluoride-deficient areas, that a minimal dosage be considered, consistent with other fluoride intake by the child; (2) institute standardized labeling of soft drinks and bottled water to indicate fluoride content; (3) place cautionary labeling on dentifrice containers indicating fluoride content, and to stress the need for parental supervision of toothbrushing for children under 6 years of age. Consideration should possibly also be given to providing fluoride supplementation for high-risk adults in fluoride-deficient areas to aid in the prevention of root and coronal root caries. Because of the widespread office and home use of fluoride products, it is often forgotten that *fluoride can be lethal,* especially to young children. Thus, there is the concurrent ethical and legal need for office safety programs. Such programs should include (1) an in-depth understanding of the toxicity of fluoride by all appropriate office personnel and a well-publicized office policy that includes the preplanned first aid measures to be taken to minimize systemic toxicity in case of an accident; and (2) a realization that when the amount of fluoride ingested approaches or exceeds the probable toxic dose, the survival of the patient can depend on securing immediate emergency hospital care. To minimize the need for

emergency care, all parents should be appraised of the need for security of all home fluoride dental products. One of the objectives for the year 2000 is to have 75% of the American people with fluoridated water supplies. This will require many more political battles for fluoridation. Various strategies are necessary; above all truth, motivation, and an informed and involved citizenry are vital.

ANSWERS AND EXPLANATIONS

1. B, C, E
   A—incorrect. McKay *started* the search for the cause of mottling; Churchill *associated* fluoride with mottling; and Smith and Smith *proved* it was the cause.
   D—incorrect. Fluoride has the same effect on adult crystalline structure as for children's.
2. D, E
   A—incorrect. Maximal values are reached within 60 minutes.
   B—incorrect. Above 10 mg/kg is of great concern; an over 15 mg/kg intake based on amount ingested per kilogram of weight can be fatal. Age is not a factor.
   C—incorrect. Instructions about the treatment of fluoride toxicity are not often emphasized in the office manual.
3. A, B, D, E
   C—incorrect. It is the consensus after well-conducted studies that fluoride has no effect on the course of osteoporosis.
4. A, C, E
   B—incorrect. The interest of parents quickly lags after a period of time.
   D—incorrect. The principal function of fluoride is to aid in remineralization of demineralized tooth structure.
5. A, C, E
   B—incorrect. Teeth are not at risk of fluorosis at any time after eruption, regard-

less of fluoride intake; all teeth of adults are past that stage.

D—incorrect. In a water fluoridation campaign, the poor, the uneducated, the aged, and the minorities usually cast a negative vote.

SELF-EVALUATION QUESTIONS

1. _Trendly_ (US Public Health Service Officer) was the first to demonstrate the inverse relationship between dental caries and water fluoride levels.

2. *In the earlier days* when water was fluoridated, a caries decrease on the order of ___50___ to ___60___ percent could be expected; it is now ___20___ to ___40___ percent.

3. The *beneficial effect* of fluoride in a *nonfluoridated area* that is due to the importation of food and drinks packaged with fluoridated water is known as the "___Halo___ effect."

4. The national *annual* cost per person for water fluoridation is ___5 / ¢ nat avg___ (amount); the cost of one amalgam restoration is about $ ___5/___ .

5. The majority of long term storage of fluoride in the body is in the ___Skeletal___ (organ system).

6. A hypercalcemia and a hyper ___Kalemia___ often precede coma, convulsions, and cardiac arrhythmias in acute fluoride toxicity.

7. A high intake of fluoride during tooth formation causes *dental* fluorosis; a high chronic intake over many years causes ___Skeletal___ fluorosis.

8. Four major sources of ingested fluoride are: ___Fl. H₂O___ , ___Soft drinks___ , ___dentifrices___ , and ___f. supp___ .

9. Children swallow from 35% to ___50___ % of the dentifrice they use in toothbrushing.

10. The bleach usually used to remove the stains of dental fluorosis is ___hydrochloric Acid h. ether___ ___Superoxol___

11. Each fluoride drop has 0.1 ppm. If the water of an area has 0.6 ppm, and 1.0 is considered optimal, _____ drops are needed.

12. According to the Food and Drug Administration, a fluoride dentifrice must have at least ___650___ ppm to be advertised that it prevents decay.

13. The Supreme Court has accepted ___∅___ (number) of cases of referendum appeals since the beginning of water fluoridation.

REFERENCES

1. Dodge CH. Fluoridation of public drinking water: Issues of health benefits and risks. In: Congressional Research Service, *Report for Congress*, 1992.

2. McNeil DR. *The Fight for Fluoridation*. New York, NY. Oxford University Press; 1957.

3. Eager JM. Denti de chiaie (Chiaie Teeth). *Public Health Rep*. 1901; 16:2576.

4. Hunstadbraten K. Fluoridation in caries prophylaxis at the turn of the century. *Bull Hist Dent*. 1982; 30:117–120.

5. Dean HT. Endemic fluorosis and its relation to dental caries. *Public Health Rep*. 1938; 53:1443–1452.

6. Backer Dirks O. The benefits of water fluoridation. *Caries Res*. 1974; 8(suppl):2–15.

7. Department of Health and Human Services. US Public Health Service, Centers for Disease Control. Letter: FL-139, May 1992.

8. Department of Health and Human Services. *Healthy People 2000—National Health Promotion and Disease Prevention Objectives*. Washington, D.C., September 1990; 68:108–109.

9. Newbrun E. Effectiveness of water fluoridation. *J Public Health Dent*. 1989; 49:279–289.

10. Horowitz HS. Appropriate uses of fluoride: Considerations for the '90s. *J Public Health Dent*. 1991; 51:20–22.

11. Stookey GK. Review of benefits vs. fluorosis risk of self-applied topical fluorides (dentifrices, mouth rinses and gels). *Community Dent Oral Epidemiol*. 1994; 22:185–190.

12. Kaminsky LS, Mahoney MC, Leach J, et al. Fluoride: Benefits and risks of exposure. *Crit Rev Oral Biol Med*. 1990; 1:261–281.

13. Whitford GM. The metabolism and toxicity of fluoride. Monograph in Oral Science. Vol 13. Myers HM, series ed. Basel, Switzerland. Karger; 1989.

14. Department of Health and Human Services. U.S. Public Health Service. Young FE, ed. *Review of Fluoride: Benefits and Risks*. 1991: I + 134.

15. Stamm JW, Banting DW, Imrey PB. Adult root caries survey of two similar communities with contrasting natural water fluoride levels. *J Am Dent Assoc*. 1990; 120:143–149.

16. Atchison KA. The ethical issues of fluoridation. *J Am Coll Dent*. 1992; 59:14–17.

17. Carmichael CL, Rugg-Gunn AJ, Ferrell RS. The relationship between fluoridation, social class and caries experience in 5-year-old children in Newcastle and Northumberland in 1987. *Br Dent J*. 1989; 167:57–61.

18. Brunelle JA, Carlos JP. Recent trends in dental caries in U.S. children and the effect of water fluoridation. *J Dent Res*. 1990; 69 (special issue):723–727.

19. Ripa LW, Leske GS, Sposato A. The surface-specific caries pattern of participants in a school-based fluoride-mouthrinsing program with implications for the use of sealants. *J Public Health Dent*. 1985; 45: 90–94.

20. Clark DC, Hann HJ, Williamson M et al. The benefits from the use of fluoridated water. *J Dent Res*. 1992; 71 (special issue): 703. Abstract 1504.

21. Newbrun E. Current regulations and recommendations concerning water fluoridation, fluoride supplements, and topical fluoride agents. *J Dent Res*. 1992; 67:1255–1265.

22. Burt BA, Ismail AI, Eklund SA. Root caries in an optimally fluoridated and a high-fluoride community. *J Dent Res*. 1986; 65: 1154–1158.

23. Horowitz HS. The future of water fluoridation and other systemic fluorides. *J Dent Res*. 1990; 69 (special issue): 760–764.

24. Department of Health and Human Services. US Public Health Service. Report of the ad hoc subcommittee to coordinate environmental health and related programs. Review of fluoride benefits and risks. Washington, DC: US Department of Health and Human Services, 1991.

25. Blair KP. Fluoridation in the 1990's. *J Am Coll Dent*. 1992; 59:3.

26. Cecil JC, Cohen ME, Schroeder DC, et al. Longevity of amalgam restorations: A retrospective view. *J Dent Res*. 1982; 61:185. Abstract 56. 2-1990-564

27. Ismail A, Brogan H, Kavanagh M. Placement and replacement of restorations in a military population. *J Dent Res*. 1990; 69 (special issue):236. Abstract 1018.

28. Qvist J, Qvist V, Mjor IA. Placement and longevity of amalgam restorations in Denmark. *J Dent Res*. 1990; 69 (special issue): 236. Abstract 1018.

29. Lemke CW, Doherty JM, Arra MC. Controlled fluoridation: The dental effects of discontinuation in Antigo, Wisconsin. *J Am Dent Assoc*. 1970; 80:782–791.

30. Stephen KW, McCall DR, Tullis JI. Caries prevalence in northern Scotland before, and 5 years after, water defluoridation. *Br Dent J*. 1987; 163:324–326.

31. Trautner K, Siebert G. An experimental study of bio-availability of fluoride from dietary sources in man. *Arch Oral Biol*. 1986; 31:223–228.

32. Whitford GM. The physiological and toxicological characteristics of fluoride. *J Dent Res*. 1990; 69 (special issue):539–549.

33. Hodge HC. Fluoride metabolism: Its significance in water fluoridation. *J Am Dent Assoc*. 1956; 52:307–314.

34. Whitford GM. The physiological and toxicological characteristics of fluoride. *J Dent Res*. 1990; 69 (special issue):539–549.

35. Bowen WH, Geddes DAM. Summary of session III: Fluoride in saliva and dental plaque. *J Dent Res.* 1990; 69 (special issue): 637.

36. Bayless JM, Tinanoff N. Diagnosis and treatment of acute fluoride toxicity. *J Am Dent Assoc.* 1985; 110:209–211.

37. Heifetz SB, Horowitz HS. The amounts of fluoride in current fluoride therapies; safety considerations for children. *J Dent Child.* 1986; 77:876–882.

38. McIvor ME. Delayed fatal hyperkalemia in a patient with acute fluoride intoxication. *Ann Emerg Med.* 1987; 16:1165–1167.

39. Whitford GM. Fluoride in dental products: Safety considerations. *J Dent Res.* 1987; 66: 1056–1060.

40. Keels MA, Osterhout S, Vann WF Jr. Incidence and nature of accidental fluoride ingestions. *J Dent Res.* 1988; 67 (special issue):335. Abstract 1778.

41. Whitford GM. Acute and chronic fluoride toxicity. *J Dent Res.* 1992; 71:1249–1254.

42. Cutress TW, Suckling GW. Differential diagnosis of dental fluorosis, *J Dent Res.* 1990; 69: 714–720; discussion 721.

43. Horowitz HS. Indexes for measuring dental fluorosis. *J Publ Health Dent.* 1986; 46:179–183.

44. Fejerskov O, Manji F, Baelum V. The nature and mechanisms of dental fluorosis in man. *J Dent Res.* 1990; 69(special issue): 692–700; discussion 721.

45. Limeback H. Enamel formation and the effects of fluoride. *Community Dent Oral Epidemiol.* In press.

46. Clark DC, Hann HJ, Williamson MF, et al. Esthetic concerns of children and parents in relation to the different classifications of the tooth surface index of fluorosis. *Community Dent Oral Epidemiol.* 1993; 21: 360–364.

47. Brunelle JA, Carlos JP. Changes in the prevalence of dental caries in U.S. schoolchildren, 1961–1980. *J Dent Res.* 1982; 61: 1346–1351.

48. Dean HT. Classification of mottled enamel diagnosis. *J Am Dent Assoc.* 1934; 105: 1421–1426.

49. Thylstrup A, Fejerskov O. Clinical appearance of dental fluorosis in permanent teeth in relation to histologic changes. *Community Dent Oral Epidemiol.* 1978; 6:315–328.

50. Horowitz HS, Driscoll WS, Meyers RJ, et al. A new method for assessing the prevalence of dental fluorosis—The Tooth Surface Index of Fluorosis. *J Am Dent Assoc.* 1984; 109:37–41.

51. Pendrys DG. The fluorosis risk index: A method for investigating risk factors. *J Public Health Dent.* 1990; 50:291–298.

52. Fédération Dentaire Internationale. Commission on Oral Health, Research and Epidemiology. An epidemiological index of developmental defects of dental enamel (DDE) index. *Int Dent J.* 1982; 32:159–167.

53. Cleaton JP, Hargreaves JA. Comparison of three fluorosis indices in a Namibian community with twice optimum fluoride in the drinking water. *Tydskrif Van Die Tandheelkundige Vereniging Van Suid Africa.* 1990; 45:173–175.

54. Ripa LW. A critique of topical fluoride methods (dentifrices, mouth rinses, operator-, and self-applied gels) in an era of decreased caries and increased fluorosis prevalence. *J Public Health Dent.* 1991; 51: 23–41.

55. Pendrys DG, Stamm JW. Relationship of total fluoride intake to beneficial effects and enamel fluorosis. *J Dent Res.* 1990; 69:529–538.

56. Lewis DW, Banting DW. Water fluoridation—current effectiveness and dental fluorosis. *Community Dent Oral Epidemiol.* 1994; 22:153–158.

57. Clark DC. Trends in the prevalence of dental fluorosis in North America. *Community Dent Oral Epidemiol.* 1994; 22:148–152.

58. Chan J, Wei S. Optimal water fluoride level based on dietary data. *J Dent Res.* 1993; 72(special issue):109. Abstract 48.

59. Evans RW, Stamm JW. Dental fluorosis following downward adjustment of fluoride in drinking water. *J Public Health Dent.* 1991; 51:91–98.

60. Levy AM. A review of fluoride exposures and ingestion. *Community Dent Oral Epidemiol.* 1994; 22:170–180.

61. Burt BA. The changing patterns of systemic fluoride intake. *J Dent Res.* 1992; 71:1228–1237.

62. Ophaug RH, Singer L, Harland BF. Dietary fluoride intake of 6-month and 2-year-old children in four dietary regions of the United States. *Am J Clin Nutr.* 1985; 42:701–707.

63. Armstrong VC, Holliday MG, Schrecker TF. *Tap Water Consumption in Canada.* Department of National Health and Welfare, Public Affairs Directorate. 1981.

64. Ripa LW, Leske GS, Forte F, et al. Caries inhibition of mixed NaF-Na$_2$PO$_3$F dentifrices containing 1,000, 2,500 ppm fluoride: 3-year results. *J Am Dent Assoc.* 1988; 116:69–73.

65. Naccache H, Simard PL, Trahan L, et al. Factors affecting the ingestion of fluoride dentifrice by children. *J Public Health Dent.* 1992; 52:222–226.

66. Osuji OO, Leake JL, Chipman ML, et al. Risk factors for dental fluorosis in a fluoridated community. *J Dent Res.* 1988; 67: 1488–1492.

67. Bailey RW, Christen AG. Bleaching of vital teeth stained with endemic dental fluorosis. *Oral Surg.* 1968; 26:871–878.

68. Coll JA, Jackson P, Strasslet HE. Comparison of enamel microabrasion techniques: Prema compound versus a 12-fluted finishing bur. *J Esthetic Dent.* 1991; 3:180–186.

69. Rakow B, Light E. Evaluation of the acid etch technique in concealing discolorations. *Quintessence Int Rep.* November 1986:23–31.

70. Gruber HE, Baylink DJ. The effects of fluoride on bone. *Clin Orthop.* 1991; 267: 264–277.

71. Department of Health and Human Services. US Public Health Service. *Review of Fluoride Benefits and Risks.* Report of the ad hoc subcommittee on fluoride. February 1991:88.

72. Simonen O, Laitinen O. Does fluoridation of drinking water prevent bone fragility and osteoporosis? *Lancet* 1985; 2:432–434.

73. Sowers MR, Clark MK, Jannausch ML, et al. A prospective study of bone mineral content and fracture in communities with differential fluoride exposure. *Am J Epidemiol.* 1991; 133:649–660.

74. Jacobsen SJ, Goldberg J, Miles TP, et al. Regional variation in the incidence of hip fracture. *JAMA.* 1990; 264:500–502.

75. Gordon SL, Corbin SB. Summary of workshop on drinking water fluoride influence on hip fracture and bone health. *Osteoporos Int.* 1992; 286:109–117.

76. Department of Health and Human Services, MIH, NTP *Technical Report on the Toxicology and Carcinogenesis Studies of Sodium Fluoride in 344/N Rats and B6C3F1 Mice (Drinking Water Studies).* Report No. 90-2848. 1990.

77. National Research Council, Committee on Toxicology. *Health Effects of Ingested Fluoride.* National Academy Press. Washington, DC. 1993.

78. Hoover RN, DeVesa SS, et al. Fluoridation of drinking water and subsequent cancer incidence and mortality. *Report to the Director of the National Cancer Institute.* June 1990.

79. Health and Human Services News Release, US Public Health Service. Feb 19, 1991.

80. Galagen DJ. Climate and controlled fluoridation. *J Am Dent Assoc.* 1953; 47:159–170.

81. Shannon IL. The problem in maintaining the fluoride level in fluoridating water supplies. *Texas Dent J.* 1980; 98(5):6–8.

82. US Dept of Health and Human Services. US Public Health Service Centers for Disease Control Water Fluoridation. *A Manual for Engineers and Technicians.* September 1986.

83. American Dental Association. Excess fluoride in dialysate linked to patient's death. Drinking of fluoridated water not a factor. *Am Dent Assoc News.* December 10, 1979.

84. Alaska Department of Health and Social Services. Hooper Bay waterborne outbreak—*Fluoride. Interim Report #2.* June 29, 1992.

85. US Public Health Service, Centers for Disease Control. *Letter to State Dental Directors and State Drinking Water Chiefs. Late-breaking information, Fluoride Related Incident.* August 6, 1993.

86. Corbin SB. Fluoridation Symposium. Policy options for fluoride use. *J Am Coll Dent.* 1992; 59:18–23.

87. Kuthy, RA, McTigue DJ. Fluoride prescription practices of Ohio physicians. *J Publ Health Dent.* 1987; 47:172–176.

88. Mason JO. A message to health professionals about fluorosis. *JAMA.* 1991; 265:2939.

89. Whitford GM. Fluorides: Metabolism, mechanisms of action and safety. *Dent Hyg.* 1983; 57(5):16–29.

90. Murry JJ, Rugg-Gunn AJ, Jenkins GN. *Fluorides in Caries Prevention.* Oxford. Butterworth-Heinemann, Ltd; 1991.

91. Beltran ED, Burt BA. The pre- and posteruptive effects of fluoride in the caries decline. *J Public Health Dent.* 1988; 48:233–240.

92. Workshop Report—Group III. Definitive support for recommending prenatal fluoride supplements to prevent caries, still lacking. University of North Carolina at Chapel Hill, April 23–25, 1991. *J Dent Res.* 1992; 71:1224–1227.

93. DePaola PF. Reaction paper: The use of topical and systemic fluorides in the present era. *J Public Health Dent.* 1991; 51:48–52.

94. Aasenden R, Peebles TC. Effects of fluoride supplementation from birth on human deciduous and permanent teeth. *Arch Oral Biol.* 1974; 19:321–326.

95. Hargreaves JA. The level and timing of systemic exposure to fluoride with respect to caries resistance. *J Dent Res.* 1992; 71:1244–1248.

96. Thylstrup A. Clinical evidence of the role of pre-eruptive fluoride in caries prevention. *J Dent Res.* 1990; 69:742–750.

97. Groeneveld A, van Eck AAMJ, Backer Dirks O. Fluoride in caries prevention: Is the effect pre- or posteruptive? *J Dent Res.* 1990; 69:751–755.

98. Hargreaves JA. Water fluoridation and fluoride supplementation: Considerations for the future. *J Dent Res.* 1990; 69:765–770.

99. Evans R, Stamm JW. An epidemiologic estimate of the critical period during which human maxillary central incisors are most susceptible to fluorosis. *J Public Health Dent.* 1991; 51:251–255.

100. Horowitz HS. The need for toothpastes with lower than conventional fluoride concentrations for preschool-aged children. *J Dent Res.* 1992; 52:216–221.

101. Faller RV, Eversole S, Hargis DJ. Impact of orifice size and useage statements on dentifrice use. *J Dent Res.* 1993; 72:248. Abstract 1161.

102. Clarkson J. A European view of fluoride supplementation. *Br Dent J.* 1992; 172:357.

103. Clark DC, Limeback H. The Canadian workshop on the evaluation of current recommendations concerning fluorides. *Community Dent Oral Epidemiol.* 1994; 22:133–188.

104. Clark DC: Personal communication.

105. Ismail AI, Brodeur JM, Kavanagh M, et al. Prevalence of dental caries and dental fluorosis in students, 11–17 years of age, in fluoridated and nonfluoridated cities in Quebec. *Caries Res.* 1990; 24:290–297.

106. Clark DC, Hann HJ, Williamson MF, et al. The influence of exposure to various fluoride technologies on the prevalence of dental fluorosis. *J Dent Res.* In press.

107. Pendrys DG, Katz RV. Risk of enamel fluorosis associated with fluoride supplementation, infant formula, and fluoride dentifrice use. *Am J Epidemiol.* 1989; 130:1199–1208.

108. Riordan PJ, Banks JA. Dental fluorosis and fluoride exposure in Western Australia. *J Dent Res.* 1991; 70:1022–1028.

109. Evans RW, Stamm JW. An epidemiologic estimate of the critical period during which human maxillary central incisors are most susceptible to fluorosis. *J Public Health Dent.* 1991; 51:251–259.

110. Riordan PJ. Fluoride supplements in caries prevention: A literature review and proposal for a new dosage schedule. *J Public Health Dent.* 1993; 53:174–189.

111. Massler M. Geriatric dentistry: Root caries in the elderly. *J Prosthet Dent.* 1980; 44:147–149.

112. Wespi HJ. The history of salt fluoridation. In: *Salt Fluoridation,* Scientific Publication #501. Pan American Health Organization. Washington, DC. World Health Organization; 1986.

113. Organization Pan Americana de la Salud, *Primera Reunion de Expertos Sobre Fluo-*

ruracion y Yodacion de la Sal de Comsumo Humano. Antigua Guatemala, Guatemala. 17–21 Noviembre, 1986.

114. Clark RE, Sophy MM. Fluoridation: the courts and the opposition. *Wayne Law Rev.* 1967; 13:338–375.

115. Christoffel T. Fluoridation: Legal and political issues. *J Am Coll Dent.* 1992; 59: 8–13.

116. Atchison, KA. The ethical issues of fluoridation. *J Am Coll Dent.* 1992; 59:14–17.

117. Hastreiter RJ. Fluoridation conflict: A history and conceptual synthesis. *J Am Dent Assoc.* 1983; 106:486–490.

118. Newbrun E. The safety of water fluoridation. *J Am Dent Assoc.* 1977; 94:301–304.

119. Schlesinger ER, Overton DE, Chase HC, et al. Newburgh-Kingston caries-fluorine study XIII. Pediatric findings after ten years. *J Am Dent Assoc.* 1956; 52:296–306.

120. American Association of Public School Dentists. Community and school water fluoridation: Summary and recommendations. *J Public Health Dent.* 1984; 44:43–46.

121. Burt BA. The epidemiological basis for water fluoridation in the prevention of dental caries. *J Public Health Policy.* 1982; 3:391–407.

122. Clark DC, Hann HJ. A win for fluoridation in Squamish, British Columbia. *J Public Health Dent.* 1989; 49:170–171.

123. US Public Health Service, Centers for Disease Control. Knowledge of the purpose of community water fluoridation—United States, 1990. *MMWR.* 41/No. 49, 919–927, 1992.

124. Smith KG, Christen KA. A fluoridation campaign: The Phoenix experience. *J Public Health Dent.* 1990; 50:319–322.

125. Harris NO. The struggle for fluoridation: A personal and historical perspective. *Bull Hist Dent.* 1987; 35:93–100.

Appendix 8–1. Rapid Method of Calculating the Amount of Fluoride Ingested

Form	Dose	Formula	Amount to attain 50 mg*
Fluoride tablets[†]	1.0 mg F⁻/tablet	(No. tablets swallowed) (dose/tab) = mg F⁻	50 tablets
	0.5 mg F⁻/tablet		100 tablets
	0.25 mg F⁻/tablet		200 tablets
Fluoride drops[†]	0.5 mgF⁻/ml	(No. ml swallowed) (dose/ml) = mg F⁻	100 mL
	0.25 mg F⁻/drop		200 drops
	0.125 mg F⁻/drop	(No. drops swallowed) (dose/drop) = mg F⁻	400 drops
Vitamin tablets[†] with fluoride	1.0 mg F⁻/tablet	(No. tablets swallowed) (dose/tab) = mg F⁻	50 tablets
	0.5 mg F⁻/tablet		100 tablets
Vitamin drops[†] with fluoride	0.5 mg F⁻/0.6 mL		60 mL
	0.5 mg F⁻/mL	(No. ml swallowed) (dose/ml) = mg F⁻	100 mL
	0.25 mg F⁻/mL		200 mL
NaF gels and rinses	1.1% NaF		10 mL
	0.2% NaF	(4.5) (No. ml swallowed) (% NaF) = mg F⁻	56 mL
	0.05% NaF		220 mL
SnF₂ gels and rinses	1.64% SnF₂		13 mL
	0.4% SnF₂	(2.4) (No. ml swallowed) (% SnF₂) = mg F⁻	52 mL
	0.1 SnF₂		210 mL
APF gels and rinses	1.23% F⁻		4 mL
	0.5% F⁻	(10) (No. ml swallowed) (% F⁻) = mg F⁻	10 mL
	0.02% F⁻		250 mL
Toothpaste containing fluoride	1000 ppm F⁻	No. ml swallowed = mg F⁻	50 mL

*50 mg = mg/kg for an average 1- to 2-year-old child.
[†]If the dose is expressed as mg NaF instead of mg F⁻ (for example, 2.2 mg NaF), multiply by the constant 0.45 to convert the answer to mg F⁻.
(*From Bayless JM, Tinanoff N. Diagnosis and treatment of acute fluoride toxicity. J Am Dent Assoc. 1985, 110:209–211.*)

Chapter 9

Topical Fluoride Therapy

George K. Stookey
Bradley B. Beiswanger

Objectives

At the end of this chapter it will be possible to

1. Indicate the three most accepted fluoride compounds now used to control caries and indicate their relative effectiveness.
2. Discuss the possible chemical reactions associated with the topical application of sodium fluoride (NaF), stannous fluoride (SnF_2), and sodium monofluorophosphate (MFP).
3. Relate what percentages of NaF and SnF_2 are available for office, and home use (as solutions or as gels).
4. Describe how a liquid or gel topical application of fluoride is applied to the teeth.
5. Name at least four fluoride dentifrices on the market and indicate why the early dentifrices did not produce the expected caries decrements.
6. State the expected caries decrement following use of dentifrices, prophylaxis pastes, and mouth rinses containing fluoride.

RATIONALE FOR THE USE OF TOPICAL FLUORIDES

When communal water supplies are available, water fluoridation clearly represents the most effective, efficient, and economical of all known measures for the prevention of dental caries although similar results have been observed with fluoridated salt in many countries. Unfortunately, fluoridated water is available to only about 50% of the U.S. population, and alternative methods for the provision of systemic fluoride leave much to be desired. Thus additional measures are obviously needed for providing greater protection against caries to as many segments of the population as possible.

The term *topical fluoride therapy* refers to the use of systems containing relatively large concentrations of fluoride that are applied locally, or topically, to erupted tooth surfaces to prevent the formation of dental caries. This term encompasses the use of fluoride rinses, dentifrices, pastes, gels, and solutions that are applied in various manners.

MECHANISM OF ACTION

Studies of the use of topical fluoride applications for the control of dental caries began in the early 1940s. Since that time, it has been generally accepted that the fluoride content of enamel is inversely related to the prevalence of dental caries. Using in vivo enamel-sampling techniques and improved analytic methods developed during the past decade, investigators have been better able to quantitate this relationship. For example, Keene and coworkers[1] explored this relationship in young naval recruits 17 to 22 years of age; their observations are summarized in Table 9–1. These data suggest that the presence of elevated

TABLE 9–1. RELATIONSHIP BETWEEN SURFACE ENAMEL FLUORIDE CONTENT AND CARIES PREVALENCE IN YOUNG ADULTS*

Number of Subjects	Caries Prevalence (DMFT)	Enamel Fluoride Content (ppm)
47	0	3459
31	5–11	2229
29	12–26	1944

*Calculated from data presented by Keene et al.[1]

levels of fluoride in surface enamel is associated with minimal caries experience.

A much more extensive investigation of this relationship was reported by DePaola and coworkers.[2] These investigators similarly examined 1447 subjects, 12 to 16 years of age, who were lifetime residents of selected fluoridated and nonfluoridated communities; again the inverse relationship between enamel fluoride content and caries prevalence is apparent.

At the time of tooth eruption, the enamel is not yet completely calcified and undergoes a posteruptive period, approximately 2 years in length, during which enamel calcification continues. Throughout this period, called the period of *enamel maturation,* fluoride, as well as other elements, continues to accumulate in the more superficial portions of enamel. This fluoride is derived from the saliva as well as from the exposure of the teeth to fluoride-containing water and food. Following the period of enamel maturation, relatively little additional fluoride is incorporated from such sources into the enamel surface.[3] Thus most of the fluoride that is incorporated into the developing enamel occurs during the preeruptive period of enamel formation and the posteruptive period of enamel maturation.

The continued deposition of fluoride into enamel during the later stages of enamel formation, and especially during the period of enamel maturation, results in a concentration gradient of fluoride in enamel. Invariably the highest concentration of fluoride occurs at the very outermost portion of the enamel surface, with the fluoride content decreasing as one progresses inward toward the dentin.[4,5] This decrease in fluoride concentration is extremely rapid in the outermost 5 to 10 μm of enamel and is much less pronounced thereafter. This characteristic fluoride concentration gradient has been observed in unerupted teeth as well as in erupted teeth and in both the permanent and deciduous dentition, regardless of the amount of previous exposure to fluoride.

The presence of elevated concentrations of fluoride in surface enamel serves to make the tooth surface more resistant to the development of dental caries. Fluoride ions when substituted into the hydroxyapatite crystal fit more perfectly into the crystal than do hydroxyl ions. This fact coupled with the greater bonding potential of fluoride serves to make the apatite crystals more compact and more stable. Such crystals are thereby more resistant to the acid dissolution[6,7] that occurs during caries initiation. This effect is even more apparent as the pH of the enamel environment decreases due to the momentary loss of minute quantities of fluoride from the dissolving enamel and its nearly simultaneous reprecipitation as a fluorhydroxyapatite.[8]

Most of the initial studies concerning topical fluoride applications were conducted with sodium fluoride. It was recognized at that time that prolonged exposure of the teeth to low concentrations of fluoride in the dental office was not practical. To overcome this problem, two approaches were explored: *increasing the fluoride concentration and decreasing the pH of the application solution.*

Although the ability of sodium fluoride to increase the resistance of enamel to acid dissolution had been reported on several occasions, it had also been reported that lowering the pH of the sodium fluoride solution greatly increased its protection against enamel decalcification. Five clinical caries studies were conducted to evaluate the effectiveness of acidulated sodium fluoride topical solutions. The fluoride solutions were acidulated in various manners (eg, acetic acid, acid phthalate) and used with varying conditions, but in no instance was a statistically significant caries-preventive effect observed. Thus the use of acidulated sodium fluoride systems was abandoned, at least temporarily.

On the other hand, the observed results of increasing concentrations of fluoride were very encouraging, particularly when multiple applications were used. Although it was initially postulated that the effectiveness of topically applied sodium fluoride was due to the formation of a fluorhydroxyapatite,[9,10] subsequent investigations indicated that the primary reaction product involved the transformation of surface hydroxyapatite to calcium fluoride.[11–16]

$$Ca_{10}(PO_4)_6(OH)_2 + 20F^- \rightleftharpoons$$
hydroxyapatite

$$10CaF_2 + 6HPO_4^= + 2(OH)^-$$
calcium fluoride

Question 1. Which of the following statements, if any, are correct?

A. The maturation of enamel is an occurrence that continues at a *linear* rate from eruption into adulthood.

B. The fluoride content is highest at the *outer* surface of the enamel and decreases at a *linear* rate toward the dentin.

C. As a result of acid-induced demineralization followed by remineralization, hydroxyapatite can become fluorhydroxyapatite in the presence of fluoride.

D. The enamel is relatively more protected by neutral pH fluoride solutions than acidulated solutions.

E. With higher concentrations of fluoride, the *main* reaction product is fluorhydroxyapatite.

The preceding reaction involves the breakdown of the apatite crystal into its components followed by the reaction of fluoride and calcium ions to form calcium fluoride with a net loss of phosphate ions from treated enamel. Newer fluoride systems incorporate a means of preventing such phosphate loss.

The early investigators of the reaction between soluble fluoride and enamel observed that the nature of the reaction products was markedly influenced by a number of factors, including fluoride concentration, the pH of the solution, and the length of exposure. For example, the use of acidic fluoride solutions greatly favored the formation of calcium fluoride.[11] Neutral sodium fluoride solutions with fluoride concentrations of 100 ppm or less resulted primarily in the formation of fluorapatite, whereas higher fluoride concentrations resulted in the formation of calcium fluoride.[15] Because topical applications of sodium fluoride involve the use of 2.0% solutions (slightly over 9000 ppm), it follows that the use of these solutions essentially involves the formation of calcium fluoride.[14]

The second fluoride compound developed[17,18] for topical use during the 1950s was stannous fluoride, SnF_2. Compared with that of sodium fluoride, the reaction of stannous fluoride with enamel is unique in that both the cation (stannous) and the anion (fluoride) react chemically with enamel components. This reaction is commonly depicted as follows:

$$Ca_{10}(PO_4)_6(OH)_2 + 19SnF_2 \rightarrow$$
hydroxyapatite   stannous fluoride

$$10CaF_2 + 6Sn_3F_3PO_4 + SnO \cdot H_2O$$
calcium   stannous   hydrated
fluoride   fluorophosphate   tin oxide

Note from the equation that the formation of stannous fluorophosphate prevents, at least temporarily, the phosphate loss typical of sodium fluoride applications. Incidentally, the exact nature of the tin-containing reaction products varies depending on reaction conditions, including pH, concentration, and length of exposure (or reaction time).[19,20]

A third topical fluoride system was developed during the 1960s and is widely known as APF, acidulated phosphate fluoride. This system was developed by Brudevold and coworkers[21,22] in an effort to achieve greater amounts of fluorhydroxyapatite and lesser amounts of calcium fluoride formation. These investigators reviewed the various chemical reactions of fluoride with enamel (hydroxyapatite) and concluded that (1) if the pH of the fluoride system were made acidic to enhance the rate of reaction of fluoride with hydroxyapatite and (2) if phosphoric acid were used as the acidulant to increase the concentration of phosphate present at the reaction site, it should be possible to obtain greater amounts of fluoride deposited in surface enamel as fluorhydroxyapatite with minimal formation of calcium fluoride and minimal loss of enamel phosphate. On the basis of this chemical reasoning, APF systems were developed and shown to be *effective* for caries prevention.

Subsequent independent studies of the reactions of APF with enamel indicated, however, that the original chemical objectives were only partially achieved. The major reaction product of APF with enamel is also calcium fluoride,[12,23,24] although a greater amount of fluorhydroxyapatite is formed than with the previous topical fluoride systems. The chemical reaction of APF with enamel may be written as follows:

$$Ca_{10}(PO_4)_6(OH)_2 + F^- \rightarrow$$
hydroxyapatite

$$CaF_2 + Ca_{10}(PO_4)_6(OH)_{2x}F_x$$
calcium fluoride   fluorhydroxyapatite

It is obvious from the preceding discussion that the primary chemical reaction product with all three types of topical fluoride systems (ie, NaF, SnF₂, and APF) is the formation of *calcium fluoride* on the enamel surface.

The initial deposition of calcium fluoride on the treated tooth surfaces is by no means permanent; a relatively rapid loss of fluoride occurs within the first 24 hours,[25] with some continued loss occurring during the next 15 days.[26–29] The rate of loss varies between patients and is influenced by the nature of the fluoride treatment.[30,31] Although the presence of calcium fluoride on the enamel surface increases the resistance of the enamel to decalcification, the observations relative to the loss of the fluoride make it increasingly difficult to attribute the recognized cariostatic activity of topical fluoride applications to the presence of calcium fluoride.

It has been suggested that the calcium fluoride formed on the enamel surface following a topical fluoride application has two possible fates: a portion of the initial reaction product undergoes further reaction, resulting in the formation of fluorhydroxyapatite, and the remainder is lost from the enamel surface to the dental plaque and saliva. It is also recognized that the formation of fluorhydroxyapatite in this manner is a relatively slow and inefficient process.

Data demonstrating this phenomenon are presented in Figure 9–1. In this in vitro study, a series of four fluoride treatments were performed after establishing the inherent fluoride content of the enamel surface of about 200 ppm. Immediately following the first fluoride treatment, the fluoride content of the enamel surface was about

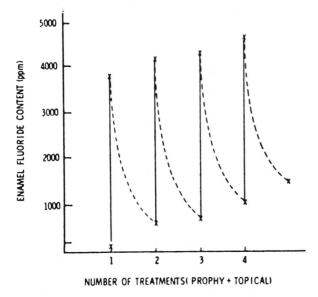

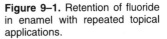

Figure 9–1. Retention of fluoride in enamel with repeated topical applications.

3700 ppm. Bathing the enamel surface in a salivalike medium, however, resulted in a rapid loss of the majority of the fluoride; after 3 days, the residual fluoride content of the enamel surface was about 500 ppm. Although much of the initial fluoride deposit was lost, the portion that remained significantly increased the fluoride content of the enamel surface by about 300 ppm. This increase in the enamel fluoride content was found to be relatively permanent in that further bathing of the enamel surface resulted in no additional loss of fluoride.

Repeating the fluoride treatments provided essentially the same amount of fluoride uptake, followed by a comparable fluoride loss as noted following the initial topical fluoride treatment. At the conclusion of the fluoride-leaching period, an additional increase in the "permanent" fluoride content of the enamel surface was observed. As can be seen from Figure 9–1, repeating this process through a series of four fluoride treatments resulted in an increase in the "permanent" fluoride content of the enamel surface of about 1300 ppm.

The foregoing in vitro data are supported by the results of a clinical study[32] in which school children were given a prophylaxis and a topical application of stannous fluoride initially and at 6-month intervals throughout a 3-year study period. Dental caries examinations were performed initially and each year thereafter. Table 9–2 summarizes the caries data as a function of the number of topical fluoride applications; it is apparent that the caries-preventive benefits increased in relation to the number of treatments.

These findings suggest that the cariostatic influence of topical fluoride applications may be due to that portion of the fluoride that is more or less permanently retained, presumably as a fluorhydroxyapatite, rather than the transient surface accumulation of calcium fluoride. It is also apparent that topical fluoride applications are relatively inefficient in that each treatment results in a rather small increase in the amount of fluorhydroxyapatite in the superficial portion of the enamel surface. Thus it follows that maximal patient benefits can only be derived from a repeated series of applications. Although the data presented in Figure 9–1 and Table 9–2 were obtained with stannous fluoride systems, the same phenomenon appears to be true with both acidulated phosphate fluoride (APF) and sodium fluoride. Mellberg[33] and coworkers[34] have also indicated the need for repeated topical APF applications. The original sodium fluoride topical application procedure developed by Knutson[35] specified a series of four treatments during a 2-week period.

It was noted earlier that the reaction of stannous fluoride with enamel resulted in the formation of tin-containing compounds. Although much less is known regarding the precise nature and ultimate fate of these

TABLE 9–2. CLINICAL REDUCTIONS IN INCREMENTAL CARIES AS A FUNCTION OF THE NUMBER OF TOPICAL FLUORIDE APPLICATIONS*

Study Period (Years)	Total Number of Topical Applications	Caries Reduction (%)	
		DMF Teeth	*DMF Surfaces*
1	2	2.8	12.6
2	4	29.2	34.1
3	6	47.4	51.5

*Calculated from Beiswanger et al.[32]

compounds, it appears that they contribute significantly to the cariostatic activity of stannous fluoride. The tin reaction products formed on sound enamel surfaces appear to be leached from the enamel in a manner similar to that for calcium fluoride.[36] The greatest accumulation of stannous complexes occurs in circumscribed areas of enamel defects; typically such areas are hypomineralized and are frequently the result of decalcification associated with the initiation of the caries process. Extremely high concentrations of tin, about 20,000 ppm, have been reported in these locations.[37] Clinically these areas, which have been described as frank carious areas, become pigmented (presumably due to the presence of the tin complexes) and appear to be more calcified following the application of stannous fluoride. This pigmentation has thus been suggested as being indicative of the arrest of carious lesions and is typically retained for 6 to 12 months or longer, suggesting that these stannous reaction products are of considerably greater significance than those formed on sound enamel.

One additional fluoride compound, sodium monofluorophosphate, has been approved as an effective agent and thereby merits consideration here. This compound has the empirical formula Na_2PO_3F and is commonly identified as MFP. It has been evaluated and approved for use in dentifrices. Though evaluated in one study as an agent for topical fluoride application, its use in this manner has received little consideration. Although the mechanism of action of sodium monofluorophosphate is thought to involve a chemical reaction with surface enamel, the precise nature of this reaction is poorly understood. Some investigators have suggested that the fluorophosphate moiety, $PO_3F^=$, may undergo an exchange reaction with phosphate ions in the apatite structure but the presence of $PO_3F^=$ in enamel has

never been demonstrated, and such a reaction mechanism appears unlikely. Others have suggested that the $PO_3F^=$ complex is enzymatically dissociated by phosphatases present in saliva and dental plaque into PO_3^- and F^- with the ionic fluoride reacting with hydroxyapatite in a manner similar to that described earlier. The fact that the treatment of enamel with sodium monofluorophosphate results in less fluoride deposition and less protection against enamel decalcification than is observed with simple inorganic fluoride compounds such as sodium fluoride, while yet imparting nearly comparable cariostatic activity, is indicative of a more complex mechanism of action.

For the most part, the foregoing discussion of the chemical reactions of concentrated fluoride solutions with enamel suggests that the reactions occur on the outer enamel surface and serve to make that surface more resistant to demineralization. It is apparent that this process is particularly predominant in newly erupted teeth that are undergoing continued enamel maturation (calcification) for the first 2 years following eruption into the oral cavity. In such instances some of the applied fluoride readily penetrates the relatively permeable enamel surface to depths of 20 to 30 μm and readily reacts with the calcifying apatite to form a fluorhydroxyapatite. Furthermore, the dissolution of the calcium fluoride deposited on the enamel surface provides additional fluoride ions, which become incorporated in maturing enamel.

It has become increasingly apparent, however, during the last decade that very little fluoride deposition lasting more than 24 hours occurs when fluoride is applied to sound, fully maturated enamel. This situation apparently occurs regardless of the nature of the fluoride compound, the concentration of fluoride, or the manner of application. Thus there appears to be no preventive benefits from the application of fluoride to maturated sound enamel.

As noted in Chapter 3, the caries process begins with a demineralization of the apatite adjacent to the crystal sheaths. This permits the diffusion of weak acids into the subsurface enamel, and because the subsurface enamel has a lower fluoride content and is less resistant to acid demineralization, it is preferentially dissolved, forming an incipient, subsurface lesion. As this process continues, it becomes clinically apparent as a so-called "white spot" that, in reality, is a rather extensive subsurface lesion covered by a relatively intact enamel surface. Thus enamel surfaces that clinically appear to be sound or free of demineralization frequently have areas that have been slightly decalcified with minute subsurface lesions that are not yet detectable clinically. This situation is particularly likely to exist in patients with clinical evidence of caries activity on other teeth.

It now appears that the predominant mechanism of action of fluoride involves its ability to facilitate the remineralization of these demineralized areas. Topically applied fluoride clearly diffuses into these demineralized areas and reacts with calcium and phosphate to form fluorhydroxyapatite in the remineralization process. It is also noteworthy that such remineralized enamel is more resistant to subsequent demineralization than was the original enamel. This process has been shown to occur with all forms and concentrations of fluoride, including concentrations as low as 1 ppm such as is found in optimally fluoridated drinking water. Studies conducted in our laboratories, however, have clearly shown that the amount of fluoride deposition in subsurface lesions following a topical fluoride application is much greater than that occurring following the use of lesser concentrations of

fluoride provided by fluoride rinses or dentifrices. As a result, topical fluoride applications appear to be an effective means of inducing the remineralization of incipient lesions.

Question 2. Which of the following statements, if any, are correct?

A. On demineralization, more *phosphate* is lost from the hydroxyapatite crystal in the presence of sodium fluoride than when stannous fluoride is present.

B. The loss of calcium fluoride from the tooth is at a *linear* rate for approximately 2 weeks.

C. As the number of treatments with topical fluoride increases, so does the caries *decrement* increase.

D. Stannous fluoride is deposited in greatest concentration where the enamel is least perfectly mineralized.

E. The use of MFP results in *less* cariostatic action than other neutral fluorides, even though a *higher* concentration is usually found on the tooth surface.

EFFECTS OF FLUORIDE ON PLAQUE AND BACTERIAL METABOLISM

Thus far we have assumed that the cariostatic effects of fluoride are mediated through a chemical reaction between this ion and the outermost portion of the enamel surface. The preponderance of data supports this view. A growing body of information suggests, however, that the caries-preventive action of fluoride may also include an inhibitory effect on the oral flora involved in the initiation of caries. The ability of fluoride to inhibit glycolysis by interfering with the enzyme enolase has long been known; concentrations of fluoride as low as 50 ppm have been shown to interfere with bacterial metabolism. Moreover, fluoride *may accumulate in dental plaque* in concentrations above 100 ppm. Although the fluoride normally present in plaque is largely bound (and thus unavailable for antibacterial action), it dissociates to ionic fluoride when the pH of plaque decreases (ie, when acids are formed). Thus, when the carious process starts and acids are formed, plaque fluoride in ionic form may serve to interfere with further acid production by plaque microorganisms. In addition, it may react with the underlying layer of dissolving enamel, promoting its remineralization as fluorhydroxyapatite. The end result of this process is a "physiologic" restoration of the initial lesion (by remineralization of enamel) and the formation of a more resistant enamel surface. The ability of fluoride to promote the reprecipitation of calcium phosphate solutions in apatitic forms has been repeatedly demonstrated.

In addition to these possible effects of fluoride, several investigators have reported that the presence of tin, especially as provided by stannous fluoride, is associated with significant antibacterial activity, which has been reported to decrease both the amount of dental plaque and gingivitis in experimental animals. Existing evidence suggests that these antibacterial effects of fluoride and tin may also contribute to the observed cariostatic activity of topically applied fluorides.

TOPICAL FLUORIDE APPLICATIONS

The use of concentrated fluoride solutions applied topically to the dentition for the prevention of dental caries has been studied extensively during the past 50 years although few studies have been conducted since the 1970s. This procedure results in a significant increase in the resistance of the exposed tooth surfaces to the development of dental caries and, as a result, has become a standard procedure in most dental offices.

At present three different fluoride systems have been adequately evaluated and approved for use in this manner in the United States. These three systems are 2% sodium fluoride, 8% stannous fluoride, and acidulated phosphate fluoride systems containing 1.23% fluoride.

Available Forms

When topical fluoride applications became available to the profession, the fluoride compounds (sodium fluoride and stannous fluoride) were obtained in powder or crystalline form, and aqueous solutions were prepared immediately prior to use. Subsequently it was realized that sodium fluoride solutions were stable if stored in plastic containers, and this compound became available in liquid and gel, as well as powder, form. With continued research of different types of agents and recognition by the dental profession of their inherent disadvantages with regard to patient acceptance and stability, as well as the need to use professional time more efficiently, the trend has been toward the use of ready-to-use, stable, flavored preparations in gel form.

Sodium Fluoride (NaF). This material is available in powder, gel, and liquid form. The compound is recommended for use in a 2% concentration, which may be prepared by dissolving 0.2 g of powder in 10 mL distilled water. The prepared solution or gel has a basic pH and is stable if stored in plastic containers. Ready-to-use 2% solutions and gels of sodium fluoride are commercially available; due to the relative absence of taste considerations with this compound, these solutions generally contain little flavoring or sweetening agents.

Stannous Fluoride (SnF$_2$). This compound is available in powder form either in bulk containers or preweighed capsules. The recommended and approved concentration is 8%, which is obtained by dissolving 0.8 g of the powder in 10 mL of distilled water. Stannous fluoride solutions are quite acidic, with a pH of about 2.4 to 2.8. Aqueous solutions of stannous fluoride are not stable due to the formation of stannous hydroxide and, subsequently, stannic oxide, which is visible as a white precipitate. As a result, solutions of this compound must be prepared immediately prior to use. As will be noted later, stannous fluoride solutions have a bitter, metallic taste. To eliminate the need to prepare this solution from the powder and to improve patient acceptance, a stable, flavored solution can be prepared with glycerine and sorbitol to retard hydrolysis of the stannous fluoride and with any of a variety of compatible flavoring agents. Ready-to-use solutions or gels with the proper SnF$_2$ concentration are not commercially available, however.

Acidulated Phosphate Fluoride (APF). This treatment system is available as either a solution or gel, both of which are stable and ready to use. Both forms contain 1.23% fluoride, generally obtained by the use of 2.0% sodium fluoride and 0.34% hydrofluoric acid. Phosphate is usually provided as orthophosphoric acid in a concentration of 0.98%. The pH of true APF systems should be about 3.5. Gel preparations feature a greater variation in composition, particularly with regard to the source and concentration of phosphate. In addition, the gel preparations generally contain thickening (binders), flavoring, and coloring agents.

Another form of acidulated phosphate fluoride for topical applications, namely thixotropic gels, has recently become available. The term *thixotropic* denotes a solution that sets in a gellike state but is not a true gel. On the application of pressure, thixotropic gels behave like solutions; it has been suggested that these preparations are more easily forced into the interproximal spaces than conventional gels. The active fluoride system in thixotropic gels is identical to conventional APF solutions. Although the initial thixotropic gels exhibited somewhat poorer biologic activity in in vitro studies, subsequent formulations were at least equivalent to conventional APF systems. Even though few clinical efficacy studies have been reported,[38] the collective data were considered adequate evidence of activity; these preparations have been approved by the American Dental Association.

Application Procedure

In essence there are two procedures for administering topical fluoride treatments. One procedure, in brief, involves the isolation of teeth and continuously painting the solution onto the tooth surfaces. The second, and currently more popular, procedure involves the use of fluoride gels applied with a disposable tray.

Until recently it was assumed that it was necessary to administer a thorough dental prophylaxis prior to the topical application of fluoride. Although the need for this measure was poorly documented, early investigations presumed that the presence of pellicle and oral debris would reduce or interfere with the reaction of the fluoride with the underlying enamel. This hypothesis was supported by the results of an early study that suggested that topically applied sodium fluoride was more effective if a prophylaxis preceded the treatment.[39] The results of four clinical trials,[40–43] have indicated that a prophylaxis immediately prior to the topical application of fluoride is not necessary. In these studies the children were given topical applications of APF in the conventional manner except that three different procedures were used to clean the teeth immediately prior to each treatment; these procedures were either a dental prophylaxis, toothbrushing and flossing, or no cleaning procedure. The results indicated that the cariostatic activity of the APF treatment was not influenced by the different preapplication procedures. *Thus the administration of a dental prophylaxis prior to the topical application of fluoride must be considered optional; it should be performed if there is a general need for a prophylaxis, but it need not be performed as a prerequisite for topical fluoride applications.*

Figures 9–2 through 9–7 illustrate the major steps recommended for applying topical fluoride solutions. The essential armamentarium for the application of concentrated fluoride solutions consists of cut cotton rolls, suitable cotton roll holders, cotton applicators, and treatment solution. If a prophylaxis is performed, the patient is al-

lowed to rinse thoroughly, and then the cotton rolls and holders are positioned so as to isolate the area to be treated. It is a common practice when using fluoride solutions to isolate both right or left quadrants at one time so as to be able to treat *one half* of the mouth simultaneously. The isolated teeth are then dried with compressed air, and the fluoride solution is applied using cotton applicators. Care should be taken to be certain that all tooth surfaces are treated. The application is performed by merely swabbing or "painting" the various tooth surfaces with a cotton applicator thoroughly moistened with the fluoride solution. The swabbing procedure is repeated continuously and methodically with repeated "loading" of the cotton applicator so as to keep the tooth surfaces moist throughout the treatment period. At the conclusion of this period, the cotton rolls and holders are removed, the patient is allowed to expectorate, and the process is repeated for the remaining quadrants.

It should be stressed that various precautions should be routinely taken to minimize the amount of fluoride that is inadvertently swallowed by the patient during the application procedure. A number of recent reports[44-50] have shown that 10 to 30 mg of fluoride may be inadvertently swallowed during the application procedure, and it has been suggested that the ingestion of these quantities of fluoride by young children may contribute to the development of dental fluorosis in those teeth that are unerupted and in the developmental stage. Precautions that should be undertaken include (1) using only the required amount of the fluoride solution or gel to perform the treatment adequately; (2) positioning the patient in an upright position; (3) using efficient saliva aspiration or suctioning apparatus; and (4) requiring the patient to expectorate thoroughly on completion of the fluoride application. The use of these procedures

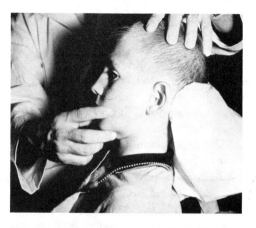

Figure 9–2. It is advisable to seat the patient in an upright position to help minimize the flow of topical solution down the child's throat.

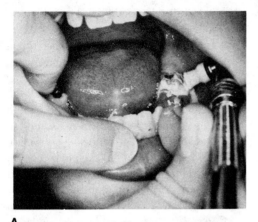

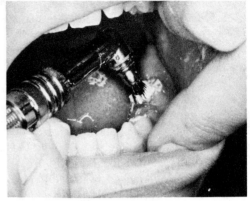

A

B

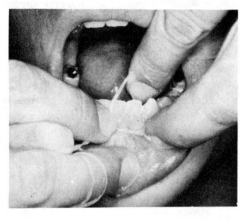

C

Figure 9–3. If desired, the topical application may be preceded by a thorough prophylaxis. The smooth tooth surfaces are cleaned with a prophylactic paste applied with a prophy cup, **A,** following the gross removal of heavy exogenous deposits (calculus) with hand instruments. A prophy brush is similarly used on the occlusal surfaces, **B,** while unwaxed dental floss is used to draw the paste interproximally to clean the proximal surfaces, **C.**

has been shown to reduce the amount of inadvertently swallowed fluoride to less than 2 mg, which may be expected to be of little consequence.[51]

After the topical application is completed, the patient is advised not to rinse, drink, or eat for 30 minutes. The necessity of the latter procedure has not been substantiated; the fact that it has been followed in most of the prior clinical studies serves as the primary basis for this recommendation. This recommendation is also supported, however, by a recently completed study[52] that measured the amount of fluoride deposition in incipient lesions (subsurface enamel demineralization) in patients who

either were, or were not, permitted to rinse, eat, or drink during this 30-minute posttreatment period. It was found that significantly greater fluoride deposition occurred when the patients were not permitted to rinse, eat, or drink following the fluoride treatment.

Whatever fluoride system is used for topical fluoride applications, the teeth should be exposed to the fluoride for 4 minutes for maximal cariostatic benefits. This treatment time has consistently been recommended for both sodium fluoride and acidulated phosphate fluoride. Some confusion has arisen, however, with regard to stannous fluoride, because shorter applica-

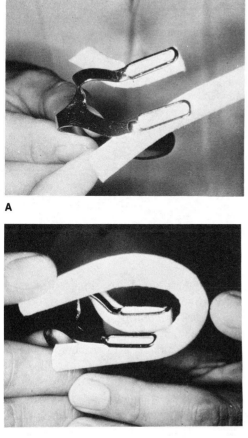

A

B

Figure 9–4. A six-inch and four-inch roll are placed in a Garmer holder in such a manner that, **A,** the lingual roll extends across the midline to isolate an area beyond the central incisors, and **B,** the long buccal roll is bent so as to isolate both the upper and lower vestibules.

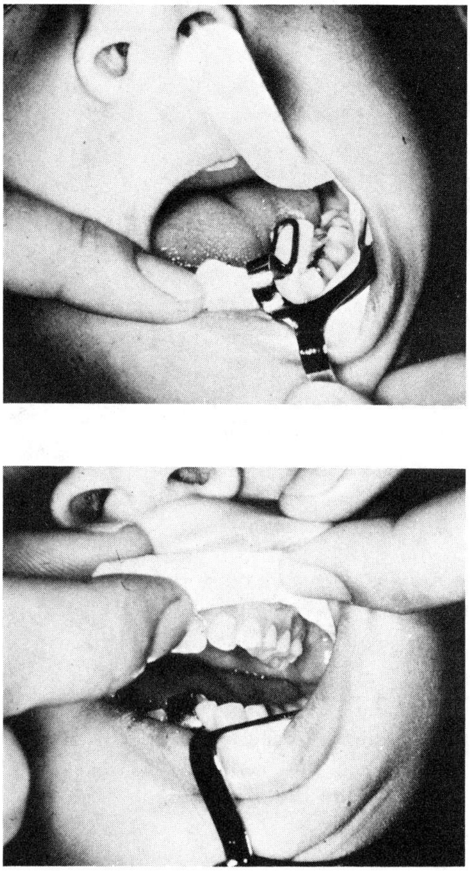

Figure 9–5. The cotton roll holder is placed in the mouth, thereby isolating both an upper and lower quadrant from the retromolar to a point beyond the central incisors.

tion periods of 15 or 30 seconds with stannous fluoride have been reported to result in significant cariostatic benefits. Nevertheless, the collective results of these and subsequent clinical investigations indicate that maximum caries protection is achieved only with the use of the longer exposure period. Thus although reduced exposure periods of 30 to 60 seconds might be appropriate as a fluoride maintenance or preventive mea-

sure in patients with very little caries activity, the use of the longer, 4-minute application should be required for patients with existing or potential caries activity.

Application Procedure— Fluoride Gels

A slightly different technique is commonly suggested for providing treatments with flu-

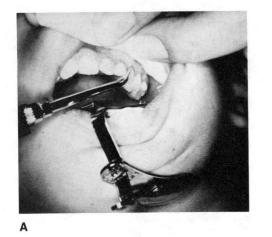

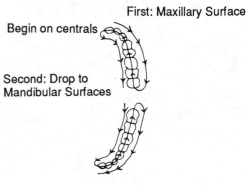

PROCEDURE FOR DRYING TEETH

First: Maxillary Surface

Begin on centrals

Second: Drop to
Mandibular Surfaces

A   **B**

Figure 9–6. The isolated teeth are, **A,** dried with an air syringe in a systematic manner, **B,** so as to avoid missing any tooth surface.

oride gels. Although these preparations may be applied by using the same basic procedure as described for solutions, the use of plastic trays has been suggested as a more convenient procedure. As with the use of topical fluoride solutions, the treatment may be preceded by a prophylaxis if indicated by existing oral conditions. With the so-called tray application technique, the

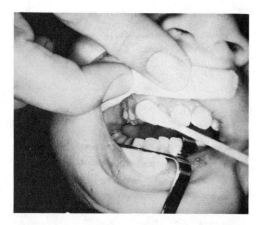

Figure 9–7. Using the same application pattern as in Figure 9–6B, fluoride solution is applied with a cotton applicator, with continual reapplications to maintain all tooth surfaces moist with the solution for a 4-minute period.

armamentarium consists simply of a suitable tray and the fluoride gel.

Many different types of trays are available; selection of a tray adequate for the individual patient is an important part of the technique. Most manufacturers of trays offer sizes to fit patients of different ages. An adequate tray should cover all the patient's dentition; it should also have enough depth to reach beyond the neck of the teeth and contact the alveolar mucosa to prevent saliva from diluting the fluoride gel. Some of the trays used in the past did not meet these requirements. Some were made of vinyl and frequently either did not reach the mucosa or impinged on the tissue, thus forcing the dentist to cut the flanges of the tray. At present, disposable soft styrofoam trays are available and seem to be adequate. These trays can be bent to insert in the mouth and are soft enough to produce no discomfort when they reach the soft tissues. With these trays, as well as with some of the previous types of trays, it is possible to treat both arches simultaneously.

If a prophylaxis is given, the patient is permitted to rinse, and the teeth of the arch to be treated are dried with compressed air.

A ribbon of gel is placed in the trough portion of the tray and the tray seated over the entire arch. The method used must ensure that the gel reaches all of the teeth and flows interproximally. If, for instance, a soft pliable tray is used, the tray is pressed or molded against the tooth surfaces, and the patient may also be instructed to bite gently against the tray. Some of the early trays contained a sponge-like material that "squeezed" the gel against the teeth when the patient was asked to bite lightly or simulate a chewing motion after the trays were inserted. It is recommended that the trays be kept in place for a 4-minute treatment period. As noted previously, the patient is advised not to eat, drink, or rinse for 30 minutes following the treatment.[52] Figure 9–8 illustrates the tray technique of fluoride gel application.

Question 3. Which of the following statements, if any, are correct?

A. Assuming that less than 1 ppm of F is in the saliva (true), the dental plaque may have 100 times this level.

B. Stannous fluoride is quite *stable* when stored in *aqueous* phase. *goes to hydroxide then wht oxide*

C. A thixotropic gel looks like a gel, acts like a gel, and is a gel. *→ not a gel*

D. After a topical application of fluoride, a patient should not eat or drink for a half hour.

E. A liquid topical solution should be maintained on the teeth for the same time as a gel tray treatment: 4 minutes.

Application Frequency

As previously mentioned, although a single, topical application is accepted as not being able to impart maximal caries protection, considerable confusion has arisen regarding the preferred frequency for administering

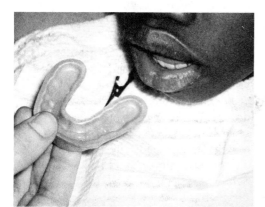

A

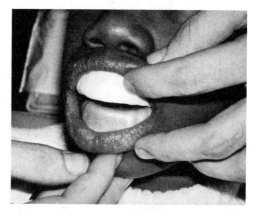

B

Figure 9–8. Appropriate sized soft styrofoam trays are used to avoid pinching the soft tissues. A ribbon of gel is dispensed into the trough of the tray. Enough gel should be used to cover all tooth surfaces, but care should be used to avoid an excess which will flow into the mouth. (Experience will teach the operator how much gel to use.) The patient is shown the loaded mandibular tray, **A,** which is ready for insertion, **B.** The maxillary tray is inserted after the mandibular is in place. The patient is then asked to bite together so as to be more comfortable and, at the same time, to force the gel against the teeth. The use of thixotropic gels facilitates the wetting of all tooth surfaces. The trays should be maintained in place for 4 minutes.

topical fluoride treatments. Much of this confusion is due to the absence of controlled, clinical evaluations of this variable, particularly with the most commonly used agent, acidulated phosphate fluoride.

The original Knutson technique[35] for the topical application of sodium fluoride consisted of a series of four applications provided at approximately 1-week intervals with only the first application preceded by a prophylaxis. It was further suggested that this series of applications be administered at ages 3, 7, 10, and 13 years, with these ages selected, or varied, in accordance with the eruption pattern of the teeth.[53] The objective of the timing was to provide protective benefits to "the permanent teeth during the period of changing dentition." Because this treatment sequence did not coincide with the common patient-recall pattern in the dental office, Galagan and Knutson[54] explored the possible use of longer intervals of 3 or 6 months between the individual applications constituting each treatment series. The results of their work indicated that although significant benefits were obtained with single applications provided at 3- or 6-month intervals, maximal benefits were obtained only with a series of treatments. Nevertheless, the administration of single applications of sodium fluoride at 3- to 6-month intervals became a common practice, because these intervals were more convenient to the dentist and his or her normal recall system.

When stannous fluoride and acidulated phosphate fluoride were subsequently developed and evaluated, apparently little if any attempt was made to determine the optimal treatment frequency. Instead, the treatments were administered as single applications provided at 6- or 12-month intervals, which were convenient to the normal office schedules. Because these treatment intervals resulted in significant cariostatic

benefits, the procedure that was ultimately approved and recommended involved this application frequency.

In view of this background, it seems that *the frequency of topical applications should be dictated by the conditions and needs presented by each patient* and not by the convenience of the dental office. This conclusion is supported by the data cited earlier that a series of applications is required to impart maximal caries resistance to the tooth surface.

Thus it is recommended that new patients, regardless of age, with active caries be given an initial series of four topical fluoride applications within a period of 2 to 4 weeks. If desired, the initial application may be preceded by a thorough prophylaxis, the remaining three applications constituting the initial treatment series should be preceded by toothbrushing to remove plaque and oral debris. It should be obvious that this series of treatments may be very conveniently combined with the plaque control, dietary counseling, and initial restorative programs that the dentist has devised for these patients. Following this initial series of treatments, the patient should be given single, topical applications at intervals of 3, 6, or 12 months, depending on his or her caries status. Patients with little evidence of existing or anticipated caries should be given single applications every 12 months as a preventive measure.

Special effort should be made by the dentist to schedule topical fluoride applications so as to provide the treatment to newly erupted teeth within at most 12 months after eruption, and preferably as close to eruption as possible. As noted earlier, an approximate 2-year enamel maturation period occurs immediately following tooth eruption. As illustrated in Table 9–3, the preventive benefits of fluoride are invariably much greater on newly erupted teeth than on pre-

TABLE 9–3. COMPARATIVE EFFECTIVENESS OF TOPICAL FLUORIDE APPLICATIONS
ON PREVIOUSLY ERUPTED AND NEWLY ERUPTED TEETH

Clinical Investigation	Topical Agent	Caries Reduction (%)	
		Previously Erupted Teeth	*Newly Erupted Teeth*
Averill (1967)[53]	NaF	22.9	37.1
Horowitz (1969)[55]	SnF$_2$	20.7	61.3
Muhler (1960)[56]	SnF$_2$	44.2	84.0
Szwejda (1972)[57]	SnF$_2$	20.4	44.4
Szwejda (1972)[57]	APF	22.5	63.0

viously erupted teeth. This finding is apparent regardless of the fluoride system used and is presumably due to the greater reactivity, permeability, and ease of formation of fluorhydroxyapatite in enamel still undergoing calcification (or maturation).

Efficacy of Topical Fluoride Therapy

Well over 100 human clinical studies demonstrate that topical fluoride therapy contributes significantly to the partial control of dental caries. Unfortunately, the practitioner is frequently concerned, and sometimes confused, about which procedure or agent should be employed in a given situation to provide a maximal degree of dental caries protection for the patient. Such concern and confusion is understandable when it is realized that dental caries investigators themselves frequently do not agree on these matters.

The results of the numerous clinical investigations with various topical fluoride agents and treatment procedures have been the subject of several reviews.[58–66] Therefore no attempt is made to repeat these reviews here.

As noted earlier, three different types of fluoride systems (ie, sodium fluoride, stannous fluoride, and acidulated phosphate fluoride) have been evaluated and approved as safe and effective for topical fluoride

applications by both the American Dental Association (ADA)[67] and the Food and Drug Administration (FDA).[68] To determine which of these systems may be the most effective, it would be desirable to compare the results of independent clinical studies in which all three systems have been tested when used in the recommended manner. Unfortunately such data are not available, and alternative procedures must be sought.

Different approaches have been taken to estimate the magnitude of the cariostatic benefits that may be expected from topical applications of the different approved fluoride systems. One approach is simply to list all of the pertinent clinical trials and then determine the arithmetic mean of the reported caries reduction. This approach has been utilized by several investigators,[63–65] and the results observed for children residing in a nonfluoridated community are summarized in Table 9–4. Another approach is to utilize an empirically based procedure with existing clinical data to predict the efficacy of different systems[69]; these data are also shown in Table 9–4. Whatever the approach, study designs varied in a number of ways, such as the number and frequency of topical applications and the study duration. These variations serve to confound estimates of cariostatic efficacy. Nevertheless, it is apparent from Table 9–4 that all three types of topical fluoride systems result in ap-

TABLE 9–4. COMPARATIVE EFFECTIVENESS OF DIFFERENT TOPICAL FLUORIDE SYSTEMS (AVERAGE PERCENTAGE REDUCTION IN CARIES INCIDENCE)

Fluoride System (%)	Form Used	Ripa[63] 1981	Mellberg & Ripa[64] 1983	Stookey[65] 1987	Clark, et al[69] 1985
NaF (2.0)	Solution	29	29	27	NA
SnF$_2$ (8.0)	Solution	32	32	36	NA
APF (1.2)	Solution	28	28	36	38
APF (1.2)	Gel	19	19	25	26

preciable cariostatic benefits of comparable magnitude with percentage reductions ranging from 27% to 36%. Furthermore, the data suggest that fluoride applied in gel form may be slightly *less* effective than solutions.

Considerably less information is available to document the efficacy of topical fluoride applications in adults. A total of 14 clinical trials were conducted in adults during the period 1944 through 1974, but the studies utilized a wide variety of experimental conditions, including the type of topical fluoride system, frequency of applications, and duration of the test period.[70–83] Although most of the methods resulted in a significant cariostatic benefit, the magnitude of this effect varied considerably, as might be expected. Furthermore, none of these studies used the application frequency suggested earlier for children.

It is generally recognized by dental scientists, however, that the dental caries process is fundamentally the same in both children and adults, although the rate of progression in young and middle-aged adults is frequently much slower due to a variety of factors, including more efficient oral hygiene and fewer between-meal snacks. Conversely, in older adults the rate of progression may increase due to the use of *medications* that reduce salivary flow. It is commonly assumed, therefore, that topical fluoride applications are effective for coronal caries prevention *regardless of the age of the patient.* Once again the frequency of ap-

plication should be dictated by the needs of the patient; in the presence of frank or incipient caries activity, *an initial series of applications should be given followed by maintenance applications at 3, 6, or 12 months,* depending on patient needs (ie, evidence and extent of caries activity). Similarly, the choice of the fluoride system (NaF, APF, SnF$_2$) may be at the discretion of the dentist because there appears to be *little, if any, difference in their efficacy.*

On occasion it has been suggested that present topical fluoride treatment systems involve the use of excessive concentrations of fluoride. For example, some have suggested that the use of 0.4% rather than 8.0% stannous fluoride is adequate to obtain maximal benefits from topical applications of this compound. The basis for such suggestions invariably rests with the results of in vitro studies, quite commonly enamel-solubility studies, in which maximal effects are achieved with lesser concentrations of fluoride. Unfortunately in vitro data do not necessarily predict clinical effects, and the results of a clinical investigation[84] clearly contradict these suggestions. As shown in Table 9–5, the use of lower concentrations of stannous fluoride resulted in smaller caries-preventive benefits in children. Thus until considerably more clinical data to the contrary become available, there is no legitimate basis for using concentrations of fluoride for topical applications other than those that have been adequately evaluated clinically and approved by review groups.

TABLE 9–5. CLINICAL EFFECTIVENESS OF VARYING CONCENTRATIONS OF TOPICALLY APPLIED STANNOUS FLUORIDE*

		Caries Reduction (%)	
SnF$_2$ Concentration (%)	Number Subjects	*DMF teeth*	*DMF surfaces*
8	135	54.7	57.2
4	140	44.1	43.5
0.4	138	29.0	27.4

*From Mercer and Muhler, 1972.[84]

Question 4. Which of the following statements, if any, are correct?

A. The *semiannual* application of fluoride to the teeth has proved to be the *most effective* time interval to reduce caries incidence.

B. There are no documented studies in which sodium fluoride, stannous fluoride, and acidulated phosphate fluoride have been tested in the same study.

C. Stannous fluoride is better than acidulated fluoride and sodium fluoride in nonfluoridated areas.

D. Both stannous fluoride and APF are effective on children, but neither is effective on adults.

E. A liquid topical of a 0.4% solution of stannous fluoride is as effective as an 8% solution.

The relative superiority of acidulated phosphate fluoride gel or solution systems is a frequent topic for research. Five clinical trials directly investigated this question, and the results are summarized in Table 9–6. Four of these studies[57,85–87] involved single annual applications; another one[38] involved semiannual treatments. These data suggest that the two forms are quite comparable, particularly when applied semiannually. In practice the gels are greatly preferred due to their ease of application and reduced chair time when trays are used.

Root Surface Caries

As noted elsewhere, the increased retention of the teeth during adulthood due to various caries-preventive measures and the increase in life expectancy in many countries has resulted in an increased prevalence of root surface caries in adults. According to the 1985–1986 United States Public Health Service (USPHS) survey of adults,[88] about one-half of U.S. adults are afflicted with root surface caries by age 50, with an average prevalence of about 3 lesions by age 70. Thus, this form of caries has received increased attention of dental scientists during the past decade, with investigations covering both its cause and measures for prevention.

Quite clearly, fluoride is very effective for the prevention of root surface caries as evidenced by a limited number of clinical trials and numerous in vitro as well as in situ

TABLE 9–6. COMPARATIVE EFFECTIVENESS OF TOPICALLY APPLIED APF GELS AND SOLUTIONS

	Reduction in Caries Incidence	
Clinical Trial	*APF solution (%)*	*APF gel (%)*
Ingraham & Williams[85]	11	41
Cons et al[86]	0	22
Horowitz & Doyle[87]	28	24
Szwejda[57]	28	4
Cobb et al[38]	34	35

studies. For example, the results of several epidemiologic studies have demonstrated that the presence of fluoridated drinking water throughout the lifetime of an individual prevents the development of root surface caries.[89–92] The magnitude of this effect is consistently greater than 50%. Furthermore, it has been observed[93] that the use of a NaF dentifrice results in a significant decrease in root surface caries of *more than 65%.*

Much less information is available, however, to document the effect of topical fluoride applications on the prevention of root caries and particularly the relative efficacy of different fluoride systems. Nyvad and Fejerskov[94] reported the arrestment of root surface caries following the topical application of 2% NaF and the daily use of a fluoride dentifrice. To obtain some perspective on the potential efficacy of different topical fluoride systems[95,96] we have utilized an established animal root caries model. The results of this investigation are summarized in Table 9–7. From these data it is apparent that all three approved topical fluoride systems decreased the formation of root caries by 63% to 76% in this preclinical model. In the absence of the results of similar clinical data and with the recognition that the application of 8% SnF_2 imparts a brown pigmentation to exposed dentin, it seems appropriate to recommend the topical use of *2% NaF* for the prevention of root caries.

RECOMMENDATIONS—TOPICAL FLUORIDE TREATMENTS

On the basis of the foregoing discussion, it is apparent that although periodic topical applications of any of the three approved agents provide protection against dental caries, maximal patient benefits may be expected only through the use of selected procedures. These recommended procedures include the following:

- Accepting the relative inefficiency of single, topical applications of fluoride solutions, patients with existing evidence of caries activity, whatever their age, should be given an initial series of topical fluoride treatments followed by quarterly, semiannual, or annual treatments as required to maintain cariostasis. The initial series of treatments should consist of four applications administered during a 2- to 4-week period, with the first treatment preceded by a thorough prophylaxis if indicated.
- Whatever fluoride system is selected, the application period (ie, the time the teeth are kept in contact with the fluoride system) should be 4 minutes in all patients with existing caries activity. Shorter treatment periods may be permissible in the performance of treatments to maintain cariostasis.

TABLE 9–7. EFFECT OF PROFESSIONAL TOPICAL FLUORIDE SYSTEMS ON ROOT CARIES IN HAMSTERS[96]

Topical Fluoride System	Root Caries Score	Percent Reduction
Control (H_2O)	8.2	—
SnF_2 (0.4%) + APF (0.3%)	4.9*	40.2
APF (1.2%)	3.0	63.4
NaF (2.0%)	2.3	72.0
SnF_2 (8.0%)	2.0	75.6

*Values within brackets do not differ significantly.

Initiation of Therapy

Practitioners frequently wonder when they should recommend and initiate a topical fluoride application program. All too frequently the tendency is to defer such treatments until the child is 8 to 10 years of age and a majority of the permanent dentition has already erupted.

As discussed earlier, it is well established that the enamel surface of a newly erupted tooth is not completely calcified and therefore that the period when the tooth is most susceptible to carious attack is the first few months after eruption. Furthermore, it has been shown that topical fluoride treatments are effective for both the deciduous and permanent dentitions. Thus it follows that topical fluoride therapy should be initiated when the child reaches about 2 years of age, when most of the deciduous dentition should have erupted. The treatment regimen should be maintained at least on a semiannual basis throughout the period of increased caries susceptibility, which persists for about 2 years after eruption of the permanent second molars (ie, until the child is about 15 years of age).

It should be added that *the susceptibility of the dentition to dental caries does not end at age 15*. It is probable, however, that the gradual decrease in caries susceptibility with increasing age will permit a less frequent topical application program to maintain cariostasis in many patients, and annual fluoride treatments may suffice.

Problems and Disadvantages

Some clinical situations may alter the selection of the treatment agent. For example, the use of stannous fluoride may be contraindicated for aesthetic reasons in specific instances. The reaction of tin ions with enamel, particularly carious enamel, results in the formation of tin phosphates, some of which are brown in color. Thus the use of

this agent produces a temporary brownish pigmentation of carious tooth structure. This stain may exaggerate existing aesthetic problems when the patient has carious lesions in the anterior teeth that will not be restored. Stannous fluoride, however, has not been found to discolor composite restorative materials.

Another problem frequently raised, particularly by pedodontists, concerns the strong, unpleasant, metallic taste of stannous fluoride. Although experienced practitioners can handle this problem, there is no question that flavored, acidulated phosphate fluoride preparations are much better accepted by children. Experimental, flavored, stannous fluoride preparations that diminish but by no means eliminate the taste problem have been evaluated clinically but are not yet commercially available.[32] Until the taste problem of stannous fluoride is solved, most pedodontists agree that the agent of choice for children is APF.

Acidulated phosphate fluoride systems have the disadvantage of possibly etching ceramic or porcelain surfaces. As a result, porcelain veneer facings and similar restorations should be protected with cocoa butter, vaseline, or isolation *prior* to applying APF. Alternatively, NaF may be used instead of APF.

Without doubt, the tendency in many dental offices is to use a specific topical fluoride system and treatment regimen for every patient. It should be emphasized, however, that the specific needs of the patient should be ascertained initially and a specific treatment program developed to fulfill those needs. For example, the use of a series of four or more topical fluoride applications within a 4-week period followed by repeated single applications at 3- to 6-month intervals should be considered for a patient with a severe caries problem. Likewise, a reduced topical application time of 30 seconds as opposed to 4 minutes may be adequate to maintain a patient with little or no current caries activity. In other words, the practitioner should be familiar with the indications and contraindications for using various approaches and select the treatment system and conditions that best meet the needs of the patient.

Fluoride-containing Prophylactic Pastes

The major functions of dental prophylactic pastes are to (1) clean the tooth surface through the removal of all exogenous deposits and (2) polish the dental hard tissues, including restorations. The fulfillment of these functions by all present-day prophylactic pastes is a mechanical process in which the abrasive particles present in the paste simply abrade the deposits and debris from the tooth surface.

In most instances the exogenous deposits are predominantly accumulations of dental pellicle that have not been removed by toothbrushing and have subsequently become calcified to various degrees due to their continual exposure to saliva. Although some portion of these deposits is removed during the scaling aspect of the prophylaxis, a prophylactic paste is typically relied on to remove the remainder of the deposit.

Due to the calcified nature of these exogenous deposits, their removal is not easily accomplished. Many of the early prophylactic pastes used relatively soft materials (eg, talc, calcite, aragonite) as abrasives, but in many patients these pastes performed inefficiently and inadequately. As a result, the use of harder materials (eg, pumice, silica, alumina, zircon) became quite common, and today *pumices* are the most widely used abrasives in prophylactic pastes.

Table 9–8 lists several types of abrasives used in prophylactic pastes and indicates their hardness relative to that of enamel and dentin. From this list, it is apparent that all of the materials listed are physically harder than dentin and that the commonly used abrasives are harder than enamel. It is well known that when two materials are placed in contact in a nonstationary manner, the harder material scratches or abrades the other. Although the degree or rate of abrasion is greatly influenced by the *particle size* of the material, it should be apparent that the use of prophylactic pastes

TABLE 9–8. HARDNESS OF ENAMEL, DENTIN, AND VARIOUS ABRASIVES USED IN DENTAL PROPHYLACTIC PASTES

Material Considered		Physical Hardness	
Name	*Major Component*	*Mohs Scale*	*Knoop Number*
Dentin	$Ca_{10}(PO_4)_6(OH)_2$	3.0–3.5	65–70
Calcite	$CaCO_3$	3	135
Aragonite	$CaCO_3$	3.5–4.0	200–260
Enamel	$Ca_{10}(PO_4)_6(OH)_2$	5.0–5.5	300
Apatite	$Ca_{10}(PO_4)_6F_2$	5	430
Pumice	Al, K, Na Silicates	5–6	450–600
Feldspar	Al, Ca, K, Na Silicates	6	560–650
Quartz	SiO_2	7	820
Zircon	$ZrSiO_4$	7.5	
Emery	$Fe_3O_4 + Al_2O_3$	8–9	2000
Alumina	Al_2O_3	9	2100

containing abrasives harder than enamel or dentin inevitably causes some finite amount of abrasion to these tissues.

The fact that enamel abrasion is inevitable with the use of the prophylactic pastes has caused some concern about the safety of using these materials. Misinformed overreactions based on these concerns have led some to recommend that these pastes not be used. Actual attempts to measure the amount of abrasion resulting from the use of pastes containing pumice have indicated that such abrasion is very superficial, with an enamel thickness of about 0.1 to 1.0 μm being removed in 10 seconds.[97,98] From a clinical viewpoint, this loss of enamel structure does not constitute a safety problem.

Reports from other investigators,[99,100] as well as studies by the author, have shown that the use of nonfluoride prophylactic paste results in a significant decrease in the fluoride content of the enamel surface. This is understandable if one recalls that the greatest concentration of fluoride in enamel occurs at the exposed enamel surface, with deeper layers of enamel containing decreasing concentrations of fluoride. The removal of even a fraction of a micron of the enamel surface would thus be expected to result in a newly exposed surface containing less fluoride than the original surface. In view of this phenomenon it has been suggested that a third function of prophylactic pastes should be to *replenish the fluoride lost from enamel by abrasion* during a prophylaxis. Thus it is not surprising that the majority of commercially available prophylactic pastes contain some type of added fluoride. In most instances this added fluoride does achieve the desired objective and thereby provides a cleaned enamel surface with a fluoride concentration comparable to that originally present. Unfortunately the presence of added fluoride in prophylactic pastes has been the source of much confusion due to the implied or stated claims that the use of such formulations may also increase the resistance of the teeth to dental caries.

The early fluoride-containing prophylactic pastes were prepared immediately prior to use in the dental office by simply adding a quantity of abrasive to a small amount of fluoride solution. For convenience, however, the majority of the pastes used during the past decade have been commercially available, ready-to-use formulations. All of the fluoride systems approved for topical fluoride applications have been used in prophylactic pastes, with formulations containing APF being most widely used at the present time.

Many investigators involved in the development of these pastes felt that these compositions might also provide caries-preventive benefits due to the promising results observed in laboratory studies. Consequently a number of clinical investigations were conducted, and the results of these efforts are summarized in Table 9–9.

Question 5. Which of the following statements, if any, are correct?

A. The first active programs for topical fluoride therapy should be initiated following the eruption of the *first permanent molar.*

B. After age 15 the need for topical applications of fluoride ceases.

C. A prophylaxis increases the effectiveness of the topical application of fluorides.

D. From *0.1 to 1.0* μm of enamel is removed during a prophylaxis.

E. The most widely used fluoride for prophylaxis is APF.

Considered collectively, the clinical data presented in Table 9–9 indicate that the use of fluoride-containing prophylactic pastes results in a very modest increase in

TABLE 9–9. SUMMARY OF RESULTS OF CLINICAL STUDIES EVALUATING FLUORIDE-CONTAINING PROPHYLACTIC PASTES

Nature of Paste					Caries Reduction (%)	
Fluoride Source	Fluoride Content (%)	Abrasive System	Treatment Frequency (mos)	Number of Studies	Range	Mean
SnF$_2$	8.9*	Pumice	6	4	12–35	28
SnF$_2$	8.9*	Pumice	12	5	0–20	13
SnF$_2$	9.0*	Zircon	6	2	0–15	8
APF	0.4†	Silica	6	3	0–2	12
APF	1.2†	Pumice	12	2	0–18	8
APF	2.1†	Pumice	12	1	6–18	12
APF	1.2†	Pumice	6	1	—	9

*% of fluoride compound.
†% of fluoride ion.

the resistance of the teeth to the development of caries. The magnitude of this effect, of about *10%*, is of questionable significance from either a practical or statistical viewpoint. Thus the broad use of fluoride-containing prophylactic pastes for caries prevention is not to be recommended.

In view of these data it is not surprising that no commercially available fluoride-containing prophylactic pastes are approved as safe and effective by either the ADA or the FDA. Although there is no apparent need for concern regarding the safety of these preparations, no formulations have consistently imparted significant cariostatic benefits. Efforts to develop compositions that not only satisfy the cleaning and polishing requirements but also impart significant amounts of caries protection are continuing. Until these formulations become available, fluoride-containing prophylactic pastes should not be considered as caries-preventive measures. However, such pastes should be used rather than their nonfluoride counterparts.

The preceding statement is based on the conclusions of a considerable amount of research with fluoride-containing prophylactic pastes. Such conclusions state that (1) these preparations may replenish enamel

fluoride lost during tooth cleaning and polishing and (2) they may have a modest cariostatic value. Obviously the present stage of development of fluoride prophylactic pastes is such that the clinician is left somewhat in limbo. Should the clinician use these products? In summary, the following recommendations are proposed:

- When a simple prophylaxis is administered, which will not be followed by a topical fluoride application, fluoride-containing prophylactic pastes should be used to replenish the fluoride lost during the procedure.
- When a topical fluoride application is given to a caries-susceptible patient, it is advisable to administer the preceding prophylaxis with a fluoride-containing paste. Although no definitive proof of the additive benefits of both procedures exists as yet, an increased benefit has been shown in some studies. Even when doubt exists, it is preferable to give the patient the possible benefit of any increased protection.

Dentifrices

Through the years dentifrices have been defined as preparations intended for use with a toothbrush to clean the accessible tooth surfaces. They have been prepared in a variety of forms, including pastes, powders, and liquids. The history of dentifrices dates back several centuries. The earliest writings concerning measures to achieve oral cleanliness refer to the use of toothpicks, chewsticks, and sponges; suggested dentifrice ingredients were dried animal parts, herbs, honey, and minerals.

Materials actually detrimental to oral health were used for many years; these materials included excessively abrasive materials, lead ores, and sulfuric and acetic acids. With the appreciation for the need of safe and efficient dentifrices came the research and development that have led to the dentifrices available today and the development of a major industry. In the United States alone dentifrice sales approached $1.2 billion during 1991, and major manufacturers have invested millions of dollars, particularly during the past two decades, to improve them further and to expand their capacities to promote oral health. Without question the dental profession and the scientific community, as well as the general population, have profited immeasurably, both directly and indirectly, from the efforts of the dentifrice industry.

As a result, the functions of present-day dentifrices have been considerably expanded to include the following: (1) cleaning accessible tooth surfaces, (2) polishing accessible tooth surfaces, (3) decreasing the incidence of dental caries, (4) promoting gingival health, and (5) providing a sensation of oral cleanliness, including the control of mouth odors. These functions should be accomplished in a safe manner without undue abrasion to the oral hard tissue, particularly dentin, and without irritation to the oral soft tissues.

This chapter makes no attempt to review the components and functions of dentifrices. For information on these topics as well as a review of the early attempts to develop therapeutic dentifrices using agents other than fluoride, the reader is referred to several excellent reviews.[101–106] (See also Chapter 6.)

Fluoride Dentifrices. At present fluoride is the only dentifrice additive with significant caries-preventive value. The initial studies with fluoride-containing dentifrices were only modestly encouraging. The results of two clinical trials indicated a significant beneficial effect with formulations containing fluorapatites and rock phosphates. However, studies using products containing sodium fluoride at concentrations of 0.01% to 0.15% failed to indicate any beneficial effect.[101] In retrospect it is probable that these and later failures were largely due to the use of an incompatible abrasive system (ie, calcium carbonate) in the formulations. In the 40-year period since the initial clinical trials with fluoride-containing dentifrices, the results of more than 140 controlled clinical studies have been published. For a complete review of all of these studies, the reader is referred to a recent report.[106]

In 1954, the first report was published concerning the use of a dentifrice containing stannous fluoride (0.4%); this study indicated a significant beneficial effect attributable to this agent.[107] Since then the results of more than 60 clinical investigations with stannous fluoride-containing dentifrices have been reported; the vast majority of this work has been performed with formulations containing calcium pyrophosphate as the abrasive agent, although insoluble sodium metaphosphate and hydrated silica have also been used.

Without doubt, the most extensive documentation of the cariostatic benefits of fluoride dentifrices was generated with the original stannous fluoride–calcium pyrophosphate formulation (ie, Crest) with supportive information using this fluoride compound with other abrasive systems. The results of these investigations not only indicated that the normal home use of the stannous fluoride dentifrice resulted in a significant decrease in the incidence of dental caries in children but that similar benefits were derived by adults. Furthermore, these effects were found to be additive to those provided by communal fluoridation and by topical fluoride treatments. As a result of these findings, the Council on Dental Therapeutics of the ADA first awarded complete acceptance to a fluoride dentifrice, specifically the stannous fluoride–calcium pyrophosphate formulation (Crest), in 1964.

Primarily because of the identification of a formal mechanism by the ADA to recognize dentifrices on the basis of clinical documentation of a cariostatic activity, much effort was devoted by dentifrice manufacturers to the development and documentation of effective formulations during the past four decades. A number of effective products subsequently became available.

During the 1960s a number of reports of clinical trials indicated that the use of sodium monofluorophosphate, Na_2PO_3F, in a dentifrice likewise contributed significantly to the control of dental caries. The first product, Colgate MFP, used insoluble sodium metaphosphate as the abrasive system, and this formulation was shown to reduce the incidence of caries in children by as much as 34%. On the basis of these studies this dentifrice was approved as safe and effective by the Food and Drug Administration in 1967 and accepted by the ADA in 1969.

An interesting and unique characteristic of sodium monofluorophosphate is its compatibility with a wide variety of dentifrice abrasive systems. In contrast to other fluoride compounds, such as sodium fluoride and stannous fluoride, which are almost completely dissociated in aqueous solution to yield fluoride ions that readily react with available cations, the fluoride in sodium monofluorophosphate remains largely complexed as $PO_3F^=$ in solution. This fluoride complex is compatible with a wide variety of abrasive systems and therefore may be readily incorporated into a variety of different dentifrice formulations while continuing to provide cariostatic activity.

Additional studies with dentifrices containing sodium fluoride have indicated that this agent is also effective in contributing to the control of dental caries in children. The first of the sodium fluoride dentifrices to be substantiated in this regard included sodium metaphosphate as the abrasive agent. On the basis of three favorable clinical trials, this product (Durenamel) was given provisional acceptance by the ADA Council on Dental Therapeutics; however, this product is no longer available. Another sodium fluoride dentifrice has been the subject of several clinical trials during recent years. This formulation (Gleem) contains calcium pyrophosphate as the abrasive agent and has been found to exert a significant beneficial effect on the incidence of dental caries in children in both low-fluoride and optimal fluoride areas.

In 1981, the formulation of Crest was changed by replacing stannous fluoride with sodium fluoride and using hydrated silica in place of calcium pyrophosphate as the abrasive system. Interestingly these changes and the resultant increase in the amount of available and biologically active fluoride in the product resulted in the revised formulation being significantly more effective than the formulation originally approved.[108,109] Since that time, several additional products containing sodium fluoride have been approved by the ADA (Appendix 9–1). One reason for the increased use of sodium fluoride is that it is the preferred agent for use in tartar control formulations containing soluble pyrophosphates. Furthermore, as noted later in this section, there is evidence that sodium fluoride formulated in a highly compatible abrasive system may be a superior anticaries agent. In terms of fluoride concentration, most dentifrices currently marketed in the United States contain 1000 ppm fluoride, with two exceptions. The Crest family of products contain a hydrated silica abrasive system which is less dense than other conventionally used abrasive systems. Because dentifrice is dispensed by the consumer on the basis of volume, not weight, the concentration of fluoride was increased to 1100 ppm so that the dose delivered would be comparable to nonsilica-based products. On the other hand, Extra Strength Aim, which contains 1500 ppm fluoride from sodium monofluorophosphate, has an elevated fluoride content in an attempt to enhance its anticaries efficacy. Several controlled clinical trials have shown that, in dentifrices employing silica abrasive systems and sodium monofluorophosphate as the fluoride source, 1500 ppm of fluoride is statistically significantly more effective than 1000 ppm, with a margin of superiority of about 15%.[110–112]

The potential role of fluoride dentifrices in the etiology of dental fluorosis needs to be mentioned. Several recent reports have indicated a trend toward an increasing prevalence of fluorosis in the United States.[113,114] A national survey of U.S. children conducted between 1986 and 1987 indicated that about 22% displayed some evidence of dental fluorosis; however, it is important to note that, in terms of severity, 21% had either *very mild* or *mild fluorosis*, and only about 1% were classed as moderate or severe.[115,116] Certainly a number of sources of fluoride may be responsible, individually or collectively, for causing fluorosis. In evaluating the role fluoride toothpastes may play, however, the practitioner should consider several important factors. First, for fluorosis to occur, excessive levels of fluoride must be ingested during the time of enamel formation.[117] For practical purposes, the anterior teeth are of most concern aesthetically, and these are only susceptible to becoming fluorotic during the first 3 years of life.[118] Of course, the risk of toothpaste ingestion is increased in younger children, and some studies have shown that very young children may ingest enough toothpaste to be at risk of dental fluorosis.[119] In fact, one study found that children who brush with a fluoride toothpaste before 2 years of age have an *11-fold* greater risk of developing fluorosis than children who begin brushing later.[120] These considerations have prompted the ADA to recommend that children under age 3 should be advised to use only a *"pea-sized"* quantity of a fluoride dentifrice for brushing and that this quantity be gradually increased with age so that not until age 6 is the child using a *"full-strip"* of dentifrice on the brush head. In making recommendations, the practitioner must consider what other sources of fluoride the child may be ingesting, such as fluoride or fluoride–vitamin supplements, fluoridated communal water supplies, and infant formula prepared with fluoridated water.[120]

Not infrequently, the practitioner is asked if all fluoride dentifrices provide the same amount of caries-preventive benefits. In an attempt to answer this question, a review[106] examined the results of all published studies involving fluoride dentifrices. It was concluded on the basis of a considerable body of information that the use of sodium fluoride with highly compatible abrasive systems, such as hydrated silica or acrylic particles, is the most effective dentifrice system for caries prevention at this time.

Two subsequent literature reviews compared all available clinical data regarding the relative efficacy of compatible sodium fluoride dentifrices and those containing sodium monofluorophosphate.[121,122] Using different statistical procedures, both of these reviews concluded that *sodium fluoride was significantly more effective than sodium monofluorophosphate.* Based on a meta analysis, Johnson[123] concluded that the magnitude of this difference was 7.0%. It is interesting that many fluoride dentifrices marketed outside the United States contain mixtures of NaF and Na_2PO_3F with a total fluoride content of 1500 ppm. Clinical efficacy data of these latter systems have also been reviewed recently[122,123] with the conclusion that they are numerically less effective than an equivalent concentration of bioavailable sodium fluoride.

It is significant that the extensive research with fluoride dentifrices has resulted in the regular use of these products by a major segment of our population. In terms of total dentifrice sales, nearly 95% consists of the accepted or approved formulations listed in Appendix 9–1. The widespread acceptance and use of these products by the general public has been considered one of the primary factors contributing to the apparent decrease in the prevalence of dental caries observed in the United States.[124,125]

In general it should be apparent from this brief review that the use of approved fluoride dentifrices results in a significant decrease in the incidence of dental caries. In view of this, the use of such preparations should be routinely recommended.

Question 6. Which of the following statements, if any, are correct?

A.   The use of fluoride prophylactic pastes has yielded equivocal results as caries control agents when used as the sole method of fluoride application.

B.   Fluoride dentifrices appear to reduce caries in a range of approximately 20% to 45%.

C.   The safety of a new dentifrice containing *new fluoride compounds* must be approved by the FDA before it is accepted by the ADA.

D.   In 1981, Crest changed the fluoride in the formula from sodium fluoride to stannous fluoride.

E.   Despite the fact that several dentifrices contain fluoride, approximately 40% of the population prefers nonfluoride-containing brands.

MULTIPLE FLUORIDE THERAPY

From the prior discussions of various measures to apply fluoride to erupted teeth, it is apparent that no single fluoride treatment provides total protection against dental caries. Recognition of this fact led early investigators to evaluate the use of combinations of fluoride measures.

Multiple fluoride therapy is a term that has been used to describe these fluoride combination programs. As originally developed, this program included the application of fluoride in the dental office in the form of both a fluoride-containing prophylactic paste and a topically applied fluoride solution and the home use of an approved fluoride dentifrice. In addition, some form of systemic fluoride ingestion, preferably communal water fluoridation, was included.

The only published reports of clinical investigations that attempted to assess the total effect of this type of multiple fluoride therapy on dental caries involved the use of stannous fluoride topical systems.[126-131] In each of these studies the topical fluoride treatments were administered semiannually; the results are summarized in Table 9–10. The results of these investigations in-

TABLE 9–10. RESULTS OF CLINICAL STUDIES USING MULTIPLE FLUORIDE THERAPY INVOLVING SNF$_2$-CONTAINING PROPHYLACTIC PASTE, TOPICAL FLUORIDE, AND DENTIFRICE

Clinical Investigation	Study Population	Fluoride in Water	Study Duration	Caries Reduction (%)
Gish & Muhler[127]	Children	Yes	3 years	55
Bixler & Muhler[126]	Children	No	3 years	58
Muhler et al[128]	Adults	Yes	30 months	64
Scola & Ostrom[130]	Adults	No	2 years	58*
Scola[131]	Adults	No	2 years	56*
Obersztyn et al[129]	Adults	No	1 year	60

*Average reduction for multiple similar groups.

dicate that the combination of topical fluoride applications and home use of a fluoride dentifrice resulted in about 59% fewer carious lesions.

The fact that the magnitude of this benefit is somewhat less than that of the components evaluated individually indicates that the caries-protection effects of the individual components (ie, prophylactic paste, topical solution, and dentifrice) are only partially additive. Nevertheless, it is important to note that the combination of stannous fluoride treatments not only reduced the incidence of caries by more than 50% in both children and young adults but did so in both the presence and absence of communal fluoridation. If one accepts a 50% caries reduction attributable to water fluoridation and another 50% reduction of the remaining caries from the use of multiple fluoride treatments, it is apparent that the use of multiple fluoride therapy, including communal fluoridation, results in an overall reduction in caries of about 75%.

During the past few years clinical investigators have explored combinations of fluoride treatments using agents other than stannous fluoride with variable success. For example, Beiswanger and coworkers[132] reported that additive benefits were observed with topical applications of acidulated phosphate fluoride and the home use of a stan-

nous fluoride dentifrice. Neither Downer and associates[133] nor Mainwaring and Naylor,[134] however, were able to demonstrate additive benefits from the combined use of a sodium monofluorophosphate dentifrice and topical application of acidulated phosphate fluoride.

The available data relating to multiple fluoride therapy thus suggest additive benefits from the use of either stannous fluoride or acidulated phosphate fluoride in the dental office and the home use of dentifrices containing fluoride. This does not necessarily mean that other combinations of fluoride treatments may not provide additive benefits but merely that they have not yet been evaluated; hopefully the results of future investigations will clarify this matter. In the meantime the dental practitioner is strongly advised to use combinations of fluoride treatments to provide maximal caries protection for patients.

Fluoride Rinses

In 1960, reports began to appear indicating that the regular use of neutral sodium fluoride solutions decreased the incidence of caries. In an attempt to identify topical fluoride measures especially appropriate for use in dental public health programs, this approach was studied extensively during the subsequent 15 years. Whereas these studies employed a wide variety of experimental conditions, a number of investigations involved either the daily use of solutions containing 200 to 225 ppm or the weekly use of solutions containing about 900 ppm fluoride. The majority of these studies were conducted in schools with supervised use of the rinse throughout the school year.

The results of these investigations have been summarized on several occasions and will not be repeated here.[67,104,135-138] In general, both types of fluoride rinses resulted in significant caries reduction of about 30% to 35%. On the basis of these findings, the simplicity of administration, and the lack of need for professional dental supervision, weekly fluoride rinse programs in schools are becoming increasingly popular and are being aggressively promoted by dental public health agencies. Fluoride rinses were approved as safe and effective by the FDA in 1974[68] and by the Council of Dental Therapeutics of the ADA in 1975.[137] A "Guide to the Use of Fluoride" was published in the September 1986 issue of the *Journal of the American Dental Association*. The composition and recommended use of approved products is shown in Table 9–11.

Nearly all of the early investigations using fluoride rinses involved children residing in areas in which the drinking water was deficient in fluoride. As a result, the ap-

provals given to fluoride rinses were related to their use in nonfluoridated communities. Two reports[139,140] indicated, however, significant benefits from fluoride rinses used in the presence of an optimal concentration of fluoride in the drinking water. Three additional reports have appeared relative to the use of fluoride rinses in children residing in fluoridated communities. The results of all three studies indicate that cariostatic benefits provided by fluoride rinses are additive to those derived from communal fluoridation.[141-143] In view of these collective observations there appears to be no reason to restrict the use of fluoride rinses to nonfluoridated communities.

The approval of fluoride rinses by the FDA and the ADA's Council on Dental Therapeutics for use in public health programs opened the door for the home use of these products as a component of multiple fluoride preventive programs. Although the approved preparations were intended to be available strictly by prescription, a 0.05% neutral sodium fluoride rinse (Fluorigard) was subsequently introduced for over-the-counter sale. Ultimately, approval was given to fluoride rinses distributed over the counter for home use, although some restrictions were required. These restrictions included the distribution of quantities containing no more than 300 mg fluoride in a single container, a cautionary label to avoid swallowing, and an indication that the preparations should not be used by children younger than 6 years of age. At present there are several fluoride rinses distributed in this manner; these products contain about 225 ppm fluoride and are intended for daily usage.

The question of additivity of the effects of fluoride rinses to those obtained using fluoride with other vehicles has received contradictory answers. Ashley and associates[144] found a modest additivity of benefits

TABLE 9–11. COMPOSITION AND USAGE OF APPROVED FLUORIDE RINSES

Source of Fluoride	Fluoride Content		Recommended Usage
	Percent	*ppm*	
NaF	0.20	900	Weekly
NaF	0.02	100	Twice daily
NaF	0.05	225	Daily
APF	0.02	200	Daily
SnF_2	0.10	243	Daily

from the supervised daily rinsing in school with an acidulated phosphate fluoride rinse coupled with supervised brushing in school plus normal home use of a sodium monofluorophosphate dentifrice. A similar observation was reported by Triol and coworkers.[145] On the other hand, Blinkhorn and coworkers[146] failed to observe any indication of additive caries protection between the similar supervised daily use of a neutral 0.05% sodium fluoride and the home use of this same dentifrice. Likewise, Ringelberg and associates[147] failed to find additivity between a daily sodium fluoride rinse and home use of a stannous fluoride dentifrice. Similarly Horowitz and coworkers,[148] in a study involving the supervised weekly use of a sodium fluoride rinse and daily fluoride tablets plus the home use of approved fluoride dentifrices, observed a caries reduction comparable in magnitude to that reported earlier by these investigators with fluoride tablets or rinses used individually.

Additive effects can also be inferred from the numerous school fluoride rinse studies in which caries reductions from 30% to 35% were observed. Because the majority of these children in both the control and experimental groups used fluoride-containing dentifrices, it follows that the benefits observed in those studies were obtained above those provided by the fluoride dentifrices. The same conclusion can be reached from the data reported by Birkeland and coworkers[135] in Norway, a country where over 90% of the children use fluoride dentifrices. After 10 years of a mouth-rinsing program, these authors found a caries reduction of over 50% and reduction in the need for restoration of more than 70%.

It can thus be concluded that fluoride rinses have a place as a component of a preventive program along with, but not as substitutes for, other modalities of fluoride use. Their main use is for patients with a high risk of contracting caries. Although existing evidence may lead some to doubt whether additional benefits for the patients accrue from the use of rinses, *it is preferable in these instances to give the patients the benefit of the doubt.* Examples of patients for whom fluoride rinses should be recommended include

- Patients who, because of the use of medication, surgery, radiotherapy, and so on, have reduced salivation and increased caries formation.
- Patients with orthodontic appliances or removable prostheses, which act as traps for plaque accumulation.
- Patients unable to achieve acceptable oral hygiene.
- Patients with extensive oral-rehabilitation and multiple restorative margins, which represent sites of high caries risk.
- Patients with gingival recession and susceptibility to root caries.
- Patients with rampant caries, at least as long as the high caries activity persists.

As a general rule, daily rinses should be recommended rather than a weekly regimen; not only does the daily procedure appear to be slightly more effective, but, as a practical consideration, it is easier for patients to remember and comply with a daily procedure. In all these instances, it is important to remember that the rinses should not be used in place of any of the other modalities of fluoride use but as part of a comprehensive, preventive program that should also comprise plaque control, frequent fluoride topical applications, the home use of a fluoride dentifrice, diet control, and testing to determine if and when the oral environment is no longer conducive to caries. For children living in nonfluoride areas, the prescription of fluoride supplements may also be considered.

Fluoride Gels for Home Use

During the past decade a number of fluoride gels have become available as additional measures that may be used to help achieve caries control. These products contain 0.4% stannous fluoride (1000 ppm fluoride) or 1.0% NaF (5000 ppm) and are formulated in a nonaqueous gel base that does not contain an abrasive system. Their recommended manner of usage involves toothbrushing with gel (similar to using a dentifrice), allowing the gel to remain in the oral cavity for 1 minute, and then expectorating thoroughly.

Even though no controlled clinical trials have been conducted of these products used in this manner, a number of them have been approved by the ADA's Council on Dental Therapeutics as an additional caries-preventive measure for use in patients with rampant caries. The basis for the approval of these products has been the numerous prior clinical caries studies using dentifrices containing the same amount of stannous fluoride coupled with analytic data demonstrating the stability of these preparations.

From a practical point of view, the recommended use of fluoride gels is generally similar to that cited earlier for fluoride rinses. In other words, they may be considered as an alternative to the use of fluoride rinses and an adjunct to the use of professional, topical fluoride applications and fluoride dentifrices as a collective means of achieving caries control in patients who are especially prone to caries formation. Like fluoride rinses, the use of these gels is generally restricted to the period required to achieve caries control. Compared with fluoride rinses, however, fluoride gels appear to have an advantage in terms of patient compliance. Because these preparations are *only distributed to patients by their dentists,* it is commonly thought that patients

are more likely to use them in compliance with the recommendations of their dentist.

It should be stressed that fluoride gels should not be used in place of fluoride dentifrices. Because the gels contain no abrasive system to control the deposition of pellicle, their use in place of a dentifrice results in the accumulation of stained pellicle in the majority of patients within a few weeks. Nevertheless, the proper use of these preparations in combination with professional topical fluoride applications and the home use of fluoride dentifrices may be expected to help achieve caries control in caries-active patients.

Question 7. Which of the following statement, if any, are correct?

A. If a 20% reduction in caries occurs from water fluoridation and then another 25% from topical fluoride therapy, the total reduction is 45%.

B. Fluoride rinses are of little value in fluoridated areas.

C. A fluoride rinse container should not contain more than *300 mg* of fluoride.

D. A school rinse program can be expected to produce caries reduction on the order of *30%.*

E. It is more practical to have people use a daily rinse than a weekly rinse.

SUMMARY

A number of different aspects of topical fluoride therapy have been reviewed in the foregoing material. Without doubt, the use of topical fluoride therapy contributes significantly to the control of dental caries; however, *one cannot expect to control dental caries completely through the use of fluorides alone.* Furthermore, because no single fluoride treatment procedure provides the maximal degree of caries protection possible with fluoride, the use of *multiple fluoride therapy* is advocated. In particular the dentist should identify the needs of each patient and institute a multiple fluoride treatment program designed specifically to fulfill those needs.

ANSWERS AND EXPLANATIONS

1. C

A—incorrect. It is very rapid the first month, slows down over the next year or so, and then remains relatively stable.

B—incorrect. It decreases very rapidly in the first 10 μm and then more slowly, until the dentinoenamel junction is reached.

D—incorrect. As the pH falls, the fluoride becomes more effective in protecting; at a neutral pH no protection is needed.

E—incorrect. The main reaction product is calcium fluoride.

2. A, C, D

B—incorrect. It is not at a linear rate; the greatest loss is during the first few days and finally tapers off after about 2 weeks.

E—incorrect. There is a lesser concentration on the tooth and about the same cariostatic action as for other inorganic fluorides.

3. A, D, E

B—incorrect. Stannous fluoride in water goes to a hydroxide and then a white oxide.

C—incorrect. It looks like a gel, acts like a gel, but is not a gel.

4. B

A—incorrect. A series within a short period appears best.

C—incorrect. There appears to be little, if any, difference in their efficacy.

D—incorrect. The first part is correct; the second part is incorrect; *both* are effective, but the amount of difference between the SnF_2 and APF is debatable.

E—incorrect. In the critical field studies, the 8% wins easily.

5. D, E

A—incorrect. Too late; it should have started as soon as possible after the eruption of the first deciduous tooth.

B—incorrect. Fluoride is a lifelong adjunct for dental health.

C—incorrect. Recent studies have shown that it is not necessary to give a prophylaxis prior to a fluoride application.

6. A, B, C

D—incorrect. Vice versa. Crest started with SnF_2 but now has NaF.

E—incorrect. People use the fluoride dentifrices—up to 90%.

7. A, C, D, E

B—incorrect. The effects of fluoride are additive; the more often it is applied, the better.

SELF-EVALUATION QUESTIONS

1. There is an (inverse) (direct) relationship between the amount of fluoride (F) in the surface of the enamel and the number of caries. It requires about ___2 yrs___ (time) for the enamel surface to mature following eruption. The greatest amount of F in the enamel is located in the outer ___5-10 μm___ (distance) of the enamel.

2. The reaction of elevated concentrations of fluoride with hydroxyapatite (HA) is accompanied by the formation of ___Ca Floride___ (on the surface) (in the apatite crystal) and a loss of ___Phosphate___ (one of the key elements of HA). This

element is not lost when SnF_2 is one of the reactants, in which case, the compound ___phosphate___ (name) is formed. Along with this compound, _____ (another F compound) is formed on the surface.

3. The calcium fluoride (CaF_2) formed on the surface of the tooth with neutral sodium fluoride, APF or SnF_2, is lost relatively rapidly for ___24 hrs___ (time) and almost completely lost in ___15 days___ (time). During this period, the *calcium fluoride* (is) (is not) protective. Along with the formation—then loss of—CaF_2, there is a slow change in the apatite crystal from ___hydroxy___ (apatite) to ___fluorohydrox___ (name of crystalline form), which is more permanent. Because studies indicate that the CaF_2 is leached from the tooth, the long-term benefit must be from the ___fluorohydrox___ (crystalline form). Thus, if the buildup of the crystalline form is slow, (multiple) (single) applications of fluoride probably provide the best long-term prevention.

4. Fluoride accumulates to a greater extent in demineralized areas (true); two fluoride compounds with a low pH that demineralize enamel (and thus increase F uptake) are _____ and _____. Two times when the tooth is not optimally mineralized are just after ___erupt^n___ (event) of the tooth and just after bacterial ___d-min___ (event) of enamel; in either event, F aids in the mineralization or remineralization process.

5. The three different solutions of fluoride used in office applied topical applications are NaF, ___2%___ percent; APF, ___1.23%___ percent; and SnF_2, ___8%___ percent. The APF is made acidic by adding two acids, ___.34% hydrofluric acid___ and ___orthophospho...___ to a ___.98___ %.

REFERENCES

1. Keene HJ, Mellberg JR, Nicholson CR. History of fluoride, dental fluorosis, and concentrations of fluoride in surface layer of enamel of caries-free naval recruits. *J Public Health Dent.* 1973; 33:142–148.

2. DePaola PF, Brudevold F, Aasenden R, et al. A pilot study of the relationship between caries experience and surface enamel fluoride in man. *Arch Oral Biol.* 1973; 20:859–864.

3. Weatherall JA, Hallsworth AS, Robinson C. The effect of tooth wear on the distribution of fluoride in the enamel surface of human teeth. *Arch Oral Biol.* 1973; 18:1175–1189.

4. Aasenden R, Moreno EC, Brudevold F. Fluoride levels in the surface enamel of different types of human teeth. *Arch Oral Biol.* 1973; 18:1403–1410.

5. Brudevold F. Fluoride therapy. In: Bernier JL, Muhler JC, eds. *Improving Dental Practice Through Preventive Measures.* St Louis, Mo. Mosby; 1975.

6. Isaac S, Brudevold F, Smith FA, et al. Solubility rate and natural fluoride content of surface and subsurface enamel. *J Dent Res.* 1958; 37:254–263.

7. Thylstrup A. A scanning electron microscopical study of normal and fluorotic enamel demineralized by EDTA. *Acta Odont Scand.* 1979; 37:127–135.

8. Brudevold F, McCann HG. Enamel solubility tests and their significance in regard to dental caries. *Ann NY Acad Sci.* 1968; 153:20.

9. Bibby BG. Use of fluorine in the prevention of dental caries. I. Rationale and approach. *J Am Dent Assoc.* 1944; 31:228–236.

10. Phillips RW, Muhler JC. Solubility of enamel as affected by fluorides of varying pH. *J Dent Res.* 1947; 26:109–117.

11. Fischer RB, Muhler JC. The effect of sodium fluoride upon the surface structure of powdered dental enamel. *J Dent Res.* 1952; 31:751–755.

12. Frazier PD, Engen DW. X-ray diffraction study of the reaction of acidulated fluoride with powdered enamel. *J Dent Res.* 1966; 45:1144–1148.

13. Gerould CH. Electron microscope study of the mechanisms of fluoride deposition in teeth. *J Dent Res.* 1945; 24:223–233.

14. Joost-Larsen M, Fejerskov O. Structural studies on calcium fluoride formation and uptake of fluoride in surface enamel in vitro. *Scand J Dent Res.* 1978; 86:337–345.

15. McCann HG, Bullock FA. Reactions of fluoride ion with powdered enamel and dentin. *J Dent Res.* 1955; 34:59–67.

16. Scott DB, Picard RG, Wyckoff WG. Studies of the action of sodium fluoride on human enamel by electron microscopy and electron diffraction. *Public Health Rep.* 1950; 65:43–56.

17. Muhler JC, Van Huysen G. Solubility of enamel protected by sodium fluoride and other compounds. *J Dent Res.* 1947; 26: 119–127.

18. Muhler JC, Boyd TM, Van Huysen G. Effects of fluorides and other compounds on the solubility of enamel, dentin, and tricalcium phosphate in dilute acids. *J Dent Res.* 1950; 29:182–193.

19. Jordan TH, Wei SHY, Bromberger SH, et al. Sn₃F₃PO₄: The products of the reaction between stannous fluoride and hydroxyapatite. *Arch Oral Biol.* 1971; 16:241–246.

20. Wei SHY, Forbes WC. Electron microprobe investigations of stannous fluoride reactions with enamel surfaces. *J Dent Res.* 1974; 53:51–56.

21. Brudevold F, Savory A, Gardner DE, et al. A study of acidulated fluoride solutions. *Arch Oral Biol.* 1963; 8:167–177.

22. Wellock WD, Brudevold F. A study of acidulated fluoride solutions. II. The caries inhibition effect of single annual topical applications of an acidic fluoride and phosphate solution, a two year experience. *Arch Oral Biol.* 1963; 8:179–182.

23. DeShazer DO, Swartz CJ. The formation of calcium fluoride on the surface of hydroxyapatite after treatment with acidic fluoride-phosphate solution. *Arch Oral Biol.* 1967; 12:1071–1075.

24. Wei SHY, Forbes WC. X-ray diffraction and analysis of the reactions between intact and powdered enamel and several fluoride solutions. *J Dent Res.* 1968; 47:471–477.

25. Mellberg JR, Laakso PV, Nicholson CR. The acquisition and loss of fluoride by topically fluoridated human tooth enamel. *Arch Oral Biol.* 1966; 11:1213–1220.

26. Bruun C. Uptake and retention of fluoride by intact enamel in vivo after application of neutral sodium fluoride. *Scand J Dent Res.* 1973; 81:92–100.

27. Lovelock DJ. The loss of topically applied fluoride from the surface of human enamel in vitro using ¹⁸F. *Arch Oral Biol.* 1973; 18: 27–29.

28. Mellberg JR. Topical fluoride controversy symposium. Enamel fluoride uptake from topical fluoride agents and its relationship to caries inhibition. *J Am Soc Prev Dent.* 1973; 3:53–54.

29. Rinderer L, Schait A, Muhlemann HR. Loss of fluoride from dental enamel after topical fluoridation. Preliminary report. *Helv Odont Acta.* 1965; 9:148–150.

30. Ahrens G. Effect of fluoride tablets on uptake and loss of fluoride in superficial enamel in vivo. *Caries Res.* 1976; 10:85–95.

31. Wei SHY, Schulz EM Jr. In vivo microsampling of enamel fluoride concentrations after topical treatments. *Caries Res.* 1975; 9:50–58.

32. Beiswanger BB, Mercer VH, Billings RJ, et al. A clinical caries evaluation of a stannous fluoride prophylactic paste and topical solution. *J Dent Res.* 1980; 59:1386–1391.

33. Mellberg JR. Enamel fluoride and its anticaries effects. *J Prev Dent.* 1977; 4:8–20.

34. Mellberg JR, Nicholson CR, Miller BG, et al. Acquisition of fluoride in vivo by enamel from repeated topical sodium fluoride applications in a fluoridated area: final report. *J Dent Res.* 1970; 49:1473–1477.

35. Knutson JW. Sodium fluoride solution: Technique for applications to the teeth. *J Am Dent Assoc.* 1948; 36:37–39.

36. Puttnam NA, Bradshaw F. X-ray fluorescence studies on the effect of stannous fluoride on human teeth. *Adv Fluorine Res Dent Caries Prev: (ORCA).* 1964; 3:145–150.

37. Hoermann KC, Klima JE, Birks LS, et al. Tin and fluoride uptake in human enamel in situ: Electron probe and chemical mi-

croanalysis. *J Am Dent Assoc.* 1966; 73: 1301–1305.

38. Cobb HB, Rozier RG, Bawden JW. A clinical study of the caries preventive effects of an APF solution and an APF thixotropic gel. *Pediatr Dent.* 1980; 2:263–266.

39. Knutson JW, Armstrong WD, Feldman FM. Effect of topically applied sodium fluoride on dental caries experience. IV. Report of findings with two, four, and six applications. *Public Health Rep.* 1947; 62: 425–430.

40. Houpt M, Koenigsberg S, Shey Z. The effect of prior toothcleaning on the efficacy of topical fluoride treatment. Two-year results. *Clin Prev Dent.* 1983; 5(4):8–10.

41. Katz RV, Meskin LH, Jensen ME, et al. Topical fluoride and prophylaxis: A 30-month clinical trial. *J Dent Res.* 1984; 63(Prog. & Abstracts). Abstract 771.

42. Ripa LW, Leske GS, Sposato A, et al. Effect of prior toothcleaning on biannual professional APF topical fluoride gel-tray treatments. Results after two years. *Clin Prev Dent.* 1983; 5(4):3–7.

43. Bijella MFTB, Bijella VT, Lopes ES, et al. Comparison of dental prophylaxis and toothbrushing prior to topical APF applications. *Community Dent Oral Epidemiol.* 1985; 13:208–211.

44. Ekstrand J, Koch G. Systemic fluoride absorption following fluoride gel application. *J Dent Res.* 1980; 59:1067.

45. Ekstrand J, Koch G, Lindgren LE, et al. Pharmacokinetics of fluoride gels in children and adults. *Caries Res.* 1981; 15:213–220.

46. LeCompte EJ, Whitford GM. Pharmacokinetics of fluoride from APF gel and fluoride tablets in children. *J Dent Res.* 1982; 61:469–472.

47. LeCompte EJ, Doyle TE. Oral fluoride retention following various topical application techniques in children. *J Dent Res.* 1982; 61:1397–1400.

48. LeCompte EJ, Rubenstein LK. Oral fluoride rentention with thixotropic and APF gels and foam-lined and unlined trays. *J Dent Res.* 1984; 63:69–70.

49. McCall DR, Watkins TR, Stephan KW, et al. Fluoride ingestion following APF gel application. *Br Dent J.* 1983; 155:333–336.

50. Pourbaix S, Desager JP. Fluoride absorption: A comparative study of 1% and 2% fluoride gels. *J Biol Buccale.* 1983; 11:103–108.

51. LeCompte EJ, Doyle TE. Effects of suctioning devices on oral fluoride retention. *J Am Dent Assoc.* 1985; 110:357–360.

52. Stookey GK, Schemehorn BR, Drook CA, et al. The effect of rinsing with water immediately after a professional fluoride gel application on fluoride uptake in demineralized enamel: An in vivo study. *Pediatr Dent.* 1986; 8(3):153–157.

53. Averill HM, Averill JE, Ritz AG. A two-year comparison of three topical fluoride agents. *J Am Dent Assoc.* 1967; 74:996–1001.

54. Galagan DF, Knutson JW. Effect of topically applied sodium fluoride on dental caries experience. VI. Experiments with sodium fluoride and calcium chloride. Widely spaced applications. Use of different solution concentrations. *Public Health Rep.* 1948; 63:1215–1221.

55. Horowitz HS, Heifetz SB. Evaluation of topical fluoride applications of stannous fluoride to teeth of children born and reared in a fluoridated community: Final report. *J Dent Child.* 1969; 36:355–361.

56. Muhler, JC. The anticariogenic effectiveness of a single application of stannous fluoride in children residing in an optimal communal fluoride area. II. Results at the end of 30 months. *J Am Dent Assoc.* 1960; 61:431–438.

57. Szwejda LF. Fluorides in community programs: A study of four years of various fluorides applied topically to the teeth of children in fluoridated communities. *J Public Health Dent.* 1972; 32:25–33.

58. Brudevold F, Nanjoks R. Caries preventive fluoride treatment of the individual. *Caries Res.* 1978; 12(suppl 1):52–64.

59. Forrester DJ. A review of currently available topical fluoride agents. *J Dent Child.* 1971; 38:52–58.

60. Horowitz HS, Heifetz SB. The current status of topical fluorides in preventive dentistry. *J Am Dent Assoc.* 1970; 81:166–177.

61. Forrester DJ, Shulz EM, eds. International workshop of fluorides and dental caries reductions. Baltimore, Md: University of Maryland; 1974.

62. Stookey GK. Fluoride therapy. In: Bernier JL, Muhler JC, eds. *Improving Dental Practice Through Preventive Measures,* 2nd ed. St. Louis, Mo. Mosby; 1970.

63. Ripa LW. Professionally (operator) applied topical fluoride therapy: A critique. *Int Dent J.* 1981; 31:105–120.

64. Mellberg JR, Ripa LW. Professionally applied topical fluoride. In: *Fluoride in Preventive Dentistry. Theory and Clinical Applications.* Chicago, IL. Quintessence; 1983:181–214.

65. Katz S, McDonald JL, Stookey GK. *Preventive Dentistry in Action,* 3rd ed. Upper Montclair, NJ. DCP Publishing Company; 1979.

66. Ripa LW. Review of the anticaries effectiveness of professionally applied and self-applied topical fluoride gels. *J Public Health Dent.* 1989; 49:297–309.

67. Council on Dental Therapeutics. Fluoride compounds. In: *Accepted Dental Therapeutics,* 40th ed. Chicago, Ill. American Dental Association; 1984.

68. Fine SD. Topical fluoride preparations for reducing incidence of dental caries. Notice of status. *Federal Register.* 1974; 39:17245.

69. Clark DC, Hanley JA, Stamm JW, et al. An empirically based system to estimate the effectiveness of caries-preventive agents. A comparison of the effectiveness estimates of APF gels and solutions, and fluoride varnishes. *Caries Res.* 1985; 19:83–95.

70. Arnold FA Jr, Dean HT, Singleton DC Jr. The effect on caries incidence of a single topical application of a fluoride solution to the teeth of young adult males of a military population. *J Dent Res.* 1944; 23:155–162.

71. Frank R. Research and clinical evaluation of local applications of sodium fluoride. *Schweiz Mschr Zahnh.* 1950; 60:283–287.

72. Driak F. Kariesprophlaxe mit besonderer Berücksichtigung der Impragnierungsmethoden. *Oester Ztschr Stomat.* 1951; 48: 153–168.

73. Klinkenberg E, Bibby BG. Effect of topical applications of fluorides on dental caries in young adults. *J Dent Res.* 1950; 29:4–8.

74. Rickles NH, Becks H. The effects of an acid and a neutral solution of sodium fluoride on the incidence of dental caries in young adults. *J Dent Res.* 1951; 30:757–765.

75. Kutler B, Ireland RL. The effect of sodium fluoride application on dental caries experience in adults. *J Dent Res.* 1953; 32:458–462.

76. Carter WJ, Jay P, Shklair IL, et al. The effect of topical fluoride on dental caries experience in adult females of a military population. *J Dent Res.* 1953; 34:73–76.

77. Muhler, JC. Effect on gingiva and occurrence of pigmentation on teeth following the topical application of stannous fluoride or stannous chlorofluoride. *J Periodont.* 1957; 28:281–286.

78. Muhler, JC. The effect of a single topical application of stannous fluoride on the incidence of dental caries in adults. *J Dent Res.* 1958; 37:415–416.

79. Protheroe DH. A study to determine the effect of topical application of stannous fluoride on dental caries in young adults. *Roy Can D Corps Q.* 1961; 3:18–23.

80. Harris NO, Hester WR, Muhler JC, et al. Stannous fluoride topically applied in aqueous solution in caries prevention in a military population. SAM-TDR-64-26. Brooks Air Force Base, Tex: United States Air Force School of Aerospace Medicine; 1964.

81. Obersztyn A, Kolwinski K, Trykowski J, et al. Effects of stannous fluoride and amine fluorides on caries incidence and enamel solubility in adults. *Aust Dent J.* 1974; 24:395–397.

82. Viegas Y. The caries inhibiting effect of a single topical application of an acidic phosphate solution in young adults. A one year experience. *Rev Saude Publica.* 1970; 4:55–60.

83. Curson I. The effect on caries increments in dental students of topically applied acidulated phosphate fluoride (APF). *J Dent* 1973; 1:216–218.

84. Mercer VH, Muhler JC. Comparison of single topical application of sodium fluoride and stannous fluoride. *J Dent Res.* 1972; 51:1325–1330.

85. Ingraham RQ, Williams JE. An evaluation of the utility of application and cariostatic effectiveness of phosphate-fluorides in solution and gel states. *J Tenn Dent Assoc.* 1970; 50:5–12.

86. Cons NC, Janerich DT, Senning RS. Albany topical fluoride study. *J Am Dent Assoc.* 1970; 80:777–781.

87. Horowitz HS, Doyle J. The effect on dental caries of topically applied acidulated phosphate-fluoride: Results after three years. *J Am Dent Assoc.* 1971; 82:359–365.

88. USPHS. Oral health of United States adults. The national survey of oral health in U.S. employed adults and seniors: 1985–1986. National findings. *NIH Publ. No. 87-2868,* August, 1987.

89. Burt BA, Ismail AI, Eklund SA. Root caries in an optimally fluoridated and a high-fluoride community. *J Dent Res.* 1986; 65:1154–1158.

90. Brustman BA. Impact of exposure to fluoride-adequate water on root surface caries in elderly. *Gerodontics.* 1986; 2:203–207.

91. Hunt RJ, Eldredge JB, Beck JD. Effect of residence in a fluoridated community on the incidence of coronal and root caries in an older adult population. *J Pub Health Dent.* 1989; 49:138–141.

92. Stamm JW, Banting DW, Imrey PB. Adult root caries survey of two similar communities with contrasting natural water fluoride levels. *J Am Dent Assoc.* 1990; 120:143–149.

93. Jensen ME, Kohout FJ. The effect of a fluoridated dentifrice on root and coronal caries in an older adult population. *J Am Dent Assoc.* 1988; 117:829–832.

94. Nyvad B, Fejerskov O. Active root surface caries converted into inactive caries as a response to oral hygiene. *Scand J Dent Res.* 1986; 94:281–284.

95. Stookey GK. Critical evaluation of the composition and use of topical fluorides. *J Dent Res.* 1990; 69:805–812.

96. Stookey GK, Rodlun CA, Warrick JM, et al. Professional topical fluoride systems vs root caries in hamsters. *J Dent Res.* 1989; 68: 372. Abstract 1521.

97. Biller IR, Hunter EL, Featherstone MJ, et al. Enamel loss during a prophylaxis polish in vitro. *J Int Assoc Dent Child.* 1980; 11: 7–12.

98. Stookey GK. In vitro estimates of enamel and dentin abrasion associated with a prophylaxis. *J Dent Res.* 1978; 57:36.

99. Vrbic V, Brudevold F, McCann HG. Acquisition of fluoride by enamel from fluoride pumice pastes. *Helv Odont Acta.* 1967; 11:21–26.

100. Vrbic V, Brudevold F. Fluoride uptake from treatment with different fluoride prophylaxis pastes and from the use of pastes containing a soluble aluminum salt followed by topical application. *Caries Res.* 1970; 4:158–167.

101. Bibby BG. Test of the effect of fluoride-containing dentifrices on dental caries. *J Dent Res.* 1945; 24:297–303.

102. Gershon SD, Pader M. Dentifrices. In: Balsam H, Sagarin E, eds. *Cosmetics, Science and Technology,* 2nd ed. New York, NY. Wiley; 1972; 423–531.

103. Muhler JC, Hine MK, Day HG. *Preventive Dentistry.* St. Louis, Mo. Mosby; 1954.

104. Volpe AR. Dentifrices and mouth rinses. In: Caldwell RC, Stallard RE, eds. *A Textbook of Preventive Dentistry.* Philadelphia, Penn. W. B. Saunders; 1977.

105. Wei SHY. The potential benefits to be derived from topical fluorides in fluoridated communities. In: Forrester DJ, Schulz EM Jr, eds. *International Workshop on Fluoride and Dental Caries Reductions.* Baltimore, Md: University of Maryland; 1974.

106. Stookey GK. Are all fluoride dentifrices the same? In: Wei SHY, ed. *Clinical Uses of Fluorides.* Philadelphia, Penn. Lea & Febiger, 1983.

107. Muhler JC, Radike AW, Nebergall WH, et al. The effect of a stannous fluoride-containing dentifrice on caries reduction in children. *J Dent Res.* 1954; 33:606–612.

108. Beiswanger BB, Gish CW, Mallatt ME. Effect of a sodium fluoride-silica abrasive

dentifrice upon caries. *Pharmacol Ther Dent.* 1981; 6:9–16.

109. Zacherl WA. A three-year clinical caries evaluation of the effect of a sodium fluoride-silica abrasive dentifrice. *Pharmacol Ther Dent.* 1981; 6:1–7.

110. Fogels HR, Meade JJ, Griffith J, et al. A clinical investigation of a high-level fluoride dentifrice. *ASDC J Dent Child.* 1988; 55(3):210–215.

111. Conti AJ, Lotzkar S, Daley R, et al. A 3-year clinical trial to compare efficacy of dentifrices containing 1.14% and 0.76% sodium monofluorophosphate. *Community Dent Oral Epidemiol.* 1988; 16(3):135–138.

112. Stephen KW, Russell JI, Creanor SL, et al. Comparison of fiber optic transillumination with clinical and radiographic caries diagnosis. *Community Dent Oral Epidemiol.* 1987; 15(2):90–94.

113. Szpunar SM, Burt BA. Trends in the prevalence of dental fluorosis in the United States: A review. *J Public Health Dent.* 1987; 47:71–79.

114. Heifetz SB, Driscoll WS, Horowitz HS, et al. Prevalence of dental caries and dental fluorosis in areas with optimal and above-optimal water fluoride concentrations. *J Am Dent Assoc.* 1988; 116:490–495.

115. Brunelle JA. The prevalence of dental fluorosis in U.S. children. *J Dent Res.* 1989; 68(special issue):995. Abstract.

116. U.S. Department of Health and Human Services. Oral health of United States children. The national survey of dental caries in U.S. schoolchildren: 1986–1987 national and regional findings. *NIH Pub. No. 89-2247, 1989.*

117. Larsen MJ, Richards A, Fejerskov O. Development of dental fluorosis according to age at start of fluoride administration. *Caries Res.* 1985; 19:519–527.

118. TenCate AR. Oral histology—development, structure and function. St. Louis, Mo. Mosby; 1985.

119. Beltran ED, Szpunar SML. Fluoride in toothpaste for children: Suggestion for change. *Pediatr Dent.* 1988; 10:185–188.

120. Osuji OO, Leake ML, Chipman G, et al. Risk factors for dental fluorosis in a fluori-

dated community. *J Dent Res.* 1988; 67:1488–1492.

121. Beiswanger BB, Stookey GK. The comparative clinical cariostatic efficacy of sodium fluoride and sodium monofluorophosphate dentifrices: A review of trials. *J Dent Child.* 1989; 56:337–347.

122. Stookey GK, DePaola PF, Featherstone JDB, et al. A critical review of the relative anticaries efficacy of sodium fluoride and sodium monofluorophosphate dentifrices. *Caries Res.* 1993; 27:337–360.

123. Johnson MF. Comparative efficacy of NaF and MFP dentifrices in caries prevention: A meta-analytic overview. *Caries Res.* 1993; 27:328–336.

124. Glass RL, Scheinin A, Barmes DE. Changing caries prevalence in two cultures. *J Dent Res.* 1981; 60(special issue A): 361. Abstract 202.

125. Zacherl WA, Long DM. Reduction in caries attack rate—nonfluoridated community. *J Dent Res.* 1979; 58(special issue A): 227. Abstract 535.

126. Bixler D, Muhler JC. Effect on dental caries in children in a nonfluoride area of combined use of three agents containing stannous fluoride: A prophylactic paste, a solution, and a dentifrice. II. Results at the end of 24 and 36 months. *J Am Dent Assoc.* 1966; 72:392–396.

127. Gish CW, Muhler JC. Effect on dental caries in children in a natural fluoride area of combined use of three agents containing stannous fluoride: a prophylactic paste, a solution, and a dentifrice. *J Am Dent Assoc.* 1965; 70:914–920 (and personal communication).

128. Muhler JC, Spear LB Jr, Bixler D, et al. The arrestment of incipient dental caries in adults after the use of three different forms of SnF_2 therapy: Results after 30 months. *J Am Dent Assoc.* 1967; 75:1402–1406.

129. Obersztyn A, Piotrowski Z, Kowinski K, et al. Stannous fluoride in the prophylaxis of caries in adults. *Czas Stomat.* 1973; 26:1181–1187.

130. Scola FP, Ostrom CA. Clinical evaluation of stannous fluoride when used as a constituent of a compatible prophylactic paste,

as a topical solution, and in a dentifrice in naval personnel. II. Report of findings after two years. *J Am Dent Assoc.* 1968; 77: 594–597.

131. Scola FP. Self-preparation stannous fluoride prophylactic technique in preventive dentistry: Report after two years. *J Am Dent Assoc.* 1970; 81:1369–1372.

132. Beiswanger BB, Billings RJ, Sturzenberger OP, et al. Effect of an $SnF_2Ca_2P_2O_7$ dentifrice and APF topical applications. *J Dent Child.* 1978; 45:137–141.

133. Downer MC, Holloway PJ, Davies TGH. Clinical testing of a topical fluoride caries prevention program. *Br Dent J.* 1976; 141: 242–247.

134. Mainwaring PJ, Naylor NM. A three-year clinical study to determine the separate and combined caries-inhibitory effects of sodium monofluorophosphate toothpaste and an acidulated phosphate fluoride gel. *Caries Res.* 1978; 12:202–212.

135. Birkeland JM, Broch L, Jorkjend J. Benefits and prognoses following 10 years of a fluoride mouthrinsing program. *Scand J Dent Res.* 1977; 85:31–37.

136. Birkeland JM, Torrell P. Caries-preventive fluoride mouthrinses. *Caries Res.* 1978; 12(suppl 1):38–51.

137. Reports on Councils and Bureaus, Council on Dental Therapeutics, American Dental Association. Council classifies fluoride mouthrinses. *J Am Dent Assoc.* 1975; 91: 1250–1252.

138. Torell P, Ericsson Y. The potential benefits to be derived from fluoride mouth-rinses. In: Forrester DJ, Schulz EM Jr, eds. *International Workshop on Fluorides and Dental Caries Reductions.* Baltimore, Md: University of Maryland; 1974.

139. Hagglund O. Annual report of the first dental officer of Vasterhotten County 1969. In: Forrester DJ, Schulz EM, eds. *International Workshop on Fluorides and Dental Caries Reduction.* Baltimore, Md: University of Maryland; 1974.

140. Radike AW, Gish CW, Peterson JK, et al. Clinical evaluation of stannous fluoride as an anticaries mouthrinse. *J Am Dent Assoc.* 1973; 86:404–408.

141. Driscoll WS, Swango PA, Horowitz AM, et al. Caries-preventive effects of daily and weekly fluoride mouthrinsing in an optimally fluoridated community: Findings after 18 months. *Pediatr Dent.* 1981; 3: 316–320.

142. Jones JC, Murphy RF, Edd PA. Using health education in a fluoride mouthrinse program: The public health hygienist's role. *Dent Hyg.* 1979; 53:469–473.

143. Kawall K, Lewis DW, Hargreaves JA. The effect of a fluoride mouthrinse in an optimally fluoridated community—final two year results. *J Dent Res.* 1981; 60(special issue A): 471. Abstract 646.

144. Ashley FP, Mainwaring PF, Emslie RD, et al. Clinical testing of a mouthrinse and a dentifrice containing fluoride. A two-year supervised study in school children. *Br Dent J.* 1977; 143:333–338.

145. Triol CW, Kranz SM, Volpe AR, et al. Anticaries effect of a sodium fluoride rinse and an MFP dentifrice in a nonfluoridated water area. A thirty-month study. *Clin Prev Dent.* 1980; 2:13–15.

146. Blinkhorn AS, Holloway PJ, Davies TGH. The combined effect of a fluoride mouthrinse and dentifrice in the control of dental caries. *J Dent Res.* 1977; 56(special issue D): D111.

147. Ringelberg ML, Webster DB, Dixon DO, et al. The caries-preventive effect of amine fluorides and inorganic fluorides in a mouthrinse or dentifrice after 30 months of use. *J Am Dent Assoc.* 1979; 98:202–208.

148. Horowitz HS, Heifetz SB, Meyers RJ, et al. Evaluation of a combination of self-administered fluoride procedures for the control of dental caries in a nonfluoride area: findings after four years. *J Am Dent Assoc.* 1979; 98:219–223.

Appendix 9–1 Listing of ADA-accepted Dentifrices Being Marketed in the United States as of June, 1992.

Sodium Fluoride

Aquafresh Tartar Control Toothpaste—SmithKline Beecham Consumer Brands
Colgate Fluoride Gel—Colgate-Palmolive Company
Colgate Fluoride Toothpaste—Colgate-Palmolive Company
Colgate Tartar Control Formula Gel—Colgate-Palmolive Company
Colgate Tartar Control Formula Toothpaste—Colgate-Palmolive Company
Crest Tartar Control Formula Toothpaste, Mint, Regular—Procter & Gamble Company
Crest Toothpaste, Mint, Regular—Procter & Gamble Company
Crest Toothpaste for Kids, Fun Fruit, Sparkle Fun—Procter & Gamble Company
Gel Formula Crest—Procter & Gamble Company
Muppets Fluoride Toothpaste, Bubble Gum, Mild Mint—Oral-B Laboratories, Inc.
Prevent Tartar Prevention Toothpaste with Fluoride—Johnson & Johnson Consumer Products, Inc.
Sesame Street Fluoride Toothpaste—Oral-B Laboratories, Inc.
Shane Fluoride Toothpaste—Jerome Milton, Inc.

Sodium Monofluorophosphate

Anti-Tartar Aim Plus Fluoride Toothpaste—Chesebrough-Pond Inc.
Aquafresh Fluoride Toothpaste—SmithKline Beecham Consumer Brands
Aquafresh for Kids Toothpaste—SmithKline Beecham Consumer Brands
Colgate Junior with MFP Fluoride Gel—Colgate-Palmolive Company
Colgate with MFP Fluoride Gel—Colgate-Palmolive Company
Colgate with MFP Fluoride Toothpaste—Colgate-Palmolive Company
Dentagard Fluoride Toothpaste—Colgate-Palmolive Company
Extra-Strength Aim Gel—Chesebrough-Pond Inc.
Extra-Strength Aim Toothpaste—Chesebrough-Pond Inc.
Macleans Fluoride Toothpaste, Mildmint, Peppermint—SmithKline Beecham Consumer Brands
Regular-Strength Aim Toothpaste, Mint, Regular—Chesebrough-Pond Inc.
Topol Smoker's Fluoride Gel, Peppermint-Spearmint—DEP Corporation
Topol Smoker's Toothpaste with Fluoride, Peppermint-Spearmint—DEP Corporation

Chapter 10

Pit-and-Fissure Sealants

Franklin García-Godoy
Norman O. Harris

Objectives

At the end of this chapter it will be possible to

1. Explain how sealants can provide a primary preventive means of reducing the need for operative treatment for up to 95% of all carious lesions of the mouth.
2. Name the criteria for selecting teeth for sealant placement and the four essentials for maximum retention of sealants on teeth.
3. Describe the steps in the placement of either light cured or auto-polymerizing sealants, and discuss corrective actions to be taken in case excess sealant is placed on a tooth.
4. Discuss the different options for preventive dentistry restorations and how they involve sealants.
5. Cite five reasons given for the underuse of sealants by practitioners.
6. List and explain the different methods used to maintain a dry field.

Introduction

Fluorides are highly effective in reducing the number of carious lesions occurring on the smooth surfaces of enamel and cementum. Unfortunately fluorides are *not* equally effective in protecting the occlusal pits and fissures, where 95% of all carious lesions occur.[1] Considering the fact that the occlusal surfaces constitute only 12% of the total number of tooth surfaces, it means that

235

the pits and fissures are approximately eight times as vulnerable as the smooth surfaces.

Historically several solutions have been tried to deal with the deep pits and fissures on occlusal surfaces.

- In 1895, Wilson reported the placement of cement in pits and fissures to prevent caries.[2] Bödecker[3] in 1929 suggested that deep fissures could be broadened with a large round bur to make the occlusal areas more self-cleansing, a procedure that is called *enameloplasty*.[4] Two major disadvantages however, accompany enameloplasty. First, it requires a dentist, which immediately limits its use. Second, in modifying a deep fissure by this method, it is often necessary to remove more sound tooth structure than would be required to insert a small restoration.
- In 1923 and again in 1936, Hyatt[5] advocated the early insertion of small restorations in deep pits and fissures before carious lesions had the opportunity to develop. He termed this procedure "prophylactic odontotomy." Again, this operation is more of a treatment procedure than a preventive approach, because it requires the cutting of tooth structure.
- Several methods have been unsuccessfully used in an attempt either to seal or to make the fissures more resistant to caries. These attempts have included the use of topically applied zinc chloride and potassium ferrocyanide[6] and the use of ammoniacal silver nitrate[7]; they have also included the use of copper amalgam packed into the fissures.[8]
- Fluorides that protect the smooth surfaces of the teeth are less effective in protecting the occlusal surfaces.[9] Following the use of fluo-

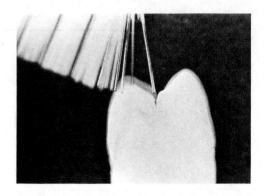

Figure 10–1. One of the reasons that 50% of the carious lesions occur on the occlusal surface. Note that the toothbrush bristle has a greater diameter than the width of the fissure. (*Courtesy of Dr J. McCune, Johnson & Johnson*).

rides, there is a large reduction of incidence in smooth-surface caries but a smaller reduction in occlusal pit-and-fissure caries. This results in an *increased proportion* in the ratio of occlusal to interproximal lesions, even though the total number may be less.

- A final course of action to deal with pit-and-fissure caries is one that is often used: do nothing; wait and watch. This option avoids the need to cut good tooth structure until a definite carious lesion is identified. It also results in many teeth being lost when individuals do not return for periodic checkups.

In the late 1960s and early 1970s, another option became available—the use of pit-and-fissure sealants.[10] With this option, a liquid plastic is flowed over the occlusal surface of the tooth where it penetrates the deep fissures to fill areas that cannot be cleaned with the toothbrush (Fig 10–1).[11] The hardened sealant presents a barrier between the tooth and the hostile oral environment.

CRITERIA FOR SELECTING TEETH FOR SEALANT PLACEMENT

Following are the criteria for selecting teeth for sealing. Because no harm can occur from sealing, *when in doubt, seal.*

A sealant is indicated if

- A deep occlusal fissure, fossa, or lingual pit is present.

A sealant is *contraindicated* if

- Patient behavior does not permit use of adequate dry-field techniques throughout the procedure.
- An open occlusal carious lesion exists.
- Caries exist on other surfaces of the same tooth.
- A large occlusal restoration is already present.

A sealant is *probably* indicated if

- The fossa selected for sealant placement is well isolated from another fossa with a restoration.
- The area selected is confined to a fully erupted fossa, even though the distal fossa is impossible to seal due to inadequate eruption.
- An intact occlusal surface is present where the contralateral tooth surface is carious or restored; this is because teeth on opposite sides of the mouth are usually equally prone to caries.
- An incipient lesion exists in the pit and fissure.

OTHER CONSIDERATIONS IN TOOTH SELECTION

All teeth meeting the previous criteria should be sealed and resealed as needed. Where the cost benefit is critical and priori-

ties must be established, such as occurs in many public health programs, ages 3 and 4 years are the most important times for sealing the eligible deciduous teeth; ages 6 to 7 years for the first permanent molars; and ages 11 to 13 years for the second permanent molars and premolars.[12] Sealants appear to be equally retained on occlusal surfaces in primary,[13] as well as permanent teeth. They should be used in fluoride areas, as well as in nonfluoride areas.[14] Sealants should be placed on the teeth of adults if there is evidence of existing or impending caries susceptibility, as would occur following excessive intake of sugar or as a result of a drug- or radiation-induced xerostomia. In all cases *it is the disease susceptibility of the tooth that should be addressed, not the age of the individual.*

The following are two good illustrations of this philosophy. After a 3-year study, Ripa and colleagues[15] concluded that the time the teeth had been in the mouth (some for 7 to 10 years) had no effect on the vulnerability of occlusal surfaces to caries attack. Also, Arthur and Swango[16] have reported that the incidence of occlusal caries in young Navy recruits, who are usually in their late teens or early 20s, is relatively high.

BACKGROUND ON SEALANTS

Three different kinds of plastics have been used as occlusal sealants: (1) *polyurethanes,* (2) *cyanoacrylates,* and (3) *bisphenol A-glycidyl methylacrylate* (Bis-GMA).

The polyurethanes were among the first to appear on the commercial market. They proved to be too soft and totally disintegrated in the mouth after 2 or 3 months. Despite this problem, their use was continued for some time—not as a sealant but as a vehicle with which to apply fluoride to the teeth.[17] In this technique fluoride was mixed with the polyurethane and then painted over all surfaces of the teeth. During the time that the plastic adhered to the tooth, fluoride continually leached out to increase the concentration of fluoride in the enamel. This function has been superseded by the use of fluoride varnishes, which are easier to apply.[18]

The cyanoacrylates have also been tried as sealants, but they too disintegrated after a slightly longer time.[19]

Bisphenol A-glycidyl methylacrylate (Bis-GMA) is now the sealant of choice. It is a mixture of Bis-GMA and methyl methacrylate.[20] Its successful use was first reported by Buonocore[10] in the late 1960s. Some of the first commercial products to use this plastic, and which are classified as *accepted* or *provisionally accepted* by the ADA, were the following.[21]

- Concise Brand White Sealant (3M Company)
- Delton, clear and tinted (Johnson & Johnson)
- Helioseal, white (Vivadent)
- Nuva-Seal, Nuva-Cote, and Prisma-Shield (L. D. Caulk)
- Oralin Pit and Fissure Sealant, clear and tinted (S.S. White)
- Visio-Seal (ESPE)

This endorsement by the ADA indicates that sufficient research data supports each of these products being considered "safe and effective as a caries preventive procedure."[22] Classified sealants may carry the statement: "[Product name] has been shown to be acceptable as an agent for sealing off an anatomically deficient region of the tooth to supplement the regular professional care in a program of preventive dentistry."[22]

In 1972, Nuva-Seal was the first successful commercial sealant to be placed on the market. Since then more effective second- and third-generation sealants have be-

come available. Some of them contain *fillers,* which makes it desirable to classify the commercial products into *filled* and *unfilled* sealants. In addition to the Bis-GMA, the filled sealants contain microscopic glass beads, quartz particles, and other fillers used in composite restorations. The fillers make the sealant more resistant to abrasion. The fillers are coated with products such as *silane,* to facilitate their combination with the Bis-GMA plastic.

Some investigators have evaluated glass ionomer cements as fissure sealants.[23] Currently, new resin-reinforced glass ionomer cements are also being investigated for their effectiveness as pit-and-fissure sealants. The preliminary 1-year results revealed that although clinically the glass ionomer wears at a faster rate than a conventional resin sealant, in the scanning electron microscopic evaluation, the material could be seen at the deep recesses of the pits and fissures with no carious lesion present.[24] Little documentation is available at present, however, to recommend them on a routine basis.

POLYMERIZATION OF THE SEALANTS

The liquid plastic is called the *monomer.* When the monomer is acted on by the catalyst, repeating chemical bonds begin to form, increasing in number and complexity as the hardening process (*polymerization*) proceeds. Finally, the resultant hard product is known as a *polymer.* Two methods have been employed to catalyze polymerization: (1) light curing by use of a visible blue light (synonyms: photocure, photoactivation, light activation) and (2) self-curing, in which a monomer and a catalyst are mixed together (synonyms: cold cure, autopolymerization, and chemical activation). The two original Caulk products, Nuva-Seal and Nuva-Cote, were the only sealants in the United States requiring ultraviolet light for activation. They have been replaced by other light-cured sealants that require visible blue light. In the manufacture of these latter products, a catalyst, such as camphoroquinone, which is sensitive to visible blue light frequencies, is placed in the monomer at the time of manufacture. Later, when the monomer is exposed to the visible blue light, polymerization is initiated (Fig 10–2).

With the autopolymerizing sealants, the catalyst is incorporated with the monomer; in addition, another bottle contains an *initiator*—usually *benzoyl peroxide.* When the monomer and the initiator are mixed, polymerization begins.

The High-Intensity Light Source

The light-emitting device consists of a high-intensity white light, a blue filter to produce the desired blue color, usually between 400 to 500 nm, and a light-conducting rod. Of two types of lights, one is a hand-held model with a short conducting rod, the other a desktop model with a long fiberglass cable to conduct the light to the light rod. Most have timers for automatically switching off the lights after a predetermined time interval. In use, the end of the rod is held only a few millimeters above the sealant during the first 10 seconds, after which it can be rested on the hardened surface of the partially polymerized sealant. The time required for polymerization is set by the manufacturer and is usually around 20 to 30 seconds. The depth of cure is influenced by the intensity of light, which can differ greatly with different products and length of exposure. Often it is desirable to set the automatic light timer for longer than the manufacturers' instructions.[25] Even after cessation of light exposure, a final, slow polymerization can continue over a 24-hour period.[26]

It is not known whether long-term exposure to the intense light can damage the eye. Staring at the lighted operating field is uncomfortable and does produce afterimages. This problem is circumvented by the use of a round 4-in. dark yellow disk, which fits over the light housing. The disk filters out the intense blue light in the 400 to 500-nm range as well as being sufficiently dark to subdue other light frequencies.

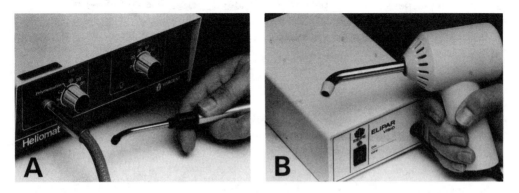

Figure 10–2. Two kinds of lights used for polymerization of a pit-and-fissure sealant. **A.** The heavier unit with a light wand at the end of a fiberoptics bundle, and **B,** a hand-held unit for direct, intraoral exposure.

by dep' Incipient lesions not invaded by bacteria & Sealent ideal preventive measure!

PHOTOCURED VERSUS SELF-CURED SEALANTS

The main advantage of the photocured sealant is that the operator can initiate polymerization at any suitable time. Polymerization time is shorter with the photocured products than with the self-curing sealants. The photocured process does require the purchase of a light source, which adds to the expense of the procedure. This light, however, is the same one that is used for polymerization of composite restorations, so is available in all offices. When using a photocured sealant in the office, it is prudent to store the product away from bright office lighting, which can sometimes initiate polymerization.

Conversely, the self-curing resins do not require an expensive light source. They do, however, have the great disadvantage that once mixing has commenced, if some minor problem is experienced in the operating field, the operator must either continue mixing or stop and make a new mix. For the autopolymerizing resin, the time allowed for sealant manipulation and placement *must not* be exceeded, even though the material might still appear liquid. Once the hardening begins, it occurs very rapidly, and any manipulation of the material during this critical time jeopardizes retention.

The light-cured sealants have a higher compressive strength and a smoother surface[27], which is probably due to air being introduced into the self-cure resins during mixing.[28] Despite these differences, both the photocured and the autopolymerizing products appear to be *equal* in retention.[29]

Question 1. Which of the following statements, if any, are correct?

A.   In an area with fluoridated water, a *lower incidence* of caries can be ex-

pected, along with a *lower proportion* of occlusal to smooth-surface lesions. > proportn p≠F

B.   Sealants should *never* be flowed over incipient caries.

C.   Bis-GMA are the initials used to specify the chemical family of plastics containing bisphenol A-glycidyl methacrylate.

D.   A monomer can polymerize, but a polymer cannot monomerize.

E.   Sealants are contraindicated for adults.

REQUISITES FOR SEALANT RETENTION

For sealant retention the surface of the tooth must (1) have a maximum surface area, (2) have deep, irregular pits and fissures, (3) be clean, and (4) be *absolutely dry* at the time of sealant placement and uncontaminated with saliva residue. *These are the four commandments for successful sealant placement, and they cannot be violated.*

INCREASING THE SURFACE AREA

Sealants do not bond directly to the teeth. Instead, they are retained mainly by adhesive forces.[30] To increase the surface area, which in turn increases the adhesive potential, *tooth conditioners* (also called etchants), which are composed of a 30% to 50% concentration of phosphoric acid, are placed on the occlusal surface prior to the placement of the sealant.[31] The etchant may be either in liquid or gel form. The former is easier to apply and easier to remove. Both are equal in abetting retention.[32,33] If any etched areas on the tooth surface are not covered by the sealant or if the sealant is not retained, the normal appearance returns to the tooth within 1 hour to a few weeks due to a remineralization from constituents in the saliva.[34] The etchant should be carefully applied to avoid contact with the soft tissues. If not confined to the occlusal surface, the acid may infrequently produce a mild inflammatory response. It also produces a sharp acid taste that is often objectionable to children.

PIT-AND-FISSURE DEPTH

Deep, irregular pits and fissures offer a much more favorable surface contour for sealant retention compared with broad, shallow fossae (Fig 10–3). The deeper fissures protect the plastic sealant from the shear forces occurring as a result of masticatory movements. Of parallel interest is the possibility of caries development increasing as the slope of the inclined planes increases.[35,36] Thus, *as the potential for caries increases, so does the potential for sealant retention.*

SURFACE CLEANLINESS

don't polish before placing sealant

The need and method for cleaning the tooth surface prior to sealant placement are controversial. Usually the acid etching alone is sufficient for surface cleaning. This is attested to by the fact that two of the most cited and most effective sealant longevity studies by Simonsen[37] and Mertz-Fairhurst[38] were accomplished without use of a prior prophylaxis; however, some advocate the use of a pumice and water slurry to clean the occlusal surface, which adds an extra time-consuming operation. If this extra procedure is believed necessary to remove heavy stains or is accomplished as part of a routine prophylaxis in a preventive dentistry program, the slurry must be a *nonfluoride, oil-free* mixture to avoid contamination of the tooth surface. Recently, however, it was shown that cleaning teeth with the newer prophylaxis pastes with or without fluoride (NuPro, Topex) did not affect the bond strength of sealants,[39] composites[40] or orthodontic brackets. The use of an air-polisher is another cleaning option.[41,42] Hydrogen peroxide has also been tried as a cleaning agent but has the disadvantage that it produces a precipitate on the enamel surface.[43] Whatever the cleaning preferences—either by acid etching or other methods—all heavy stains, deposits, and debris should be off the occlusal surface before applying the sealant.

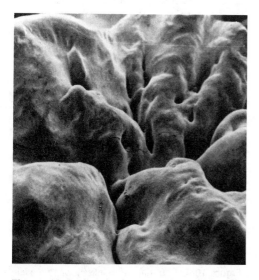

Figure 10–3. An electron scanning microscope view of the deep pits and fissures of the occlusal surface of a molar. (*Courtesy of Dr A. J. Gwinnett, State University of New York at Stony Brook.*)

DRYNESS

The teeth *must* be dry at the time of sealant placement because the present sealants are hydrophobic. The presence of saliva on the tooth is even more detrimental than water because its organic components interpose a barrier between the tooth and the sealant. Whenever the teeth are dried with an air syringe, the air stream should be checked to ensure that it is not moisture-laden. Otherwise, sufficient moisture can be sprayed on the tooth to prevent adhesion of the sealant to the enamel. A check for moisture can be accomplished by directing the air stream onto a cool mouth mirror; any fogging indicates the presence of moisture.

A dry field can be maintained in several ways, including use of a rubber dam, employment of cotton rolls, and the placement of bibulous pads over the opening of the parotid duct. The rubber dam provides an ideal way to maintain dryness for an extended time. Because a rubber dam is usually employed in accomplishing quadrant dentistry, sealant placement for the quadrant should also be accomplished during the operation. Under most operating conditions, however, it is not feasible to apply the dam to the different quadrants of the mouth; instead it is necessary to employ cotton rolls, combined with the use of an effective high-volume, low-vacuum aspirator. Under such routine operating conditions, cotton rolls, with and without the use of bibulous pads, can usually be employed as effectively as the dam for the relatively short time needed for the procedure. The most successful sealant studies have used cotton rolls for isolation.[37] In one study in which retention was tested using a rubber dam versus cotton rolls, the sealant retention was approximately equal.[44]

In programs with high patient volume where cotton rolls are used, it is best to have two individuals do the procedure—the operator, whose main task is to prepare the tooth and to apply the sealant, and the assistant, whose task is to maintain dryness. An operator working alone, however, can maintain a maximum dry field for the time needed to place the sealants. For the maxilla, there should be little problem with the placement of cotton rolls in the buccal vestibule and, if desirable, the placement of a bibulous pad over the parotid duct. For the mandible, a 5-in. segment of a 6-in. cotton roll should be looped around the last molar and then held in place by the patient using the index and third fingers of the opposite hand from the side being worked on (Fig 10–4). With this aid from the patient and with appropriate aspiration techniques, the cotton rolls can usually be kept dry throughout the entire procedure. Cotton roll holders may be used, but they can be cumbersome when using the aspirator or when attempting to manipulate or remove a roll. If a cotton roll does become *slightly* moist, many times another short cotton roll can be placed on top of the moist segment and held in place for the duration of the procedure. In the event that it becomes necessary to replace a wet cotton roll, it is essential that *no* saliva contacts the etched tooth surface; if there is *any* doubt, it is necessary to repeat all procedures up to the time the dry field was compromised.

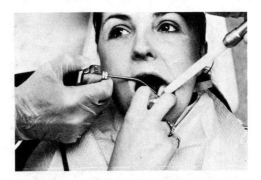

Figure 10–4. Four-handed dentistry with no assistant: The patient holds the cotton rolls with the index and third finger, thumb under chin. Patient also holds aspirator with other hand when it is not being used by operator.

This includes a 15-second etch to remove any residual saliva, in lieu of the original 1-minute etch.

Another promising dry-field isolating device that can be used for single operator use, especially when used with cotton rolls, is the VAC ejector moisture control system.[a] In one study comparing the Vac-Eject versus the cotton roll for maintaining dryness, the two were found to be equally effective.[45]

PREPARING THE TOOTH FOR SEALANT APPLICATION

The preliminary steps for the light-activated and the autopolymerized resins are similar up to the time of application of the plastic to the teeth. After the selected teeth are isolated, they are thoroughly dried for approximately 10 seconds. This can be mentally estimated by counting off the seconds—1000, 2000—until 10,000 has been reached. The liquid etchant is then placed on the tooth with a small plastic sponge or cotton pledget

---

[a] Whaledent International, 236 Fifth Ave, New York, NY.

held with cotton pliers. Traditionally, the etching solution is gently daubed, *not rubbed,* on the surface for 1 minute for permanent teeth and for 1½ minutes for deciduous teeth.[46] Other clinical studies, however, have shown that acid etching the enamel of both primary and permanent teeth for only 20 seconds produced similar sealant[47] and composite[48] retention rates as those etched for 1 and 1½ minutes. Alternatively, acid gels are applied with a supplied syringe and left undisturbed. Another 15 seconds of etching is indicated for fluorosed teeth to compensate for the greater acid resistance of the enamel. The etching period should be timed with a *clock.* At the end of the etching period, the aspirator tip is positioned with the bevel interposed *between the cotton roll and the tooth.* For 10 seconds the water from the syringe is flowed over the occlusal surface and thence into the aspirator tip. Again, this 10-second period can be mentally counted. Care should be exercised to ensure that the aspirator tip is close enough to the tooth to prevent any water from reaching the cotton rolls but yet not so close that it diverts the stream of water directly into the aspirator (Fig 10–5).

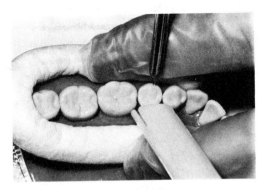 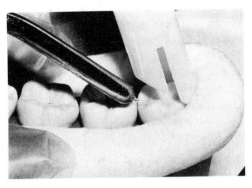

A   **B**

Figure 10–5. Showing position of aspirator tip between the bicuspid and cotton roll during flushing, **A,** and between water flow and cotton roll looped around second molar, **B.** *Complete* dryness of the cotton rolls can be maintained with this technique.

Following the water flush, the tooth surface is dried for 10 seconds. The dried tooth surface should have a white, dull, frosty appearance. This is due to the etching having removed approximately 5 to 10 μm of the original surface,[49] although at times interrod penetrations of up to 100 μm may occur.[50] The etching does not always involve the interrod areas; sometimes the central portion of the rod is etched, and the periphery is unaffected. The pattern on any one tooth is unpredictable.[51] In any event, the surface area is greatly increased.

Question 2. Which of the following statements, if any, are correct?

A. Autopolymerizing sealants and photocured sealants have approximately the same record for longevity.

B. A 40% phosphoric acid etchant should be satisfactory for both etching and cleaning the average tooth surface.

C. Fossae with deep inclined planes tend to have more carious fissures; fossae with deep inclined planes tend to retain sealants better.

D. In studies in which a rubber dam was used to maintain a dry field for sealant placement, the retention of sealants was greater than when cotton rolls were used.

E. In placing a sealant, 10 seconds are devoted to each of the drying and etching phases and 1 minute to the flushing of the etchant from the tooth.

APPLICATION OF THE SEALANT

When the plastic sealant flows over the prepared surface, it penetrates the fingerlike depressions created by the etching solution. These projections of plastic into the etched areas are called tags[52] (Fig 10–6). The tags are essential for retention. Scanning electron studies of sealants that have not been retained have demonstrated large areas devoid of tags or incomplete tags due to saliva contamination. If a sealant is forcefully separated from the tooth by masticatory pressures, many of these tags are retained in the etched depressions.

With either the photocured or the autopolymerized sealants, the material should first be placed in the fissures where there is the maximum depth. At times penetration of the fissure is negated by the presence of debris, air entrapment, narrow orifices, and excessive viscosity of the sealant.[53] The sealant should not only fill the fissures but should have some bulk over the fissure. After the fissures are adequately covered, the material is then brought to a knife edge, approximately halfway up the inclined plane.

Following polymerization, the sealants should be examined carefully *before* discontinuing the dry field. If any voids are evident, additional sealant can be added without the need for any additional etching. The hardened sealant has an oily residue on the surface. This is unreacted monomer that can be either wiped off with a gauze sponge or can be left. If a sealant requires repair at any time after the dry field is discontinued, it is prudent to repeat the same etching and drying procedures as initially used. Because all the commercial sealants—both the photocured and self-cured—are of the same Bis-GMA chemical family, they easily bond to one another.[54]

Question 3. Which of the following statements, if any, are correct?

A. The etchant *predictably* attacks the center of the enamel prism, leaving the periphery intact.

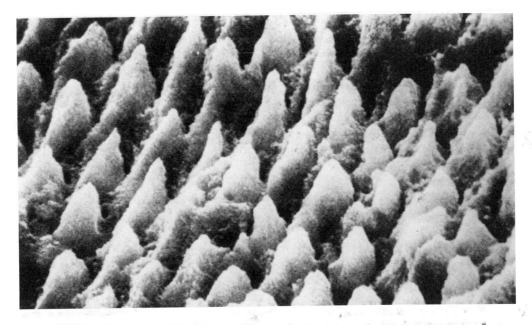

Figure 10–6. Tags, 30 μm. Sealant was flowed over etched surface, allowed to polymerize, and tooth surface subsequently dissolved away in acid. (*Courtesy, Silverstone LM, Dogon IL. The Acid Etch Technique. St. Paul, MN: North Central Publishing Co; 1975.*)

B. When the data of a study indicate that 65% of the original sealants are retained for 7 years, it is the same as saying that 5% are lost each year.

[handwritten: T / 7]

C. Bis-GMA products by different manufacturers are incompatible with one another.

[handwritten: F]

D. An etched area that is not rapidly sealed will retain its rough, porous surface indefinitely.

[handwritten: F] *[handwritten: R min occurs Rapidly hrs – days]*

E. The cleansing and etching of the occlusal surface with phosphoric acid is accomplished by *rubbing* the surface during the etching process.

[handwritten: F] *[handwritten: dabbed]*

OCCLUSAL AND INTERPROXIMAL DISCREPANCIES

At times an excess of sealant may be inadvertently flowed into a fossa or into the adjoining interproximal spaces. To remedy the first problem, the occlusion should be checked visually or, if indicated, with articulating paper. Usually any minor discrepancies in occlusion are rapidly removed by normal chewing action. If the occlusal contact is unacceptable, a large, no. 8, round *cutting* bur may be used to rapidly create a broad plastic fossa.

The integrity of the interproximal spaces can be checked with the use of dental floss. If any sealant is present, the use of scalers may be required to accomplish removal. These corrective actions are rarely needed once proficiency of placement is attained.

RETENTION OF SEALANTS

The finished sealant should be checked for retention without using undue force. In the event that the sealant does not adhere, the placement procedures should be repeated, with only about 15 seconds of etching needed to remove the residual saliva before again flushing, drying, and applying the sealant. If two attempts are unsuccessful, the sealant application should be postponed until remineralization occurs.

Plastic sealants are retained better on recently erupted teeth than in teeth with a more mature surface; they are retained better on first molars than on second molars. They are better retained on mandibular than on the maxillary teeth. This latter finding is possibly due to the fact that the lower teeth are more accessible, direct sight is possible, isolation of the teeth is easier, and gravity aids the flow of the sealant into the fissures.[55,56]

Teeth that have been sealed and then have lost the sealant have had fewer lesions than control teeth.[57] This is possibly due to the tags that are retained in the enamel after the bulk of the sealant has been sheared from the tooth surface.

The number of retained sealants decreases at a *curvolinear rate*.[55] Over the first 3 months, the rapid loss of sealants is probably due to faulty technique in placement. The fallout rate then begins to plateau, with the ensuing sealant loss probably being due to abnormal masticatory stresses. After a year or so, the sealants become very difficult to see or to discern tactilely, especially if they are abraded to the point that they fill only the fissures. In research studies this lack of visibility often leads to underestimating the effectiveness of the sealants that remain but cannot be identified. Because the most rapid falloff of sealants occurs in the early stages, an initial 3-month recall following placement should be routine for determining if sealants have been lost. If so, the teeth should be resealed. Teeth successfully sealed for 6 or 7 years are likely to remain sealed.[58]

In a review of the literature, Mertz-Fairhurst[58] cited studies in which 90% to 100% of the original sealants were retained over a 1-year period (Table 10–1). One 10-

TABLE 10–1. A COMPARISON OF RETENTION OF FIRST- AND SECOND-GENERATION SEALANTS FROM SEVERAL STUDIES*

Sealant		Months after Placement							
Generation	*Product*	6	12	24	36	48	60	72	84
First	Nuva-Seal		87	73	59	42			
	Nuva-Seal†		**84**	**58**	**60**		**35**	**37**	**35**
	TOTAL		85	65	60	42	35	37	35
Second	Concise		100						
	Concise		96	95	94				
	Delton		95						
	Delton		92		80				
	Delton		96						
	Delton				80				
	Delton†		**95**	**84**	**80**		**72**	**68**	**65**
	Nuva-Cote	100	100						
	Oralin		98		78				
	Oralin		97		95				
	Prisma-Shield	94	95						
	Prisma-Shield		94						
	TOTAL	97	95	89	84		72	68	65

* Bold lettering is from study of Mertz-Fairhurst[58]
† Direct 7-year comparison of first- and second-generation sealants.
Courtesy Dr Linda Scheirton, Department Dental Hygiene, University of Texas Health Science Center, San Antonio, TX.

year study using 3M Concise Sealant had a 57% complete retention and a 21% partial retention of sealant, all with no caries. Another study, using Delton, registered a 68% retention after 6 years[59] (Fig 10–7). These are studies in which the sealant was placed and then observed at periodic intervals; there was no resealing when a sealant was lost. Where resealing is accomplished as needed, a higher and more continuous level of protection is achieved.

COLORED VERSUS CLEAR SEALANTS

Both clear and colored sealants are available. They vary from translucent to white, yellow, and pink. Some manufacturers sell both clear and colored sealants in either the photocuring or autopolymerizing form. The selection of a colored versus a clear sealant is a matter of individual preference. The colored products permit a more precise placement of the sealant, with the visual assurance that the periphery extends halfway up the inclined planes. Retention can be more accurately monitored by both the patient and the operator placing the sealant. On the other hand, a clear sealant may be considered more esthetically acceptable.

THE PLACEMENT OF SEALANTS OVER CARIOUS AREAS

Sealing over a carious lesion is important because of the professional concern about the possibility of caries progression under the sealant sites.

In teeth that have been examined in vivo and then later subjected to histologic examination following extraction for orthodontic reasons, it has been found that areas of incipient or overt caries often occur under many fissures, which cannot be detected with the explorer.[60] In some studies sealants have been purposely placed over small, overt lesions.[58,61] When compared with control teeth, many of the sealed carious teeth have been diagnosed as sound 3 years and 5 years later.[62] Handelman has indicated that sealants can be considered a viable modality for treatment of pit-and-fissure caries.[63] In other studies of sealed lesions, the number of bacteria recovered from the sealed area decreased rapidly.[61,63,64] This decrease in bacterial population is probably due to the integrity of the seal of the plastic to the etched tooth surface[65]—a seal that does not permit the movement of fluids or tracer isotopes between the sealant and the tooth.[66]

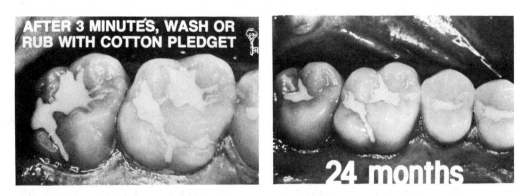

Figure 10–7. Showing how pit-and-fissure sealants are abraded over time but yet protect the vulnerable fissures. (*Courtesy of Dr R. Simonsen, University of Minnesota Dental School*).

Sealants have been place over more extensive lesions in which carious dentin is involved.[67] Even with these larger lesions, there is a decrease in the bacterial population and an arrest of the carious process as a function of time. In another study, clinically detectable lesions into the dentin were covered for 5 years with Nuva-Seal. After that time the bacterial cultures were essentially negative, and an apparent 83% reversal from a caries-active to a caries-inactive state was achieved.[61] Jordan and Suzuki[68] sealed small lesions in 300 teeth. During clinical and x-ray observations over a 5-year period, they found no change in size of the carious lesion, so long as the sealant remained intact. More recently Mertz-Fairhurst and colleagues[69] demonstrated that sealed lesions became inactive bacteriologically, with the residual carious material suggesting decay cessation. This ability to arrest incipient and early lesions is highlighted by the statement in the 1979 publication of the ADA Council on Dental Therapeutics: "Studies indicate that there is an apparent reduction in microorganisms in infected dentin covered with sealant . . . These studies appear to substantiate that there is no hazard in sealing carious lesions." The statements ends with the cautionary note: "However, additional long term studies are required before this procedure can be evaluated as an alternative to traditional restorative procedures.[70] There have been reports of sealants being used to achieve penetration of incipient smooth-surface lesions of facial surfaces.[71]

Question 4. Which of the following statements, if any, are correct?

A. Tags can be easily determined by their rough feel when checking the *surface* of a sealant with an explorer.

B. Teeth that lose a sealant are more susceptible than ones that retain a sealant but less caries-prone than a control tooth that was never sealed.

C. The falloff of sealants is linear as a function of time.

D. A study in which the periodic resealing of fissures occurs would be expected to have a *lesser* caries rate than a long-term study in which the same annual falloff is experienced, but where no resealing is accomplished.

E. Following placement of a sealant over a fissure with an undetectable carious lesion, the size of the subsurface lesion gradually *increases*.

SEALANTS VERSUS AMALGAMS

Comparing sealants and amalgams is not an equitable comparison because sealants are used to prevent occlusal lesions, and amalgam is used to treat occlusal lesions that could have been prevented. Yet, the comparison is necessary. One of the major obstacles to more extensive use of sealants has been the belief that amalgams, and not sealants, should be placed in anatomically defective fissures; this belief stems from misinformation that amalgams can be placed in less time and that once placed they are a permanent restoration. Several studies have addressed these suppositions. For instance, sealants require approximately 6 to 9 minutes to place initially, amalgams 13 to 15 minutes.[72,73]

Many studies on *amalgam* restorations have indicated a longevity from only a few years to an average life span of 10 years.[74-77] Equally perturbing is the fact that in one large study of school children, 16.2% of all surfaces filled with amalgam had marginal leakage and needed replacement.[78] The life span of an amalgam is shorter with younger children than with adults.[79]

The retention data from the earlier sealant studies were discouraging. In recent years, using later-generation sealants, along with the greater care in technique used for their insertion, much longer retention periods have been reported. In five long-term studies from 3 to 7 years, the average sealant loss per year ranged from 1.3% to 7%.[58] If the yearly loss of these studies is extrapolated, the average life of these sealants compares favorably or exceeds that of amalgam. When properly placed, sealants are no longer a temporary expedient for prevention; instead, they are the only effective *predictable* clinical procedure available for preventing occlusal caries.

The commonest cause for sealant replacement is loss of material, which mainly occurs during the first 6 months; the commonest cause for amalgam replacement is marginal decay,[80] with 4 to 8 years being the average life span.[78] To replace the sealant, only resealing is necessary. No damage occurs to the tooth. Amalgam replacement usually requires cutting more tooth structure with each replacement. Even if longevity merits were equal, the sealant has the advantage of being painless to apply, aesthetic, as well as emphasizing the highest objectives of the dental profession—prevention and sound teeth.

THE PREVENTIVE DENTISTRY RESTORATION

The use of sealants has spawned an entirely different concept of conservation of occlusal tooth structure in the management of deep pits and fissures early in caries involvement. The preventive dentistry restoration embodies the concepts of both prophylactic odontotomy (enameloplasty) and extension for prevention, yet requires only a minimum or no cutting of tooth structure at the carious site. Pain and apprehension are slight,

and aesthetics and tooth conservation are maximized.[81] Several options are available in selecting preventive dentistry restorations, depending on the professional's judgment.

The first option is simply to place a conventional sealant over the incipient lesion as well as over the remaining occlusal fissure system.

The second option, reported by Simonsen in 1978,[82] advocates the use of the smallest bur to remove the carious material from the bottom of a pit or fissure and then using an appropriate instrument to tease either sealant or composite into the cavity preparation. Following this operation, sealant is then placed over the polymerized material as well as flowed over the remaining fissures. Aside from protecting the fissures from future caries, it also possibly protects the composite from abrasion.[83]

A third option, reported by Garcia-Godoy in 1986 involves the use of a glass ionomer cement as the preventive glass ionomer restoration (PGIR).[84] The glass ionomer cement is used only in the cavity preparation involving dentin (Fig 10–8).

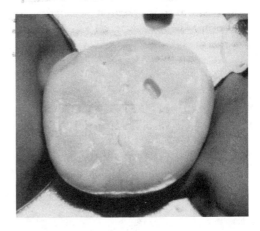

Figure 10–8. Preventive glass ionomer restoration (PGIR). Cavity preparation for reception of glass ionomer cement. (*Courtesy of Dr. Franklin Garcia-Godoy, University of Texas Dental School, San Antonio, TX.*)

The occlusal surface is then etched with a gel etchant, (avoiding if possible etching the glass ionomer). The conventional resin sealant is placed over the glass ionomer and the entire occlusal fissure system. In the event sealant is lost, the fluoride content of the glass ionomer helps prevent future primary and secondary caries formation.

Each of these options requires a judgment decision by the dentist. That judgment can well be based on the criterion that if an overt lesion cannot be *visualized,* it should be sealed; if it can be visualized, the smallest possible preventive dentistry restoration should be used along with its required sealant "topping."[85] Mertz-Fairhurst and associates[69] has pointed out that the first option could provide the preferred model for conservative treatment of *incipient* and *minimal, overt,* pit-and-fissure caries. It could also serve as an interim treatment for larger lesions. These options would be especially valuable in areas of the world with insufficient professional dental personnel and where preventive dentistry auxiliaries have been trained to place sealants under supervision. In all cases the preventive dentistry filling should be considered as an alternative to the traditional class I amalgam with its accompanying extension for prevention that often includes the entire fissure system.

THE SEALANT AS PART OF A TOTAL PREVENTIVE PACKAGE

The sealant is used to protect the occlusal surface. A major effort should be made to incorporate the use of sealants along with other primary preventive dentistry procedures, such as plaque control, fluoride therapy, and sugar discipline. Whenever a sealant is placed, a topical application of fluoride should follow if at all possible. In this way the whole tooth can be protected. Ripa and colleagues[86] completed a 2-year study for children in second and third grades assessing the effectiveness of a 0.2% fluoride mouth rinse used alone compared with a rinse plus sealants. Twenty-four occlusal lesions developed in the 51 rinse subjects, and only three in the 84 subjects receiving the rinse plus sealants. The conclusion was that caries could be almost completely eliminated by the use of these two preventive procedures. In many public health programs, however, it is not possible to institute full-scale prevention programs, either because of apathy or lack of time and money. In such cases there is some consolation in knowing that at least the most vulnerable of all tooth surfaces is being protected.

MANPOWER

The *cost* of sealant placement *increases* directly with the level of professional education of the operator. Dental hygienists, assistants, and even lesser trained auxiliaries can place sealants.[87,88]

In view of the cost effectiveness, dental auxiliaries should be considered as the logical individuals to place sealants. All states permit dental hygienists to apply sealants, whereas 15 states permit dental assistants to accomplish the procedure.[89] Deuben and coworkers[90] found that 77% of the schools of dental hygiene included the placement of sealants as part of the curriculum. Often auxiliaries who have received sealant instruction, either through continuing education courses or as part of a curriculum, are stymied either because of state laws interdicting their placing sealants or by the nature and philosophy of the practice of the employing dentist. Because many dentists consider the placement of sealants to be a relatively simple procedure, few are returning for continuing education programs to learn the exacting and precise process necessary to ensure maximum sealant retention. Even when the dental professional desires to participate in such continuing education, a 1990 survey found relatively few courses available.[89] In only 4 of the states in which hygienists were permitted to place sealants—Texas, Florida, New Jersey, and New Mexico—must they be *certified* by the State Board of Dental Examiners for the procedure.

ECONOMICS

Bear in mind that not every tooth receiving a sealant would necessarily become carious; hence the cost of preventing a single carious lesion is greater than the cost of a single application. For instance, Leverett and colleagues calculated that five sealants would need to be placed on sound teeth to prevent one lesion over a 5-year period,[91] and Rock and Anderson estimated one in three are prevented from becoming carious.[92] Sealants would be most cost-effective if they could be placed over only those teeth that are destined to become carious, such as option one type preventive-dentistry restorations. Unfortunately, we do not have a caries predictor test of such exactitude. Instead it is necessary to rely on professional judgment, based on the severity of the caries activity indicators: number of "sticky" fissures,[b] level of plaque index, number of incipient and overt lesions, and microbiologic test indications.

In an office setting, it is estimated that it costs 1.6 times more to treat a tooth than to seal.[37] Under public health conditions,

the cost of sealing a tooth in a New Mexico program was $1.37 per tooth, in Tennessee $1.20.

BARRIERS TO SEALANT USAGE

Sealant usage has been strongly supported by the ADA "as a safe and effective means for caries control."[21] The United States Public Health Service in a recent request for a proposal for a school pit-and-fissure study, states "*This combination of preventive techniques (combined use of fluoride and sealants) is expected to essentially eliminate caries in teeth erupting after the initiation of the study.*"[93]

Despite the support from the two largest organizations most interested in the dental health of the nation, the rank-and-file of the dental profession have not accepted sealants as a routine method for prevention. For example, one report indicates that 70% of the dentists in the United States use sealants.[94] Yet, only 6% to 8% of the school children in the United States have sealants.[95] At the same time 92% of the children's lesions are located on the occlusal surface. Possibly the incongruity of numbers is due to the fact that although the majority of dentists use sealants, the *frequency* of use is low.[96] Reasons for this apathy have ranged from economic considerations, to lack of technical skill, and to need for more research before acceptance. Probably the salient factor in the underuse of sealants is that most dentists are treatment-oriented. Rarely do they explain to patients the advantages of sealant over dental restorations.[97]

Regardless of increased rhetoric about prevention, the concepts and actions of prevention are not being fully implemented in dental schools.[98] Dental school faculties need to be educated about the effectiveness and methods of applying sealants.[99,100] Possi-

---

[b] A "sticky" fissure is one that catches the tine of the explorer but that may or may not be carious.

bly the acceptance of a model curriculum for teaching sealant usage would help.[101] Even though the students are inculcated with a preventive philosophy, there is concern that the staggering debts accrued by recent dental graduates will divert their efforts from prevention to treatment.[102] The dental community must develop a consensus about the value and economic effect of preventive measures.[99] Other barriers to effective delivery include state board restrictions on auxiliary placement of sealants, lack of consumer knowledge of the effectiveness of sealants, and, resultantly, a lack of demand for the product.[87] Economics and education of the profession and of the public are the prime requisites for sealant acceptance.[103]

Question 5. Which of the following statements, if any, are correct?

A. The longevity expectation for a properly placed amalgam restoration is approximately twice that of a properly placed sealant.

B. Sealants should be placed only on permanent teeth of children up to age 16.

C. The most conservative preventive dentistry restoration involves the most cost-effective use of a sealant.

D. Following the graduation of students presently in dental schools, a large increase in the use of sealants can be expected.

E. Hygienists and dentists in most states do not need to demonstrate sealant placement proficiency for certification.

SUMMARY

Approximately 90% of all carious lesions that occur in the mouth occur on the occlusal surfaces. Which teeth will become

carious cannot be predicted; however, if the surface is sealed with a pit-and-fissure sealant, no caries will develop as long as the sealant remains in place. Recent studies indicate an approximate 90% retention rate of sealants 1 year after placement. Even when sealants are eventually lost, most studies indicate that the caries incidence for teeth that have lost sealants is less than that of control surfaces that had never been sealed. Research data also indicate that many incipient and small overt lesions are arrested when sealed. Not one report has shown that caries developed in pits or fissures when under an intact seal. Sealants are easy to apply, but the application of sealants is an extremely sensitive technique. The surfaces that are to receive the sealant *must be completely isolated from the saliva during the entire procedure, and etching, flushing, and drying procedures must be timed to ensure adequate preparation of the surface for the sealant.* Sealants are competitive with amalgam restorations for longevity and do not require the cutting of tooth structure. Sealants do not cost as much to place as amalgams. Despite their advantages, the use of sealants has not been embraced by the dental profession, even though endorsed by the ADA and the US Public Health Service. Even when incipient pit-and-fissure lesions exist, they can be dealt with conservatively by use of preventive dentistry restorations. What now appears to be required is that the dental schools teach sealant usage, the dental profession use them, the hygienists and the auxiliary personnel be permitted to apply them, and the public demand them.

ANSWERS AND EXPLANATIONS

1. C, D

   A—incorrect. Because the fluorides protect the smooth surface, there will be a greater proportion of pit and fissure lesions.

B—incorrect. By definition, an incipient lesion has not been invaded by bacteria; thus the use of a sealant is an ideal preventive measure.

E—incorrect. Remember, it is the caries susceptibility of the teeth that is important—not the age of the individual.

2. A, B, C

D—incorrect. All the major, successful, long-term retention studies have used cotton-roll isolation; in the one study of rubber dam versus cotton rolls, the rolls were equal to, or better than, the dam.

E—incorrect. Ten seconds are used for the drying and flushing procedures, and 1 minute for the etching.

3. A, B

C—incorrect. Bis-GMA plastics are of the same chemical family, hence will bond to each other, regardless of manufacturer.

D—incorrect. Remineralization from saliva constituents occurs rapidly in a period of hours to days.

E—incorrect. Cleansing and etching do occur; however, rubbing tends to obliterate the delicate etching pattern and reduce retention potential.

4. B, D

A—incorrect. The tags of the sealant cannot be felt with the explorer; they extend into the enamel from the underneath side of the plastic.

C—incorrect. The curvolinear falloff is greatest at 3 months, less at 6 months, after which it gradually plateaus.

E—incorrect. The literature is unanimous that caries does not progress under an intact sealant.

5. C, E

A—incorrect. There is little difference between the longevity of a well-placed amalgam compared with a well-placed sealant.

B—incorrect. If a tooth is susceptible to caries, it should be sealed, whatever the patient's age.

D—incorrect. All signs indicate that the teaching of sealant placement is greatly neglected in dental schools.

SELF-EVALUATION QUESTIONS

1. Approximately ___95___ % of all carious lesions occur on the occlusal surfaces; the continual use of fluorides (increases) (decreases) this percentage.

2. Four different methods used prior to the advent of polyurethane, cyanoacrylate, and Bis-GMA sealants, were _enamel cement_, _Prophy odontotomy_, _do nothing_, _plasty_ and _Floride_.

3. One condition that *indicates the use of a sealant is* _deep occ P&F_; *four conditions that contraindicate* the use of sealants are _Pat, Br_, _Open Occ Caries_, _caries on other surfs same tooth_ and _lg occ Rest_; three conditions that *probably indicate* the use of sealants are _fossa well isolated from fully erupted fossa_, _to rest_, and _incipient lesion_.

4. Two photoactivated, and two chemically activated sealants that have been accepted, or provisionally accepted, by the ADA are (photoactivated) _photocure light act'n_, and (chemically activated) _self curing_ and _autopolymerize_.

5. The liquid plastic in a sealant kit is known as the _monomer_; when it is catalyzed the hardening process is known as _polymerizat'n_. The catalyst used for the polymerization of chemically activated sealants is _benzy peroxide_ and for visible photoactivation, _camphoroquinone_.

6. Two advantages to light-cured sealants are _initiate poly any time_ and _shorter_; and two advantages of autopolymerized sealants are _no exp. light_ and _____.

7. _adhesive_ forces, not chemical bonding causes retention of the sealant to the tooth; the four commandments to ensure maximum retention are _dry_, _max surf-area_, _irreg p & fiss_, and _surf-clean_.

8. Three methods by which a dry field can be established are _dent dam_, _cotton rolls_, and _HVS_.

9. The placement of sealants is extremely technique-sensitive; after selection of the tooth for sealant placement, it should be dried for _10 sec_ (time); then etched for _1 min_ (time), followed by a water flush of _10 sec_ (time), and finally, dried for _10 sec_ (time) before placing the sealant.

10. Excessively high sealants that interfere with occlusion can be reduced by use of a number _____ (cutting) (finishing) bur.

11. The fall off of sealants is (linear) (curvalinear); long-term studies where 65% of the sealants are retained after 7 years indicate an average yearly loss of _5_ %. After 10 years, _50_ % would be retained. This contrasts to an average life expectancy of an amalgam of approximately _4-8_ (years).

12. To protect the total tooth, the application of a sealant should be followed by an application of _fluoride_.

13. To ensure that sealant placement techniques have been perfected in dental and dental hygiene schools, it should be necessary for _____ (state dental-regulating agency) to require a demonstration of proficiency for all candidates prior to state licensure.

14. The three key components of a light source for polymerizing sealants are _high intensity wht. ligh_, _blue filter_, and _light wand_ (which results in the blue color).

15. There are three basic options for a preventive dentistry restoration; they are _place sealant over incipt les._, _sm. burr cut_, and _carious tus, menseal_. _prev. glass Iam. Rest_

REFERENCES

1. Mertz-Fairhurst EJ. Pit-and-fissure sealants: A global lack of science transfer? [editorial] *J Dent Res.* 1992; 71:1543–1544.

2. Wilson IP. Preventive dentistry. *Dent Dig.* 1895; 1:70–72.

3. Bödecker CF. The eradication of enamel fissures. *Dent Items Int.* 1929; 51:859–866.

4. Sturdevant CM, Barton RE, Brauer JC, et al. *The Art and Science of Operative Dentistry.* New York, NY. McGraw-Hill; 1968:93.

5. Hyatt TP. 1982, Prophylactic odontotomy: The ideal procedure in dentistry for children. *Dent Cosmos.* 1936; 78:353–370.

6. Ast DB, Bushel A, Chase CC. A clinical study of caries prophylaxis and zinc chloride and potassium ferrocyanide. *J Am Dent Assoc.* 1950; 41:437–442.

7. Klein H, Knutson JW. Studies on dental caries. XIII. Effect of ammoniacal silver nitrate on caries in the first permanent molar. *J Am Dent Assoc.* 1942; 29:1420–1426.

8. Miller J. Clinical investigations in preventive dentistry. *Br Dent J.* 1951; 91:92–95.

9. Backer-Dirks O, Houwink B, Kwant GW. The results of 6½ years of artificial fluoridation of drinking water in the Netherlands. The Tiel-Culemborg experiment. *Arch Oral Biol.* 1961; 5:284–300.

10. Buonocore MG. Caries prevention in pits and fissures sealed with an adhesive resin polymerized by ultraviolet light: A two-year study of a single adhesive application. *J Am Dent Assoc.* 1971; 82:1090–1093.

11. Gillings B, Buonocore M. Thickness of enamel at the base of pits and fissures in human molars and bicuspids. *J Dent Res.* 1961; 40:119–133.

12. Simonsen RJ. Pit and fissure sealant in individual patient care programs. *J Dent Educ.* 1984; 48(suppl 2):42–44.

13. Simonsen RJ. The clinical significance of a colored pit and fissure sealant at 36 months. *J Am Dent Assoc.* 1981; 102:323–327.

14. Bohannan HM. Caries distribution and the case for sealants. *J Public Health Dent.* 1983; 33:200–204.

15. Ripa LW, Leske GS, Varma AO. Ten to 13-year-old children examined annually for three years to determine caries activity in the proximal and occlusal surfaces of first permanent molars. *J Public Health Dent.* 1988; 48:8–13.

16. Arthur JS, Swango P. The incidence of pit-and-fissure caries in a young Navy population: Implication for expanding sealant use. *J Public Health Dent.* 1987; 47:33. Abstract.

17. Lee H, Stoffey D, Orolowski J, et al. Sealing of developmental pits and fissures. III. Effects of fluoride on adhesion of rigid and flexible sealers. *J Dent Res.* 1972; 51:191–201.

18. Seppä L. Fluoride varnishes in caries prevention. *Proc Finn Dent Soc.* 1982; 78(suppl 8).

19. Pugnier VA. Cyanoacrylate resins in caries prevention: a two-year study. *J Am Dent Assoc.* 1972; 84:829–831.

20. Bowen RL. Dental filling material comprising vinyl silane treated fused silica and a binder consisting of the reaction product of bis-phenol and glycidyl acrylate. US Patent #3,006,112. November 1962.

21. Council on Dental Materials, Instruments and Equipment. Clinical products in dentistry. *J Am Dent Assoc.* 1983; 107:876.

22. Council on Dental Materials, Instruments, and Equipment. Pit and fissure sealants. *J Am Dent Assoc.* 1983; 107:465.

23. Widmer RP, Jayasekera TR. Fissure sealing with a glass ionomer cement: 2 year results. *J Dent Res.* 1989; 68:539 (Abstract 8).

24. Torppa-Saärinen E, Seppä L. Short-term retention of glass ionomer fissure sealants. *Caries Res.* 1990; 24:412 (Abstract 63).

25. Leung R, Fan PL, Johnston WM. Exposure time and thickness on polymerization of visible light composite. *J Dent Res.* 1982; 61:248. Abstract 623.

26. Leung R, Fan PL, Johnston WM. Post-irradiation polymerization of visible light-activated composite resin. *J Dent Res.* 1983; 62:363–365.

27. Blankenau RJ, Cavel WT, Kelsey WP, et al. Wavelength and intensity of seven systems for visible light curing composite resins: A comparison study. *J Am Dent Assoc.* 1983; 106:471–474.

28. Council on Dental Materials, Instruments, and Equipment. Visible light-cured composites and activating units. *J Am Dent Assoc.* 1985; 110:100–103.

29. Houpt M, Fuks A, Shapira J, et al. Auto-polymerized versus light-polymerized fissure sealant. *J Am Dent Assoc.* 1987; 115:55–56.

30. Buonocore MG. Principles of adhesive retention and adhesive restorative materials. *J Am Dent Assoc.* 1963; 67:382–391.

31. Gwinnett AJ, Buonocore MG. Adhesion and caries prevention. A preliminary report. *Br Dent J.* 1965; 119:77–80.

32. Garcia-Godoy F, Gwinnett AJ. Penetration of acid solution and high and low viscosity gels in occlusal fissures. *J Am Dent Assoc.* 1987; 114:809–810.

33. Brown MR, Foreman FJ, Burgess JO, et al. Penetration of gel and solution etchants in occlusal fissures sealing. *J Dent Child.* 1988; 55:26–29.

34. Arana EM. Clinical observations of enamel after acid-etch procedure. *J Am Dent Assoc.* 1974; 89:1102–1106.

35. Bossert WA. The relation between the shape of the occlusal surfaces of molars and the prevalence of decay. II. *J Dent Res.* 1937; 16:63–67.

36. Konig KG. Dental morphology in relation to caries resistance with special reference to fissures as susceptible areas. *J Dent Res.* 1963; 42:461–476.

37. Simonsen RJ. Retention and effectiveness of a single application of white sealant after 10 years. *J Am Dent Assoc.* 1987; 115:31–36.

38. Mertz-Fairhurst EJ. Personal communication, 1984.

39. Bogert TR, Garcia-Godoy F. Effect of prophylaxis agents on the shear bond strength of a fissure sealant. *Pediatr Dent*. 1992; 14: 50–51.

40. Garcia-Godoy F, O'Quinn JA. Effect of prophylaxis agents on shear bond strength of a resin composite to enamel. *Gen Dent*. 1993; 41:557–559.

41. Scott L, Brockmann S, Houston G, et al. Retention of dental sealants after airpolishing. *J Dent Res*. 1988; 67:382. Abstract 2151.

42. Garcia-Godoy F, Medlock JW. An SEM study of air polishing on fissure surfaces. *Quint Int*. 1988; 19:465–467.

43. Titley KC, Torneck CD, Smith DC. The effect of concentrated hydrogen peroxide solution on the surface morphology of human tooth enamel. *J Dent Res*. 1988; 67(special issue):361. Abstract 1989.

44. Straffon LH, More FG, Dennison JB. Three year clinical evaluation of sealant applied under rubber dam isolation. *J Dent Res*. 1984; 63:215. IADR Abstract 400.

45. Wood AJ, Saravia ME, Farrington FH. Cotton roll isolation versus Vac-Ejector isolation. *J Dent Child*. 1989; 56:438–440.

46. Council on Dental Materials and Devices. American Dental Association. Status report on acid etching procedures. *J Am Dent Assoc*. 1978; 97:505–508.

47. Nordenvall KJ, Brannstrom M, Malgrem O. Etching of deciduous teeth and young and old permanent teeth. A comparison between 15 and 60 seconds etching. *Am J Orthod*. 1980; 78:99–108.

48. Eidelman E, Shapira J, Houpt M. The retention of fissure sealants using twenty-second etching time: Three-year follow-up. *J Dent Child*. 1988; 55:119–120.

49. Pahlavan A, Dennison JB, Charbeneau GT. Penetration of restorative resins into acid-etched human enamel. *J Am Dent Assoc*. 1976; 93:1070–1076.

50. Silverstone LM. Fissure sealants, laboratory studies. *Caries Res*. 1974; 8:2–26.

51. Bozalis WB, Marshall GW. Acid etching patterns of primary enamel. *J Dent Res*. 1977; 56:185.

52. Myers CL, Rossi F, Cartz L. Adhesive tag-like extensions into acid-etched tooth enamel. *J Dent Res*. 1974; 53:435–441.

53. Powell KR, Craig GG. An in vitro investigation of the penetrating efficiency of Bis-GMA resin pit and fissure coatings. *J Dent Res*. 1978; 57:691–695.

54. Silverstone LM. Fissure sealants: The enamel-resin interface. *J Public Health Dent*. 1983; 43:205–215.

55. Harris NO, Moolenaar L, Hornberger N, et al. Adhesive sealant clinical trial: Effectiveness in a school population of the U.S. Virgin Islands. *J Prev Dent*. 1976; 3: 27–37.

56. Garcia-Godoy F. Retention of a light-cured fissure sealant (Helioseal) in a tropical environment. *Clin Prevent Dent*. 1986; 8:11–13.

57. Hinding J. Extended cariostasis following loss of pit and fissure sealant from human teeth. *J Dent Child*. 1974; 41:41–43.

58. Mertz-Fairhurst EJ. Current status of sealant retention and caries prevention. *J Dent Educ*. 1984; 48:18–26.

59. Mertz-Fairhurst EJ, Fairhurst CW, Williams JE, et al. A comparative clinical study of two pit and fissure sealants: Six year results in August, Ga. *J Am Dent Assoc*. 1982; 105:237–239.

60. Miller J, Hobson P. Determination of the presence of caries in fissures. *Br Dent J*. 1956; 100:15–18.

61. Going RE, Loesche WJ, Grainger DA, et al. The viability of organisms in carious lesions five years after covering with a fissure sealant. *J Am Dent Assoc*. 1978; 97:455–467.

62. Mertz-Fairhurst EJ, Richards EE, Williams JE, et al. Sealed restorations: 5-year results. *Am J Dent*. 1992; 5:5–10.

63. Handelman SL, Washburn F, Wopperer P. Two year report of sealant effect on bacteria in dental caries. *J Am Dent Assoc*. 1976; 93:976–980.

64. Jeronimus DJ, Till MJ, Sveen OB. Reduced viability of microorganisms under dental sealants. *J Dent Child*. 1975; 42: 275–280.

65. Theilade E, Fejerskov O, Kannikar M, et al. Effect of fissure sealing on the microflora in occlusal fissures of human teeth. *Arch Oral Biol.* 1977; 22:251–259.

66. Jensen OE, Handelman SL. In vitro assessment of marginal leakage of six enamel sealants. *J Prosthet Dent.* 1978; 36:304–306.

67. Handleman S. Effects of sealant placement on occlusal caries progression. *Clin Prevent Dent.* 1982; 4:11–16.

68. Jordan RE, Suzuki M. Unpublished report, quoted by Going, R.E. Sealant effect on incipient caries, enamel maturation and future caries susceptibility. *J Dent Educ.* 1984; 48(suppl) 2:35–41.

69. Mertz-Fairhurst EJ, Shuster GS, Fairhurst CW. Arresting caries by sealants: Results of a clinical study. *J Am Dent Assoc.* 1986; 112:194–203.

70. *Accepted Dental Therapeutics*, 39th ed. American Dental Association, Chicago, Ill. 1982.

71. Micik RE. Fate of in Vitro Caries-like Lesions Sealed within Tooth Structure. *IADR Program*, March 1972. Abstract 710.

72. Burt BA. Fissure sealants: Clinical and economic factors. *J Dent Educ.* 1984; 48 (suppl) 2:96–102.

73. Dennison JB, Straffon LH. Clinical evaluation comparing sealant and amalgam after seven years—final report. *J Dent Res.* 1984; 63(special issue):215. Abstract 401.

74. Allen DN. A longitudinal study of dental restorations. *Br Dent J.* 1977; 143:87–89.

75. Cecil JC, Cohen ME, Schroeder DC, et al. Longevity of amalgam restorations: A retrospective view. *J Dent Res.* 1982; 61:185. Abstract 56.

76. Healey HJ, Phillips RW. A clinical study of amalgam failures. *J Dent Res.* 1949; 28:439–446.

77. Lavell CL. A cross-sectional, longitudinal survey into the durability of amalgam restorations. *J Dent.* 1976; 4:139–143.

78. Robinson AD. The life of a filling. *Br Dent J.* 1971; 130:206–208.

79. Hunter B. The life of restorations in children and young adults. *J Dent Res.* 1982; 61:537. Abstract 18.

80. Dennison JB, Straffon LH. Clinical evaluation comparing sealant and amalgam—4 years report. *J Dent Res.* 1981; 60(special issue A):520. Abstract 843.

81. Swift EJ. Preventive resin restorations. *J Am Dent Assoc.* 1987; 114:819–821.

82. Simonsen RJ. Preventive resin restorations. *Quintessence Int.* 1978; 9:69–76.

83. Dickinson G, Leinfelder KF, Russell CM. Evaluation of wear by application of a surface sealant. *J Dent Res.* 1988; 67:362. Abstract 1999.

84. Garcia-Godoy F. Preventive glass ionomer restorations. *Quint Int.* 1986; 17:617–619.

85. Mertz-Fairhurst EJ, Call-Smith KM, Shuster GS, et al. Clinical performance of sealed composite restorations placed over caries compared with sealed and unsealed amalgam restorations. *J Am Dent Assoc.* 1987; 115:689–694.

86. Ripa LW, Leske GS, Forte F. The combined use of pit and fissure sealants and fluoride mouthrinsing in second and third grade children: Final clinical results after two years. *Pediatr Dent.* 1987; 9:118–120.

87. Harris NO, Lindo F, Tossas A, et al. *The Preventive Dentistry Technician: Concept and Utilization.* Monograph, Editorial UPR, University of Puerto Rico. October 1, 1970.

88. Leske G, Cons N, Pollard S. Cost effectiveness considerations of a pit and fissure sealant. *J Dent Res.* 1977; 56:B–71. Abstract 77.

89. American Dental Association, Department of Educational Surveys. *Legal Provisions for Delegating Functions to Dental Assistants and Dental Hygienists*, 1990. Chicago, Ill. April 1991.

90. Deuben CJ, Zullos TG, Summer WL. Survey of expanded functions included within dental hygiene curricula. *Educ Direc.* 1981; 6(3):22–29.

91. Leverett DH, Handelman SL, Brenner CM, et al. Use of sealants in the prevention and early treatment of carious lesions: Cost analysis. *J Am Dent Assoc.* 1983; 106:39–42.

92. Rock WP, Anderson RJ. A review of published fissure sealant trials using multiple regression analysis. *J Dent.* 1982; 10:39–43.

93. National Institute of Dental Research. RFP No., NIH-NIDR-5-82, IR. Washington, DC: National Institutes of Health; May 1982.

94. Cohen I, Labelle I, Rosenberg E. The use of pit and fissure sealants in private practice; a national survey. *J Publ Health Dent.* 1988; 48:26–35.

95. Brunnelle J. Prevalence of dental sealants in U.S. school children. *J Dent Res.* 1989; 68(special issue):183. Abstract.

96. Gonzalez CD, Frazier PJ, Messer LB. Sealant knowledge and use by pediatric dentists. 1987, Minnesota survey. *J Dent Child.* 1988; 55:434–438.

97. Silverstone LM. The use of pit and fissure sealants in dentistry: Present status and future developments. *Pediatr Dent.* 1982; 4:16–21.

98. Terkla LG. The use of pit and fissure sealants in United States dental schools. In: *Proceedings of the Conference on Pit and Fissure Sealants: Why Their Limited Usage.* Chicago, Ill: American Dental Association; 1981:31–36.

99. Frazier, PLJ. Public health education and promotion for caries: The role of the dental schools. *J Public Health Dent.* 1983; 43:28–42.

100. McLeran JH. Current challenges and response of the College of Dentistry. *Iowa Dent Bull.* 1981; 12:21.

101. American Association of Public Health Dentistry. Recommendations for teaching pit and fissure sealants. *J Public Health Dent.* 1988; 48:112–114.

102. American Dental Association. *Interim Report of the American Dental Association Special Committee on the Future of Dentistry.* Chicago, Ill: 1981:45.

103. Cohen L, BaBelle A, Romberg E. The use of pit and fissure sealants in private practice: A national survey. *J Public Health Dent.* 1988; 48:26–35.

Chapter 11

Oral Biologic Defenses and the Demineralization and Remineralization of Teeth

James S. Wefel
Michael W. J. Dodds

Objectives

At the end of this chapter it will be possible to

1. Explain how a three-compartment model consisting of saliva, plaque, and the tooth enamel cap can help provide a basis for understanding the caries process.
2. List the various methods by which saliva contributes to the defense of the tooth in preventing caries.
3. Explain the concept of supersaturation of saliva as it applies to demineralization and remineralization.
4. Name at least eight functions that fluoride performs in helping to prevent caries.
5. Explain the role of dental plaque in the development of caries.
6. Describe how glyco- and proline-rich proteins can influence ecologic niche formation.
7. Give the sequence of biochemical and physiologic events that occur in plaque and the enamel cap following a cariogenic challenge that results first in demineralization and then remineralization.
8. Explain why a remineralized lesion is usually more caries-resistant than the original enamel.

Introduction

The mouth is the gateway for food and drink destined for the gastrointestinal (GI) tract. The teeth function to break up the food in preparation for continuing digestion in the stomach and intestine. To help ensure the integrity of the oral tissues exposed to harsh, abrasive, and possibly dangerous foods as well as to potential pathogens, two unique defensive systems exist in the mouth: *saliva* and *taste*. The complex physical and chemical composition of salivary secretions performs a considerable number of protective functions, and taste enables the host to reject food considered obnoxious.

The salivary defensive system functions continuously, but it is most active during eating periods and least operational during inactive or sleeping periods of the daily cycle. The defensive functions of the saliva are part of the total body's ability to maintain *homeostasis* (ie, the ability to resist routine daily challenges of physical and bacterial agents and to repair limited amounts of damage). It is only when the challenges exceed the capabilities of the body's defensive systems that disease ensues. For example, the secretory defense system functions efficiently as long as the dental plaque is composed largely of nonpathogenic bacteria with infrequent access to sucrose; it is only when the defensive capabilities of the system are exceeded by more frequent exposure to sucrose that pathogenic bacteria (eg, *Streptococcus mutans* and other opportunistic organisms) begin to dominate the ecologic niches and disease ensues.

The salivary secretions have several other nonantimicrobial functions, the scope of which is still unfolding. Without continual flushing of the teeth by saliva, pathogenic plaque can accumulate, resulting in a prolonged low pH following the intake of refined carbohydrates. The mucus component of the saliva serves to *lubricate* and to prevent desiccation of both the soft and hard tissues of the mouth. The moistening of food by the saliva *facilitates chewing and swallowing.* Other essential but less considered salivary functions are the initial *dissolution of food,* which enables *taste,* and the facilitation of *speech* by reducing friction between the tongue and soft tissues. Accordingly, a lack of saliva (xerostomia) results in a greatly *increased risk of caries and stomatitis,* as well as an extremely *annoying dry-mouth* sensation. Chewing, swallowing, and speaking can all be difficult and uncomfortable with dry-mouth syndrome and often require a frequent ameliorating sip of water.

To provide the conceptual background for caries development in this defensive environment, it is desirable to consider the multiplicity of events that occur in a three-compartment system that includes *saliva, plaque,* and the *tooth enamel cap.*[a]

THE SALIVA COMPARTMENT

The fluid found in the mouth is derived from the *major* and *minor* salivary glands. The major glands are the *parotid, submandibular,* and *sublingual.* Of these, the parotid elaborates a serous secretion containing electrolytes but is relatively low in mucoid organic substances. The submandibular has both a serous and a mucus secretion; the sublingual has a greater proportion of mucus output than the other major glands. The minor *palatal, lingual, buccal,* and *labial* salivary glands empty onto

---

[a] The enamel cap is that part of the tooth composed of enamel; its outer surface is exposed to the saliva and oral environment, and its inner surface approximates and is attached to the coronal dentin.

the lining mucous membrane of the mouth in many places: on the palate, under the tongue, and on the inner sides of the cheeks and lips. These minor glands are mainly mucus-secreting glands.

The *pure* saliva secreted by the oral glands is sterile until it is discharged onto the mouth. When it mixes with saliva from other glands, it becomes known as *pooled,* or *whole,* saliva. Whole saliva is further altered by additions from the periodic ingestion of food, oxygen from the air, carbon dioxide from the lungs, tissue fluids entering via the gingival crevice, and release of a great variety of intracellular organics from lysed bacteria, sloughed oral epithelial cells, and dissolved food fragments. It becomes even more complex by the inclusion of *living* cells, for example, bacteria from the mouth that produce enzymes and other chemicals, epithelial cells sloughing from the mucous membrane, and leukocytes derived from the gingival crevice and tonsils. Both of the latter also release proteins, ions, and even radicals into the pooled saliva.

Flow Rate

The composition of saliva varies, depending on whether it is *stimulated* or *unstimulated* (*resting*).[1] During the day the submandibular gland secretes the greatest proportion of the unstimulated saliva, although the flow rate of resting saliva is very slow for *all* of the three major glands, being as low as 0.26 mL/minute for the submandibular, 0.12 mL/minute for the sublingual, and 0.11 mL/minute for the parotid gland. Approximately 69% of the unstimulated saliva is from the submandibular gland, 26% from the parotid, and 5% from the sublingual gland.[1] The minor glands secrete about 8% of the total amount of saliva.[2] This unstimulated flow rate is subject to a circadian rhythm, with the highest flow in midafternoon and the lowest around 4 AM.[3,4] Flow

varies considerably among individuals under resting conditions. The flow is exceedingly low, or nonexistent, during sleep.

Upon moderate stimulation, the submaxillary and parotid glands secrete approximately equal amounts of saliva, whereas at full stimulation the parotid has the greatest output. When salivary flow is stimulated by the chewing of gum or paraffin, from 1 to 2 mL/minute can be collected. The minimum level of stimulated salivary flow necessary to maintain hard- and soft-tissue health is not known, but when it is as low as *1 mL/minute,* there is cause for concern. Once it is below 0.7 mL/minute, the condition qualifies as xerostomia.[5] In the course of a day, up to a liter of saliva is secreted.[1]

Flow rate is less for females than for males. Seasonal variations also occur, with flow being lower in warm weather and higher in cold. The act of smoking increases flow rates; light deprivation, such as when blindfolded, decreases flow. Flow is greater while standing than when sitting; and the flow is greater when sitting than when recumbent. These changes parallel the changes in blood pressure in subjects in these different postures. Flow of resting saliva appears to increase from age 8 years to 29 years.[6] A decrease of saliva is not inevitably a part of aging, per se;[7] most of the apparent decreases that occur with age are due to the medications used by aging populations.[8,9]

Under physiologic conditions, the stimulant may be *mechanical,* such as during chewing. It may be *gustatory* (taste), resulting from the stimulation of taste buds, or it may be *psychologic,* as when an increased flow of saliva (hypersalivation) is evoked while anticipating that first delicious bite of a well-cooked steak. Conversely, the flow of saliva can be greatly depressed (hypoptyalism, xerostomia) by fear; head and neck radiation that irreversibly destroys the salivary glands; tumors of the salivary glands; thyroid deficiencies; Sjögren's syndrome; or the use of antisialagogic drugs.[b] A great variety of commonly used drugs are able to either increase or, especially, decrease saliva flow.[10] The three most encountered xerogenics causing the most severe, long-term xerostomic effects are the neuroleptics, tricyclic antidepressants, and antihypertensive drugs.[9]

The concentration of the various components secreted by the glands is closely related to the flow rate. Increasing the rate of flow by stimulation increases the concentration of *some* constituents and decreases it for others.[11] Stimulation of the parotid gland causes an increase in calcium, sodium, chloride, bicarbonate, and pH. The same saliva demonstrates a decrease in phosphate and potassium.[2] In addition to the secretion of different proportions of electrolytes, organic molecules are secreted that can be categorized into five major groups: amylases, mucins, phosphoproteins, glycoproteins, and immunoglobulins.[12]

The concentration of the various constituents of saliva also changes with a circadian rhythm. For instance, parotid inorganic phosphate in one study reached a peak at 8:30 AM and was at a minimum level at midnight.[3] In fibrocystic disease, the calcium and phosphate output is much greater than for normal individuals. This along with the higher pH of the saliva, probably accounts for the greater amount of calculus experienced by these individuals.[13]

Protective Functions of Saliva

The protective functions of saliva are due to its *physical*, *chemical*, and *antibacterial* properties.[14] The physical effect is mainly dependent on the water content and the

flow rate of saliva.[15] Saliva, in sufficient quantity, serves a cleansing function. The fluid dilutes and removes acid components in the dental plaque. A viscous saliva is not as effective as a more fluid saliva in clearing carbohydrates. If saliva does not have access to all tooth surfaces, the cleansing and dilution potential is diminished.

Chemical Protection. Bacterial acidogenesis in the dental plaque causes the pH to fall and to remain low. Tooth damage results from a drop of pH in the plaque compartment. The chemical protection afforded by the saliva minimizes the pH drop, accelerates the return of the pH to normal, and provides the ionic environment that facilitates repair of the enamel following acidogenesis.

Sodium bicarbonate is the main buffering and neutralizing constituent of the saliva.[16] Other components serving a similar function are the phosphates, amphoteric proteins, and urea.[17] The last of these compounds is broken down by the bacteria to form ammonia. Its neutralizing effectiveness probably accounts for the fact that patients with renal transplants or on hemodialysis have both an increased salivary urea level and a reduced caries prevalence.[18]

Another mechanism for pH control is the secretion of a protein known as *sialin,* or pH *rise factor.*[19] This protein tends to minimize the drop in the Stephan curve and to reduce the time necessary for the pH to return to more neutral levels.

The cations and anions of saliva most associated with increasing the resistance of enamel to acid attack are calcium, phosphate, and fluoride. At the time of secretion, saliva is supersaturated (with calcium and phosphate) in relation to hydroxyapatite.[20] Supersaturated solutions have a potential for precipitation of calcium salts. In the case of saliva, however, the calcium and

---

[b] Antisialagogue = An agent that diminishes or arrests the flow of saliva.

phosphates do not precipitate because of the presence of a proline-rich phosphoprotein in the saliva called *statherin*.[21] Statherin acts to stabilize the calcium and phosphates in the supersaturated saliva and plaque fluid. In turn, the supersaturated fluids aid in preventing demineralization, as well as promoting remineralization.[22] Furthermore, as the fluid-phase calcium and phosphate ions fall, statherin may release its bound calcium. As the secretion of calcium increases on stimulation, so does the flow of statherin.[23] Other *proline-rich proteins* also aid in maintaining supersaturation.

Question 1. Which of the following statements, if any, are correct?

A. Pooled saliva contains more components than the combined secretions of pure saliva.

B. In the course of a day, the resting submandibular gland secretes *more* fluid than the resting parotid gland.

C. The concentration of *all* chemical components of saliva varies *directly* with the flow rate (ie, the more flow, the greater the concentration).

D. The neutralizing and buffering effects of saliva are due to its high dilution capability.

E. Sialin is related to *pH* control, whereas statherin is related to maintaining the calcium and phosphate supersaturation of saliva in relation to hydroxyapatite.

Antibacterial Properties of Saliva. The subject of saliva's antibacterial properties gained considerable attention in the news media when the National Institutes of Health announced that saliva inhibits human immunodeficiency virus (HIV) infectivity.[24] The antibacterial properties of whole saliva are due either to substances secreted by the glands or to humoral components of the body's defense system that enter the saliva via the gingival crevice.

The most easily understood antibacterial function is performed by the secreted sulfated glycoproteins—the mucins—that trap, or *aggregate, bacteria,* which are eventually swallowed. The same mucins provide a thin lubricating film over the mucous membrane and teeth to serve as lubricants.[14]

Four important proteins found in saliva are bacteriostatic or bacteriocidal: lysozyme, lactoferrin, salivary peroxidase, and secretory immunoglobulin A (sIgA).[25] Lysozyme activity is depressed by the presence of iron and copper. Lactoferrin, however, combines with iron and copper to protect the lysozyme action while depriving bacteria of some of their essential needs for those two metals. Salivary peroxidase[26] reacts with salivary thiocyanate in the presence of hydrogen peroxide to form the antimicrobial compound, hypothiocyanite,[27] which, in turn, inhibits the capability of the bacteria to use glucose fully. Interestingly, the hydrogen peroxide is mainly a product of the plaque bacterial metabolism.

Lactoperoxidase strongly adsorbs to hydroxyapatite.[28] As a component of the acquired pellicle, it can influence the qualitative and quantitative characteristics of the microbial population of plaque. The sIgA is derived mainly from the *minor salivary glands* located strategically near and on all sides of the teeth.[29]

The role of the body's cellular and immunologic defense systems in moderating the course of the plaque diseases needs clarification. The main access that phagocytic cells and their antibacterial products have to the oral cavity is through the *gingival crevice.* This route may prove to have important implications on the onset and progress of periodontal disease.[30] Conceivably, once the cellular and immunologic components are in the gingival crevice, they can influence the subgingival plaque organisms responsible for root caries and periodontal disease. It is more difficult to conceive of the humoral defense system operating in supragingival plaque. Yet low levels of leukocytes flow into the saliva continually.[31] About 500 leukocytes per second are estimated as emigrating from the tissues to the crevice.[30] The majority of these soon disintegrate in the saliva,[32] a phenomenon which may be related to the fact that more intact polymorphs occur in caries-free than in caries-susceptible individuals.[33]

The immunologic defenses, despite theoretic limitations, may have an influence on dental caries. Individuals with major immunologic deficiencies have more caries than normal persons.[34] In the vaccination of monkeys against *S mutans*, serum IgA, serum IgG, and serum IgM all increase as the caries incidence decreases.[35] Perhaps these three serum immunoglobulins may prove important in the control of caries.[36] Thus, on a research basis there is reason to believe that a linkage exists between normal defenses and the plaque diseases. How the cells and immunoglobulins exercise this potential is unclear. The development of a successful caries and possibly a periodontal disease vaccine will ultimately depend on such a clarification.

THE PLAQUE COMPARTMENT

The plaque compartment includes the acquired pellicle, which is an acellular protein layer of saliva components that is adsorbed to the surface of the enamel. For several hours after the initial sorption, a steady change occurs in quantity and composition of the pellicle as new proteins are added.[37] The proline-rich proteins (PRPs), which make up approximately 40% of the pellicle,[38] and the glycoproteins appear to mediate the attachment sites of the subsequent, colonizing plaque bacteria.[39] Mucins are a minor component of the pellicle and can be quite *protective against acid diffusion.*[40,41] In the case of the glycoproteins, adherence can occur in the saliva, as manifested by bacterial agglutination.[12] Some of the PRPs, however, do not bind with bacteria in the saliva but do form attachment sites after they have been adsorbed onto the enamel. This latter phenomenon is probably due to conformational changes after the PRPs are adsorbed onto the enamel, which unmasks binding sites. Gibbons has termed these unmasked attachment sites *cryptitopes* (hidden places).[42]

To understand the effect that plaque has on teeth, it is necessary to focus on the action of acid in demineralizing teeth. To reduce the potential of demineralization, it is necessary to (1) reduce the *number* of bacteria producing the acid, (2) reduce the *amount of acid produced* by the existing bacteria, or (3) *negate the effect* of the produced acids.

Reducing Bacterial Population

Toothbrushing and flossing are prime means of plaque control. At least three oral-defense mechanisms exist, however, that do not depend on the frailties of human motivation and technique:

1. Great numbers of bacteria in the saliva are eliminated by agglutination and *swallowing.*
2. The bacterial populations in the saliva and plaque are continually exposed to the *antibacterial elements of the saliva.*
3. The *flow of saliva* prevents many bacteria from being adsorbed to the plaque covering the teeth.

Reducing Acid Production

The reduction of the amount of acid produced by the bacteria is mainly a function of reducing the intake of refined carbohydrates (ie, sugar discipline). This subject is discussed in detail in later chapters dealing with sugars, nutrition, and clinical preventive dentistry.

Reducing Acid Damage

The plaque pH can drop to 4.0 after a glucose mouth rinse.[43] Buffering of acid in the plaque, as in the saliva, is achieved by dilution, chemical buffering, neutralizing, and by increasing the protective ions in the environs of the teeth. The water content of the saliva and plaque aids greatly in diluting the acid generated and in transporting it into saliva, where it is further diluted and swallowed. This dilution effect is supplemented by the buffering capacity of the plaque, which is 10 times higher than for saliva.[44] This higher buffering level is due to the ability of plaque to adsorb and to concentrate bicarbonates, phosphates, and ammonia from the saliva. These neutralizing and buffering actions serve as a brake on the rapidity of and extent to which the pH can drop during periods of acidogenesis.

Each individual has a different potential for modifying the drop and recovery of the pH in the Stephan curve. For instance, if a group of individuals is given a glucose mouth rinse, each person demonstrates a different but reproducible Stephan curve. Once the pH has started to fall, the availability of sialin helps to shorten the time that the pH is at its minimum and most dangerous level.

Supersaturation of Saliva

The concentration of calcium and phosphate ions in the fluid bathing the tooth at the plaque–tooth interface is extremely important, because these are the same elements composing the hydroxyapatite crystal. *If the fluid adjacent to the tooth is supersaturated with calcium and phosphorus ions at a given pH, the enamel certainly cannot undergo demineralization at its surface.*

The saliva bathing the teeth is normally supersaturated with respect to the calcium and phosphate of enamel.[15] The continued supersaturation of the tooth's environs is possible because the plaque can concentrate both calcium and phosphate to a higher level than in saliva. The phosphate in the plaque is three times greater than the level occurring in the saliva. This is of practical importance because the calcium and phosphate in plaque tend to be inversely related to caries score.[45] With these higher levels of calcium and phosphate, spontaneous precipitation would probably occur were it not for the influence of statherin and other PRPs that enter the plaque compartment and adsorb onto the enamel surface.

As the pH drops, the level of supersaturation also drops, and the possibility of demineralization increases. There is no exact pH at which the demineralization of enamel begins, only a general range of 5.5 to 5.0. This range is rather large because demineralization is a function of both pH and duration of exposure of the enamel surface to the acid environment. Also, different plaques have different initial pHs, buffering potentials, and concentrations of calcium and phosphorus in different parts of the mouth. A change in any of these variables results in a different level of supersaturation in the tooth environment.[46]

The maintenance of the supersaturated state is not absolute, however, as demonstrated by the fact that deposits of calcium and phosphate salts occur in all plaques. These deposits may range from amorphous precipitations to microcrystals to visible, gross calculus—often containing other elements such as fluoride.[47] Some plaques contain calculus deposits with five to eight times the amount of fluoride seen in enamel.[48]

Calcium also is bound to proteins in the plaque. As the pH of the plaque drops following acidogenesis, dissolution of the enamel occurs, and calcium and phosphate are liberated, along with other bound ions in the plaque. In this way all minerals that are more soluble than hydroxyapatite serve to protect the apatite crystal by increasing the ionic saturation of the threatened area. The fluoride that is released from the dissolving mineral serves to lower the pH at which demineralization occurs. Fortunately plaque can accumulate fluoride to concentrations higher than in the saliva. This effect is enhanced by municipal water fluoridation; a greater amount of fluoride occurs in plaques where the water supplies contain fluoride compared with those that do not.[49]

Question 2. Which of the following statements, if any, are correct?

A. Bacteria requiring iron and copper have less possibility of survival in the presence of lactoferrin.

B. The minor glands are responsible for a major output of secretory IgA.

C. The receptor sites of the glycoproteins and PRPs can aid in determining bacterial occupants of ecologic niches.

D. If the product of calcium and phosphate ions is relatively low, the pH in the environs of the tooth must be relatively high to prevent demineralization.

E. The presence of calcium phosphate salts in the dental plaque is protective because these salts dissolve before hydroxyapatite; their dissolution provides a higher level of supersaturation in the environs of the teeth.

PHYSICAL CHARACTER OF PLAQUE

A major consideration in the defense of the tooth is the physical character of the plaque itself. For fluids and chemical components of the saliva and plaque to function, they must be able to diffuse freely throughout the plaque. This diffusion requires time, which is contingent on several factors. (1) If the water content in the plaque is relatively high, incoming and exiting constituents diffuse rapidly. (2) If the colloid and glucan content of the plaque is high, the diffusion is slower. (3) If the plaque is thick, it takes longer for ions to diffuse from the saliva–plaque interface to the plaque–tooth interface and vice versa.

Probably the most unpredictable factor relating to plaque diffusion is the character of the microbial population. Variations in species from one plaque to another or in different parts of the same plaque result in different diffusion patterns. In other words, the bacterial components can act as either a barrier or as a gate to the passage of selected anions and cations. For example, the bacteria use phosphate in their metabolism—a metabolism that is accentuated during periods of acidogenesis. Thus, their need for phosphate from the plaque metabolic pool occurs at a time when the same phosphate is required to maintain the supersaturation at the plaque–tooth interface.[50] Yet not all bacteria are bad. *Veillonella*, if present, can metabolize lactic acid generated by *S mutans*, lactobacilli, actinomycetes, and other acidogenic organisms. Presumably this action decreases the amount of acid available to demineralize teeth. Several studies indicate that the presence of *Veillonella* does decrease the caries risk. Thus the varieties, metabolic characteristics, and interrelationships of the plaque bacteria at any one time, or at different times, are important in determining whether caries will occur.

TOOTH COMPARTMENT

Enamel is more mineralized than bone or dentin. It is estimated that enamel is approximately 96% mineral by weight and an average of 87% by volume.[51] The enamel contains millions of rods that run from the dentinoenamel junction to the tooth surface. The rods are approximately 4 to 7 μm and 6 to 8 μm in diameter for primary and permanent teeth, respectively.[51] The length of the enamel rod is established by the thickness of the enamel cap, usually about 1 to 3 mm. In cross sections they resemble keyholes more than rods (Fig 11–1A, B). *Between each rod is a protein matrix.* During formation of the crown, the organic matrix is almost certainly involved in determining crystal size and orientation.

The inorganic phase of enamel is based on the mineral hydroxyapatite, $Ca_5(OH)(PO_4)_3$. We say *based on* because although the mineral of enamel has the crystal structure and general composition of hydroxyapatite, it is never stoichiometric,[c] always having a lower calcium to phosphorus ratio than is indicated for the theoretic formula. It also contains ions other than calcium, phosphate, and hydroxyl; in fact, many elements may be substituted in the crystal. More than 40 elements have been identified in an analysis of enamel.[52]

Each rod is made up of crystals that are shaped much like a carpenter's hexagonal lead pencil, which is slightly flattened on two opposite sides (Fig 11–1C). Each of the millions of crystals in each rod (Fig 11–1C) has three axes, an *a*- and a *b*-axis represent-

ing the longest and shortest cross sections, respectively, of the basal face,[d] and a *c*-axis that parallels the long axis (Fig 11–1C). Between the crystals along the *c*-axis in a parallel array in the head of the rod, are *submicroscopic amounts of matrix.* To this point, the details of the tooth structure can be visualized with the electron microscope. Beyond this stage it is the world of molecules, atoms, and ions, where more sophisticated methods are required to establish spatial and structural relationships.

The theoretic description of the substructure of the crystal is based on x-ray diffraction studies and other methods of crystal identification. The main elemental components making up a crystal of hydroxyapatite—calcium, phosphate, and hydroxyl group—are arranged in repeating configurations known as *unit cells* (Fig 11–1D). A unit cell is the smallest subdivision of a crystalline substance that is entirely representative of the stoichiometric structure of the crystal. This means that all crystals of any macroscopic dimension can be constructed by adding additional unit cells much as a building can be increased in size by adding additional bricks.[53] It is important to recognize that the unit cells, unlike the bricks, have no physical meaning as such; they are just a convenient means of conceptualizing the atomic structure at the simplest level.

If one column of molecules could be detached from the *c*-axis of the unit cell, it would resemble wind chimes on a string, with each successive segment being a grouping of calcium, phosphate, oxygen, and hydrogen ions equidistant from adjacent groupings (Fig 11–1E). When looking at the atomic arrangement of the ions *from the top* of the column, the center position is

---

[c] Stoichiometric = Always having a fixed proportion of its component elements.

[d] Basal face = The area at the ends of the crystal encompassed by the *a* and *b* axes.

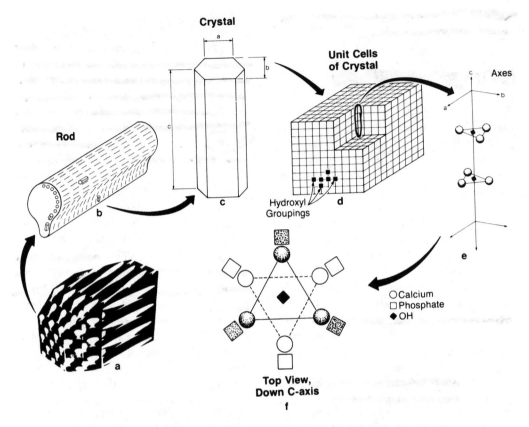

Figure 11–1. Enamel, from the microscopic to the molecular. **A.** Model of human dental enamel prepared by cementing together individual prisms (rods). Note the variety of patterns formed by milling the surfaces of the model at different angles to the prism axis. (*From Meckel AH, Griebstein WJ, Neal RJ. Structure of mature human dental enamel as observed by electron microscopy. Oral Biol. 1965; 10:775–783.*) **B.** Individual enamel rod, showing different crystallite orientations in head and tail. **C.** Illustration of a crystallite with labeled a, b, and c axes. (Also see Fig 11–3B). **D.** Theoretic presentation of unit cells that make up the crystallite. **E.** Vertical arrangement of molecules of hydroxyapatite along C axis making up unit cell. **F.** Looking down on Fig 11–1e, showing how every other molecular configuration is rotated 180° as illustrated by first the solid and then the dotted lines. (*Courtesy of Dr N. O. Harris, University of Texas Dental School, San Antonio, TX.*)

occupied by a hydroxyl ion, surrounded by a triangular configuration with a calcium ion at each point of the triangle. Immediately peripheral to each calcium atom is a phosphate grouping (Fig 11–1F). Each successive grouping along the *c*-axis is rotated 180° from the ones above and below, as illustrated by the solid and the dotted lines in Figure 11–1F.

Each of these atoms can be replaced by other atoms. For instance a hydroxyl group can be substituted by fluoride, a calcium ion can be replaced by strontium, and a phosphate group can be replaced by a carbonate ion. Not all original ions are replaced, nor are all replacements permanent. Ionic exchange is continual throughout life. When a great number of random hydroxyl groupings are replaced by fluoride ions, the hydroxyapatite crystal becomes *fluorhydroxyapatite*. If *all* hydroxyls were replaced with fluoride, the crystal would be termed *fluorapatite*. As each crystal acquires more fluoride, it becomes increasingly more resistant to acid; conversely, if the fluoride is later replaced with hydroxyl, it becomes more soluble. Similarly, replacement of the calcium and phosphate by other ions can result in a more or less stable crystal.

If the serum fluoride level is higher during the formation of the teeth, as occurs when there is a fluoridated water supply, more of the hydroxyl sites are occupied by fluoride than occurs for people living in a nonfluoride area. Once the enamel is formed, it is much more difficult to replace the hydroxyls with fluoride, because such an ion exchange requires a diffusion of the fluoride into, and the hydroxyl ions out of, the solid crystal.

After the tooth erupts into the oral cavity, however, and becomes exposed to the fluoride and other ions present in the saliva, in drinking water and foods, and in the plaque, the concentrations of fluoride in the outermost layers of enamel increases to as high as 2000 ppm, whereas the fluoride concentration in deeper layers may be as low as 50 ppm.[54] This suggests that fluoride substitutions in the crystalline lattice do occur *following* the period of enamel formation, and account for the majority of reactive surface fluoride.

Permeability of the Enamel

It is the inorganic phase of enamel that is lost during demineralization; however, it is the organic matrix that hastens the demineralization by providing the invasion channels for the acid. In a demineralized tooth, the matrix appears as a network that permeates the entire enamel volume. Between the rods, the matrix is a few hundred angstroms in width. Between the parallel apatite crystals of the rod, the intercrystalline matrix is approximately 17 Å (1.7 nm).[55] Interconnecting the matrices of the rods and crystals are the hypomineralized areas occupied by the incremental lines and the strial of Retzius. In addition, the interrod and intercrystalline matrices extend into the less mineralized areas along the dentinoenamel junction. Finally, the various matrices contact the relatively hypomineralized areas making up the lamellae, spindles, and tufts. Ions can freely diffuse through this watery network. If they are hydrogen ions, the results can be damaging because of the intimate contact between the organic and inorganic phases of the enamel. Conversely, if the ions are calcium, phosphate, or fluoride, the resistance of the enamel may be upgraded.

Enamel, especially recently erupted enamel, is permeable to many ions. In young monkeys it only takes 5 hours for radioactive iodine to go from the outside of the tooth to the pulp and thence to the thyroid gland, where it can be quantitated. Radioactive phosphorus is able to move in the reverse direction, from the pulp to the outside, in the same amount of time.[56] In another study, when extracted teeth with class V cavities were placed in solutions with several radioactive elements—sulfur, sodium, rubidium, and calcium—all reached the pulp within 24 hours.[57] The velocity of water flow through enamel is estimated at 0.1 mm/hour.[14] Free water constitutes about 3% of the enamel mass but 10% to 11% of enamel volume. This water is important for many of the characteristics of enamel: *permeability, ion exchange capacity,* and *elasticity*.[58] The movement of water through the enamel cap is probably via the same channels of diffusion that transport ions during demineralization and remineralization (Fig 11–2). After eruption, many of the

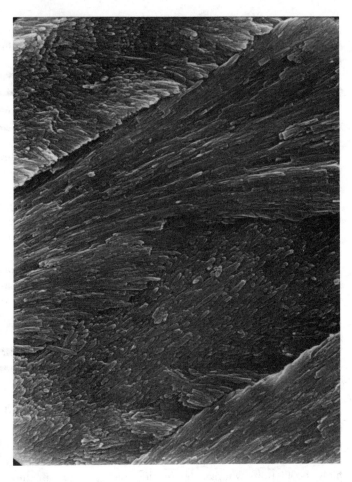

Figure 11–2. Cleaved enamel surface, showing original and remineralized crystals in adjacent prisms (×16,500). (*Courtesy of Dr WL Jongebloed, University of Gröningen, The Netherlands.*)

crystals are not fully matured, and time is needed to add the missing ions from the saliva.[59,60] During the immediate posteruptive period—at least in humans—caries susceptibility is high. When fluoride is applied to the teeth immediately after eruption, it penetrates the enamel for about 100 μm; later, when the enamel has matured, the fluoride does not penetrate further than 20 μm. Eventually, there is a gradient of mineralization from the surface toward the dentinoenamel junction, with calcium, phosphate, and fluoride being greatest on the surface and decreasing in concentration as

the dentinoenamel junction is approached. Other ions, such as carbonate, bicarbonate, magnesium, and sodium, increase toward the dentinoenamel junction.

Question 3. Which of the following statements, if any, are correct?

A. Bacteria can reduce the amount of phosphate in the environs of the teeth.

B. The enamel *rod* resembles a hexagonal pencil that has been flattened on opposing sides, whereas the enamel *crystal* resembles a keyhole.

C. In the unit cell, hydroxyl groupings are surrounded by a triangular configuration of calcium atoms.

D. Enamel is permeable to the movement of ions other than hydrogen (acid).

E. The same channels of diffusion that transport ions and fluids *outward* during demineralization transport ions and fluids *inward* during remineralization.

IN VITRO DEMINERALIZATION

Demineralization is the loss of mineral apatite from the enamel. There is no preferential site for acid attack on the enamel *prism.* Following surface etching of the enamel, the rod core may be initially attacked, leaving a raised periphery. In other areas on the same tooth surface, the core remains intact and the periphery dissolves. Finally, at times there is no consistent pattern. These three possibilities have been designated as type I, II, and III etchings, respectively.[61]

The initial morphologic changes occurring on the enamel surface following carious dissolution in vivo was studied by Holmen and colleagues,[62] using the SEM. These investigators showed a direct dissolution of the surface itself causing an enlargement of intercrystalline pathways when viewed at high magnifications. Lower power shows little surface change at this early stage of dissolution. Arends and coworkers[63] concluded that the mineral loss after an initial caries attack comes from the interprismatic areas and from the prism peripheries. The interprismatic demineralization does not contribute significantly to mineral loss in the initial stages of lesion formation. Focal pits or holes can often be observed as the dissolution continues. This increase in space as the mineral dissolves results in enlarged pathways for diffusion of mineral out of the enamel and for acid penetration into the subsurface.

Typically, in vitro demineralization of the crystal occurs in two stages: (1) dissolution of the *cores* of the individual apatite crystals,[55] and (2) subsequent dissolution of the remaining "shell" of the crystal. The dissolution of the crystal cores has been associated with both an increased carbonate content and the presence of crystalline imperfections. The destruction of the crystal begins with the formation of *etch* pits (Fig 11–3A), small indentations in the center of the terminal ends of the apatite crystal, which progressively deepen as the dissolu-

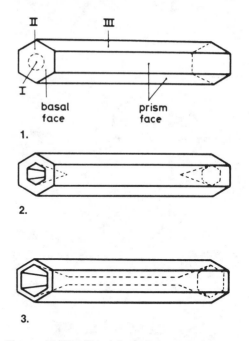

Figure 11–3A. Dissolution of the crystal, schematic: Each enamel prism is made up of parallel crystals of hydroxyapatite that have a slightly flattened hexagonal appearance. **1.** The initial etching of the crystal begins at the ends, **2.**, with the formation of etchpits. These etchpits deepen along the c-axis to eventually produce a hollow core, **3.** (*From Arends J, Jongebloed WL. Ultrastructure studies of synthetic apatite crystals. J Dent Res. 1979; (special issue B) 58:837–843.*)

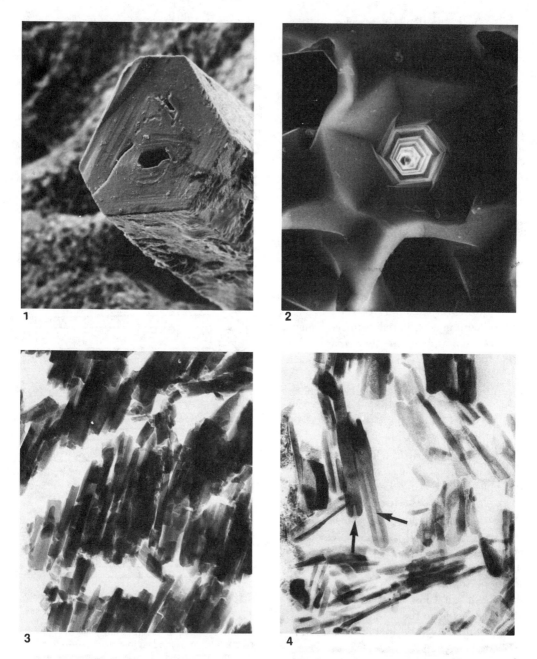

Figure 11–3B. Dissolution of the crystal, photographic. **1.** Artificially grown apatite crystal with etchpit on basal face, original magnification ×500; **2.** A hexagonal etchpit in fluorapatite, original magnification ×2500; **3.** TEM-picture of sound enamel crystallites, original magnification ×100,000; and **4.** TEM-picture of etched enamel crystallites that are partially hollowed out, original magnification ×100,000. (*Courtesy of Dr WL Jongebloed, I Molenaar, and L Arends, University of Gröningen, The Netherlands; and Joel News, Japan. 1976; 13e(2):14–19.*)

tion continues down the center of the crystal.[64,65] Again, if the crystal is compared to a pencil, the dissolution follows the path of the lead.[66] The preferential dissolution of the crystal core (Fig 11–3B) is demonstrated by in vitro experiments in which the cores are completely dissolved in a few minutes by dilute lactic acid, whereas dissolution of the remaining shell requires several hours.

THE SUBSURFACE LESION

Caries development is the result of alternating episodes of demineralization and remineralization (Fig 11–4). It can take 2 years or more for some carious lesions to develop.[59] In other cases, such as seen in the xerostomia that follows head and neck radiation, the enamel appears to almost melt away over a 6-month period. It has long been noted that the outer enamel surface is more resistant to dissolution than the subsurface area making up the incipient enamel lesion.[67] The maturity of surface enamel was believed to result from the addition of ions such as fluoride from the saliva. A second and possibly more dominant mechanism is that the mineral diffusing outward from the subsurface lesion replaces that which had been lost on the surface. Possibly the pellicle acts as a template for this reconstruction, because no additional thickness of the enamel cap is observed. This provides a damage

control system by maintaining a minimal pore size until later remineralization of the deeper layers can be accomplished, provided an adequate remineralization environment exists. Such a remineralizing environment can be produced by good plaque control, vigorous fluoride therapy, and restricted sugar intake—*the same requirements that prevent demineralization.*

If an extracted tooth is simply placed in an acid, the external surface is removed layer by layer. This surface dissolution of enamel does not resemble in vivo caries, in which a mature layer occurs with pores connecting the surface to the subsurface lesion. In attempting to duplicate the subsurface lesion, Silverstone[68] submerged extracted teeth in acid-buffered cellulose gels. With this technique, he was able to produce lesions similar to those seen in vivo. In the course of the experimentation, it appeared that the calcium and phosphate salts were transported from the subsurface area to the surface, where they accumulated, became saturated, and then precipitated between the gel and the tooth. In carrying this experiment further, the entire mature layer of the enamel was ground off before placing the tooth in the buffered gel. When the tooth was eventually recovered from the gel, an entire new mature layer had formed. When an extracted tooth with a carefully preserved plaque is immersed in an acid, the same buildup of calcium and phosphates occurs beneath the pellicle. These experiments highlight the fact that the intact surface is a unique protective layer overlying the subsurface demineralization.

The sodium, magnesium, and carbonate that is first liberated by the demineralization serves briefly as a buffer to limit damage.[69] The dissolution of the hydroxyapatite also tends to neutralize the hydrogen ions. Then, with a return of the pH to normal, the damaged crystals may be repaired,

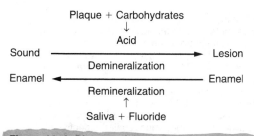

Plaque + Carbohydrates
↓
Acid

Sound ———————————→ Lesion
Demineralization
Enamel ←——————————— Enamel
Remineralization
↑
Saliva + Fluoride

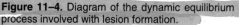

Figure 11–4. Diagram of the dynamic equilibrium process involved with lesion formation.

or new crystals may be formed from the previously dissolved mineral. If fluoride is present, the reassembly occurs with many of the hydroxyl spaces being occupied by fluoride.[70] A later ion exchange reaction may occur after the hydroxyapatite has formed, which also results in the formation of fluorhydroxyapatite.

The extent of demineralization can be slowed by the presence of the acquired pellicle,[16,71,72] which serves much as Silverstone's gel in retaining the subsurface ions against the tooth surface. Older pellicles are more effective than those recently formed.[73]

This decelerating action in the transport of ions through the acquired pellicle is four to five times more efficient if the pellicle is adsorbed onto fluorapatite, as compared with hydroxyapatite.[74] The fluoride necessary for the multiple protective actions can be derived either from the fluoride contained in the dissolving fluorhydroxyapatite crystals, or it can come from the plaque. Thus, in the presence of fluoride, a previously demineralized site that remineralizes can become more acid-resistant than the original apatite (Fig 11–5). This increased resistance probably extends to crystals located along the or-

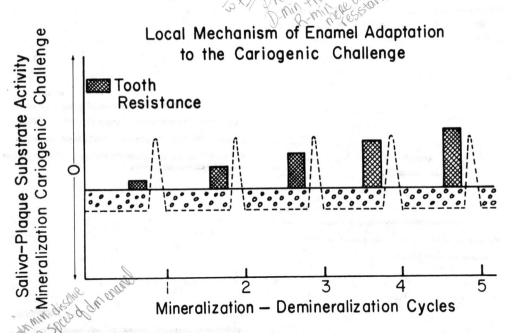

Local Mechanism of Enamel Adaptation to the Cariogenic Challenge

Figure 11–5. The reactions leading to enamel adaptation are diagrammatically illustrated. The fluid in contact with the tooth surface becomes unsaturated due to the low pH generated by the microbial plaque and supersaturated when salivary flow neutralizes the acid. During the unsaturation phase, tooth mineral dissolves. During the supersaturation phase, minerals precipitate within the microspaces of the partially demineralized enamel. Many cycles of unsaturation and supersaturation lead to enamel adaptation because the most soluble mineral dissolves and is replaced by a less soluble mineral if proper ionic components are present in the fluid environment. Preferential mineral retention is evidenced by the high level of fluoride present in areas of arrested caries. As in other adaptation reactions, the magnitude and frequency of the periods of challenge and repair are critical. By minimizing challenge and enhancing repair the dentist can shift the equilibrium towards caries arrest with development of resistant, or adapted, areas of enamel. Fluoride treatments and improved oral hygiene are instrumental in attaining adaptation. (From Koulourides TI. Proceedings of Symposium on Incipient Caries of Enamel, ed. NH Rowe, University of Michigan. November 11–12, 1977:51–68.)

ganic invasion channels where the pore space and interrod volume would be expected to decrease.

REMINERALIZATION

Remineralization is the repair of enamel rod structure following acidogenic episodes. When teeth erupt, they are anatomically complete but crystallographically incomplete.[75] Following eruption, the missing ions are supplied from the saliva, a process termed *posteruptive maturation*. Throughout life ions from the saliva are used in the same way to repair acid-damaged tooth structure. This repair process can range from an almost immediate replacement of daily ion losses from the enamel surface to a slow repair (under proper conditions) of extensive subsurface lesions that are due to a long-term negative caries balance.[76] Without specific knowledge of the caries process, one is likely to envision the development of a carious lesion as a continuous process, accompanied by an ever-increasing loss of tooth mineral until the stage is reached when a clinically discernible cavity is present. Fortunately this conception is incorrect. The process of demineralization is *not* irreversible or inevitably progressive. If damage has not progressed beyond a certain ill-defined point, lost mineral *can* be replaced (Fig 11–6).

There is considerable clinical evidence for remineralization. Head,[77] a physician and a dentist, pointed out in 1912 that teeth underwent cycles of softening and hardening. By 1933 Boedecker[78] advocated the use of Andresen's method of remineralizing "soft" teeth and white spots. Andresen's mineralizing powder consisted of tartaric acid, gelatin, calcium, phosphate, calcium carbonate, magnesium carbonate, sodium bicarbonate, and sodium chloride. Boedecker comments as follows: "The purpose

that this powder is to fulfill is to go into solution in the saliva and in this state permeate and recalcify the porous area in the enamel . . . and after the remineralizing powder had been used for six weeks redecay around fillings will come to a standstill."

Muhler, in several clinical studies of the anticaries effectiveness of stannous fluoride, often found that the experimental subjects had more sound teeth later in the study than at the initial examination.[79] Invariably the number of these *reversals* was greater in the fluoride treatment groups than in the controls. Von der Fehr and colleagues[80] were able to induce white spots with sucrose mouth rinses and then reverse the process. Backer-Dirks,[59] in a long-term study, noted that 50% of the interproximal lesions seen at the initial examination did not progress, indicating an arrestment phenomenon due to remineralization. Additional support for remineralization is derived from the frequent observations of teeth that are acid-etched prior to placement of pit-and-fissure sealants, composite resin restoratives, or orthodontic brackets.[81] For those etched areas not covered with the resin, the chalky white appearance disappears over a period of a few days, and the enamel regains its initial, translucent, glossy appearance.

Except under unusual circumstances such as occur following the destruction of the salivary glands during cancer radiotherapy or diseases of the glands, deviations from remineralizing conditions in the mouth are transient. For example, the local pH may be lowered to where enamel demineralization occurs during the ingestion of acid foods or from the production of acid by the plaque bacteria following the ingestion of refined carbohydrates. If the insults are *brief* and *widely separated* in time, remineralizing conditions can be restored in the intervening periods and the slight damage repaired. On the other hand, frequent or

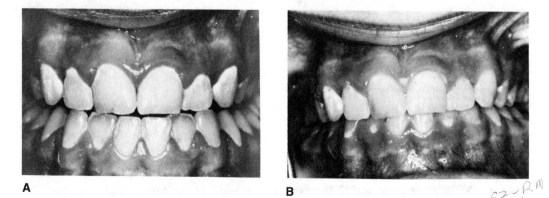

A   **B**

SZ -RM
BL -dm
DZ -RM
TZ -dm

Figure 11–6. A. Teeth before treatment that show incipient caries along the gingival margin. **B.** Remineralization is evident after two months of treatment, with the treatment consisting of plaque control, 1.1% NaF (Thera-Flur) followed by 0.05% APF (Phos-Flur) for the second month. (*Courtesy of Dr N Tinanoff, University of Connecticut School of Dental Medicine.*)

protracted periods of acidogenesis, with insufficient time intervals for remineralization, ultimately lead to the development of overt caries. For example, following the ingestion of sucrose, bacterial metabolic activity immediately increases as does the subsequent production of acid. If the acid attack is short, the demineralization of enamel that follows is limited. Any acid that is produced is immediately buffered by the plaque and saliva while the teeth are protected by the high concentration of calcium and phosphates in the plaque. If the insult is protracted, the availability of protective plaque minerals and the local high buffering capacity are exhausted; any further acid produced is available for demineralizing the enamel.

Crystal Size in Demineralization and Remineralization

Silverstone has contributed much to the understanding of the details of the remineralization process. In his review of remineralization,[82] he pointed out that crystal sizes differ *predictably* in each of the zones of the incipient lesion and in remineralized carious areas. In the incipient carious lesions, the crystals in the two zones of *de*mineraliza-tion—the *body of the lesion* and the *translucent zone*—were smaller than in sound enamel (Fig 11–7). The crystals in the two zones of *remineralization*—the *dark* and the *surface zones*—were equal to or greater in size than those found in normal enamel. Predictably, when a remineralizing solution

Lesion of Enamel Caries

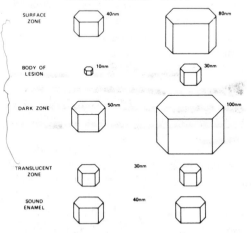

Figure 11–7. Illustration of the relative crystal diameters in sound enamel (bottom) and in the four histologic zones of the enamel lesions. (*From Silverstone LM. The significance of remineralization in caries prevention. J Can Dent Assoc. 1984; 50:157–164.*)

when a remineralizing solution with fluoride is used to remineralize the subsurface lesion, the crystal sizes in all zones are greater than for normal enamel[82] (Fig 11–8).

Remineralizing Solutions

Remineralizing dentifrices have been proposed but not accepted by the American Dental Association (ADA).[83,84] Several ADA-accepted artificial salivas have been accepted for use by patients with hyposalivation but not as remineralizing solutions.[85,86] In vitro it has been demonstrated that solutions containing calcium and phosphate ions may result in remineralization and that the remineralization can be enhanced by the presence of fluoride. The lack of evidence that the mineral content of dentifrices or mouth rinses is effective in vivo is probably due to the short contact time between the teeth and the agent.[87]

An ideal artificial remineralizing medium should be (1) hydrophilic, (2) of low viscosity to permit penetration into the subsurface lesion, (3) antibacterial, (4) supplemental to the saliva, (5) rapid-acting, and (6) dependable. The elements used in most remineralizing formulations include calcium, phosphates, and fluoride. Ions such as tartrates may promote the complexing and transport of calcium ions into the subsurface lesion for repair.[88] Sodium chloride is often added to stabilize the solution and to prevent the spontaneous precipitation of the calcium and phosphate.[89] Other compounds may be added at physiologic levels to simulate saliva more closely.

The amount of remineralization that occurs varies according to the (1) total *time* the teeth (or sections of teeth) are immersed in the remineralizing solution, (2) *reactants*, (3) the extent of *supersaturation* of the solution in relation to the teeth, (4) *rate of precipitation* of the reactants, and (5) *pH* of the solution.

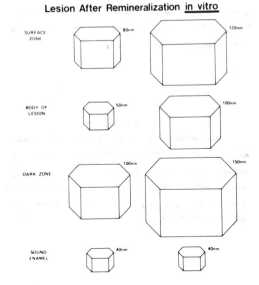

Figure 11–8. Crystal diameters in a lesion after exposure to low calcium calcifying fluid containing fluid ions. (*From Silverstone LM. The significance of remineralization in caries prevention. J Can Dent Assoc. 1984; 50:157–164.*)

Of these limiting factors, *time* is probably the most critical. It is possible to accelerate in vitro remineralization by changing formulas, pH, and temperature, but it has been found that as these are changed, so does the *quality* of the remineralized enamel. The eventual objective should be to produce both *optimal* and *maximal* remineralization.

The importance of the concentration of the reactants and speed of reaction is illustrated by two different experiments. If *tooth sections* are exposed to remineralizing solutions with relatively high calcium and phosphate concentrations, the entire subsurface lesion remineralizes. If an extracted *intact tooth* with a subsurface lesion is exposed to a similar remineralizing solution, however, the subsurface lesion does not completely remineralize. The difference between the two in vitro results is due to the pores of the intact tooth connecting the surface to the subsurface enamel becoming clogged with precipitate,[90] whereas the tooth sections that were broadly exposed to the reactants did not require the remineralizing solution to penetrate the pores. This same self-limiting action is also seen when saliva is used. This suggests the possibility that higher concentrations might be used to remineralize very early surface alterations that remineralize rapidly,[76] whereas lower concentrations might be used to facilitate deeper penetration, once the subsurface lesion develops.

The role of supersaturation, kinetics, and precursor phases were used to explain the limited remineralization of 3 mM calcifying fluids as opposed to 1 mM Ca calcifying fluids during in vitro experiments. The higher concentrated calcifying fluid produced less overall remineralization and was surface-limited. The 1 mM Ca fluid was effective throughout the entire lesion depth.[91]

Studies by Silverstone[91] of the subsurface lesion indicate that the dark zone is a site of active remineralization. This zone occurs in the majority of lesions seen in sections with incipient caries. In some cases, it is absent, presumably due to the fact that no remineralization was occurring in the tooth at the time of extraction. When these sections are placed in remineralizing solutions, the dark zone appears in its expected position between the translucent zone and the main body of the lesion (Fig 11–9). Early studies of in vitro remineralization, either using saliva or artificial solutions, indicated that the process was rapid over the first 24 hours; then it slowed over the next 48 hours.[87] In more recent studies, Silverstone[82] exposed demineralized specimens to ten 6-minute exposures to a remineralizing solution. Maximal remineralization had occurred at the end of the tenth exposure, with approximately 80% of the final degree

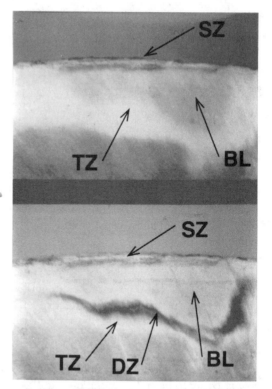

Figure 11–9. A polarized light photomicrograph of a section from an artificial white spot lesion that has been imbibed in quinoline to show the translucent and dark zones. The top photo is prior to remineralization. Note surface zone (SZ), a body of the lesion (BL), and the translucent zone (TZ). Bottom photograph is after remineralization. Note the remineralizing dark zone (DZ) and the clearly defined translucent and surface zones. (*Courtesy of Dr James S. Wefel, College of Dentistry, University of Iowa.*)

of remineralization being found at the end of the fifth exposure.

When using saliva as the remineralization solution, the ability to remineralize tooth sections in vitro varies with the saliva of different individuals but is consistent for the saliva for each individual. This indicates that some people have a greater capacity for remineralization (host resistance) than others.

Fluoride has considerable influence on both demineralization and remineralization.

Fortunately, only small concentrations of fluoride are needed to inhibit demineralization or to enhance remineralization. As little as 0.1 ppm fluoride can reduce the amount of enamel dissolution in vitro.[92] The presence of fluoride at the remineralizing site can accelerate rehardening by a factor of four to five.[93] Silverstone[82] found that 1 ppm of fluoride reduced the area of the body of the lesion from 22% to 72% when using 1 mM calcifying fluids. No additional benefit was observed by the addition of 10 ppm fluoride. Wefel[94] has described the effects of fluoride on caries development when using intraoral models. The presence of fluoride *in solution* is more critical than fluoride in enamel, because fluoride acts to affect the rates of reaction as one of its major mechanisms. Thus, greater caries reduction can be expected if fluoride was present in low concentrations at the time of active demineralization and remineralization. In the mouth, the required small amounts of fluoride can come from four sources: (1) transitory contact with fluoridated drinking water; (2) the continual low fluoride output of the *salivary glands;* (3) the bound fluoride occurring in the *plaque,* which is released when the pH drops to around 5.0; or (4) from the fluoride contained in the *mature enamel layer* following demineralization. The ingested amount of fluoride required to elevate salivary concentrations would be prohibitive as a practical method of fluoride delivery. Fluoride in enamel is redistributed during lesion formation such that the body of the lesion increases in fluoride content while the sound enamel is reduced.[95] The use of enamel-bound fluoride, however, requires the dissolution of the tooth structure to liberate fluoride to the fluid phase. Thus, a fluoride reservoir or slow-release fluoride agent seems the most preferable for continuous caries protection. Both fluoride rinses and fluoride dentifrices are low-concentration/high-frequency agents that supply fluoride to the oral environment. These exposures to fluoride are also transient, and further work needs to be done on new vehicles for the delivery of fluoride. One such system is the intraoral fluoride-releasing system, which provides continuous fluoride release into the oral environment.

Intraoral Fluoride Slow-release Device

Silverstone pointed out that at *all times* the great majority of tooth surfaces have in situ incipient lesions, which are present at the histologic level but cannot be seen at the clinical level.[82] These in situ lesions must be prevented from progressing. It is accepted that frequent or continuous exposure to fluoride reduces caries and enhances remineralization. In the absence of water fluoridation, which helps fulfill this requisite, fluoride supplements have been used. The use of fluoride tablets, however, results in a once-a-day *spiking* of the fluoride levels in blood, urine, and saliva, that is, the fluoride levels rapidly increase about an hour after ingestion and then the concentration of the fluoride rapidly decreases as it is being eliminated by the kidneys. The problem is how to maintain an optimum and constant level of fluoride in the oral environment.

In the case of a slow-release intraoral device being developed for caries control, the therapeutic fluoride compound is sealed within a kidney-shaped copolymer capsule that permits a *predetermined* amount of fluoride to diffuse *continually* to the surface and into the oral environment (Fig 11–10). The rate of delivery can be altered by changes in the formulation of the copolymer. The device is approximately 8 mm long, 3 mm wide, and 2 mm thick. This is attached to the bilateral upper first or second molars with a sealant (Fig 11–11).

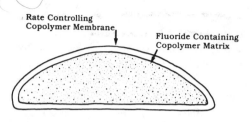

Figure 11–10. Cross section of intraoral device for controlled release of fluoride. (*Courtesy of Dr Ralph A. Frew.*)

A study of its effectiveness found that salivary fluoride increased by one to two times, and the plaque level was 20 to 50 times higher.[96–98] If eventually approved by the Food and Drug Administration, the device will be applicable to individuals at high risk for coronal or root caries, such as encountered in xerostomia, high sugar intake, orthodontic cases, and for mentally and physically disabled individuals. The same approach could probably be used for the controlled delivery of remineralization salts to the site of an incipient lesion. The main disadvantage is the need to replace the device at periodic intervals.

Review of the Many Roles of Fluoride

Fluoride functions in several roles to protect the tooth by reducing the challenge to the tooth surface, in preventing demineralization, and by enhancing remineralization:

- Immediately following eruption, the presence of fluoride accelerates the maturation of the tooth enamel, as fluoride, calcium, and phosphate are taken up by the outermost surface layers of enamel.
- The outward diffusion of minerals from the subsurface lesion is better contained by a pellicle formed on fluorhydroxyapatite than one formed on hydroxyapatite.
- The presence of fluoride in the environment during development, maturation, or remineralization increases the amount of fluoridated hydroxyapatite (eg, fluorhydroxyapatite) in the crystal.
- The replacement of the hydroxyl ion of the crystal by fluoride tends to stabilize the crystal and make it more resistant to demineralization.
- The presence of fluoride in the subsurface lesion results in the forma-

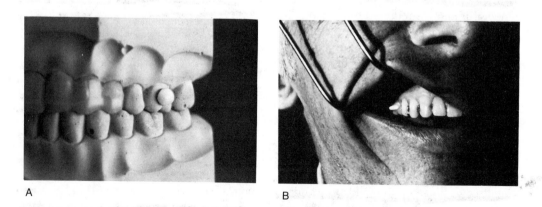

Figure 11–11. Photographs of intraoral device on stone model, **A,** and in human mouth, **B.**

tion of larger, better formed, and more insoluble crystals along the avenues of diffusion.

- In remineralization of the subsurface lesion, fluoride enhances the nucleation of calcium phosphate.
- Fluoride blocks glycolysis of plaque organisms, thus reducing the amount of acid formed.
- The presence of fluoride lowers the pH at which enamel demineralizes.

Question 4. Which of the following statements, if any, are correct?

A. The in vitro development of caries-like lesions is usually accomplished by placing extracted teeth in a *solution* buffered to a pH of 5.0 for a sufficient time.

B. An acquired pellicle adsorbed to hydroxyapatite is less permeable to ions from the subsurface lesions than is one adsorbed to fluorhydroxyapatite.

C. More time is involved in demineralizing a tooth site than remineralizing the site after acidogenesis.

D. Present plaque control measures would probably slow the loss of calcium and phosphate ions from the subsurface lesion.

E. The *dark zone* of the subsurface lesion is the initial site for remineralization.

SUMMARY

It has been emphasized that oral disease, in fact *all* disease, *occurs when the challenge posed by pathogens exceeds the body's capability for defense and repair.* In the case of dental caries, the defense and self-repair mechanisms of the body operate continuously in the saliva, in the plaque, and in the

enamel cap. Aside from the host's usual humeral and cellular defense functions to destroy pathogens, the saliva, too, is essential to the protection of the teeth. Normally the saliva is supersaturated with calcium and phosphate in relation to the crystalline structure of the enamel. During a meal or snack, the psychologic, gustatory, and masticatory stimuli of eating are sufficient to evoke an increased flow of saliva to help clear foods from the mouth. With the increase in saliva, the buffering due to the contained carbonate of the saliva also increases. Calcium concurrently increases thereby helping to maintain the high saturation of elements that help protect the teeth against demineralization and improving the possibility of remineralization. To avoid precipitation of the calcium and phosphate, the secretion of statherin increases, which serves to maintain the supersaturated level of minerals. Muscular action by the cheeks during chewing serves to pump this supersaturated saliva into the interproximal areas. During this period of eating with its concomitant intense salivary activity, the tooth is less at risk than a short time later when flow rate and buffering are not available to cope with retained foods and plaque pHs that have not yet returned to normal.

In the plaque compartment, the acquired pellicle presents as a thin layer of proteins, mainly glyco- and proline-rich proteins (PRPs). Initially the pellicle provides a welcome mat (literally) for the attachment of noncariogenic organisms that help to establish their etiologic niches in the plaque. Once formed, the pellicle can act as a barrier to the back-and-forth diffusion of demineralizing hydrogen ions as well as ions from a demineralization attack during a challenge period or as a reservoir for calcium, phosphates, and fluoride to be used for remineralization during the repair phase. The plaque has the ability to imbibe and to concentrate ions to approximately one order of magnitude higher than the saliva. Fluoride ions are usually found in higher concentrations in the plaque but are bound at near-neutral pH. Following an exposure to a fermentable carbohydrate, a dynamic series of reactions occurs, *with the drop in pH being the main triggering factor.* As the pH drops, the bound fluoride is released, thus ensuring a lower pH before demineralization can occur. The presence of sialin also slows the drop in pH. An increased amount of salivary buffering minimizes the acidogenic end products of the bacteria. The increased flow of saliva, with its high fluid content, enhances the removal of cariogenic foods as well as establishes an osmotic environment favorable for the more rapid diffusion of hydrogen ions toward the saliva rather than toward the tooth. As the pH drops, the supersaturation of the plaque fluids decreases. Ions, such as magnesium and carbonate, that are adsorbed onto the tooth or crystals dissolve preferentially and add to the buffering of the environment. When undersaturation occurs, somewhere between pH 5.0 and 5.5, the crystals of the fluorhydroxyapatite begin to dissolve. Even then, the ions of calcium and phosphate that are released from the enamel act as buffers and become available for remineralization when the pH begins to return to normal. At that time, the demineralization process reverses. The fluoride, calcium, and phosphate, and probably other ions, available to any submicroscopic damaged site on the tooth surface take part in the remineralization process. The ions in excess of the repair needs are again bound into the organic components of the plaque or participate in the remineralization process—to be available at the next acidogenic cycle.

This dynamic equilibrium process is set into action every time food is eaten. If the period of acidogenesis is prolonged, as when food is retained, acid production continues long after the major flow of saliva—with its cleansing, neutralizing, and buffering action—has ceased. Supersaturation of the plaque and its buffering capacity is largely exhausted after prolonged acidogenesis. The acid attack from this time on is directly on the apatite crystal. Even the repair process is impeded by the fact that the glucans of a cariogenic plaque can slow the dilution and buffering of the acids in the plaque as well as slow the diffusion of the remineralization ions from the saliva, through the plaque, to the tooth surface. Thus, homeostasis can only be maintained if (1) the acidogenic challenge can be minimized in time and pH drops, and (2) the saliva is normal in flow, ion content, and buffering capacity. The balance between caries resistance and caries susceptibility can often be tipped by the presence of fluoride, which increases the resistance of the apatite crystal to acid attack, attenuates the affect of pH drop, and accelerates the remineralization process.

ANSWERS AND EXPLANATIONS

1. A, B, E
   C—incorrect. Phosphate concentration, for instance, decreases as flow rate increases.
   D—incorrect. Neutralizing and buffering are due to chemical constituents of saliva; the dilution and cleaning effect is due to the high fluid content of saliva.
2. A, B, C, D, E
3. A, C, D, E
   B—incorrect. In cross section, the rod resembles a keyhole, whereas the cross section of the crystal resembles a flattened hexagonal pencil much like a carpenter uses.

4. E

A—incorrect. Usually a gel (not a solution) is used to form the subsurface lesion.

B—incorrect. The more fluoride, the more adsorption takes place.

C—incorrect. It only takes a few minutes with the sugar to do the damage; it takes much longer to repair the damage.

D—incorrect. If no pellicle or just a recent plaque is present, the calcium and phosphate ions from the subsurface can be rapidly cleared.

SELF-EVALUATION QUESTIONS

1. Three types of physiologic stimuli that increase the flow of saliva are _mechanical_, _taste, gustatory,_ and _psychologic_. Three conditions that slow salivary flow are _H & N Rad. Therapy_, _Medicuts_, and _Tumors, Thyroid deficiency_.

2. As flow rate increases, calcium (increases) (decreases), whereas phosphate (increases) (decreases). The main buffer in the saliva and plaque is _Sodium Bicarbonate_; two lesser effective buffers are _Phosphate PO_ and _Proteins & Urea_.

3. The name of the protein that is also known as the pH rise factor is _Sialin_, whereas the protein that stabilizes the saliva to prevent precipitation is known as _statherin_. In remineralizing solutions, the element _Sodium Chloride_ is often added to the phosphorous and calcium to prevent in vitro precipitation. It requires (more) (less) ions to maintain a supersaturation of saliva at a high pH, compared with a low pH.

4. The (bacteriocidal) (agglutinating) properties of saliva account for the continual major loss of oral bacteria.

5. Tooth enamel begins to demineralize between pH _5.5_ and _5.0_. The element _Sodium Fluoride_ (name) depresses the pH at which dissolution of enamel begins; also, the presence of an increased number of _Ca & PO4_ in the area results in a supersaturation in relation to the apatite crystal.

6. One element that is critical to both bacterial energy metabolism and remineralization of apatite is _Ca or Fluoride_.

7. An enamel crystal may be portrayed as a _Carp. Hexag. pencil_ (common object) with two flattened sides. The c-axis of this crystal is comparable to the _lead_ of the previous common object.

8. The building blocks for the hydroxyapatite crystal are called _unit cells_. Around the central hydroxyl grouping is a triangular configuration of _Calcium_ (element) atoms, and peripheral to these are _phosphate_ groupings. During the formation of the crystal, if fluoride is available, it is deposited (central) (peripheral) to the calcium atoms. The long axis of the hydroxyapatite crystal is known as the _C_ axis. The longest axis of the basal face of the hydroxyapatite crystal is the _ab_ axis, and the shortest axis is the _a_ axis. The more mature surface layer of teeth is probably due to (accumulation of fluoride) (limited remineralization) (both). Dissolution of the apatite crystal begins in the (core) (periphery). On the other hand, the rod may be initially attacked at the _core_ (site), the _shell_ (site), or combinations of the two, thus providing the basis for type _____, _____, and _____ etchings, respectively. The carbonate that is initially dissolved serves to protect the tooth by its limited ability to _buffer_.

(action) the acid. The ___Surface___ and
___Dark___ zones of the classic white
spot lesion described by Silverstone are
due to remineralization. Four attributes
(of a possible six) of a good remineralizing solution are: ___hydrophilic___,
___low viscosity___, ___antibacterial___, and
___rapid acting___.

9. Three elements usually in remineralizing solutions to aid in reconstruction of
the crystal are ___Calcium___, ___phosphates___
and ___Flouride___. The compound,
___Sodium Chloride___ is often added to prevent
precipitation of the three previous reactants. A (high) (low) concentration of
reactants in a remineralizing solution is
indicated for a surface repair only,
whereas a (high) (low) concentration of
reactants is indicated for subsurface
remineralization.

REFERENCES

1. Schneyer LS, Levin LK. Rate of secretion by
individual gland pairs of man under conditions of reduced exogenous stimulation. *J
Appl Phy.* 1955; 7:508–512.

2. Dawes C, Wood CM. The contribution of
oral minor mucous glands secretion to the
volume of whole saliva in humans. *Arch
Oral Biol.* 1973; 18:337–342.

3. Ferguson DB, Fort A. Circadian variations
in calcium and phosphate secretion from
human parotid and submandibular glands.
Caries Res. 1973; 7:19–29.

4. Ferguson DB, Botchway CA. Circadian variations in flow rate and composition of
human stimulated submandibular saliva.
Arch Oral Biol. 1979 24:433–437.

5. Osterberg T, Landahl S, Hedegard B. Salivary flow, saliva, pH and buffering capacity
in 70-year old men and women. *J Oral Reha-
bil.* 1984; 11:157–170.

6. Becks H, Wainwright WW III. Rate of flow
of resting saliva of healthy individuals. *J
Dent Res.* 1943; 22:391–396.

7. Ben-Aryeh H, Miron D, Szargel R, et al.
Whole-saliva secretion rates in old and
young health subjects. *J Dent Res.* 1984;
63:1147–1148.

8. Council on Dental Therapeutics. Consensus: Oral health effects of products that increase salivary flow rate. *J Am Dent Assoc.*
1988; 116:757–759.

9. Parvinen T, Parvinen I, Larmas M. Stimulated salivary flow rate, pH and lacto-bacillus
and yeast concentrations in medicated
persons. *Scan J Dent Res.* 1984; 92:524–
532.

10. Sreebny LM, Schwartz SS. A reference
guide to drugs and dry mouth. *Gerontology.*
1986; 5:75–99.

11. Dawes C. The effects of flow rate and duration of stimulation on the concentrations of
protein and the main electrolytes in human
submandibular saliva. *Arch Oral Biol.* 1974;
19:887–895.

12. Levin MJ, Reddy MS, Tabak LA, et al.
Structural aspects of salivary glycoproteins.
J Dent Res. 1987; 66:436–441.

13. Chauncey HH, Levine DM, Kass G, et al.
Parotid gland secretory rate and electrolyte
concentration in children with cystic fibrosis. *Arch Oral Biol.* 1962; 7:707–713.

14. Boackle RJ, Suddick RP. Salivary proteins
and oral health. In: L Menaker, ed. *The Biologic Basis of Dental Caries,* Hagerstown,
Md. Harper and Row; 1980: 113–131.

15. Suddick RP, Hyde RJ, Reller RP. Salivary
water and electrolytes and oral health. In: L
Menaker, ed. *The Biologic Basis of Dental
Caries.* Hagerstown, Md. Harper and Row;
1980: 132–143.

16. Kreusser W, Heidland A, Hanneman H, et
al. Mono- and divalent electrolyte patterns,
PCO_2 and pH in relation to flow rate in normal parotid saliva. *Europ J Clin Invest.* 1972;
2:398–406.

17. Biswas SD, Kleinberg I. Effect of urea concentration on its utilization on the pH and
the formation of ammonia and carbon dioxide in a human salivary sediment system.
Arch Oral Biol. 1971; 16:759–780.

18. Renson CE, Mercer CE. Dental caries
prevalence in hemodialysis and renal trans-

plant patients. *J Dent Res.* 1975; 54(special issue A):L85. Abstract L339.

19. Kleinberg I, Craw D, Komiyama K. Effect of salivary supernatant on the glycolytic activity of the bacteria in salivary sediment. *Arch Oral Biol.* 1973; 18:787–798.

20. Gron P. Saturation of human saliva with calcium phosphates. *Arch Oral Biol.* 1973; 18:1385–1392.

21. Schlesinger DH, Hay DI. Complete covalent structure of statherin, a tyrosine-rich acidic peptide which inhibits calcium phosphate precipitation from human parotid saliva. *J Biol Chem.* 1977; 252:1689–1695.

22. Hay DI, Moreno ED. Monomolecular inhibitors of calcium phosphate precipitation in human saliva. Their roles in providing a protective environment for the teeth. In: Kleinberg I, Ellison SA, Mandel ID, eds. *Proceedings of Saliva and Dental Caries.* Special Supp *Microbiology Abstracts.* 1979; 45–58.

23. Gron P, Hay DI. Inhibition of calcium phosphate precipitation by human salivary secretions. *Arch Oral Biol.* 1976; 21:201–205.

24. Fox PC, Wolff A, Yeh CK, et al. Saliva inhibits HIV-1 infectivity. *J Am Dent Assoc.* 1988; 116:635–637.

25. O'Brien T. Rationale for continued investigations on a vaccine as an approach to dental caries prevention. Immunologic aspects of dental caries (Special Suppl to *Immunology Abstract*). In: Bowen WH, Genco RJ, O'Brien TC, eds. *Proceedings of workshop on selection of immunogens for a caries vaccine and cross reactivity of antisera to oral microorganisms with mammalian tissues.* Washington. National Institutes of Health, Information Retrieval Inc., January 1976:3–10.

26. Slowey RR, Eidelman S, Klebanoff SJ. Antibacterial activity of the purified peroxidase from human saliva. *J Bacteriol.* 1968; 97:575–579.

27. Pruitt KM, Mansson-Rahemtulla B, Tenovuo J. Detection of hypothiocyanite (OSCN⁻) ion in the human parotid saliva and the effect of pH on OSCN⁻ generation in the salivary peroxidase antimicrobial system. *Arch Oral Biol.* 1983; 28:517–525.

28. Pruitt KM, Adamson M. Enzyme activity of salivary lactoperoxidase adsorbed to human enamel. *Infect Immun.* 1977; 17:112–116.

29. Crawford JM, Taubman MA, Smith DJ. Minor salivary glands as a major source of secretory IgA in the human oral cavity. *Science.* 1975; 190:1206–1208.

30. Sharry JJ, Krasse B. Observations of the origin of salivary leucocytes. *Acta Odont Scand.* 1960; 18:347–348.

31. Schiött CR, Löe H. The origin and variation in number of leukocytes in the human saliva. *J Periodont Res.* 1970; 5:36–41.

32. Taichman NS, Tasai C, Baehni PC, et al. Interaction of inflammatory cells and oral microorganisms. *Infect Immun.* 1977; 16:1013–1028.

33. Wright DE, Jenkins GN. Leukocytes in the saliva of caries-free and caries-active subjects. *J Dent Res.* 1953; 32:511–523.

34. Cole MF, Arnold RR, Rhodes MJ, et al. Immune dysfunction and dental caries: A preliminary report. *J Dent Res.* 1977; 56:198–204.

35. Lehner T, Challacombe SJ, Caldwall J. Immunologic basis for vaccination against dental caries in rhesus monkeys. *J Dent Res.* 1976; 55:C166–80.

36. Arnold RR, Pruitt KM, Cole MF, et al. In: Kleinberg I, Ellison SA, Mandel ID, eds. *Proceedings on Saliva and Dental Caries* (Special Suppl *Microbiology Abstracts*), 1979; 449–462.

37. Lie T. Scanning and transmission electron microscope study of pellicle morphogenesis. *Scan J Dent Res.* 1977; 217–231.

38. Bennick A, Chau G, Goodlin R, et al. The role of human salivary acidic proline-rich proteins in the formation of acquired dental pellicle in vivo and their fate after adsorption to the human enamel surface. *Arch Oral Biol.* 1988; 28:19–27.

39. Nieuw Amerongen AV, Oderkerk CH, Driessen AA. Role of mucins from human whole saliva in the protection of tooth enamel against demineralization in vitro. *Caries Res.* 1987; 21:297–309.

40. Eggen KH, Rölla G. Further studies on the composition of the acquired pellicle. *Scan J Dent Res.* 1983; 91:439–446.

41. Tabak LA, Levine MJ, Mandel ID, et al. Role of salivary mucins in the protection of the oral cavity. *J Oral Pathol.* 1982; 11:1–17.

42. Gibbons RJ. Bacterial adhesion to oral tissues: A model for infectious disease. *J Dent Res.* 1989; 68:750–760.

43. Shields WF, Mühlemann HR. Simultaneous pH and fluoride telemetry from the oral cavity. *Helv Odont Acta.* 1975; 19:18–26.

44. Edgar WM. The role of saliva in the control of pH changes in human dental plaque. *Caries Res.* 1976; 10:241–254.

45. Ashley FP. Calcium and phosphorous concentrations of dental plaque related to dental caries in 10–14 year old male subjects. *Caries Res.* 1975; 9:351–362.

46. Ashley FP. Calcium and phosphorous levels in human dental plaque—variations according to site of collection. *Arch Oral Biol.* 1975; 20:167–170.

47. Kaufman HW, Leinberg I. X-ray diffraction examination of calcium phosphate in dental plaque. *Calcif Tissue Res.* 1973; 11:97–104.

48. Hellström I. Fluoride uptake in intact enamel, calculus deposits and silicate fillings. *Caries Res.* 1970; 4:168–178.

49. Dawes C, Jenkins GN, Hardwick JL, et al. The relation between the fluoride concentrations in the dental plaque and in drinking water. *Br Dent J.* 1965; 119:164–167.

50. Luoma H. The appearance of the ^{32}P of tooth origin among phosphorus taken up by caries-inducing streptococci in rats. *Arch Oral Biol.* 1970; 15:509–522.

51. Mortimer KV. The relationship of deciduous enamel structure to dental disease. *Caries Res.* 1970; 4:206–223.

52. Losee FL, Cutress TW, Brown R. Natural elements of the periodic table in human dental enamel. *Caries Res.* 1974; 8:123–134.

53. McLean FC. Bone. *Sci Am.* 1955; 192:84.

54. Weatherell JA, Deutsch D, Robinson C, et al. Assimilation of fluoride by enamel throughout the life of the tooth. *Caries Res.* 1977; 11(Suppl 1):85–115.

55. Scott DB, Nygaard V. Mineralization of dental enamel. In: Rowe MH, ed. *Symposium on Chemistry and Physiology of Enamel.* Ann Arbor. University of Michigan. September 1976: 6–24.

56. Sognnaes RF, Shaw JH, Bogorach R. Radiotracer studies on bone, cementum, dentin and enamel of rhesus monkeys. *Am J Physiol.* 1955; 180:408–420.

57. Going RE, Massler M, Dute HL. Marginal penetration of dental restorations by different radioactive isotopes. *J Dent Res.* 1960; 39:273–284.

58. LeGeros RZ, Bonel G, LeGros R. Types of H_2O in human enamel and in precipitated apatites. *Calcif Tissue Res.* 1978; 26:111–118.

59. Backer-Dirks O. Posteruptive changes in dental enamel. *J Dent Res.* 1966; 45 (Suppl):503–511.

60. Beltran ED, Burt BA. The pre- and posteruptive effects of fluoride in the caries decline. *J Publ Health Dent.* 1988; 48:233–240.

61. Silverstone LM, Saxton CA, Dogon IL, et al. Variation in the pattern of acid etching of human dental enamel examined by scanning electron microscopy. *Caries Res.* 1975; 9: 373–387.

62. Holmen L, Thylstrup A, Ögaard B, et al. A scanning electron microscopic study of progressive stages of enamel caries in vivo. *Caries Res.* 1985; 19:355–367.

63. Arends J, Jongebblood WL, Ögaard B, et al. SEM and microradiographic investigation of initial enamel caries. *Scand J Dent Res.* 1987; 95:193–201.

64. Hamilton WJ Jr, Judd G, Ansell GS. Mechanisms of acid attack in human enamel as determined by electron optical instrumentation analysis. *J Dent Res.* 1972; 51:1407–1420.

65. Arends J, Jongebblood WL. Mechanism of enamel dissolution and its prevention. *J Biol Buccale.* 1977; 5:219–237.

66. Jongebblood WL, Vandenberg PJ, Arends J. The dissolution of single crystals of hydroxyapatite in citric and lactic acids. *Calcif Tissue Res.* 1974; 15:1–9.

67. Pincus P. Caries: Attack on enamel protein in an alkaline medium. *Br Dent J.* 1937; 63: 511–514.

68. Silverstone LM. The surface zone in caries and in caries-like lesions produced in vitro. *Br Dent J.* 1968; 125:145–157.

69. Driessens FC, Heijligers HJ, Borggreven JM, et al. Posteruptive maturation of tooth enamel studied with the electron microprobe. *Caries Res.* 1985; 19:390–395.

70. Weatherell JA, Robinson C, Strong MMRC. Future possibilities for increased tooth resistance to dental caries. *J Can Dent Assoc.* 1984; 50:149–156.

71. Moreno EC, Zahradnik RT. Demineralization and remineralization of dental enamel. *J Dent Res.* 1979; 58(special issue B):896–902.

72. Zahradnik RT. Modification by salivary pellicles of in vitro enamel remineralization. *J Dent Res.* 1979; 58:2066–2073.

73. Zahradnik RT, Propoas D, Moreno EC. Effect of salivary pellicle formation time on in vitro attachment and demineralization by *Streptococcus mutans. J Dent Res.* 1985; 19: 507–511.

74. Moreno EC, Kresak M. Effect of salivary pellicles on diffusion through hydroxy- and fluorhydroxyapatite discs. *J Dent Res.* 1978; 57(special issue A):284. Abstract 838.

75. Mandel ID. The functions of saliva. *J Dent Res.* 1987; 66(special issue):623–627.

76. Arends J, Gelhard T. In vivo remineralization of human enamel. In: Leach SA, Edgar WM, eds. *Demineralization and Remineralization of the Teeth.* Oxford: IRL Press LTD; 1983:1–16.

77. Head JA. A study of saliva and its action on tooth enamel in reference to its hardening and softening. *J Am Med Assoc.* 1912; 59: 2118–2122.

78. Boedecker CF. Dental erosion, its possible cause and treatment. *Dent Cosmos.* 1933; 75:1056–1062.

79. Muhler JC. A practical method of reducing dental caries in children not receiving the established benefits of communal fluoridation. *J Dent Child.* 1961; 28:5–12.

80. von der Fehr FR, Löe H, Theilade F. Experimental caries in man. *Caries Res.* 1970; 4:131–148.

81. Albert M, Grenoble DE. An in vivo study of enamel remineralization after acid etching. *J S Calif Dent Assoc.* 1971; 39:747–751.

82. Silverstone LM. The significance of remineralization in caries prevention. *J Can Dent Assoc.* 1984; 50:157–167.

83. Council on Dental Therapeutics. American Dental Association. Eff-remin dentifrice—Not acceptable for ADR. *J Am Dent Assoc.* 1939; 26:1887–1889.

84. Reports of Councils and Committees. The status of dentifrices. *J Am Dent Assoc.* 1945; 32:750.

85. Council on Dental Materials, Instruments and Equipment. List of certified dental materials, instruments, and equipment. *J Am Dent Assoc.* 1983; 107:880.

86. Shannon IL, Trodahl JN, Starcke EN. Remineralization of enamel by a saliva substitute designed for use by irradiated patients. *Cancer.* 1978; 41:1746–1750.

87. Johansson B. Remineralization of slightly etched enamel. *J Dent Res.* 1985; 44:64–70.

88. Featherstone JDB, Cutress TW, Rodgers BE, et al. Remineralization of artificial caries-like lesion in vitro by a self-administered mouth rinse or paste. *Caries Res.* 1982; 16:235–242.

89. Koulourides T, Feagin F, Pigman W. Effect of pH, ionic strength and cupric ions on the rehardening rate of buffer-softened human enamel. *Arch Oral Biol.* 1968; 13:335–341.

90. Briner WW, Gray JA, Francis MD. Significance of enamel remineralization. *J Dent Res.* 1974; 53:239–243.

91. Silverstone LM, Wefel JS. The effect of remineralization on artificial caries-like lesions and their crystal content. *J Crystal Growth.* 1981; 53:148–159.

92. Mainly RS, Harrington DP. Solution rate of tooth enamel in an acetate buffer. *J Dent Res.* 1959; 38:910–919.

93. Feagin F, Patel PR, Koulourides T, et al. Study of the effect of calcium, phosphate, fluoride and hydrogen ion concentrations on the remineralization of partially demineralized human and bovine enamel surfaces. *Arch Oral Biol.* 1971; 16:535–548.

94. Wefel JS. Effects of fluoride on caries development and progression using intraoral models. *J Dent Res.* 1990; 69(special issue): 626–633.

95. Clarkson BII, Wefel JS, Feagin FF. Fluoride distribution in enamel after in vitro caries-like lesion formation. *J Dent Res.* 1986; 65:963–966.

96. Mirth DB, Adderly DD, Monell-Torrens E, et al. Comparison of the cariostatic effect of topically and systemically administered controlled-release fluoride in the rat. *Caries Res.* 1985; 19:466–477.

97. Mirth DB, Shern RJ, Emilson CG, et al. Clinical evaluation of an intraoral device for the controlled release of fluoride. *J Am Dent Assoc.* 1982; 105:791–797.

98. Kula K, Kula T, Davidson W, et al. Pharmacological evaluation of an intraoral fluoride-releasing device in adolescents. *J Dent Res.* 1987; 66:1538–1542.

Chapter 12

Caries Activity Testing

Kichuel K. Park
David W. Banting

Objectives

At the end of this chapter, it will be possible to

1. State the purpose of caries activity tests and indicate their limitations and advantages.
2. Cite two essential specifications for an accurate caries activity test.
3. Delineate between risk factor, risk indicator, risk marker, and risk assessment.
4. Differentiate between prevalence and incidence.
5. Differentiate between sensitivity and specificity.
6. Identify the two bacteria most often measured in caries activity tests to determine the magnitude of the bacterial challenge to the teeth.
7. Name two high-tech diagnostic units that better identify incipient lesions of smooth surfaces and of pits and fissures.

Introduction

The term *dental caries* has been applied to a heterogeneous collection of conditions including active caries, arrested caries, treated caries either in the form of restora-tions or missing teeth, caries on the crowns of teeth, caries on the roots of teeth, and preclinical conditions such as white spot lesions. Several investigators have advocated the subdivision of active dental caries in adults into incipient and cavitated categories, which serves to distinguish between early and advanced lesion development.[1–4] This delineation can be useful when estimating treatment needs or recommending specific therapies. It also acknowledges that there is a natural progression of dental caries that can be categorized into increasing levels of severity of the disease. In children, researchers are now recording non-cavitated colored, and noncavitated white spot lesions on enamel and including these in the definition of active dental caries.[5] The introduction of more sophisticated diagnostic technology may allow for the detection of even earlier lesion formation.

During the past decade some interesting and important contrasts have emerged concerning the nature and distribution of dental caries in adults, particularly older adults, as compared with children. For instance, adults continue to experience *primary caries*, but they also experience a significant amount of *secondary caries* around existing restorations.[6] Children today have comparatively few, if any, restorations and experience mostly primary caries of the noncavitated type.[5] Between 40% and 76% of dental caries lesions in adults are arrested,[3,7] a condition uncommonly observed in children. Furthermore, loss of epithelial attachment, which is rarely found before age 30, predisposes the roots of adult teeth to dental caries. It is estimated that 21% of employed U.S. adults, and 63% of U.S. adults over age 65 have experienced root caries.[8]

The caries process begins with the loss of ions from the apatite crystal and ends with cavitation of the tooth surface. Between these two events, many dynamic reactions take place as part of a fluctuating process of demineralization and remineralization of teeth.[9,10] If the demineralization is matched in extent by the ensuing remineralization, no carious lesions occur. Whenever demineralization outstrips remineralization, however, caries eventually occur.

In diagramming the course of the caries process (Fig 12–1), two landmarks are of great clinical significance. These two events are (1) the initiation of the incipient lesion and (2) overt cavitation when the caries process ceases to be reversible. It is between these two landmarks that primary preventive practices should be vigorously and continuously applied to arrest and reverse the progress of caries.

In the initial stages of caries, each day, many microscopic loci of demineralization exist.[11] In these cases a physiologic remineralization can occur within a few hours. If the loss of tooth mineral continues, micropores eventually develop in the surface enamel, to be followed by subsurface involvement. This is the beginning of the incipient carious lesion that appears as a *white spot*. At

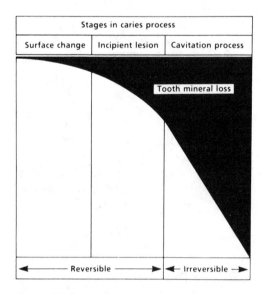

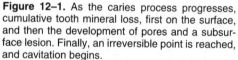

Figure 12–1. As the caries process progresses, cumulative tooth mineral loss, first on the surface, and then the development of pores and a subsurface lesion. Finally, an irreversible point is reached, and cavitation begins.

2nd *caries* 1/2

this stage, the progress of the caries process still can be reversed.[12] If appropriate steps are not taken, an increasing number of bacteria, mainly lactobacilli and *mutans streptococci*[a] begin to mobilize at the site of the future lesions.[13] Eventually, the subsurface lesion becomes irreversible. The irreversible stage may be due to such events as (1) destruction of the enamel matrix, (2) changes in the acid diffusion patterns in the subsurface lesion, resulting in longer and lower pH changes, or possibly, (3) bacterial invasion of the subsurface lesion.

Dental caries is a multifactorial disease, and its many contributing factors can be grouped into three categories: (1) those microorganisms that constitute a *challenge* to the integrity of the tooth, (2) tooth and host *resistance,* and (3) *remineralization* capacity (biologic repair). The objective of caries activity testing is to identify some parameter(s) of the triad of challenge, defense, and repair that indicate impending or existent caries formation. Such information can be used to help estimate the probability of caries development, but more importantly, to formulate strategies for the prevention of disease.[9,14,15]

Diagnosis of dental caries has become more difficult as our knowledge of the disease has changed.[1] So far, most research effort on caries activity tests has focused on primary caries. The issue of secondary caries, which accounts *for as much as one*

half of all caries-related treatments, is only beginning to be examined.[16]

CLINICAL DIAGNOSIS

Clinical diagnosis is the process of recognizing diseases by their characteristic signs and symptoms. It is an imperfect process because considerable subjective variation occurs both in the signs and symptoms of disease in individual subjects and in the subjective interpretation of those signs and symptoms by different clinicians. Nevertheless, clinical observations are powerful determinants of diagnosis.

For instance, if all the teeth are noncarious, an individual is considered to be caries-resistant. The probability for future caries activity is further decreased if the teeth are well aligned. The presence of deep fissures and other retentive sites can predispose to caries. The presence of plaque over a long period is usually a reliable prognostic sign of a higher caries risk. A high and frequent intake of refined carbohydrates also increases the risk of caries. Or, if a tooth on one side of the mouth has a lesion, the probability that the contralateral tooth will also develop a similar lesion increases. *Probably the most predictive visible sign of impending caries is the incipient lesion in the form of a white spot.*[1] Because the subsurface lesion (ie, the white spot) represents the last stage of the carious process preliminary to cavitation, it has a high probability of becoming an irreversible lesion, unless decisive professional intervention takes place.

All of these clinical observations are subjective and are based on professional experience. As Newbrun noted, consideration of various factors in a patient's history, as well as clinical and laboratory examinations,

---

[a] The term *mutans steptococci* includes several species of streptococci, which historically were often collectively referred to as *Streptococci mutans.* Based on generic, serologic, and biochemical studies, the species include *S mutans, S sobrinus, S cricetus, S. rattis, S ferus,* and *S macacae.* These can be differentiated in the laboratory. Factors such as ecology, acid formation, and cariogenicity under experimental conditions are so similar, however, that it is appropriate to have the common designation, "mutans streptococci" (MS).

assist the dental clinician in making difficult diagnostic decisions.[17]

Given a general lack of uniformity regarding the clinical description of dental caries, it is natural to question the accuracy of clinical diagnoses. *Accuracy* reflects the closeness of a clinical observation to the true condition. It is measured against a standard which, in the case of coronal caries, is usually a radiograph, an explorer survey, or a histologic assessment. Unfortunately, there is *no* similar standard against which to measure the accuracy of clinical *root caries* diagnoses.

Clinical disagreement in dental caries diagnosis can be attributed to several factors. Variation in an examiner's visual acuity (eg, presbyopia, color blindness) can affect the interpretation of the presence or absence of cavitation or color change. Disagreement between examiners concerning the relative softness or hardness of the area examined due to differences in tactile sensitivity can also have a profound effect, especially if this sign is considered to be confirmatory of the presence of dental caries.

Direct and indirect lighting, the use of magnifying eyewear, patient position, the use of compressed air to dry the teeth, the sharpness of the explorer used, the position of the recorder, the quietness of the examination area and malfunction of equipment can all contribute to examiner disagreement. Unfortunately, the collective effect of these conditions on disagreement is not readily measurable.

Recognizing that at least these potential sources of examiner disagreement exist, strategies can be implemented to enhance *reliability* and *accuracy* of dental caries diagnosis, including (1) provision of a suitable diagnostic environment, (2) establishment of a standard classification scheme that uses objective criteria based on clinical signs, (3) intensive instruction and calibration of den-

tal examiners, and (4) a standardized reporting method.[18]

Despite these clinical limitations, reliability measures for the diagnosis of dental caries by experienced investigators have been quite good.[19–24] The recent trend of diminishing prevalence of caries in the Western world, however, increases the problem of false-positive diagnoses. This situation may be corrected by developing more objective diagnostic methods having lower false-positive rates.[25]

CARIES DIAGNOSTIC TESTS

Development

To improve the *validity*[b] of caries diagnostic tests (CDT), new and better, noninvasive, and more accurate devices need to be continually developed to measure caries. Parallel to this is the need to develop and improve on *diagnostic and predictor tests* that permit early identification of *impending* cariogenicity.

The main reason for employing new and better diagnostic technology and predictor tests is to improve patient care. Can a diagnosis be made early enough to permit sealant placement and remineralization strategies in lieu of treatment? Is the need for a particular treatment more clearly defined? Does it lead to a better clinical outcome for the patient? Are there cost savings? Unless these kinds of questions can be answered affirmatively, diagnostic tests are only marginally useful. Most often, clinical data and professional judgment are still far more powerful than laboratory tests or sophisticated technology and are usually quite sufficient to establish a definitive diagnosis.[26]

---

[b] Valid = Sufficiently supported by actual fact, sound, good, or effective.

At present, the dental office-based CDT for dental caries activity are generally limited to determining the presence or absence of specific microorganisms in saliva and plaque, salivary secretion rate, salivary components, salivary buffer effect, and oral sugar clearance time. Researchers and clinicians look for new diagnostic tests in the hope that they will perform better, that is, be more reliable and therefore be used to evaluate disease status more *accurately*.

Three concerns surround the development and evaluation of new diagnostic technology in general, and caries activity tests in particular: the technical considerations of *validity* and *reproducibility*[c] and the clinical decision of whether the test can replace the present method of *diagnosis*[d] or *prediction*.[e]

As an example let us apply these concerns to the development of a new diagnostic *device*. At present it is difficult for a dentist to use an explorer to determine *accurately* if a "sticky" occlusal fissure is carious. This has resulted in many sound teeth being unnecessarily restored, and other carious lesions have gone without care. With this *actual* problem in mind, imagine that a hypothetical dental supply manufacturer places a new high-tech electronic device on the market, which it claims is much more accurate than the explorer in delineating between sound and carious occlusal surfaces.

The validity of the new test instrument is established by studying its performance to determine if it can differentiate between sound and carious teeth. Reproducibility is assessed by making a series of replicate measurements of the the same carious and noncarious teeth to determine if the results are consistent.[29]

Once theses critical basic requirements are satisfied, the results attained with this new instrument are compared with those of a parallel *explorer examination*, which is the *standard* used by the profession to detect caries. The paradox of this comparison is that the performance report of the new instrument depends on the accuracy of a clinical diagnosis made with the explorer. If the data attained with the new device is compared with the standard (ie, the explorer) the test results may appear worse, *even when they are actually better*. For instance, if the new device is *truly* more accurate than the explorer, the additional lesions identified will incorrectly be classified as being *falsely positive*.[f] Similarly, if the new diagnostic test is more often truly correct in identifying the *absence* of disease (than with the explorer), more apparently *false-negative* findings will occur. Therefore, if an inaccurate clinical standard (in this case the explorer) is used, *any new diagnostic test will appear inferior, even when it actually approaches the truth more closely*.[28]

Evolution of a Caries Diagnostic Test

The development of a CDT for the dental office occurs in two phases. The first centers on the *research and development* needed to validate and establish standardized procedures for the test; the second is the *application* of the final, validated technology to

---

[c] Reproducibility, also referred to as reliability = The ability to replicate chemical or microbiologic test results when run under standardized conditions. Lack of reliability may arise because of divergence between observers, or instruments of measurement, or instability or the variable being measured.

[d] Diagnosis = A clinical decision about the presence or absence of disease(s), based on available information and professional experience.

[e] Prediction = A clinical decision about the outcome of a disease process, based on available information and professional experience.

---

[f] False positive = A sound tooth that is diagnosed as carious.

False negative = A carious tooth that is diagnosed as sound.

the day-to-day practice of preventive dentistry. Much of the validation occurs in dental school research programs. Most of the technology transfer to the profession can be credited to the dental industry in its development of convenient test kits and instruments.

The best way to introduce the subject of CDTs is to introduce several terminologies applying to test development. One variable of every caries diagnostic test involves either a *risk factor* or a *risk indicator*. A risk factor is a physiologic compound (in saliva) or an oral microorganism that is known or believed to *cause* caries (ie, etiologic agents). On the other hand, the risk indicator (sometimes referred to as a *risk marker*) is a variable *associated* with caries, but over which preventive or treatment control is not possible. These variables include factors, such as age and economic or social status, each of which can greatly influence caries status.

In planning a CDT a risk factor or a risk indicator is always one of the variables, and the other is always caries incidence. It is assumed that subjects possessing the selected risk factor should have a significantly different caries *incidence*[g] or prevalence contrasted with those not possessing it. On the other hand, if the factor contributes to the resistance or to the biologic repair of the tooth (such as fluoride, calcium, and phosphorus), fewer carious lesions should occur in its greater presence. A high *positive* correlation should occur between the number of challenge organisms and the number of carious lesions developing over the time of the study (incidence), and a strong *negative*

---

[g] Caries incidence = The number of carious lesions that occur over a given period divided by the number of subjects in the study. Two different examinations are required to determine incidence: one before and one at the end of the selected period.

correlation should arise in the case of defense and repair factors.

The research protocol used in the continual search for new risk factors is relatively uncomplicated. The first level of sophistication is usually in the form of a pilot study. The selected risk factor might be a newly discovered compound in the saliva. To assess its potential value, a caries examination is performed on a limited number of individuals prior to collecting a sample of saliva from each. After the chemical tests have been completed, classic statistical analysis can be employed to determine whether a significant relationship (ie, a correlation) exists between the potential new risk factor and caries *prevalence*. If the *risk factor–prevalence* study proves fruitful, a more time-consuming (year or longer) and expensive *risk factor–incidence* study may be indicated.

Note that an incidence study results in a much more valid outcome than a prevalence study. Prevalence does *not* indicate the present state of caries activity. Instead, it represents the cumulative caries activity that occurred in the past. It is not known if all the decayed surfaces seen as part of the decayed, missing, or filled surfaces (DMFS) *prevalence* score have developed over the past year or represent an accumulation over several years. Similarly, a question always arises about whether all the restorations were placed following a single episode of high caries activity, or whether they were placed over a period of years, or even whether they were placed in an occlusal pit as a result of false-positive diagnosis. Despite its limitations, however, prevalence methods provide a "quick-and-dirty" means to explore hypotheses that possibly would not otherwise be addressed.

The second level of sophistication is much the same as the pilot study except that the number of subjects is sufficient to meet the requirements for a meaningful statistical analysis. Also, based on the experience gained in the pilot study, the expectation for success should be much greater. Again, an initial DMFS examination is completed to identify the caries status of each tooth, and the total number of carious lesions in the mouth. The other variable, say the number of mutans streptococci (MS), is similarly quantitated and recorded for each individual. At the end of the study, following a second DMFS examination, the caries *incidence* for each of the subjects is arrayed with the original totals of MS. Classic statistics are then applied to determine if a significant correlation might exist between the two variables.

This approach has been very successful in establishing that MS and lactobacilli are directly related to cariogenesis. A modification of the same protocol can be made by dividing the initial group of subjects into two, with the second group, for instance, using a chlorhexidine antiplaque mouth rinse daily. In this way, it is possible to determine the potential for chlorhexidine to suppress MS and possibly reduce the caries incidence. This protocol requires a second DMFS dental examination as well as a second quantitation of MS to compare with the initial data.

Advantages of Caries Activity Tests

The successful development of a valid CDT that could signal the early stages of the caries process, especially at a time *before* the incipient lesion has reached an irreversible stage, would

- Establish an initial baseline level of the cariogenic pathogens from which to follow temporal changes in caries activity status.
- Permit evaluation of patient compliance with dietary (ie, sugar) instructions—the more lactobacilli, the less compliance.
- Permit public health dental personnel to screen large segments of the population, such as school children, to determine prospective workloads; as a result, those children found to have a high probability of caries could be included in low-cost, high-volume primary preventive programs.
- Enable third-party payment groups to establish preventive dentistry policies based on the *potential* for caries activity; this permits consumers to be eligible for periodic evaluations and preventive maintenance at a lower cost than plans covering treatment only.
- Provide a patient with an objective evaluation of *risk assessment*[h] and develop a preventive program to match the severity of that assessment.
- Aid the dental researcher to better balance control and experimental groups in testing new preventive agents or techniques; this shortens testing time, reduces costs, and increases the possibility of better dental control measures.

Prediction, Risk Reduction, and Diagnostic Tests

Accomplished in much the same way as previous CDTs, the present generation of CDTs offer the possibility of successful caries *prediction—not diagnosis.* The main difference between the two is that the final handling of the statistics permits a much finer focus on the ability of the test correctly to predict sound-to-caries and sound-to-sound teeth. This ability of a CDT to iden-

---

[h] Risk assessment = A professional judgment of an individual's future risk of disease based on the best information available.

tify correctly which sound teeth *will become carious* is termed *sensitivity*. Similarly, the ability of the test to predict no change in status is termed *specificity*.

Again an example is in order. In this hypothetical study, samples of plaque were taken from 300 teeth of several institutionalized senior citizens. The objective of the study was to determine if an increasing number of MS on the root surfaces of individual teeth would enable the better prediction of site-specific root caries, as well as predicting those at minimal risk. Thus, the two variables in the study were *risk factors* and *incidence*. After 2 years, a second decayed or filled tooth surface (DFTS) examination using mouth mirror and explorer (i.e., to establish incidence) was made of the original teeth, with the results seen in Table 12–1.

Critique on Prediction

At the present stage of development of caries prediction tests, it is not possible to assign a valid predictive value for sound-to-caries and sound-to-sound sites. Instead, this general statement is in order: the higher the predictive value, the more valid the test. There are several reasons for this uncertainty. Events can occur during the study, such as major changes in diet (ie,

sugar restriction), more thorough mechanical and chemical plaque control procedures, or more intensive use of fluorides, all of which can effect the outcome. Because of such alternating or permanent changes during the study, both the incidence and the risk factors are affected.

A major problem is the fact that the most accurate test would theoretically be one that considered that all the potential sites on each tooth be sampled on a continuing basis. The sampling would also have to include every risk factor related to the development or reversal of the carious lesion. These objectives *cannot* be met; hence compromise is necessary. This compromise usually consists of the selection of one, or perhaps two variables that reflect either the challenge to or the defense of the teeth.

False-Positive and False-Negative Responses

False responses should be a minimal. Any errors in *prediction* should preferably be in the direction of being *false-positives*, because these only trigger intensified countermeasures to prevent caries. Such measures include counseling on more effective chemical and mechanical plaque control and sugar discipline at home and more frequent prophylaxes and fluoride applications at the

TABLE 12–1. THE SENSITIVITY AND SPECIFICITY OF USING MUTANS STREPTOCOCCI ON TEETH ROOTS AS A METHOD OF PREDICTING SITE-SPECIFIC ROOT CARIES.

Mutans Streptococci Test Results	Clinical Examination for Root Caries		
	Presence (Yes)	**Absence (No)**	**Total**
MS-positive	46	14	60
MS-negative	54	186	240
Total	100	200	300

*Sensitivity: 46/100 = 0.46. Specificity: 186/200 = 0.93.
Predictive: 46/60 = 0.77
False-Positive Rate = 14/60 = 0.23; False-Negative rate = 54/240

* In a second consecutive plaque sample, the sensitivity rate was 0.38 (38/100); the specificity = 0.96 (192/200), yielding a predictive value of 0.88 (38/46). The false-positive rate was 0.17 (8/46), and the false-negative rate = 0.24 (62/254).

office. None of these additional intensified measures, which should already be part of the patients day-to-day oral health care, can cause harm. On the other hand, if the same caries activity test information is to be used as part of a *diagnostic* decision, a false-positive could possibly result in an unneeded restoration. Conversely, in both predictive and diagnostic situations, a *false-negative* deprives the patient of the intensive program needed to prevent the onset of caries. We must mention that with other diseases such as cancer, either a false-positive or false-negative can have grave consequences.

Question 1. Which of the following statements, if any, are correct?

A. Secondary caries are often more prevalent in children than primary caries.

B. No new caries activity test can be better than the standard by which it is judged.

C. A caries *risk factor–incidence* test requires only *one* dental examination.

D. Caries activity tests permit an estimation of the *probability* for caries development but not an accurate prediction for cavitation.

E. For *preventive* care, a false-positive caries activity test would probably be more advantageous to the patient than a false-negative test.

ORAL MICROORGANISMS AND DENTAL CARIES

For a long time the number of lactobacilli in the saliva was used to estimate caries activity, mainly because these organisms were considered to be the major cause for dental caries. W. D. Miller, in his classic studies in 1890 leading to the chemicoparasitic theory of dental caries, demonstrated the presence of lactobacilli in the mouth and their ability to produce lactic acid. It was not until 1922, however, that Rodriguez, a dental officer in the U.S. Army, developed a reliable method of selectively culturing lactobacilli.[29,30] Up to that time every culture made from the mouth ended with an overgrowth of every type of bacteria in the saliva. After much research, Rodriguez established the relationship between the number of lactobacilli in the mouth and caries prevalence. He noted, for instance, that in the 12-to-16 age group, there appeared to be more lactobacilli and likewise more caries.[30]

Hadley and colleagues[31,32] at the University of Michigan, later developed a tomato agar that made lactobacilli counting simpler for the average small laboratory. They reported on the direct relationship of lactobacilli counts to caries scores. The examinations of 24 children, aged 9 to 16 years, revealed that the average count of lactobacilli in 14 caries-active persons was 60,000 colonies, whereas, that for the 10 caries-free children was 600. Later the development of a completely synthetic selective media for lactobacilli further simplified counting techniques.[33] In the 1960s, when the role of *S mutans* unfolded as the prime cause of caries initiation, streptococci counting replaced lactobacilli counting.[34] A critical number of streptococci probably need to be present to constitute a viable challenge.

In as much as the organisms related to caries development are acidogenic, the pH of the saliva and the plaque has been studied extensively. A significant *group* correlation exists between the numbers of any specific acidogenic bacteria and the amount of acid that appears following a sucrose or glucose rinse. If *Veillonella* or *Neisseria* or both are present in the plaque, they use the acid for their own metabolism, thus favorably modifying the pH of the bacterial ecosystem.[35] This fact illustrates another barrier to developing a completely valid caries activity test, namely, that unless the symbiotic relationships of all the plaque bacteria are considered, the extent of the cariogenic challenge can be misinterpreted. This bacterial interrelationship is further complicated by the fact that all organisms are continually competing for ecologic niches in the plaque. Organisms such as *Actinomyces viscosis/ naeslundi* are antagonistic to *S mutans*. At other times one cariogenic organism decreases as another increases. For example, following radiation therapy for head and neck cancer, the population of *S mutans* increases and then gradually decreases, being replaced by lactobacilli that have the potential of an even lower pH.[36] This shift reflects the fact that *S mutans* is related to the incipient lesion and lactobacilli more to the overt carious lesion.[37]

Once cavitation has occurred, the high lactobacilli count in the saliva is difficult to reduce unless all restorative work is completed, including dental prophylaxis, placement of pit-and-fissure sealants, or possible extraction of the carious tooth.[38] In one study the lactobacilli counts after all carious lesions were restored, dropped from levels of 74,000 colonies to below 900 colony-forming units/mL.[39]

CARIES ACTIVITY TESTS FOR THE DENTAL OFFICE

Saliva obtained from subjects with active caries usually has high numbers of lactobacilli. The saliva of caries-free subjects has either no lactobacilli or significantly fewer lactobacilli than that of a caries-prone individual.[40] When lactobacilli are detected in large numbers in caries-free individuals,

carious lesions usually develop at the site within the following year.[41] Boyar and Bowden found lactobacilli at 85% of progressing incipient lesions and no lactobacilli from nonprogressing sites.[42] A restriction of dietary carbohydrate can induce a dramatic decrease in salivary lactobacilli. In fact, the lactobacillus count is often useful in determining whether patients restrict their carbohydrate intake and if they have actively participated in preventive dentistry home care programs.[43] The salivary lactobacillus counts reflect the caries status of individuals with extremely high or extremely low caries experience.[30,31]

Lactobacilli are associated with carious lesion development of both the coronal and root surfaces of the teeth, especially recurrent caries.[44] Tests for this organism appear to be a useful tool for identifying unsuspected sources of lactobacilli, such as around restorations with poor marginal adaptation or undetected lesions. Because lactobacilli are not considered essential for the *initiation* of carious lesions,[41] they are probably inaccurate for *predicting* the onset of caries.[45] Their presence in relatively high numbers, however, should prompt an immediate preventive dentistry treatment regimen.

Lactobacilli Counts

In the 1950s, most of the caries activity tests were performed in well-equipped laboratories. The first microbiologic caries activity test that was used by practitioners was the lactobacilli count.[46] These tests were usually performed gratis by the laboratories of state health departments or academic institutions using specimens sent by mail.

The lactobacilli counts were performed by using serial dilutions of saliva that was collected by chewing a 1-g paraffin wafer or a sterilized rubber band. A 1-mL aliquot from each dilution was then placed in a series of petri dishes, to which was added approximately 10 mL (45°C) of Rogosa's lactobacilli selective medium. After incubating 4 days, the number of colonies was counted.

Counts were often scored 1 to 4, depending on whether they fell within the ranges of 0 to 1000, 1000 to 10,000, 10,000 to 100,000, or 100,000 and up. When the score increased for a group of individuals, so did the caries score increase. At times individuals had high lactobacilli scores and low DMFS. On the other hand, when a lactobacilli count was low, *the correlation between a zero count and caries resistance was usually excellent*. Few false-negatives occurred. Despite the well-established direct relationship between lactobacilli counts and DMFS scores, this method of caries activity evaluation is not widely utilized by the profession, partially because of the successive introduction of an improved series of caries activity tests that included the Alban, and dip-slide methods. Lactobacilli counts are still used in the research laboratory, however.

Alban's Test

Alban's test is an easy-to-accomplish caries activity test for routine dental office use.[47] At the time of the test, a 5-mL tube of semisolid agar[i] is removed from the refrigerator. The patient is asked to spit unstimulated saliva directly into the tube until a thin layer of saliva covers the surface of the green agar. A small funnel may be used in the specimen collection. With small children a cotton swab can be rubbed across the tooth surface and the swab inserted or stabbed just beneath the surface of the agar.[48] The tube is

then incubated for 4 days, and daily recordings are made to observe color changes produced by the acidogenic or aciduric organisms in the saliva specimen. The color changes are scored from 0 to 4, based on the amount of color change occurring from top to bottom in the tube. A zero score indicates no color change; a 1+ score is a color change to yellow in the top quarter of the tube, 2+ to the halfway mark, 3+ to the three-quarter mark, and 4+ when the entire length of the agar column has changed to yellow (Fig 12–2).

Like the lactobacilli counts, Alban's test is probably most predictive when the scores reflect either an extreme maximum or minimum challenge (ie, with scores recorded as 4+ at the end of 24 hours [very susceptible] or zero at the end of 96 hours [very resistant]). Also, like the other lactobacilli tests, the Alban test is good for indicating caries inactivity. Few false-positives occur.[30,32] In this respect, all negative lactobacilli tests can be considered highly indicative of the caries resistance of the *individual*.[49]

The Alban test is ideal for patient education. Most patients can understand the

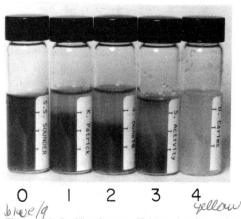

O I 2 3 4
blue/9   yellow

Figure 12–2. Alban's test. Tubes showing color change from blue-green (0) to yellow (4) with an increasing number of lactobacilli.

---

[i] BBL Microbiological Systems, Benton-Dickenson and Company, Cockeysville, MD 21030. To prepare Alban's medium, 60 g of Synder test agar mixture is used to prepare 1.0 L of the medium.The classic formula of Synder's agar per liter of purified water is pancreatic digest of casein, 13.5 g; yeast extract, 6.5 g; dextrose, 20.0 g; sodium chloride, 5.0 g; agar, 16.0 g; and, bromocresol green 0.029 g.

importance of acid in the caries process as well as the implications of the potential for acid production by bacteria taken from *their own* mouths. It is also an ideal test for following patient cooperation. Favorable changes in diet intake and plaque control procedures are reflected within a few weeks by corresponding changes in the Alban test score.[50] If a series of any of the lactobacilli test scores for the same patient are compiled over time, any change is meaningful, because it indicates a change in the patient's dietary habits.

Dip-Slide Method

The dip-slide test is more objective than Alban's test, because the latter requires a subjective evaluation of a color change that is often not clear-cut. The dip-slide test is a practical method for quantitating lactobacilli and is adaptable for day-to-day use in the dental office.[51,52] A specially designed dip-slide of plastic is coated with lactobacilli-selective (LBS) agar. Undiluted, paraffin-stimulated saliva is flowed over the agar surfaces. The amount of saliva sample on the dip-slide is relatively constant in spite of the inoculation method. The plastic slide holders are positioned vertically to ensure that both agar surfaces are totally wetted with saliva. Excessive saliva is allowed to drain onto a clean absorbent paper. The slide is then placed into a sterile tube, which is tightly closed and incubated at 37°C for 4 days. It is then removed, and the colony density is determined by comparing it with a model chart that is provided (Fig 12–3). The lactobacilli growing on the LBS agar surface form either white or transparent colonies. Readings of more than 10,000 colonies per milliliter of saliva are considered high, whereas readings of fewer than 1000 colony counts are considered low. Any results between 1000 and 10,000 are considered medium.

When the bacterial colonies are great in number, a confluent, carpetlike growth is

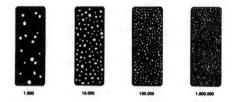

Figure 12–3. Chart used to estimate number of oral lactobacilli, using a dip-slide.

found on the agar surfaces. All agar surfaces that are negative at the time of examination should be carefully reexamined with reflected light for the appearance of colonies. Because the technique is simple, the cost reasonable, and the results easy to read, it is a practical caries activity test that can be used in a private dental office. The dip-slide method is highly correlated with conventional lactobacilli counts and with caries activity.[52,53]

Mutans Strepococci Tests

Mutans streptococci (MS) are usually associated with the initiation of caries.[54] The levels of MS in saliva and on the tooth surfaces usually reflect the number of colonized sites in the mouth.[55] Streptococci have been shown to induce transmissible caries infections in animals.[56,57] Human isolates are also highly cariogenic in animals.[58] MS have several characteristics that enhance cariogenic potential. They are acidogenic microorganisms that primarily colonize on tooth surfaces.[59] They can store *intra*cellular polysaccharides, thereby promoting chances for prolonged acid production during periods of limited carbohydrate intake by the host.

In the quantitative evaluation of the number of MS *colony-forming units* (CFUs),[j] a serial dilution is performed using

---

[j] CFU = Following incubation, each viable reproducing bacterium forms a colony that can be counted; this is the colony-forming unit (CFU).

1 mL of saliva. One-milliliter aliquots of these serial dilutions are then plated, using conventional mitis salivarius agar with the addition of sucrose and bacitracin.[59] This is followed by an incubation period of 4 days, at which time the CFUs are counted. Like the plate counts for lactobacilli, those for MS are best accomplished in the research laboratory and are not readily adaptable to the dental office.

Considerations in Evaluation. Smooth-surface and root caries rarely occur in the absence of mutans streptococci. Hence the organism appears to be essential for the initiation of this type of lesion.[60] Following stabilization of this type of plaque, if the *proportion* of MS to other plaque organisms is high or if the *total* count of MS exceeds a threshold value, the individual can be considered caries-prone. A threshold value of 2.5×10^6 CFU/mL of saliva has been suggested to select children considered to be at a high caries risk.[61] This group of high-risk patients is referred to as the "millionaires." Children who harbor MS in their dental plaque at age 2 years often become caries-active by the age of 4 years,[62] Therefore the early establishment of MS in the plaque of primary teeth is an important factor in determining later carious susceptibility.[63,64] Individuals with a superinfection of MS should be considered for special preventive attention. If the salivary levels of MS numbers are high enough, the probability exists for an intraoral spread of the infection.[61,65] A decrease in the number of tooth surfaces infected with MS or a decrease in the proportions of MS in plaque may prove to be useful indicators for determining the success of preventive therapy.

Sometimes the total number of MS can be overestimated by the presence of mutans serotypes that are benign.[66] This has been considered as only a minor problem however, and the rule still holds that low MS counts are associated with low caries probability, and high counts are associated with a high caries probability. The lesser ability to predict carious involvement on the basis of high counts may or may not be due to the presence of some of these benign MS serotypes.[67,68] The ecology of MS *and lactobacilli* appears to be similar. Both organisms preferentially colonize retentive sites on the teeth,[41,69] and their frequency of isolation is high in both carious and incipient lesions.[60,70]

Dip-Slide Method for Mutans Streptococci Count. A dip-slide test has been devised for the estimation of MS levels in saliva.[71] This method is very similar to that of the dip-slide method[k] for lactobacilli. Undiluted, paraffin-stimulated saliva is poured on a special plastic slide that is coated with mitis salivarius agar, containing 20% sucrose. The agar surface is thoroughly moistened, and the excess saliva is allowed to drain off. Two discs containing 5 μg of bacitracin are placed on the agar 20 mm apart. The slide is then tightly screwed into a cover tube and incubated at 37°C for 48 hours.

The density of MS colonies is evaluated as follows: 1 = low—colonies are discrete and can be readily counted at 15× magnification, with the total count of CFU inside the inhibition zone less than 200; 2 = medium—the colonies are discrete and the number in the zone of inhibition is more than 200 at 32×; 3 = high—the colonies are tiny and almost completely or totally cover the inhibition zone, with the number of colonies uncountable, even when using a 32× magnification.

A modification of this method proposed by Jordan and associates makes it

---

[k] Ivocar, North America, 175 Pineview Drive, Amherst, N. Y. 14228.

even easier to use. Saliva is collected in a vial containing a diluent to which bacitracin is added immediately before use. A dip-slide coated with selective growth media is dipped into this mixture. Another vial is prepared in the meantime with a CO_2 tablet, and the slide is then transferred to this second vial and incubated for 48 hours.[72] The colony density on the dip-slide is compared with a reference colony density chart, with six illustrations between the range of 10,000 to 1,000,000 counts. A significant relationship exists between dip-slide scores and conventional agar counts. The slides are commercially available, and easy to use.[73]

Question 2. Which of the following statements, if any, are correct?

A.   A valid test can be *both* accurate and reliable.

B.   Mutans streptococci are a risk marker for dental caries.

C.   A *risk assessment* requires knowledge about a *risk factor.* causes caries

D.   A better correlation usually exists between a low bacterial count and caries resistance, than between a high count and caries susceptibility.

E.   In caries, as the count for *Actinomyces viscosus/naeslundii* decreases, so does the count of MS increase.

Count MS↓   A. viscous ↑

COMMENTS ABOUT MICROBIOLOGIC CARIES ACTIVITY TESTS

Although caries prevalence has declined in some developed countries, one of the greatest needs in dental research is the development of a reliable, inexpensive, and practical method to identify individuals at high risk of dental caries before rather than after cavitation.[70] The need for such a prognostic/diagnostic caries activity test is highlighted by the fact that in a recent National Caries Study it was found that approximately 20% of the school population studied accounted for 60% of the caries problem.[74] Being able to identify this 20% at the earliest possible time would be extremely helpful. On the other hand, economic tests are available that are suitable for mass screening to identify *low*-risk populations who do not require preventive treatment.[75]

The current state of the art *does* allow placing individuals on a *statistical* susceptibility scale, a higher or lower risk for a *group* can be predicted on the basis of test results. Unfortunately the same tests cannot be used equally to predict *individual* susceptibility. The accuracy improves however, as the difference between zero counts (resistant) and high counts (susceptible) increases. Conversely, the ability to correctly predict future caries on the basis of high and low counts decreases as the difference in bacterial counts between two groups converges toward zero.[76]

It has been suggested that possibly more precision can be introduced into the area of caries activity testing by use of multiple different tests of the same sample of saliva. With the simplicity of some of the commercial dip-slide tests that are now becoming available, multiple testing has been tried as a method of refining caries activity prognosis. For instance, it is recognized that as MS increases, the number of *S sanguis* decreases for both infants and adults.[77] Being able to have the ratio as well as the total counts of the two should aid in risk assessment. Because smooth-surface caries is usually initiated by MS, only to be partially replaced by greater numbers of lactobacilli as the lesion progresses, a ratio between the two as well as absolute numbers could provide an indication of the status of the caries process.[66] One study used two dip-slide tests, one for lactobacilli and the other for yeasts. After the 3 years of the study, only 3 of 298 children who were negative for both tests had one DMF each; those who were positive for both lactobacilli and yeast had a 39-fold greater caries incidence.[78] In another study using two tests, one for MS and one for lactobacilli, it was found that when both counts were low, caries incidence was low, and when both were positive, caries development was high. Probably the greatest sensitivity and specificity could be attained by a combination of tests used in series *over time*.[79] A primary concern about caries activity tests is not whether they are reasonably predictive but whether they are even being used and if so if they are being evaluated correctly.

Plaque pH Measurements: Acid Production by Dental Plaque

Plaque and saliva pH can be directly measured intraorally using either glass or antimony electrodes.[80,81] The resting plaque pH and the plaque pH level occurring following sucrose rinses have both been found to be lower in groups of caries-active than in groups of caries-free subjects.[82] In caries-susceptible individuals, occlusal fissures have appreciably lower pH values than fissures in caries-resistant subjects.[83]

Taking a direct, in-site pH measurement to detect acidogenic changes in plaque provides a method of evaluating the environment in which caries occurs. As will be discussed in Chapter 15, the method is much more valuable in following pH changes after the intake of various foods than it is in predicting caries. The use of pH

measurements to detect the magnitude and duration of pH changes in the mouth has been facilitated by the development of indwelling electrodes[l] and telemetry system that permit the transmission of pH data to an extraoral data acquisition system.[80,83] Simultaneous transmission of data relating to both plaque and saliva pH can be recorded. With this method, continuous pH changes can be monitored as they occur while the experimental subject is eating. Special foods or confections can be introduced into the mouth to determine the extent of plaque pH drop, and the clearance time for carbohydrate substrates can be quantitated.[82–85]

DEFENSE FACTORS

Evaluating Saliva Defense

Saliva flow rate, viscosity, and buffering capacity of saliva, as well as saliva constituents, have been studied along with other systemic and oral parameters that might be related to caries. Much interest is due to the fact that saliva is responsible for diluting, neutralizing, and buffering acids, and for helping to clear bacterial substrates from the mouth.

Four theoretical mechanisms by which saliva can affect dental caries are (1) the mechanical cleansing of debris and plaque bacteria, (2) the enhancement of remineralization and inhibition of demineralization, (3) the buffering and neutralization of plaque acids, and (4) the antibacterial activity against oral microflora.[84–89]

Saliva Flow Rate. Flow rate is determined by collecting paraffin-stimulated saliva in a calibrated cylinder or test tube over a 5-minute period. Approximately 13 mL can be collected from an adult during this period. Although no defined boundary exists between normal and abnormal flow rates, values of 0.05 mL unstimulated and

---

[l] In-dwelling electrodes = These are miniature electrodes implanted at the contact point of a hollow-crown (pontic) in a removable partial denture appliance.

0.5 mL/min stimulated saliva are considered extremely low.[90,91] Normally, these low values are considered highly indicative of impaired glands. However, both a low and a high output can often be traced to medications being taken, especially among senior citizens.[92,93]

An inverse *group* relationship exists between flow rate and the number of carious lesions on a stepwise basis between 0 and 10 (ie, as the flow rate increases, the number of carious lesions decreases). Above 10 lesions no further stepwise decrease takes place in the already low flow rate.

A severely decreased flow is related to caries susceptibility.[94] Following head and neck radiation, when the salivary glands are severely damaged by the primary radiation beam, there are drastic decreases in the amount of saliva produced. At 1 week, 6 weeks, and 3 years after treatment, the output of saliva drops 57%, 76%, and 95%, respectively, below the baseline amount established prior to treatment.[95] The flow rate can be as low as 0.05 mL/minute 3 years after radiation therapy. Following this early drop in flow rate, rampant caries involving every surface of the tooth can be expected—even the incisal surfaces. The pattern is so characteristic that it is called *radiation caries*.[96] Thus a very low rate of saliva flow appears to modify caries status to a much greater extent than at a midrange flow rate.

As salivary flow rate decreases, viscosity increases. This inverse relationship is important, because saliva that is more viscous is less effective in clearing the mouth. A greater DMFS score is usually seen with individuals with viscous saliva.[97]

Viscosity of Saliva. If the saliva appears to have a ropy appearance, high salivary viscosity should be suspected, especially when the stimulated flow rate is low. The viscosity of saliva is determined by

comparing it with that of water.[98] A special Ostwald pipette with a calibrated bore is used. First, 5 mL of water is introduced into the pipette and allowed to flow by gravity from an upper mark on the pipette past a lower mark. The time in seconds needed to pass these two points is recorded. The procedure is then repeated with 5 mL of the saliva specimen. The relative viscosity is calculated by the following formula:

$$\text{Relative viscosity (RV)} = \frac{\text{time required for the saliva}}{\text{time required for the water}}$$

A normal viscosity should be somewhere in the area of 1.5.

Buffering Capacity of Saliva. The buffering capacity of saliva is directly related to flow rate. Of parallel interest is that the buffering capacity of saliva and its inverse relationship to caries have been noted by several investigators.[99] As with other caries activity tests, modifications have facilitated its use in an office practice. Two successive tests, the original Dreizen test and the modification of the original, were titration tests with the endpoint being determined by a dye color change.[100]

In 1980, Frostell introduced a much simpler method to measure the buffering capacity of saliva by using the Dentobuff system.[101] The system is readily adaptable for dental office use and is now commercially available. With this test, paraffin chewing is maintained for 2 minutes or until 5 mL of saliva has been collected. One milliliter of saliva is then added to the commercially available vial of Dentobuff solution. After shaking 10 seconds, the contained carbon dioxide is allowed to evaporate for 2 minutes. The color of the indicator in the Dentobuff solution is then compared with colors on a chart provided to determine the buffering capacity of the saliva sample. The results are interpreted as follows: final pH, 3.0 to 4.0 (yellow)—poor buffering capacity; pH 4.5 to 5.0 (green)—intermediate buffering capacity; and, pH 5.5 to 6.5 (purple)—good buffering capacity.

A recent, even more simplified modification of the Dentobuff system has been suggested by Ericson and Bratthall.[102] A small amount of acid is impregnated on a pH indicator strip. One drop of saliva is placed on the test strip (Dentobuff strip) to dissolve the acid. The final pH is compared after 5 minutes with a color chart of the pH indicator. The method identifies saliva with low-, intermediate-, and high-buffer capacity.

Question 3. Which of the following statements, if any, are correct?

A. *Specificity* is defined as the percentage of diseased sites predicted on the basis of a previous microbiologic test.

B. 1×10^4 CFU of MS is considered the threshold at which the challenge organisms overwhelm the host defenses to the point that caries can be reliably predicted.

C. An average collection of 5 mL saliva over 10 minutes is considered abnormally low.

D. The viscosity of saliva is *inversely* related to saliva flow rate (ie, the more flow, the less viscosity, or vice versa).

E. The white spot of the incipient lesion is the last opportunity for remineralization therapy before overt cavitation.

EVALUATING TOOTH DEFENSE

In the past, caries activity has focused mainly on chemical or microbial constit-uents of the *saliva or plaque or both.* The effort has always been to obtain information that could be used to better evaluate *individual* caries status, rather than *group* status. Although much information has been secured, this approach has not been completely successful. For this reason we need to shift emphasis directly to the *tooth surface* in an effort to identify the presence or absence of early carious change. The tooth surface is where the dynamic challenge and defense activities occur. If early white spot lesions on the tooth surface could be directly visualized, a 100% of certainty would exist of identifying early carious changes that could probably be reversed. For instance, after etching teeth prior to sealant placement, it is possible to directly visualize a frosty-appearing surface that indicates an early, reversible stage of demineralization.

Visualizing Incipient Lesions

Von der Fehr and colleagues in 1970[12] conducted a study in which volunteer subjects refrained from oral hygiene for a period of 23 days. During this time, the experimental group rinsed their mouths nine times a day with a sugar solution. By *visual examination alone*, developing incipient lesions could be identified, as well as their disappearance after initiation of fluoride-induced remineralization. The point was made that if a tooth was *well dried, adequately lighted, and examined under magnification, incipient white spot lesions could be detected before they developed into overt lesions.* Compare these requisites posed by Von der Fehr with the following capabilities of the intraoral video camera.

The Intraoral Video Camera

The intraoral video camera is slightly larger than the dental handpiece. The camera has its own lights and as a result, as it is moved around the mouth, the video images are of the same high quality in color and detail. Magnification up to 50× is offered by some manufacturers. The images are stored on video tape in the same manner as for a hand-held video camera. Single freeze frames can be easily stored on a computer disk for either later review on the monitor, or for feeding into a high-quality photo printer for insurance verification or patient education. By use of split screen techniques, an original white spot lesion can be placed adjacent to a later image to monitor remineralization progress.

As the video camera examination proceeds, the images are displayed on a high-resolution television screen for viewing by both the dentist and the patient. This ability is outstanding for patient education (and practice building). Probably one of the intraoral video camera's greatest contributions to preventive dentistry will be the ability to take advantage of the magnification, color, and high picture quality to better *identify white spot lesions* in time for re-mineralization and to *study fissure lesions* better as candidates for sealant placement.

Computed Dental Radiography

The exciting recent advances in computer-assisted radiographic imaging technology has made possible the development of *computed dental radiography (CDR)* for the detection of early carious lesions. The same radiograph now used in the dental office is the source of the x-ray energy. An intraoral sensor, is used to replace the x-ray film (Fig 12–4). The x-ray unit is activated by a computer-controlled timer, and the image from the sensor is loaded into a computer, where it is electronically *processed* in about 5 seconds, eliminating all need for wet chemicals. The image can be stored in the computer, available for retrieval at any time (Fig 12–5). Transmission over the telephone lines is also possible through a modem.

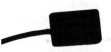

Size 0 Pedo sensor, 24 × 17 × 5 mm.

Size 1 Anterior sensor, 38 × 22 × 5 mm.

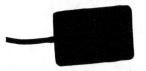

Size 2 Bitwing sensor, 40 × 28 × 5 mm.

Figure 12–4. Multisized sensors used in lieu of x-ray film in computed dental radiography. In use, the sensor corresponding to film sizes 0, 1, and 2 is placed in the mouth as for a regular radiograph. (Sensors portrayed are 0.084× normal size). The sensors are connected to a computer where the image is processed and can be immediately viewed on the monitor. (*Reproduced with permission courtesy of Schick Technologies, Inc., Long Island City, NY*).

With CDR, the dosage of x-rays needed for a quality image is markedly lower than required for even ultrahigh-speed film. Another great advantage is the ability to place the image on the screen of a television monitor, or to print out the image on a high-quality photographic printer. From a diagnostic viewpoint, one of the greatest advantages of CDR is *image enhancement*. With this technique the various shades of gray can be electronically altered as desired to provide the best presentation of selected details. Image enhancement facilitates the earlier detection of smooth-surface and pit-and-fissure caries

Another exceedingly valuable characteristic of CDR involves the ability to employ *subtraction radiography* when appropriate. This is a technique by which images

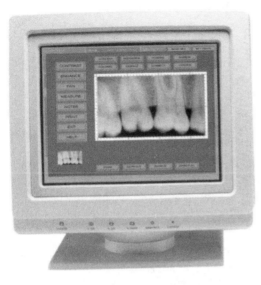

Figure 12–5. Computed dental radiograph unit. Requires only 10% of x-ray dosage required with ultra high-speed film. The electronically created image is fed into the computer where it is formed into an image that can be directed to the monitor, the photographic printer, or stored for future use. The clarity is superior to that of film, and the resolving power is comparable. Control buttons allow enhancement of images by varying contrast. Zooming for better evaluation is possible, as is the placement of tag markers (arrows) at the site(s) of interest. (*Reproduced with permission of Insight, San Carlos, CA*).

from two different times can be superimposed to determine if any change has taken place in disease status—an achievement that is in keeping with the emerging philosophy of longitudinal assessment of disease.[103,104] The requirements for the standardization and reproducibility of CDR are more rigid than in conventional visual interpretation of radiographic film.[105]

Between the intraoral video camera and the CDR, it is now possible to visualize high-contrast, high-resolution images of incipient lesions—both before and during remineralization. Because the incipient lesion is the predecessor to overt cavitation, *the camera and the CDR offer the possibility*

of identifying all developing lesions in time to avoid the need for restorations (See Chapter 21).

Fluoride Levels as a Method of Estimating Tooth Resistance

In a community with fluoridated water there is a higher level of fluoride in the enamel than in a nonfluoridated community. It would be expected that if enamel biopsies[m] were made,[106] the fluoride levels of caries-resistant teeth would demonstrate a higher level of fluoride than caries-susceptible teeth. This is not the case.[107] In all teeth, both inside and outside fluoride areas, there is a great variation of fluoride concentration at different sites of each tooth. Because fluoride has an affinity for *hypocalcified* and demineralized areas, many teeth that have experienced acidogenic episodes as part of an aborted caries process have higher localized fluoride concentrations than those that have not experienced limited demineralization. During and after these "minicarious" attacks, fluoride is incorporated into the apatite crystal through recrystallization,[108] which in turn raises the fluoride content and the resistance of the previously caries-susceptible teeth.[109]

Electric Resistance

The use of electric resistance for the detection of early carious lesions was first proposed by Pincus in 1951.[110] He used a circuit that was composed of a battery, a voltohmmeter, a wired explorer that served as one electrode, and a second electrode held by the patient. When the explorer is touched to a tooth, a low-amperage current flows. Intact enamel is more resistant to the passage of

---

[m] Enamel biopsy = A procedure by which a small amount of surface enamel is etched with a weak acid and the etching solution then collected and analyzed for fluoride or other elements.

the electric current than porous enamel that has imbibed saliva with all of its electrolytes. Thus teeth having low electric resistance have a greater probability of being carious.[111]

Teeth with over 600,000 ohms resistance are generally caries-resistant, whereas teeth with less than 250,000 ohms tend to be caries-susceptible.[112] This method appears to be considerably more sensitive in detecting pit-and-fissure lesions than is the more conventional use of an explorer.[113] In the in vitro testing of a commercially available electronic caries detector, (Fig 12–6), Plaitz and colleagues[114] found that the readings of the electronic device increased as the histologically determined depth of the lesion increased. Radiographic evidence of the same occlusal caries was not demonstrated until significant dentinal involvement occurred. In England, Rock and Kidd[115] completed a study of 50 teeth that prior to extraction were examined by explorer, by radiograph, and by use of the Vanguard electronic caries detector. After

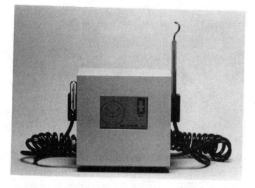

Figure 12–6. A Vanguard electronic caries detector. Note the explorerlike electrode on the right and hand-held electrode on the left. Smile on the screen (with no caries present) merges into a frown when current flow measurements on the upper left of the screen increase from 0 to 9. (*Courtesy of Vanguard, Massachusetts Manufacturing Company, Cambridge, Mass.*)

removal, the teeth were subjected to histologic examination and the results compared with the preextraction data. The explorer and radiograph failed to reveal any caries, whereas the histologic examination demonstrated evidence of *demineralization* in 37 teeth. The remaining 13 failed to demonstrate any demineralization. Compared with the histologic examination, the electronic caries detector identified demineralization of 26 of the 37 teeth, a sensitivity of 70%, while showing a zero reading for 11 of the 13 intact teeth, a specificity of 85%.

Question 4. Which of the following statements, if any, are correct?

A   The same dip-slide can be used interchangeably for lactobacillus and MS.

B.   The film used with the digitized radiograph is ultrahigh-speed.

C.   Subtraction radiography permits an electronic comparison of films taken at two different times.

D.   The intraoral video camera permits the dental examination to be stored on video tape.

E.   The electric circuit for the electronic caries detector consists of an electrode held by the patient and another electrode shaped like an explorer that is held by the operator.

SUMMARY

The most effective way to summarize this chapter is by reviewing what is known about caries development. Only then is it possible to underline the importance of microbiologic testing in a primary prevention program.

- Caries development is due to a prolonged and often oscillating negative and positive mineral balance of the teeth.

- Over a long time, not all incipient lesions progress to overt lesions, indicating that the course of the disease can be altered.
- A physiologic remineralization occurs in the mouth if the host defense and repair capability exceeds that of the challenging organisms.
- An increased use of fluorides in preventive programs can enhance the remineralization process.
- Mutans streptococci and lactobacilli are the prime cariogenic pathogens.
- Frequent sucrose exposure, either in raw form or in baked confection, accelerates the caries process.
- The number of MS and lactobacilli can be increased or decreased in number over days or weeks by placing individuals on high- or low-carbohydrate diets respectively;.
- Existing microbiologic caries activity tests can be used to monitor patient compliance with dietary counseling recommendations.
- Negative or very low counts of MS and lactobacilli are highly predictive of a caries-free state.
- The use of the intraoral video camera and computed dental radiography permits identification of all incipient lesions in time to institute remineralization strategies.

In reviewing the above mentioned facts, the only unknown factors necessary to prevent, arrest, or reverse the caries process during the long interval between the beginning of the incipient lesion and cavitation are (1) a knowledge of the extent of the microbial challenge, (2) the amount of intake of refined carbohydrates and, (3) the body's capacity for biologic self-repair.

One repeated criticism of caries activity tests has been that they are better corre-

lated with the prognosis/diagnosis of group outcomes than for individuals. This difference should not be interpreted in terms of false-positive or false-negative outcomes. Any increase in the challenge factors or decrease in the defense and repair factors at any time should be considered as a warning sign. Considering the many fluctuations of demineralization and remineralization that make up the caries process, probably these lactobacilli and MS tests *do* accurately reflect the caries activity challenge *at the time of the test.*

ANSWERS AND EXPLANATION

1. B, E

A—incorrect. For an adult this is true but not for children.

C—incorrect. Two exams are necessary to determine the number of carious lesions occurring over a given amount of time.

D—incorrect. The first part is a precarious statement, although a reliable prediction of the future is not possible.

2. A, B, C, D

E—incorrect. As the count for MS goes down, *A. viscosus/naeslundii* go up.

3. A, E

B—incorrect. 1×10^6—the millionaires club—; this is where you can expect caries.

C—incorrect. This is well above 1 mL/minute which is still normal.

D—incorrect. Flow and viscosity of the saliva are directly related.

4. C, D, E

A—incorrect. Each of the dip-slides has a different medium, one for lactobacilli and one for MS.

B—incorrect. Instead of a film, there is an electronic sensor that detects the x-rays.

SELF-EVALUATION QUESTIONS

1. Currently, in the United States, adults generally have a greater prevalence of (primary)(secondary) caries.
2. The *triad* of factors that determine the presence or absence of disease is challenge, resistance, and _____.
3. If an epidemiologic clinical caries survey is being conducted, the number of decayed teeth (D) present at that time constitutes a caries _____ study; if the same people are examined 6 months later, the number of now decayed teeth diagnosed constitutes a caries _____ study.
4. A tooth diagnosed as a false-positive could result in (restoring a *sound* tooth)(restoring a *carious* tooth).
5. With the decreasing number of caries seen in the industrial world over the last 20 years, one could expect a greater number of (false-negatives)(false-positives) to be diagnosed.
6. The risk of future disease, based on all information available, is termed risk _____.
7. For convenience, the initials _____ _____ are given to several serotypes of streptococci as a group.
8. A salivary flow of less than _____ mL/minute is cause to suspect xerostomia.
9. An incipient *white spot lesion* can be seen with the unaided eye. (True, False).
10. Two of the most prevalent MS are *Streptococcus* _____ and S _____.
11. The "millionaires club" is made up of people who have at least 1×10 _____ (superscript) MS.
12. In a population of children 6 to 18 years old, about 25% of the children account for approximately _____% of the caries.
13. Incipient (and overt) smooth-surface caries (can)(can't) be detected by use of appropriate radiographs and an intraoral video camera.

REFERENCES

1. Billings RJ, Brown LR, Kaster AG. Contemporary treatment strategies for root surface dental caries. *Gerodontology*. 1985; 1:20–27.
2. DePaola PF, Soparkar PM, Kent RL. Methodological issues relative to the quantification of root surface caries. *Gerodontology*. 1989; 8:3–8.
3. Fejerskov O, Lian WM, Nyvad B, et al. Active and inactive root caries lesions in a selected group of 60- to 80-year-old Danes. *Caries Res*. 1991; 25:385–391.
4. Nemes J, Banoczy J, Wierbicka M. Clinical study on the effect of amine fluoride/stannous fluoride on exposed root surfaces. *J Clin Dent*. 1992; 3:51–53.
5. Ismail AI, Brodeur J, Gagnon P, et al. Prevalence of non-cavitated and cavitated carious lesions in a random sample of 7–9-year-old schoolchildren living in Montreal, Quebec. *Community Dent Oral Epidemiol*. 1992; 20:250–255.
6. Chauncey HH, Garcia RI, Alman JE, et al. Resolution of restorative need in the VA longitudinal study. *J Dent Res*. 70(special issue). 1991; Abstract 481.
7. Ravald N, Birkhed D. Factors associated with active and inactive root caries in patients with periodontal disease. *Caries Res*. 1991; 25:377–384.
8. U.S. Department of Health and Human Resources. *Oral Health of United States Adults—Regional Findings*. NIH Publication No. 88-2868:13, 361, 1988.
9. Backer-Dirks O. Post-eruptive changes in dental enamel. *J Dent Res*. 1966; 45:503–511.
10. Silverstone LM. Remineralization and enamel caries: New concepts. *Dent Update*. 1983; 10:261–273.

11. Silverstone LM. Significance of remineralization in caries prevention. *J Can Dent Assoc.* 1984; 50:157–166.

12. von der Fehr FR, Löe H, Theilade E. Experimental caries in man. *Caries Res.* 1970; 4:131–148.

13. Duchin S, Van Houte J. Relationship of *Streptococcus mutans* and lactobacilli to incipient smooth surface dental caries in man. *Arch Oral Biol.* 1978; 23:779–786.

14. Federation Dentaire International: Review of methods of high caries risk groups and individuals. Technical Report No. 31, *Int Dent J.* 1988; 38:177–189.

15. Gibbons RJ, DePaola PF, Spinell DM, et al. Interdental localization of *Streptococcus mutans* as related to dental caries experience. *Infect Immun.* 1974; 9:481–488.

16. Hume R. Need for change in standards of caries diagnosis—perspective based on the structure and behavior of the carious lesion. *J Dent Educ.* 1993; 57:439–443.

17. Newbrun E. Problems in caries diagnosis. *Int Dent J.* 1993; 43:133–142.

18. Stamm JW, Disney JA, Beck JD, et al. The University of North Carolina caries risk assessment study: Final results and some alternative modeling approaches. In: Bowen WH, Tabak LA, eds. *Cariology for the Nineties.* University of Rochester Press, NY; 1993:209–234.

19. Banting DW, Ellen RP, Fillery ED. Prevalence of root surface caries among institutionalized older persons. *Community Dent Oral Epidemiol.* 1980; 8:84–88.

20. Hunt RJ. Percent agreement, Pearson's correlation, and kappa as measures of interexaminer reliability. *J Dent Res.* 1986; 65:128–130.

21. Vehkalahti MM. *Occurrence of Root Caries and Factors Related to It.* Helsinki, Finland: University of Helsinki; 1987:40. Dissertation.

22. Wallace MC, Retief DH, Bradely EL. Incidence of root caries in older adults. *J Dent Res.* 1988; 67:147. Abstract.

23. Fure S, Zickert I. Prevalence of root surface caries in 55, 65, and 75-year-old Swedish individuals. *Community Dent Oral Epidemiol.* 1990; 18:100–105.

24. Hellyer PH, Beighton D, Heath MR, et al. Root caries in older people attending a general practice in East Sussex. *Br Dent J.* 1990; 169:201–206.

25. Bader JD, Brown JP. Dilemmas in caries diagnosis. *J Am Dent Assoc.* 1993; 124:48–50.

26. Kroncke A, Navjoks R. Dental caries susceptibility tests and their significance in dental practice. *Int Dent J.* 1956; 6:174–188.

27. Socransky SS. Caries susceptibility tests. *Ann NY Acad Sci.* 1968; 153:137–146.

28. Fletcher RH, Fletcher SW, Wagner EH. *Clinical Epidemiology—The Essentials,* 2nd ed. Baltimore, Md. Williams & Wilkins; 1988:46, 94, 104.

29. Rodriguez FE. A method of determining quantitatively the incidence of *Lactobacillus acidophilus-odontolyticus* in the oral cavity. *J Am Dent Assoc.* 1930; 17:1711–1719.

30. Rodriguez FE. Quantitative incidence of *Lactobacillus acidophilus* in the oral cavity as a presumptive index of susceptibility to dental caries. *J Am Dent Assoc.* 1931; 18:2118–2135.

31. Hadley FP. A quantitative method for estimating *Bacillus acidophilus* in saliva. *J Dent Res.* 1933; 13:415–428.

32. Hadley FP, Bunting RW, Delves EA. Recognition of *Bacillus acidophilus* associated with dental caries. *J Am Dent Assoc.* 1930; 17:2041–2058.

33. Rogosa M, Mitchell JA, Wiseman RF. A selective medium for the isolation and enumeration of oral lactobacilli. *J Dent Res.* 1951; 30:682–689.

34. Loesche WJ, Rowan J, Straffon LH, et al. Association of *Streptococcus mutans* with human dental decay. *Infect Immun.* 1975; 11:1252–1260.

35. Mikx FHM, van der Hoeven JS, Konig KG, et al. Establishment of defined microbial ecosystems in germ-free rats. *Caries Res.* 1972; 6:211–223.

36. Brown L, Dreizen S, Handler S. Effects of selected caries preventive regimens and microbial changes following irradiation-induced xerostomia in cancer patients. In: Stiles HM, Loesche WJ, O'Brien TC, eds. *Proceedings on Microbial Aspects of Dental Caries.* (Special Supplement) *Microbiology Abstract.* 1976:275–290.

37. Steinle CJ, Madonia JV, Bahn AN. Relationship of lactobacilli to the carious lesion. *J Dent Res.* 1967; 46:191–196.

38. Shklair IL, Mazzarella MA. Effects of full mouth extraction on oral microbiota. *Dent Prog.* 1961; 1:275–280.

39. Kesel RG, Shklair IL, Green GH, et al. Further studies on lactobacilli counts after elimination of carious lesions. *J Dent Res.* 1958; 37:50–51.

40. Stecksén-Blicks C. Salivary counts of lactobacilli and *S mutans* in caries prediction. *Scand J Dent Res.* 1985; 93:204–212.

41. Ikeda T, Sandham HJ, Bradley EL Jr. Changes in *Streptococcus mutans* and lactobacilli in plaque in relation to the initiation of dental caries in Negro children. *Arch Oral Biol.* 1973; 18:555–566.

42. Boyar RM, Bowden GH. The microflora associated with the progression of incipient carious lesions of children living in a water-fluoridated area. *Caries Res.* 1985; 19:298–306.

43. Newbrun E. *Cariology, 1989,* 3rd ed. Chicago, Ill: Quintessence Publishing Co; 1989; 8:273–293.

44. Emilson CG, Klock B, Sanford BC. Microbial flora associated with presence of root surface caries in periodontally treated patients. *Scand J Dent Res.* 1988; 96:40–49.

45. Boyd JD, Wessels KE, Cheyne VD. The correlation between salivary lactobacillus counts and the rates of progression of dental caries: A statistical appraisal. *J Dent Res.* 1949; 28:641.

46. Sandy CE, Bulate L. The salivary lactobacillus count as an index of caries activity. *Aust J Dent.* 1950; 54:18–26.

47. Alban A. An improved Snyder test. *J Dent Res.* 1970; 49:641.

48. Grainger RM, Jarret TM, Honey FSL. Swab test for dental caries activity. An epidemiological survey. *J Can Dent Assoc.* 1965; 31:515–526.

49. Crossner CG, Holm AK. Saliva tests in the prognosis of caries in children. *Acta Odontol Scand.* 1977; 35:134–138.

50. Toto PD, Evans CL, Sawinski VJ. Reduction of acidogenic microorganisms by toothbrushing. *J Dent Child.* 1967; 34:38–40.

51. Birkhed D, Edwardsson S, Anderson H. Comparison among a dip-slide test (Dentocult), plate count, and Snyder test for estimating number of lactobacilli in human saliva. *J Dent Res.* 1981; 60:1832–1841.

52. Larmas M. A new dip-slide method for counting of salivary lactobacilli. *Proc Finn Dent Soc.* 1975; 71:31–35.

53. Rytomaa I, Tuompo H. Is the Dentocult dip-slide test useful in clinical practice? *Proc Finn Dent Soc.* 1978; 74:23–26.

54. Loesche WJ. Role of *Streptococci mutans* in human dental decay. *Microbial Rev.* 1986; 50:353–380.

55. Togelius J, Kristofferson K, Anderson H, et al. *Streptococcus mutans* in saliva: Intraindividual variations and relation to the number of colonized sites. *Acta Odontol Scand.* 1984; 42:157–163.

56. Fitzgerald RJ, Keyes PH. Demonstration of the etiological role of streptococci in experimental caries in the hamster. *J Am Dent Assoc.* 1960; 61:9–19.

57. Fitzgerald RJ. Dental caries in research in gnotobiotic animals. *Caries Res.* 1968; 2: 139–146.

58. Zinner DD, Jablon JM, Aran AP, et al. Experimental caries induced in animals by streptococci of human origin. *Proc Soc Exp Biol.* (NY) 1965; 118:766–770.

59. Krasse B, Edwardsson S, Svensson I, et al. Implantation of caries-inducing streptococci in the human oral cavity. *Arch Oral Biol.* 1967; 12:231–236.

60. van Houte J. Microbiological predictors of caries risk. *Adv Dent Res.* 1993; 7(2):87–96.

61. Zickert I, Emilson CG, Krasse B. Effect of caries preventive measures in children

highly infected with the bacterium *Streptococcus mutans*. *Arch Oral Biol*. 1982; 27: 861–868.

62. Alauusua S, Rekenon DV. *Streptococcus mutans* establishment and dental caries experience in children 2 to 4 years old. *Scand J Dent Res*. 1983; 91:453–457.

63. Kock G. Selection and caries prophylaxis of children with high caries activity. One-year result. *Odontol Rev*. 1970; 21:71–81.

64. Kohler B, Petterson GM, Bratthall D. *Streptococcus mutans* in plaque and saliva and the development of caries. *Scand J Dent Res*. 1981; 89:19–25.

65. Kohler B, Andreen I, Jonsson B. The effect of caries preventive measures in mothers and dental caries and the oral presence of the bacteria *Streptococcus mutans* and lactobacilli in their children. *Arch Oral Biol*. 1984; 29:879–883.

66. Hamada S, Slade HD. Biology, immunology, and cariogenicity of *Streptococcus mutans*. *Microbiol Rev*. 1980; 44:331–335.

67. Edwardsson S. Characteristics of caries-inducing human streptococci resembling *Streptococcus mutans*. *Arch Oral Biol*. 1968; 13:637–646.

68. Littleton NW, Kakehashi S, Fitzgerald RJ. Recovery of specific "caries-inducing" streptococci from carious lesions in the teeth of children. *Arch Oral Biol*. 1970; 15: 461–463.

69. Shklair IL, Keene HJ, Cullen P. The distribution of *Streptococcus mutans* on teeth of the two groups of naval recruits. *Arch Oral Biol*. 1974; 19:199–202.

70. Vanderis AP. Bacteriologic and nonbacteriologic criteria for identifying individuals at high risk of developing dental caries: a review. *J Public Health Dent*. 1986; 46:106–113.

71. Alaluusua S, Savolainen J, Tuompo H, et al. Slide-scoring method for estimation of *Streptococcus mutans* level in saliva. *Swed Dent J*. 1980; 4:81–86.

72. Jordan HV, Laraway R, Snirch R, et al. A simplified diagnostic system for cultural detections and enumeration of *Streptococcus mutans*. *J Dent Res*. 1987; 66:57–61.

73. Emilson CG, Krasse B. Comparison between a dip-slide test and plate count for determination of *Streptococcus mutans* infection. *Scand J Dent Res*. 1986; 94:500–506.

74. Bell RM, Klien SP, Bohanan HM, et al. *Results of Baseline Dental Examinations in the National Preventive Dentistry Demonstration Program*. Rand Publication Series No. R-2862-RWJ. Santa Monica, Calif: Rand Corp, April 1982.

75. Newbrun E, Matsukuba T, Hooever CI, et al. Comparison of two screening tests for *Streptococcus mutans* and evaluation of their suitability for mass screening and private practice. *Community Dent Oral Epidemiol*. 1984; 12:325–331.

76. Graves R, Disney J, Stamm J, et al. Relation to multiple factors to baseline caries experience in children. *J Dent Res*. 1988; 67:171. Abstract 464.

77. De Stoppelaar JO, Van Houte J, Backer Dirks O. The relationship between extracellular polysaccharide-producing streptococci and smooth surface caries in 13-year-old children. *Caries Res*. 1969; 3: 190–199.

78. Pienihäkkinen K, Schienën A, Bánáezy J. Screening of caries in children through salivary lactobacilli and yeast. *Scand J Dent Res*. 1987; 95:397–404.

79. Thorner RM, Remein OR. *Principles and Procedures in the Evaluation of Screening for Tissues*. US Public Health Service. Publication No. 846, Monograph No. 67, 1961.

80. Imfeld TN. Identification of low caries risk dietary compounds. In: Myer HM, ed. *Monograph in Oral Science*. New York, NY: Karger; 1983; 2:1–98.

81. Jensen ME, Polansky PJ, Schachtele CF. Plaque sampling and telemetry for monitoring acid production on human buccal tooth surfaces. *Arch Oral Biol*. 1982;27:21–31.

82. Imfeld TN. *Identification of Low Caries Risk Dietary Components*. Monographs in Oral Science. In: Myers HM, ed. Vol. 11, Basel, New York, Karger; 1983:195.

83. Park KK, Schemehorn BR, Bolton JW, et al. Effect of sorbitol gum chewing on plaque pH response after ingesting snacks containing predominantly sucrose or starch. *Am J Dent.* 1990; 3:185–191.

84. Schou L. Social and behavioral aspects of caries prediction. In: Johnson NW, ed. *Risk Markers for Oral Diseases, Vol. I. Dental Caries,* Cambridge, Cambridge Univ. Press; 1991:172–197.

85. Park KK, Shemehorn BR, Bolton JW, et al. The impact of chewing sugarless gum on the acidogenicity of fast-food meals. *Am J Dent.* 1990; 3:231–235.

86. Mandel ID, Wotman S. The salivary secretions in health and diseases. *Oral Sci Rev.* 1976; 8:25–47.

87. Shannon IL, Terry JM. A higher parotid flow rates in subjects with resistance to caries. *J Dent Med.* 1965; 20:128–132.

88. Park KK, Schemehorn BR, Stookey GK. Effect of time and duration of sorbitol gum chewing on plaque acidogenicity. *Pediatr Dent.* 1993; 15: 197–202.

89. Manning RH, Edgar WM, Agalamanyi EA. Effects of chewing gums sweetened with sorbitol or a sorbitol/xylitol mixture on the remineralization of human enamel lesions in situ. *Caries Res.* 1992; 26:104–109.

90. Dawes, C. Physiological factors affecting salivary flow rate, oral sugar clearance, and the sensation of dry mouth in man. *J Dent Res.* 1987; 66:648–653.

91. Ship JA, Fox PC, Baume BS. How much saliva is enough? Normal function defined. *J Am Dent Assoc.* 1991; 122:63–69.

92. Council on Dental Therapeutics. Consensus: Oral health effects of products that increase salivary flow rate. *J Am Dent Assoc.* 1988; 116:757–759.

93. Screebny LM, Swartz SWS. A reference guide to drugs and dry mouth. *Gerontology.* 1986; 5:75–99.

94. Losch PK , Weisberger D. High caries susceptibility in diminished salivation. *Am J Orthod Oral Surg.* 1940; 26:1102–1104.

95. Dreizen S, Brown LR, Daly TE, et al. Prevention of xerostomia-related dental caries in irradicated cancer patients. *J Dent Res.* 1977; 56:99–104.

96. Dreizen S, Daly TE, Drane JB, et al. Oral complication of cancer radiotherapy. *Post-Grad Med.* 1977; 61:85–92.

97. McDonald RE. *Pedodontics.* St. Louis, Mo. Mosby; 1973:183–192.

98. Katz S, McDonald JM, Stookey GK, 3rd eds. *Preventive Dentistry in Action.* Upper Montclair, NJ. DCP Publishing Co; 1979.

99. Marshall JA. The neutralizing power of saliva and its relation to dental caries. *Am J Physiol.* 1915; 36:260–279.

100. Dreizen S, Mann AW, Cline JK, et al. The buffer capacity of saliva as a measure of dental caries activity. *J Dent Res.* 1946; 25: 213–222.

101. Frostell G. A colourmetric screening test for evaluation of the buffer capacity of saliva. *Scand Dent J.* 1980; 4:81–86.

102. Ericson D, Bratthall D. A simplified method to estimate the salivary buffer capacity. *Scand J Dent Res.* 1989; 97:405–407.

103. Russell M, Pitts NB. Radiovisiographic Diagnosis of Dental Caries; Initial Comparison of Basic Mode Videoprints with Bitewing Radiography. *Caries Res.* 1993; 27: 65–70.

104. Duncan RC, Heaven TJ, Weems RA, Firestone AR, Greer DF, Patel JR. Computer-assisted Radiographic Detection of Approximal Cavitation. *JDR.* 1993; 72: Abstract #1223, 256.

105. Van der Stelt PF. Modern Radiographic Methods in the Diagnosis of Periodontal Disease. *Adv Dent Res.* 1993;7(2):158–162.

106. Brudevold F, Reda A, Aasenden A, et al. Determination of trace elements in surface enamel of human teeth by a new biopsy procedure. *Arch Oral Biol.* 1975; 20:667–673.

107. Poulsen S, Larsen MJ. Dental caries in relation to fluoride content of enamel in the primary dentition. *Caries Res.* 1975; 9:59–65.

108. Koulorides TI, Keller SE, Manson-Hing L, et al. Enhancement of fluoride of effectiveness by cariogenic priming of human enamel. *Caries Res.* 1980; 14:32–39.

109. Koulorides TI. To what extent is the incipient lesion of dental caries reversible? In: Rowe NH, ed. *Proceedings on Incipient*

Caries of Enamel. Ann Harbor, Mich.: Univ of Michigan School of Dentistry; 1977:51–68.

110. Pincus P. A new method of examination of molar tooth grooves for the presence of dental caries. *J Physiol*. 1951; 113:13–14.

111. White GE, Tsamtsouris A, Williams DL. A longitudinal study of electronic detection of occlusal caries. *J Pedodon*. 1980; 5:91–101.

112. Mayuzumi Y, Suzuki K, Sunada I. Diagnosis of incipient pit and fissure caries by means of measurement of electrical resistance. *J Dent Res*. 1964; 43:941. Abstract 12.

113. White GE, Tsamtsouris A, Williams DL. Detection of occlusal caries by measuring the electrical resistance. In: Bibby BG, Shern RJ, eds. (Special supplement.) *Proceedings on Methods of Caries Prediction. Microbiology Abstract*. 1978:267–270.

114. Plaitz CM, Hicks MJ, Silverstone LM. Clinical radiographs, histologic and electronic comparison of fissure caries. *J Dent Res*. 1985;64(special issue):365. Abstract 1714.

115. Rock WP, Kidd EAM. The electronic detection of demineralization in the occlusal fissures. *Br Dent J*. 1988; 164:243–247.

Chapter 13

Periodontal Disease—Risk Assessment and Evaluation

Kichuel K. Park
Arden G. Christen

Objectives

At the end of this chapter it will be possible to

1. Name and describe two plaque indices and one oral hygiene index that are useful for general and public health dentists to assess and monitor the pattern of plaque location in individual mouths.
2. Name and describe two of the commonest indices used for evaluating gingival inflammation.
3. Describe how the sulcus bleeding index is scored.
4. Explain the relationship between gingival crevicular fluid flow and periodontal disease, and describe two methods used for quantitating crevicular fluid.
5. Name two methods used in epidemiologic studies to determine the severity of periodontal disease in individuals or populations.
6. Describe the differences between vertical and circumferential probing methods in determining pocket depth, and explain how probes differ in design and marking.
7. Discuss how a community periodontal index of treatment need is scored and assessed.

Introduction

Dental caries in the United States is on the wane.[1] The dental profession is now beginning to shift its energies to the diagnosis and treatment of periodontal disease, which is epidemic in the United States. The perception of the nature of periodontal disease has changed over the years although it is still recognized by the public as an inflammatory disease characterized by the presence of periodontal pockets and active bone resorption.[2] In the recent literature, dental practitioners are no longer reporting that periodontal disease is the principal reason for tooth extractions at all ages.[3,4]

It is interesting to speculate on whether these findings represent a real change in its decreased severity, modified treatment philosophies, improved treatment methods, or possibly more positive public attitudes toward tooth retention. Yet, despite the more optimistic epidemiologic outlook, great numbers of people still have multiple active periodontal lesions in need of treatment.

Recognition of the signs and symptoms of early periodontal disease is the *key* requirement for its prevention and control. Marginal gingivitis and its frequent sequela, periodontitis, are extremely common among all age groups. Generally, marginal gingivitis begins in early childhood, increases in prevalence and severity to the early teen years, thereafter subsiding slightly and leveling off for the remainder of the second decade of life.[5] The prevalence of plaque-related periodontal disease, however, is *not* considered to be age-dependent.[6]

Dentists have a moral, legal, and professional responsibility to conduct a thorough intraoral examination and to report the results to their patients in a clear and understandable manner. A systematic periodontal evaluation is a necessary part of this examination and includes periodontal probing, the use of radiographs of diagnostic quality, and, where appropriate, laboratory assays.

Dentists often fail to evaluate or to take seriously early inflammatory, gingival changes. Because gingivitis is considered such a commonly occurring entity, dentists feel no need to inform their patients about its presence.[7] Patients with advanced diseases are informed more frequently, because the signs and symptoms are more easily detected. In one study 48% of patients with diagnosed, advanced periodontitis had been informed of their condition by their dentist. Only 20% of the patients with early periodontitis and 12% of those with gingivitis had been made aware of their disease.[8]

Simple and reliable periodontal disease indicators (indices) are available to help clinicians and researchers assess current periodontal status as well as evaluate the risk of developing periodontal disease. These indices are used to assign numerical scores to various parameters known to be related to the initiation or progression of periodontal diseases. A good index is reliable and reproducible, measures what it intends to measure, is simple and easy to perform, and is easily understood or explained. No single index is appropriate for all types of studies.[9] In view of a new concept that only a small group of people are highly susceptible to developing rapidly progressive periodontitis, the need for a reliable, reproducible marker of periodontal disease activity is acute. Once an acceptable marker is developed, however, it remains to be seen whether it will be practical and sufficiently cost-effective for use in epidemiologic studies as well as in private practice settings.[10]

A variety of indicators have been used in research and clinical settings to measure the prevalence and severity of periodontal disease. The most popular indices have evaluated the following parameters: extent of supragingival and subgingival plaque, gingival inflammation, bleeding, color, contour, supragingival and subgingival calculus, crevicular exudate flow rates, number of leukocytes in the saliva, histologic status, pocket depth, tooth mobility, gingival recession, radiographically observed loss of alveolar bone, and the loss of epithelial attachment as measured from the cementoenamel junction. Some of these indices, although helpful to the researcher, have little practical application for the clinician.[11]

A query on the patient's awareness of any symptoms, such as persistent halitosis; gingival bleeding that is spontaneous on brushing or flossing; perceived changes in occlusion or the altered fit of removable prostheses; or vague pressure sensations in the gingiva or alveolar bone may draw attention to possible periodontal disease activity.

Some individuals are highly susceptible to the development of an especially destructive form of periodontitis. A small percentage of these individuals appear to have an intercurrent disease or a host-defense defect. Because part of the periodontal breakdown mechanism is considered to be due to the effect of immunosuppression, some current research is focusing on the neuropeptides. The association of chronic life stresses with acute necrotizing ulcerative gingivitis and periodontitis have also been reported.[12]

The purpose of this chapter is to examine several major periodontal disease indicators that can be useful to the dentist and dental hygienist or to the scientific investigator. These include indices that measure the (1) extent of dental plaque, (2) amount of gingival inflammation (edema, bleeding, and crevicular fluid flow), and (3) extent of destructive periodontal disease.

PRESENCE OF DENTAL PLAQUE

Abundant evidence suggests that dental plaque is positively correlated to all forms of periodontal disease. Therefore it is important to note objectively the presence, amount, and pattern of plaque in the individual patient's mouth. In a large-scale study of the dental needs of adults an excellent correlation was found between sites with different dental plaque levels, calculus, and periodontal health status.[13] The investigators used the simplified oral hygiene index (OHI-S) of Greene and Vermillion, which was modified for this study. Periodontal health was graded on a continuum from healthy oral tissues through gingivitis and moderate to severe periodontitis. Probing and dental radiographs were used. In those parts of the mouth where the levels of plaque and calculus were higher, the evidence of destructive periodontal disease was also greater (Fig 13–1).

Studies have also indicated that significant differences of plaque accumulation,

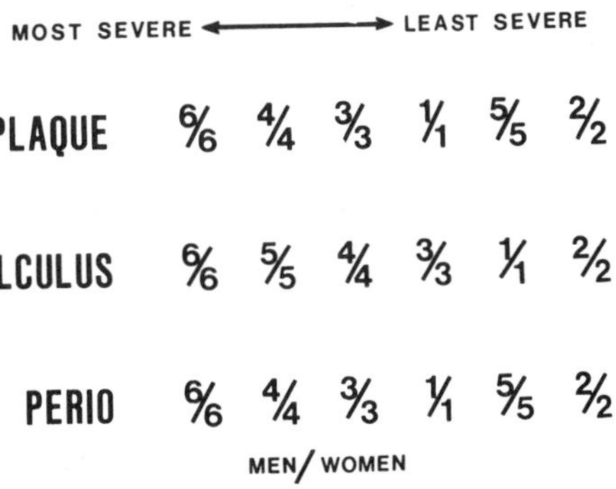

MOST SEVERE ◄──────► LEAST SEVERE

PLAQUE	$\frac{6}{6}$	$\frac{4}{4}$	$\frac{3}{3}$	$\frac{1}{1}$	$\frac{5}{5}$	$\frac{2}{2}$
CALCULUS	$\frac{6}{6}$	$\frac{5}{5}$	$\frac{4}{4}$	$\frac{3}{3}$	$\frac{1}{1}$	$\frac{2}{2}$
PERIO	$\frac{6}{6}$	$\frac{4}{4}$	$\frac{3}{3}$	$\frac{1}{1}$	$\frac{5}{5}$	$\frac{2}{2}$

MEN / WOMEN

Figure 13–1. Mean rankings of plaque, calculus, and periodontal disease, by segment in 5805 U.S. Air Force men and women, ages 17–57. (Segment 1 = right maxillary posteriors; segment 2 = maxillary anteriors; segment 3 = left maxillary posteriors; segment 4 = left mandibular posteriors; segment 5 = mandibular anteriors; and segment 6 = right mandibular posteriors. As shown in the figure, the mandibular areas in men and women (segment 6) had the most severe levels of plaque, calculus, and periodontal disease, whereas the anterior maxillary area (segment 2) had the least. (*From Christen AG, Park PR, Graves RC, et al. United States Air Force survey of dental needs, 1977: methodology and summary of findings. J Am Dent Assoc. 1979; 98:726–730.*)

calculus buildup, and destructive periodontal disease occur within the mouth (Fig 13–2). The posterior mandibular segments of the mouth have statistically greater levels of dental plaque than the rest of the mouth. These results support the viewpoint that the clinician should not use only one segment or area of the mouth as an indicator of the mouth's condition as a whole. *Except for certain large-scale epidemiologic studies, the periodontium of each tooth should initially be individually assessed for periodontal risk factors.*

The O'Leary Plaque Index

The O'Leary plaque index is ideal for monitoring the patient's oral hygiene perfor-

mance.[14] The completed charting indicates the location of plaque and allows dentists and patients to visualize progress made in mastering plaque control programs. It also helps the clinician to determine where plaque accumulates and if brushing or flossing or both should be emphasized.

The Steps for Using the O'Leary Plaque Index and Its Accompanying Chart

1. Every tooth in the mouth is divided into four sections (mesial, distal, buccal, and lingual) at the anatomic line angles (Fig 13–3).
2. Initially all missing teeth are crossed out, and the total number of remaining teeth are determined. For plaque control purposes, the pontic(s) of fixed bridge(s) should be scored in a manner similar to that of natural teeth because plaque can accumulate on any hard surface in the mouth.
3. The patient is asked to rinse vigorously with water to dislodge any loose food debris.
4. The plaque is disclosed by applying a disclosing solution to all teeth, making sure that the dentogingival junctions are reached by the agent.

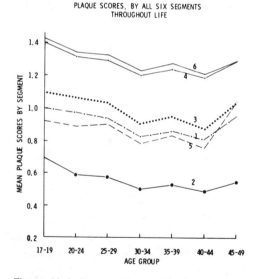

Figure 13–2. Plaque score means, by segments and age groups in 5805 men and women. Note that mandibular posterior teeth (segments 4 and 6) have statistically significant higher (0.01) plaque scores at all ages. The method used to score plaque was a modified simplified oral hygiene index (OHI-S) of Greene and Vermillion. (*From Christen AG, Park PR, Graves RC, et al. United States Air Force survey of dental needs, 1977: methodology and summary of findings. J Am Dent Assoc. 1979; 98:726–730.*)

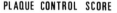
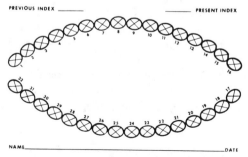

Figure 13–3. O'Leary's chart for plaque and bleeding assessment.

5. After the mouth is rinsed vigorously again with water, the operator uses an explorer or tip of a periodontal probe to confirm the presence of disclosed accumulations of plaque at the dentogingival junction. If the plaque is on a tooth surface, *in contact with the gingival margin*, a dash mark is placed in the appropriate space on the chart. Some operators fill in the entire tooth surface space with a red pen or pencil to increase visibility and enhance the form's impact. Areas having stained pellicle alone should not be scored as having plaque.

An important feature of this and some other indices is that only those surfaces with plaque *in the cervical area* approximating the gingival margin or papilla are positively diagnosed. No attempt is made to quantify the amount of plaque accumulations on the tooth surfaces. Only soft plaque deposits are scored because patients can remove these with routine oral hygiene procedures. Surfaces with no plaque or with plaque that does not approximate the soft tissues are left blank.

The total number of scored tooth surfaces are then added together, divided by the total number of available surfaces in the mouth, and multiplied by 100. This is the final plaque index for the patient. The baseline percentage can be compared with subsequent O'Leary indices to monitor a patient's progress objectively.

O'Leary and colleagues[14] have stated that a suitable goal in teaching personal oral hygiene is to reduce the plaque index to *10%* or less of the available tooth surfaces. It is suggested that surgical periodontal therapy or definite fixed prosthodontics should not be initiated until this goal has been reached. A goal of 15% to 20% reduc-

tion between each appointment period, however, is probably more realistic for most individuals.

Plaque Index of Silness and Löe

The plaque index of Silness and Löe (PLI) scores the *location* and *quantity* of plaque *immediately adjacent to gingival tissues*.[15] It is intended to be used *together* with the gingival index to help correlate the presence of dental plaque with gingival inflammation. The criteria of this plaque index are shown in Table 13–1.

This index can be used for full or partial mouth recording. The cervical area of each tooth is divided into mesial, distal, lingual, and facial parts, and each area is recorded separately. It can also be easily and rapidly performed semiquantitatively with a minimum of equipment.

This index stresses the importance of plaque located at the gingival margin and is very *sensitive to small changes in the amount of dental plaque.*

Oral Hygiene Index and Simplified Oral Hygiene Index: (The Green and Vermillion Index)

One of the most popular indicators for determining *oral hygiene status* in epidemio-

TABLE 13–1. THE CRITERIA OF THE PLAQUE INDEX OF SILNESS AND LÖE (PLI)

Score	Criteria
0	No plaque in gingival areas.
1	Film of plaque at free gingival margin, detectable only by removal with perio-probe or by disclosing solution.
2	Moderate accumulation of plaque, visible to the naked eye within the crevice, on the marginal gingiva or on the adjacent tooth surface or on both.
3	Heavy accumulation of soft matter on the gingival margin of the tooth surface. Soft debris. Soft debris fills the interdental region.

logic studies, the original OHI was developed in 1960 by Greene and Vermillion,[16] and 4 years later it was modified. The shortened, revised version can provide the same information on the oral hygiene status of large population groups; it is called the simplified oral hygiene index (OHI-S).[17]

This index can be accomplished rapidly and is very useful for large-scale epidemiologic surveys. It is *not* generally believed to be sensitive enough, however, to measure the oral hygiene status of an *individual* patient.

The OHI has two components: the *oral debris* score and the *calculus score*. The term *oral debris* includes "plaque, materia alba, and food remnants." For the OHI-S, soft and hard deposits are evaluated only on the *facial* or *lingual surfaces of six selected teeth*. They are the buccal surfaces of the upper first molars of both sides, the labial surfaces of the upper right and lower left central incisors, and the lingual surfaces of both lower first molars. The criteria for the OHI scores are shown in Table 13–2.

The criteria for determining the calculus score is essentially the same as for the debris score, *with the same area of tooth surface being evaluated* with the following exceptions: individual tooth surfaces having flecks of *supra*gingival calculus are given a score of 2, whereas a continuous heavy band of *sub*gingival calculus is scored as 3. An explorer is used to identify and score calculus deposits; results can be expressed separately for either debris or calculus scores, and the *two added together* give a total OHI or OHI-S score; both debris and calculus scores can be added and divided by the number of surfaces examined to calculate the average oral hygiene score.

Question 1. Which of the following statements, if any, are correct?

   A. Two dentists in *different parts of the world* using the same periodontal disease index can accumulate data *that can be compared statistically*.
   B. More periodontal disease indices have been developed for research studies than are used for routine clinical studies.
   C. The O'Leary plaque index considers all stain and plaque found on *all parts* of each surface of a tooth.
   D. The plaque index of Silness and Löe differs from the O'Leary index by *quantitating* the amount of plaque adjacent to or in contact with the gingival tissues.
   E. The OHI-S is an excellent method for establishing and monitoring an *individual's* periodontal disease status.

DISEASE INDICATORS FOR GINGIVAL INFLAMMATION: GINGIVAL BLEEDING, CREVICULAR FLUID FLOW

The most commonly used indicators to determine the degree of gingival inflammation are the gingival index (GI) of Löe and Silness[18] and the papillary-marginal-attached (PMA) index of Schour and Massler.[19]

Periodontal disease severity is closely related to the virulence of microorganisms

TABLE 13–2. THE CRITERIA FOR THE ORAL HYGIENE INDEX SCORES (OHI)

Score	Criteria
0	No debris or stain present.
1	Soft debris covering not more than one third of the tooth surface.
2	Soft debris covering more than one third but not more than two thirds of the tooth surface.
3	Soft debris covering more than two thirds of the tooth surface.

and the host's resistance,[20] however, the association of organisms with specific disease sites does not prove a cause-and-effect relationship.

Löe and Silness Gingival Index

The most frequently used index for evaluating gingivitis is the Löe and Silness gingival index.[18,21] With this index it is possible to measure bleeding tendencies, color, and contour changes of the gingiva; alternations in the consistency of tissue; and the presence of ulceration (Table 13–3). *Bleeding* is the most important criterion of inflammation in this index; however, the distinction between normal (0) and mild inflammation (1) is based on visual appearance of the tissues.

The gingival condition around each tooth is examined, and a score for the mesial, distal, buccal, and lingual areas is recorded. If desired, the gingival index can also be used on only selected teeth in the mouth.

The sums of scores from the four areas of each tooth are divided by the number of teeth examined to produce a gingival index for the individual. Because bleeding on probing can be scored more objectively than a visual assessment of change in color, form, and consistency of gingival tissues,

the intensity of probing with a blunt instrument must be carefully controlled. The basic intention of this index is not to assess the depth or extent of a pocket or to determine bone loss but *only* to evaluate the status of gingival health.

Papillary-Marginal-Attached Gingival Index

The PMA gingival index is based on the concept that the extent of inflammation is an indicator of the severity of the condition.[19] Gingival inflammation starts in the dental *papilla*, spreads around the gingival *margin*, and, if more severe, involves the *attached* gingival tissues. This index scores the severity of inflammation of each of these three gingival areas on a scale ranging from 0 to 4, as shown in Table 13–4.

This index may be used for a full-mouth examination or for an evaluation of

TABLE 13–3. THE CRITERIA FOR THE LÖE-SILNESS GINGIVAL INDEX (GI)

Score	Criteria
0	Normal gingiva.
1	Mild inflammation—slight change in color, slight edema, *no bleeding on probing*.
2	Moderate inflammation—redness, edema and glazing, *bleeding on probing*.
3	Severe inflammation, marked redness and edema, *ulceration, tendency toward spontaneous bleeding*.

TABLE 13–4. THE PMA GINGIVAL INDEX SCORES FOR THE INFLAMMATION OF THE DENTAL PAPILLA, GINGIVAL MARGIN, AND GINGIVAL TISSUES

Score	Criteria
0	Normal, no inflammation.
1	Mild papillary engorgement, slight increase in size, mild inflammation with slight change of color, and little loss of contour.
2	Obvious increase in size, hemorrhage on pressure, moderate inflammation with swelling, glazing, and redness. Tendency to bleed on slight pressure. Papillae or margins become blunt and rounded. Slight extension of inflammation to adjacent tissues.
3	Excessive increase in size with spontaneous hemorrhage. Severe inflammation with more swelling and redness, pocket formation, spontaneous bleeding, and involvement of adjacent tissues.
4	Necrotic changes, very severe inflammation, including ulceration and sloughing (as in acute necrotizing ulcerative gingivitis [ANUG]).

the anterior segment only. The scores for PMA units *are recorded separately* using the appropriate number to indicate severity.

The scores are then added, and the sum is divided by the number of teeth examined to give the patient's overall score. The number of affected papillary, marginal, and attached gingival areas are recorded separately. Data from this index can be presented in a number of different ways (eg, the percentage of individuals having one or more inflamed gingival units or as the average number of PMA units per person). The accuracy of this index depends on the ability of the examiner to differentiate affected from nonaffected areas and to assess severity.

Recent knowledge concerning the development of gingival inflammation has cast doubt on the validity of this index and, as a result, it has fallen into disfavor.

ASSESSMENT OF GINGIVAL BLEEDING

Sulcus Bleeding

Gingival bleeding on probing is the most significant sign of active periodontal disease. Any gingival bleeding should be viewed seriously by both the clinician and patient.

Sulcular bleeding on gentle periodontal probing is considered the most significant indicator of gingival inflammation.[22] Assessment of gingival bleeding on probing is an essential part of a periodontal examination.[23] Gingival bleeding is perhaps the *earliest* clinical sign of gingivitis, preceding discoloration and swelling. Gingival bleeding can also be easily demonstrated and understood by the patients, and some clinicians believe that it can help motivate patients to improve their oral hygiene.

The number of bleeding points is significantly increased as early as the sixth day following the termination of mechanical plaque control procedures. Because of the lag period between plaque formation, gingival bleeding, and clinically detectable inflammatory changes in gingival tissues, some adherent bacterial colonies may be *present* in areas *with clinical signs of gingival bleeding*.

The criteria for the sulcus gingival bleeding index (SBI) are shown in Table 13–5. This index may provide a sensitive measure of the gingival condition, but it is often difficult to maintain consistent, reproducible results. To partially eliminate this potential problem, *only* the presence or absence of sulcus bleeding can be recorded on a chart similar to that used for the O'Leary

TABLE 13–5. THE CRITERIA FOR THE SULCUS GINGIVAL BLEEDING INDEX (SBI)

Score	Criteria
0	Healthy gingiva, no bleeding on careful, blunt probing of the gingival sulcus.
1	Healthy gingiva, no discoloration or swelling. Small bleeding points appear within 1 to 15 seconds after probing of the sulcus or gingival pocket with blunt probe.
2	Several isolated bleeding points occur subsequent to probing of the gingival sulcus, and discoloration of the gingiva is present. No swelling or macroscopic edema is seen.
3	The interdental triangle is filled with blood subsequent to probing, discoloration, and slight edematous swelling of gingiva occurs.
4	Routine bleeding on sulcular probing; discoloration and obvious gingival swelling are present.
5	Bleeding on sulcular probing and spontaneous bleeding, discoloration, severe swelling with or without gingival ulceration.

index.[14] If bleeding is present on a particular surface of the tooth, the area is given a score of 1. The procedures are quick and sample.

The step-by-step procedures are as follows:

1. All missing teeth are crossed out, and the number of available areas to be examined is calculated by multiplying the total number of teeth present in the mouth by 4.
2. The cheek mucosa is retracted by using a mirror or gloved index finger. *Without* air drying, cleaning, or disclosing, the gingiva are systematically examined. Beginning with the most posterior tooth of the upper right or left quadrant, the tip of a periodontal probe is carefully placed into the opening of each gingival sulcus until a slight resistance is encountered. The probe tip is then gently moved mesiodistally and buccolingually.
3. The areas where bleeding *occurs* with probing are recorded for all teeth.
4. The sulcular bleeding index score is determined by counting the total number of sulci with bleeding, dividing this number by the total number of sulci obtained from step 1 above, and multiplying by 100.

CREVICULAR FLUID ASSESSMENT

Gingival Fluid Flow Measurement and Analysis

Crevicular fluid production is considered as pathologic in nature (eg, a transudate) and serves to flush out metabolic catabolites. This fluid contains not only protective elements of the host's humoral defense system

but also serves as a substrate for microorganisms of the subgingival plaque. As the gingivitis increases in severity, so does the flow of gingival crevicular fluid increase— usually *proportional* to the increase in inflammation.[24] Thus the measurement of the flow rate of crevicular fluid has been proposed as a means of monitoring the degree of gingival inflammation.

The presence of gingival crevicular fluid (GCF) as a periodontal disease indicator has numerous advantages. The evidence that periodontal destruction progresses through acute, site-specific episodes followed by periods of quiescence has stimulated investigation of the GCF components. The results from GCF analysis may provide information on the host's responses to inflammation and tissue destruction. Unlike serum and saliva, GCF is site-specific and conveniently sampled and contains components derived from both the host and the plaque. It can be in the form of plasma, connective tissue, and cell components, or the dental plaque itself.[25] A keen interest has arisen in determining the nature of collagenase activity in GCF.[26]

SAMPLING OF CREVICULAR FLUID FLOW

Sodium fluorescein, a fluorescent dye that is injected intramuscularly, can be recovered 3 minutes later on an absorbent paper strip inserted into the gingival sulcus. Similarly, when fluorescein is given orally in capsular form, it appears in the crevicular fluid. The amount recovered correlates with the clinical severity of *gingival inflammation.* but *not* necessarily with the severity of periodontitis.[27,28]

Recent advances in immunology have produced rapid, routine, diagnostic tests to evaluate crevicular fluid. Tests are available to measure polymorphonuclear (PMN) leukocyte chemotaxis and phagocytosis. The orogranulocytic migratory rate (OMR), which counts the number of leukocytes in gingival fluid, becomes a clinical tool with improvement and simplification in harvesting techniques.[19,29,30] A *direct* correlation exists between the OMR and the gingival index.[18]

Current methods of crevicular fluid collection are still crude and may themselves provoke inflammation. Crevicular fluid can be collected by means of (1) absorbent paper strips, (2) gingival washings, and (3) microcapillary pipettes.

Absorbent Paper Strip Technique

It is relatively simple to measure the crevicular fluid flow rate by using standardized absorbent paper strips. The procedure is as follows:

1. After the gingiva has been isolated with cotton rolls, the tissue is dried with a gentle stream of air for 5 seconds.
2. A paper strip is inserted in the sulcus for 5 seconds, removed, and discarded.
3. A second strip is either placed at the entrance to the gingival sulcus (extra-sulcular method) or inserted into the sulcus until a frictional bind is encountered (intrasulcular technique). The intrasulcular technique can itself irritate the crevicular epithelium and trigger the flow of crevicular fluid.
4. The strips are allowed to remain in place for 5 seconds.
5. The amount of crevicular fluid can be quantitated by using a variety of methods.

The paper strips can be presoaked with a ninhydrin solution. In the presence of crevicular fluid on the strip, a chemical reaction turns the amino acids blue. This area can be directly measured planimetrically under a magnifying glass,[a] a microscope, or by using an enlarged photograph.

The strips can also be placed in a gingival fluid meter, the *Periotron*,[b] to quantitate the gingival crevicular fluid. This meter measures the fluid collected in the absorbent paper (Periopaper) strip, using an electronic transducer (Fig 13–4).[18,24,27,31]

The manufacturer claims that this method provides an "early warning system" for the detection of gingivitis. The extent of wetness of the paper strip produced by the gingival fluid affects the flow of a current through a moisture-sensitive sensor. The current flow is displayed as a digital readout.

Other Methods

The use of micropipettes inserted into the sulcus allows the collection of gingival fluid by a microcapillary tube. The amount of gingival crevicular fluid can be determined by centrifuging the microcapillary tube. The gingival washing method uses a special plastic appliance that covers the hard palate and the vestibule. Fluid is collected by rinsing the sulci from one side to the other through palatal and facial channels with a syringe or a pump.[32] The content is later centrifuged and analyzed.[31,33,34] The gingival crevicular fluid assays determine the presence of *marker enzymes*, including aspartate aminotransferase, collagenases, β-glucuronidase, and elastase, and the inflammatory mediators, all

---

[a] Compensatory polar planimeter with tracing point (#62-0002), Keuffel & Esser Co, Morristown, NJ: A planimeter is a simple instrument for the accurate measurement of plane areas of any form. To measure an area it is only necessary to run a tracer point around the periphery of the figure and read the distance that a measuring wheel has revolved during the process.

[b] Harco Medical Electronics Devices, Inc. Tustin, CA.

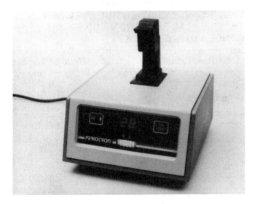

Figure 13–4. The Periotron device that determines the volume of gingival crevicular fluid sampled on an absorbent paper strip. (*Courtesy of Rex D. Bare, Harco Medical Electronic Devices, Inc.*)

of which have been correlated to periodontal disease activity.[35]

INDICES OF DESTRUCTIVE PERIODONTAL DISEASE

The most widely used indices to indicate periodontal disease activity are Russell's periodontal index[36] and the Ramfjord's periodontal disease index.[37] Both indices measure *gingival inflammation and periodontal*

destruction. The overall attachment loss gives an accurate historic picture of the patient's periodontal health status. The recording of gingival recession is as important as measuring pocket depths. These findings should be interpreted in conjunction with the presence of gingival inflammation and any previous history of periodontal therapy.

Russell's Periodontal Index

The Russell's periodontal index (PI) evaluates the progressive stages of periodontal disease, from gingival inflammation to the loss of periodontal attachment, and, eventually, bone loss.[36,38] The extent of total attachment loss on each tooth surface assesses the destruction caused by periodontal disease. Attachment loss is the *sum* of the clinical probing depth and gingival recession, the latter being measured from the cemento-enamel junction. In this index the presence or absence of gingival inflammation and its severity, pocket formation, and masticatory function are measured. Tissues around each tooth are examined with a mouth mirror and a noncalibrated periodontal probe and scored using the criteria shown in Table 13–6.

A basic rule for this index is, *when in doubt, assign a lesser score.*

TABLE 13–6. CRITERIA FOR EXAMINING AND SCORING THE TISSUE AROUND EACH TOOTH USING THE RUSSELL'S PERIODONTAL INDEX (PI)

Score	Criteria and Scoring for Field Studies
0	*Negative.* There is neither overt inflammation in the investing tissues nor loss of function due to destruction of supporting tissues.
1	*Mild gingivitis.* There is an overt area of inflammation in the free gingiva, but this area does not circumscribe the tooth.
2	*Gingivitis.* Inflammation completely circumscribes the tooth, but there is no apparent break in the epithelial attachment.
6	*Gingivitis with pocket formation.* The epithelial attachment has been breached, and there is a pocket (not merely a deepened gingival crevice due to swelling in free gingivae). There is no interference with normal masticatory function. The tooth is firm in its socket and has not drifted.
8	*Advanced destruction with loss of masticatory function.* The tooth may be loose, may have drifted, may sound dull on percussion with a metallic instrument, or may be depressible in its socket.

The total score, divided by the number of teeth examined, represents the PI score for the *individual*. When used in an epidemiologic survey, the PI score for the selected *group* is the total of all individual scores divided by the number of examinees. The findings may be reported either as (1) the mean score for a group or age group, (2) the proportion of examinees with zero scores, or (3) the proportion of examinees with one or more scores of 6 or 8.

This index is easily and quickly learned, is reproducible, and can be applied with a minimal amount of equipment and training. The criteria are clear, and the results obtained from different examiners are widely comparable. This index has been extensively used throughout the world for studies on major population groups. Because the PI assesses both reversible (gingivitis) and the more destructive irreversible changes of periodontitis, it is an epidemiologic index having a true biologic significance.

This index also accurately reflects the clinical condition by giving *greater weight to the advanced destructive stages*. It does not adequately discriminate, however, between moderate and severe gingivitis and is not sensitive to minor changes in gingival tissue status.

The relationship between the clinical condition and score ranges in the Russell's PI is summarized in Table 13–7.

Ramfjord's Periodontal Disease Index

The Ramfjord's periodontal disease index (PDI) system evaluates gingival health, depth of crevice or pocket, plaque, and calculus.[9,37,39] The gingival and pocket scores can be combined into a composite score for scoring the overall periodontal status. Provision is made for the accurate measurement of the *epithelial attachment and its relationship to the cementoenamel junction*. Six se-

TABLE 13–7. RELATIONSHIP BETWEEN THE CLINICAL CONDITION AND SCORE RANGES IN RUSSELL'S PI

Clinical Condition	Group PI Score
Clinically normal tissues*	0–0.2
Simple gingivitis*	0.3–0.9
Incipient destructive periodontal disease*	0.7–1.9
Established destructive periodontal disease†	1.6–5.0
Terminal stages of periodontal disease†	3.8–8.0

*Reversible
† Irreversible

lected teeth, the maxillary right-first molar, maxillary left-central incisor, maxillary left-first bicuspid, mandibular left-first molar, mandibular right-central incisor, and mandibular right-first bicuspid, are examined and scored. The mean score for these six teeth correlates well with the mean score for all teeth, so it is not necessary *in epidemiologic studies* to evaluate every tooth in the mouth. Training and calibration with an experienced examiner are considered essential, particularly for measuring periodontal pockets.

Increased tooth mobility can be the result of hyperfunction or loss of attachment. For this reason, if increased mobility exists, an evaluation should be made relative to the cause, such as primary or secondary occlusal trauma or perhaps both. Two instrument handles are used to check mobility, one placed on the lingual, and the other on the facial surface. Force is then applied through the handles to compare the facial–lingual mobility of one tooth against another. Considerable skill is required to achieve consistent, reproducible results.

The gingiva surrounding each tooth is scored on a scale of 0 to 3, according to the degree of inflammation. The gingival sulci on the mesial and buccal areas of the selected teeth are then probed and scored on a scale of 4 to 6. The distance from the *cementoenamel junction to the bottom of the sulcus* is determined. The criteria for the Ramfjord index are shown in Table 13–8.

The crevicular depth is scored using a Michigan No. 0 calibrated periodontal probe, which is graduated in 3-mm increments. All measurements are rounded to the nearest millimeter. The distance from (1) the cementoenamel junction to the free gingival margin is measured, as well as (2) the distance from the free gingival margin to the bottom of the gingival sulcus or pocket. The difference between the two measurements provides the gingival sulcus depth, to the epithelial attachment. This is considered an *important clinical measurement* in determining the status of the periodontium.

The crevice measurements are made at the midpoint of the buccal surface and at the mesiobuccal line angle, keeping the probe parallel to the long axis of the tooth.

This index is used in examinations of an individual patient and is, therefore, a useful tool for the general dentist and periodontist. It is also useful for descriptive and analytic epidemiologic surveys and for clinical trials that evaluate therapeutic agents and treatment procedures in which the loss of periodontal attachment is important.

Ramfjord,[40] however, indicated that none of the current periodontal indices provide data with adequate details for studies and clinical trials involving loss or gain of elements of the periodontium. It is generally conceded that the destruction of bone is still the most important criterion for assessing the severity of periodontal disease.[41]

Question 2. Which of the following statements, if any, are correct?

A. In the Löe and Silness gingival index, *bleeding* is the most important criterion of the severity of the gingivitis.

B. The PMA index emphasizes the presence but not the severity of inflammation of the papilla, marginal gingiva, and attached gingiva of each tooth.

C. The Löe and Silness gingival index and sulcular gingival bleeding index provide similar data relating to probe-induced or spontaneous bleeding of the sulcular epithelium.

D. The flow of gingival crevicular fluid is greater in gingival health than in gingival disease.

E. Russell's index is weighted to give a higher score than Ramfjord's for equally severe advanced periodontitis.

TABLE 13–8. THE CRITERIA FOR RAMFJORD INDEX (PDI)

Score	Criteria
0	Absence of signs of inflammation.
1	Mild to moderate inflammatory gingival change not extending around the tooth.
2	Mild to moderately severe gingivitis extending around the tooth.
3	Severe gingivitis characterized by marked redness, swelling, tendency to bleed, and ulceration.
4	Gingival crevice in any of four measured areas (mesial, distal, buccal, and lingual), extending apically past the cementoenamel junction but not more than 3 mm.
5	Gingival crevice in any of the four measured areas extending apically to cementoenamel junction 3 to 6 mm.
6	Gingival crevice in any of the four measured areas extending apically more than 6 mm from the cementoenamel junction.

PERIODONTAL DISEASE CAUSATION: CHANGING CONCEPTS

Until recently periodontal disease was considered to be the result of a mixed, bacterial infection of the periodontal structures. It was assumed that once a patient was "infected with periodontal disease," the condition progressed continuously and became more severe as a function of time; in other words, periodontal disease was considered a physiologic penalty for aging. Also, periodontitis was considered to be universally prevalent in adults, and the entire population was therefore considered to be at high risk. Recent studies indicate, however, that the periodontal diseases are cyclical and episodic, with varying lengths of remission periods that are followed by periods of disease activity.[42] This episodic disease pattern, characterized by bursts and remissions, has caused considerable interest because an understanding of these cyclical changes could provide important new insights into the nature of destructive periodontal disease and its treatment. Approaches to an understanding of the mechanisms associated with progressing periodontitis have changed over the past decade.[20] These newer concepts have emphasized a *bacterial specificity* in the etiology of various forms of periodontal disease.[43]

New technology involving recent advances in microbiology, molecular biology, and the other basic sciences is always exciting and always holds our hope that practical alternatives to the present methods will evolve from the research into diagnosing and treating disease.[44] Marker tests aid in determining the presence of specific periodontal pathogens, in locating sites of disease activity, and in helping develop effective treatments plans. Tests can also be useful to the clinician in evaluating the effects of treatment, in establishing timely recall visits, and in identifying those individuals who are at greater risk for the development of periodontitis. The use of immunologic tests to determine periodontal disease activity will permit the objective analysis of important aspects of the disease *process*.[45] New diagnostic methods must be both reliable and cost-effective.

Plaque from individuals with periodontitis has been associated with more than 350 microbial species. A very strong case can be made for implicating a number of specific bacteria as risk indicators for destructive periodontal disease. These bacterial species include, among others, *Porphyromonas gingivalis* (Pg) *Prevotella intermedia,* (Pi) *Actinobacillus actinomycetemcomitans, Eikenella corrodens, Fusobacterium nucleatum, Bacteroides forsythus, Campylobacter rectus,* and spirochetes or *Treponema* species.[46-48]

Patients with juvenile periodontitis have elevated antibody titers to Aa and to its leucotoxins when compared with both healthy controls and those with adult periodontitis. These titers fall after effective treatment is instituted. Likewise, those with severe adult periodontitis have shown that IgG antibody levels to the whole cells of Pg are elevated compared with control subjects.[49-50]

Microbiologic Testing

Microbiologic testing for periodontal disease activity will become increasingly valuable to the clinician in determining the presence of specific periodontal pathogens, in locating sites of active disease, and in helping develop effective treatment plans. It could also be useful to the clinician in evaluating the effects of treatment, in establishing timely recall visits, and in identifying those who are at risk for the development of periodontitis.

The DNA Probe

The DNA probe analysis appears to be the most promising diagnostic system on the horizon for the clinician.[54–56] DNA assays show a better correlation with the clinical signs of disease on an individual basis than culture techniques. They do not depend on the presence of *living* bacteria, and thus they require no special packaging. The test centers on the fact that the two molecular strands of DNA are complementary. Single-control strands of the DNA of a particular bacterial species are matched with a complementary strand of the DNA of bacteria taken from a patient sample. The sample strand is marked with a radioisotope so that it can be detected if it attaches to the control DNA complementary strand. As the number of complementary strand couplings increase in proportion to the number of Aa, Pg, and Pi, the amount of radioactivity also increases. The level of radioactivity detected forms the basis for the final report.

The American Dental Association (ADA) has granted its seal of acceptance to two DNA assay systems, the DMD$_x$ test for periodontitis and Pathotek pathogen detection system.[c] The DMD test measures individual levels of Aa, Pi, and Pg, and test results are reported as negative, low, moderate, or high for the detected level of each organism. A color-coded report form graphically illustrates periodontal risk levels. This can be used for purposes of patient education and motivation. Pathotek detects all three pathogens and reports on their levels collectively. This test informs the clinician whether significant members of pathogen bacteria are present in a pooled sample from two subgingival sites and is helpful for screening new patients and as a recall-monitoring device.

The DNA assay tests are simple to use. The site to be sampled is cleaned of supragingival plaque, and a paper point is gently inserted into the gingival site and removed after 10 seconds. It is then placed in a vial that is mailed to the laboratory for analysis. Test results are generally available within 10 days after mailing or within a few days if a telephone report is desired.

The BANA Test

The bacterium *Actinobacillus actinomycetemcomitans* (Aa) is associated with many periodontitis lesions.[49] A number of microbe derived protease enzymes have been implicated as virulence factors in the pathogenesis of periodontal diseases, particularly those associated with the black-pigmented *Bacteriodes* spp.[50] N-Benzoyl-DL-arginine-2-naphthylamide (BANA) has been found in *Treponema denticola, Porphyromonas gingivalis*, and *Bacteroides forsythus*, but not with other plaque bacterial species.[51] As these three are among those species most frequently associated with adult forms of periodontitis, and all are anaerobes, the BANA enzyme can possibly be used as a "marker" for the diagnosis of anaerobic periodontal infections.

This method can be used as a chairside diagnostic test for detecting those bacteria that produce a trypsinlike enzyme that can hydrolyze the BANA substrate. In turn, when Evans black dye is added, a positive response evokes a blue color.

Other Approaches

Clinical studies suggest a correlation between a positive response to other enzymes and the development of periodontal disease.[52,53] *Prevotella intermedia* may be identified by differences in fluorescence of their colonies under ultraviolet light, or in their trypsinlike or BANA-like activity.[52] Future efforts will focus on the level of infectious-

---

[c] Both tests have been developed by Biotechbica Diagnostics, Inc, 61 Molton St, Cambridge, MA 02138.

ness, possibly producing an assay for antigens or products that are associated with their level of virulence.[54] Other advanced diagnostic methods include the use of immunofluorescence microscopic techniques and enzyme immunosorbent assays to identify bacteria in plaque samples.[57,58] These and other tests could be useful for predicting future disease or for diagnosing a currently active disease process.

PERIODONTAL PROBING

The periodontal probe is useful for locating the dentogingival junction for measuring pocket depth and sometimes as an aid for detecting plaque and calculus (Fig 13–5).[59]

Conducting a periodontal examination in a systematic manner can be accomplished quickly with the help of an assistant. Necessary instruments include a dental mirror and a conventional or electronic periodontal probe. Probing can be influenced by various factors, such as the type of probe, angulation and force of probing, and inflammation of periodontal tissue, and all these factors can create errors in measuring attachment level changes. To limit the error, in conventional probing it has been suggested that active sites be defined as those that show a loss of attachment of at least 2 to 3 mm in two sequential measurements. Manual probes have long been part of dental instrumentation, but computer-coupled electronic probes (to be discussed later) promise to facilitate probing and more accurately recording diagnostic information.

The probing depth seldom corresponds to the microscopic (histologic) sulcus or pocket depth. The clinical pocket depth, however, does reflect the relative position of the actual histologic pocket depth. It provides the clinician with a useful estimate of the location of the most coronal insertion of connective tissue fibers along the root. Also, the clinical pocket depth, as measured to the nearest millimeter, has been shown to be a reproducible measurement.[60] Periodontists generally concur that pocket probing represents a valid estimate of the underlying bone morphology and pattern.

Chilton and Miller[61] reported several important factors that can affect probe measurements. They include:

1. Variations in probing force
2. The angle at which the probe is inserted
3. The point at which the measurement is taken
4. Inability to read the probe graduation markings accurately
5. Errors in grading of the probes
6. Size and shape of the probe

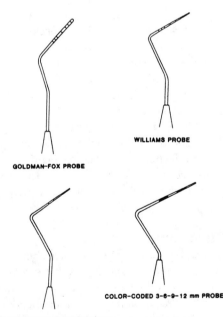

WILLIAMS PROBE

GOLDMAN–FOX PROBE

COLOR–CODED 3–6–9–12 mm PROBE

UNIVERSITY OF MICHIGAN "o" PROBE

Figure 13–5. Different types of calibrated periodontal probes useful in assessing the depth and configuration of periodontal pockets.

7. Consistency and health of the gingival connective tissues.

For example, if one uses excessive or uncontrolled force, the tip of the probe can actually penetrate through some of the underlying connective tissue fibers that are located between the most apical extent of the junctional epithelium and the coronal extension of the intact connective fibers. This is particularly true in periodontitis, where the connective tissues are already damaged.[62] Probes of smaller diameter require less force.

Methods of Probing

In the *circumferential probing method,* the probe is inserted into the sulcus at the proximal surface. It is aligned as vertically as possible but with a slight angle toward the midpoint of the tooth buccolingually. Without being withdrawn, the probe is moved along the sulcular crevice until the opposite proximal contact area is reached. In a systematic manner, the probe is then withdrawn and placed in the sulcus of the next tooth. As the sulcus is traversed, Glickman[60] recommends that a "walking" motion of the probe be used (Fig 13–6).

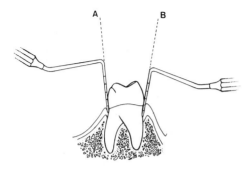

Figure 13–6. Methods of periodontal probing: **A.** Vertical probing method. **B.** Circumferential probing method. The perioprobe is illustrated along the base of the pocket from proximal contact to proximal contact.

In the *vertical probing method,* the measurements are reported as the probe is inserted at distinct separate points around a tooth.[63]

A *two-phase probing method* suggested by Easley[64] can result in a more comprehensive diagnosis. The first phase is accomplished by the circumferential method and consists of using the probe to "feel the epithelial attachment" around the tooth. If there is a deviation from the normal sulcular depth of 2 to 3 mm, a second examination is performed. The second probing, done with a local anesthetic, consists of both vertical and horizontal probing to locate and chart the level of the underlying osseous structures.

The instrument should be parallel to the long axis of the tooth when probing. An exception is when examining the interproximal areas. In this instance, slight probe angulation allows detection of an interproximal crater, which usually occurs below the contact points of adjacent teeth. This pattern of bone loss can easily remain undiagnosed if probing is performed at the proximal line angles only.

Accurate probing requires step-by-step probing around each tooth, with the recording of six clinical depth measurements per tooth. Gingival recession should be recorded as a facial and lingual reading measured from the cementoenamel junction to the gingival margin.

World Health Organization Periodontal Probe

A special periodontal probe has been developed by the World Health Organization (WHO).[65] The probe was designed for two purposes: (1) the measurement of pocket depth, and (2) the detection of subgingival calculus. The probe has a ball tip of 0.5 mm that facilitates the detection of subgingival calculus and the identification of the base of the periodontal pocket. It avoids overextension of pocket depth determination, thus minimizing the tendency for false reading by overmeasurement. The accuracy of pocket depth measurements is facilitated by color coding at the probe end. A black mark starts at 3.5 mm and ends at 5.5 mm (Fig 13–7).

If the color-coded area of the probe remains visible during gentle pocket-depth probing, the pocket is 3 mm or less. If only part of the color-coded area remains visible, the pocket depth is 4 or 5 mm, and if the colored area of the probe totally disappears into the pocket, its depth must be 6 mm or over.

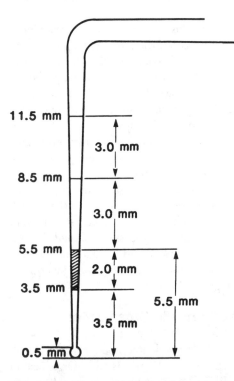

Figure 13–7. Diagram of WHO periodontal probe. It has a ball-tip end to avoid false assessment by overmeasurement and for easier detection of subgingival calculus. The color-coded part from 3.5 to 5.5 mm greatly facilitates rapid assessment of periodontal pocket depth. (*From WHO Technical Report Series 621, 1978.*)

Electronic Periodontal Probes

Active or progressive periodontal disease can best be diagnosed by monitoring changes in alveolar crestal bone and attachment levels over a specified period. At least two examinations must be compared to determine if destruction has occurred. During the past few years, improvements in detecting longitudinal changes in clinical attachment have been introduced by means of a *constant-force electronic probe.*[66,67] The probes input the automated data into a computer.

One example is the Florida Probe, which has been routinely used in the University of Florida's Disease Research Center since 1985.[66,68,69] In one well-controlled study, the Florida Probe was shown to be extremely *accurate,* and the results were *reproducible,* that is, the maximum probing error standard deviation was found to be only about 0.3 mm.[66] The usual range of accuracy of electronic probes is between 0.5 and 0.1 mm. In contrast, the resolution of the standard manual probe is 1 mm.

Other electronic probes are Bausch & Lomb's Interprobe, which uses an optical encoder attached to a disposable plastic fiber tip. Measurements are recorded on a "memory card".[69] The Toronto probe uses air pressure to extend and retract the measuring tip; this action controls the probing force. Measurements are made from the occlusal or incisal edge of the tooth to the depth of the periodontal pocket.[69,70] The Alabama Probe automatically detects the cementoenamel junction and measures the clinical attachment levels to within a 0.2-mm tolerance level.[71]

These automatic electronic probes are very promising because they can shorten the time between two sequential measurements to determine periodontal disease activity. Even when perfected for clinical practitioners, however, the conceptual problem of how to define periodontal disease will still exist.[72]

COMMUNITY PERIODONTAL INDEX OF TREATMENT NEEDS

The Federation Dentaire Internationale (FDI) in collaboration with the Oral Health Unit of the WHO developed the community periodontal index of treatment need (CPITN).[73] In this method the periodontal treatment needs are recorded for six segments (sextants) in each mouth.[74]

The system excludes the third molars, except where the third molars are functioning in the place of the second molars. The sextants involved are anterior segments (canine-to-canine) and right and left posterior segments (premolars and molars) of the upper and lower jaws. A sextant must have at least two functional teeth. The *worst* condition observed within each sextant is recorded using the criteria shown in Table 13–9.

Periodontal Screening and Recordings System

To encourage dentists to screen *individual patients* for undetected periodontal disease, a *periodontal screening and recording system (PSR)* is recommended by the American Dental Association for all patients 18 and older. Only 5 minutes is needed to accomplish the screening (probing). This probing test is somewhat similar to the CPITN, inasmuch as it too divides the mouth into sextants. Scoring is on a similar 0 to 4 basis, with the severe 4 code indicating a probing depth of over 5.5 mm. A special color-coded, beaded explorer is used that permits the PSR to be quickly accomplished.[75]

A weight force of no more than 20 to 25g is considered sufficient to detect pathologic conditions without causing pain to the

TABLE 13–9. CRITERIA USED TO RECORD THE WORST CONDITION OBSERVED IN EACH SEXTANT (CPITN)

Code	Description of the Condition
0	Healthy sextant.
1	Bleeding after gentle probing of the pockets (25g force).
2	Supragingival or subgingival calculus or other plaque retentions.
3	One or more 4 to 5 mm deep pathologic pockets.
4	One or more 6 mm, or deeper, pathologic pockets.

patient (Fig 13–8). *Between* clinicians using manual probing, however, weight-forces can range between 3 and 130g. The degree of probing force by the *same* clinician may differ from one examination to another by a ratio of 2:1.[76] A specially designed, thermoplastic probe, the Sensor Probe, permits the clinician to maintain a constant probing force of 20g that does not vary.[d]

Question 3. Which of the following statements, if any, are correct?

A. The DNA probe can identify Aa, Pg, Pi as a group but not as individual organisms.

B. The circumferential probing technique permits more sites to be sampled by the "walking technique" than does vertical probing, even though the circumferential and the probing techniques give the same results if the same sites are sampled.

C. The WHO probe is more likely to give a *deeper* pocket reading than one without the 0.5-mm ball point.

D. The community periodontal index of treatment needs represents a total score for bleeding, calculus, and pocket depth.

---

[d] Sensor Probe, Pro-Dentec, Professional Dental Technologies, Inc.

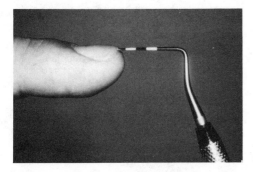

Figure 13–8. Practical test for establishing 20 to 25 g periodontal probing pressure. The periodontal probe is placed underneath the fingernail where the sensitivity approximates that of the bottom of a periodontal pocket. The correct amount of force should not cause pain to the patient on probing.

E.   About *100g* of pressure should be used with a periodontal probe.

SUMMARY

Many indices have been used by various investigators for periodontal disease assessment and evaluation. Like dental caries, periodontal disease is a multifactorial infectious disease. Gingivitis and early stages of periodontitis must be detected early and treated promptly to prevent further progression. The pool of knowledge about the numerical relationship of bacterial species to the incidence and severity of the periodontal diseases is growing. At present there appears to be no bacteriologic criteria by which the susceptibility of periodontal disease can be assessed.

Cyclical remission and exacerbations of inflammation often hinder attempts to quantify the periodontal disease progress over short periods. Therefore periodontal disease risk assessment and evaluation are currently based on the degree of plaque accumulation and its sequela, the extent of gingival crevicular exudate, gingival bleeding, or gingival inflammation. The information obtained from the O'Leary index or plaque and gingival indices of Silness and Löe can be routinely used in an office setting to monitor the effectiveness of a plaque control program. The assessment of crevicular gingival fluid flow and disease markers can often be used in the private dental clinic to indicate periodontal disease activity prior to the appearance of clinical symptoms. Probing to measure pocket depths with manual, or computer-coupled probes and apical radiographs to evaluate bone resorption can be used to assess the periodontal health of either individuals or large populations. The community periodontal index of treatment needs is also suitable for use in comprehensive care systems for adult populations. Because no single periodontal disease risk evaluation can predict the future periodontal status of an individual, the combined use of various methods of periodontal disease risk assessment is strongly suggested. In suspected sites a minimum plaque index and periodontal assessment (which is based on the combination of a gingival bleeding index and a probe depth measurement of the four sides of each tooth should be used).

ANSWERS AND EXPLANATIONS

1. A, B, D
   C—incorrect. The O'Leary index considers only the presence of plaque that is at the cervical portion of the tooth in contact with the gingiva.
   E—incorrect. The OHI is an excellent method of assessing periodontal disease status of populations but not of individuals.
2. A, C, E
   B—incorrect. The PMA considers both the presence and the severity of inflammation of each of the PMA units.
   D—incorrect. Vice versa. The more se-

vere the periodontal disease status, the more gingival crevicular fluid that flows.

3. B, D

A—incorrect. Each of the three prime suspects has its own complementary strand; thus each can be identified separately.

C—incorrect. The 0.5-mm ball point on the WHO probe prevents it from penetrating as deeply into the pocket as one without ball.

E—incorrect. About 25g of pressure should be used; this is about the amount of pressure it takes to cause pain if the probe was used under the fingernail.

SELF-EVALUATION QUESTIONS

1. A routine systematic periodontal evaluation should include the recording of a plaque index, use of a _____, examination of each tooth, as well as _____, to determine bone loss.

2. Five indicators of periodontal disease are _____, _____, _____, _____, and _____.

3. The two popular indices for determining the extent of plaque are the _____ index, and the plaque index of _____ and _____.

4. Greene and Vermillion developed the two oral hygiene indices referred to as the _____ index and the _____ index. The six surfaces sampled in using the index are the buccal surfaces of the upper right and left _____; the labial surfaces of the upper and lower _____; and the lingual surfaces of the lower right and left _____.

5. Both the _____ gingival index and the _____ index assess severity of gingival inflammation on the basis of _____.

6. In the PMA index of Massler and Schour, the P stands for _____, the M for _____, the A for _____.

7. It requires approximately _____ (time) following cessation of personal plaque control methods before gingivitis becomes manifest.

8. The method that counts the number of leukocytes in gingival fluid is known as the _____ (OMR).

9. The _____ is an instrument that is used to evaluate the amount of crevicular fluid that flows in a period of 5 seconds.

10. Two methods by which the flow of crevicular fluid can be estimated are _____ and _____.

11. The periodontal indices used to estimate present and cumulative damage to the periodontium are _____'s index and _____ index.

12. The six teeth used to assess periodontal status by Ramfjord method are _____, _____, _____, _____, _____, and _____.

13. The two generally used methods of periodontal probing are the _____ probing method and the _____ probing method. If they are combined, the resulting method is known as the _____ probing method.

14. The method developed by the Federation Dentaire International (FDI) to assess community periodontal status on the basis of bleeding, calculus presence, and pocket depth is known as the _____.

REFERENCES

1. National Institutes of Health. *Oral Health of United States Children. The National Survey of Dental Caries in U.S. School Children: 1986–1987.* Epidemiology and Oral

Disease Prevention Program, NIDR, U.S. Department of Health and Human Services, NHH Publication No. 89-2247, September, 1989.

2. Page RC, Schroeder HE. Periodontitis in Man and Other Animals. Basel. Karger; 1982.

3. Kay EJ, Blinkhorn AS. The reasons underlying the extraction of teeth in Scotland. *Br Dent J.* 1986; 160:287–90.

4. Bailit HL, Braun R, Maryniuk GA, et al. Is periodontal disease the primary cause of tooth extraction in adults? *J Am Dent Assoc.* 1987; 114:40–45.

5. Stamm JW. Epidemiology of gingivitis. *J Clin Periodontal.* 1986; 13:360–366.

6. Abdellatif HA, Burt BA. An epidemiological investigation into the relative importance of age and oral hygiene status as determinants of periodontitis. *J Dent Res.* 1987; 66: 13–18.

7. Page RC. Oral health of US adults: NIDR 1985 National survey: discussion. *J Public Health Dent.* 1987; 47:200–204.

8. Brady WF. Periodontal disease awareness. *J Am Dent Assoc.* 1984; 109:706–710.

9. Poulsen S. Epidemiology and indices of gingival and periodontal disease. *Pediatr Dent.* 1981; 3:82–88.

10. Burt BA. The distribution of periodontal destruction in the populations of industrialized counties. In: Johnson NW, ed. *Risk Markers for Oral Diseases; Periodontal Diseases*, Vol. 3. Cambridge. Cambridge University Press; 1991: 9–26.

11. Jakush J. (Compiled) Plaque: Current approaches to prevention and control. Workshop discussions on dental plaque control measures and oral hygiene practices. *J Am Diet Assoc.* 1984; 109:690–702.

12. Green LW, Tryon WW, Marks B, et al. Periodontal disease as a function of life events stress. *J Hum Stress.* 1986; 12:32–36.

13. Christen A, Park PR, Graves RC, et al. United States Air Force survey of dental needs, 1977: Methodology and summary of findings. *J Am Dent Assoc.* 1979; 98:726–730.

14. O'Leary TJ, Drake RB, Naylor JE. The plaque control record. *J Periodontal.* 1972; 43·38.

15. Silness J, Löe H. Periodontal disease in pregnancy. II. Correlation between oral hygiene and periodontal condition. *Acta Odontol Scand.* 1964; 22:121–135.

16. Greene JC, Vermillion JR. The oral hygiene index: A method for classifying oral hygiene status. *J Am Diet Assoc.* 1960; 61:172–179.

17. Greene JC, Vermillion JR. The simplified oral hygiene index. *J Am Diet Assoc.* 1964; 68:7–13.

18. Löe H, Silness J. Periodontal disease in pregnancy. I. Prevalence and severity. *Acta Odontol Scand.* 1963; 21:533–551.

19. Massler M. The PMA Index for the assessment of gingivitis. *J Periodontol.* 1969; 38: 592.

20. Genco RJ, Slots J. Host responses in periodontal diseases. *J Dent Res.* 1984; 63:441–451.

21. Löe H. The gingival index, the plaque index, and the retention index system. *J Periodontol.* 1967; 38(suppl part II):610–616.

22. Muhlemann HR, Son S. Gingival sulcus bleeding—a leading symptom in initial gingivitis. *Helv Odontol Acta.* 1971; 15:107–113.

23. Greenstein G. The role of bleeding upon probing in the diagnosis of periodontal disease. *J Periodontol.* 1984; 55:684–688.

24. Shapiro L, Goldman H, Bloom A. Sulcular exudate flow in gingival inflammation. *J Periodontol.* 1979; 50:301–304.

25. Curtis MA. Markers of periodontal disease susceptibility and activity derived from gingival crevicular fluid: Specific vs. Nonspecific analyses. In: Johnson NW, ed. *Risk Markers for Oral Diseases; Periodontal Diseases*, Vol. 3. Cambridge. Cambridge University Press; 1991:254–276.

26. Kryshtalskyj E, Sodek J, Ferrier JM. Correlation of collagenolytic enzymes and inhibitors in gingival crevicular fluid with clinical and microscopic changes in experimental periodontitis in the dog. *Arch Oral Biol.* 1986; 31:21–31.

27. Golub LM, Kleinberg I. Gingival crevicular fluid: A new diagnostic aid in managing the periodontal patient. *Oral Sci Rev.* 1976; 9: 49–61.

28. Mörmann W, Regolati B, Lutz F, et al. Gingivitis fluorescein test in recruits. *Helv Odontol Acta.* 1975; 19:27–30.

29. Woolweaver DA, Koch GG, Crawford JJ, et al. Relation of the orogranulocytic to migratory rate to periodontal disease and blood leukocyte count. *J Dent Res.* 1972; 51:929–939.

30. Hinrickes JE, Bandt CD, Smith JA, et al. A comparison of 3 systems for quantifying gingival crevicular fluid with respect to linearity and the effects of qualitative differences in fluids. *J Clin Periodontol.* 1984; 11:652–661.

31. Suppipat W, Suppipat N. Evaluation of an electronic device for gingival fluid quantitation. *J Periodontol.* 1977; 48:388–394.

32. Cimasoni G. The crevicular fluid updated, In: Myers HM, ed. *Monographs in Oral Science.* Basel, Switzerland. S Karger; 1983:152.

33. Bjorn HL, Koch G, Lindhe J. Evaluation of gingival fluid measurements. *Odont Rev.* 1965; 16:300–307.

34. Brill N. Effect of chewing on flow of tissue fluid into gingival pockets. *Acta Odontol Scand.* 1959; 17:277–284.

35. Johnson NW. Crevicular fluid-based diagnostic tests. *Curr Opin Dent.* 1991; 1:52–65.

36. Russell AL. A system of classification and scoring for prevalence surveys of periodontal diseases. *J Dent Res.* 1956; 35:350–359.

37. Ramfjord SP. Indices for prevalence and incidence of periodontal disease. *J Periodontol.* 1959; 30:51–59.

38. Russell, AL. The periodontal index. *J Periodont.* 1967; 38(suppl part II):13–19.

39. Ramfjord SP. The periodontol disease index (PDI). *J Periodontol.* 1967; 38:602–610.

40. Ramfjord SP. Design of studies or clinical trials to evaluate the effectiveness of agents or procedures for the prevention or treatment of loss of the periodontium. *J Periodontol Res.* 1974; 9(suppl 14):78–93.

41. Bakdash MB. A clinical model for monitoring patients' oral hygiene performance. *Northwest Dent.* 1981; 60:77–83.

42. Dahlen G. Role of suspected periodontopathogens in microbiological monitoring of periodontitis. *Adv Dent Res.* 1993; 7(2):163–174.

43. Slots J, Listgarten MA. *Bacteriodes gingivalis, Bacteroides intermedius,* and *Actinobacillus actinomycetemcomitans* in human periodontal diseases. *J Clin Periodontol.* 1988; 15:85–93.

44. Ciancio SG, Newman MG, Safer R. Recent advances in periodontal diagnosis and treatment: Exploring new treatment alternatives. *J Am Dent Assoc.* 1992: 123:34–43.

45. Ebersole JL, Holt SC. Immunological procedures for diagnosis and risk assessment in periodontal diseases. In: Johnson NW, ed. *Risk Makers for Oral Diseases; Periodontal Diseases,* Vol. 3. Cambridge. Cambridge University Press; 1991:203–227.

46. Wolff L, Dahlen G, Aeppli D. Bacteria as risk markers for periodontitis. *J Periodontol.* 1994; 64:498–510.

47. Beck JD, Kock GG, Zambon JJ, et al. Evaluation of oral bacteria as risk indicators for periodontitis in older adults. *J Periodontol.* 1992; 63:93–99.

48. Lai CH, Oshima K, Slots J, et al. *Wolinella recta* in adult gingivitis and periodontitis. *J Periodontol.* 1992; 27:8–14.

49. Moore WEC. Microbiology of periodontal disease. *J Periodont Res.* 1987; 22:335–341.

50. March PD. Do bacterial markers exist in subgingival plaque for predicting periodontal disease susceptibility? In: Johnson NW, ed. *Risk Makers for Oral Diseases; Periodontal Diseases,* Vol. 3. Cambridge. Cambridge University Press; 1991:365–388.

51. Loesche WJ, Bretz WA, Kerscheeensteiner D, et al. Development of a diagnostic test for anaerobic periodontal infections based on plaque hydrolysis of benzoyl-DL-arginine-naphthylamide. *J Clin Microbiol.* 1990; 28:1551–1559.

52. Beck JD, Koch GG, Rozier RG, et al. Prevalence and risk indicators for periodontal attachment loss in a population of older community-dwelling blacks and whites. *J Periodontol.* 1990; 61:521–528.

53. Slots J. Rapid identification of important periodontal microorganisms by cultivation. *Oral Microbiol Immunol.* 1986; 1:48–55.

54. Loesche WJ, Bretz WA, Lopatin D, et al. Multi-center clinical evaluation of a chairside method for detecting certain periodontopathic bacteria in periodontal disease. *J Periodontol.* 1990; 61:189–196.

55. Savitt ED, Strzempko MN, Vaccaro KK, et al. Comparison of cultural methods and DNA probe analyses for the detection of *Actinobacillus actinomy-cetemcomitans, Bacteroides gingivalis,* and *Bacteroides intermedius* in subgingival plaque samples. *J Periodontol.* 1988; 59:431–438.

56. Strzempko MN, Simon SL, French CK, et al. A cross reactivity study of whole genomic DNA probes for *Haemophilus actinomy-cetemcomitans, Bacteroides intermedius* and *Bacteroides gingivalis. J Dent Res.* 1987; 66:1543–1546.

57. Zambon JJ, Bochacki V, Genco RJ. Immunological assays for putative periodontal pathogens. *Oral Microbiol Immunol.* 1986; 1:39–44.

58. Yukna RA. HTR polymer grafts in human periodontal osseous defects. I. 6-month clinical results. *J Periodontol.* 1990; 61:633–642.

59. Proceedings of the workshop on quantitative evaluation of periodontal diseases by physical measurement techniques. *J Dent Res.* 1979; 58:547–553.

60. Glickman I. The gingiva. In: Carranza FA, ed. *Glickman's Clinical Periodontology,* 5th ed. Philadelphia, Penn. WB Saunders; 1979.

61. Chilton NW, Miller MF. Diagnostic methods and the epidemiology of periodontal disease. In: *International Conference on Research in the Biology of Periodontal Disease,* Chicago, Ill; June 12–15, 1977; 94–118.

62. Saglie R, Johansen JR, Flotra L. The zone of completely and partially destructed periodontal fibers in pathological pockets. *J Clin Periodontol.* 1975; 2:198–202.

63. Johnson NW. Detection of high-risk groups and individuals for periodontal diseases. *Int Dent J.* 1989; 39:33–47.

64. Easley JR. Methods of determining alveolar osseous form. *J Periodontol.* 1967; 38:112–118.

65. World Health Organization. *Epidemiology,* *Etiology and Prevention of Periodontal Diseases.* Geneva, Switzerland. WHO Technical Report Series, No. 621. 1978.

66. Clark WB, Yang MCK, Magnusson I. Measuring clinical attachment: Reproducibility of relative measurements with an electronic probe. *J Periodontol.* 1992; 63:831–838.

67. Yang MCK, Marks RG, Magnusson I, et al. Reproducibility of an electronic probe in relative attachment level measurements. *J Clin Periodontol.* 1992; 19:541–548.

68. Osborn J, Soltenberg J, Huso B, et al. Comparison of measurement variability using a standard and constant force periodontal probe. *J Periodontol.* 1990; 61:497–503.

69. Goodson JM. Diagnosis of periodontitis by physical measurement: Interpretation from episodic disease hypothesis. *J Periodontol.* 1992; 63:373–382.

70. Karim M, Birek P, McCulloch CA. Controlled force measurements of gingival-attachment level made with the Toronto automated probe using electronic guidance. *J Clin Periodontol.* 1990; 17:594–600.

71. Jeffcoat MK, Reddy MS. Progression of probing attachment loss in adult periodontitis. *J Periodontol.* 1991; 62:185–189.

72. Jeffcoat MK, Jeffcoat RL, Jens SC, et al. A new periodontal probe with automated cemento-enamel junction detection. *J Clin Periodontol.* 1986; 13:276–280.

73. Ainamo J, Barmes D, Beagrie G, et al. Development of the World Health Organization (WHO) community periodontal index of treatment needs (CPITN). *Int Dent J.* 1982; 32:281–291.

74. O'Leary TJ. A study of periodontal examination system. *J Dent Res.* 1964; 43:794. Abstract 118.

75. *Periodontal Screening and Recording (PSR) System.* American Dental Association and The American Academy of Periodontology. Sponsored by Procter and Gamble, Chicago, IL. 1993.

76. Lang NP, Nyman S, Sen CH, et al. Bleeding on probing as it relates to probing force and gingival health. *J Clin Periodontol.* 1991; 18:257–261.

Chapter 14

Sugar and Other Sweeteners

Bruce A. Matis
Laurence P. Crigger

Objectives

At the end of this chapter it will be possible to

1. Name the three sugars that are composed of molecules of glucose, fructose, or galactose, all of which can produce caries.
2. Describe some industrial attributes and disadvantages of sucrose.
3. Discuss statutory and regulatory safeguards on the introduction of new sweetener products to the marketplace and laws governing the withdrawal of sweeteners that are carcinogenic, teratogenic, or mutagenic.
4. List three polyols that are sweeteners and cite their advantages and disadvantages for caries incidence.
5. Defend the Food and Drug Administration (FDA) for either removing or attempting to remove saccharin and cyclamate from the marketplace.
6. Name a sweetener that has recently received FDA approval, and list three more that are candidates for approval.

Introduction

To most people the term *sugar* refers to the common household foodstuff, table sugar (sucrose). Yet sucrose is only one of many naturally occurring sugars used by humans. Sugars represent only one class of sweeteners that can satisfy our taste for sweets.

Technically the term *sugar* applies both to monosaccharides (simple sugars), of which glucose, fructose, and galactose are the commonest, and disaccharides (two simple sugar molecules linked together), of which sucrose, lactose, and maltose are the commonest. Sucrose is composed of one glucose linked to one fructose unit; lactose, of a glucose and a galactose unit; and maltose, of two glucose units.

Sweeteners can be either *caloric* or *noncaloric* (low in calories) and are interpreted by taste buds as sweet. Caloric sweeteners include monosaccharides and disaccharides, corn syrup, and other sweeteners such as the polyols ("sugar alcohols"). Noncaloric sweeteners, which are also called *intense sweeteners,* include saccharin, aspartame, acesulfame K, and a host of other lesser known products.

SENSATION OF TASTE

It is difficult to determine whether taste is genetically linked, acquired in utero, neonatal, or influenced by visual, auditory, or taste stimuli during infancy, early childhood, or even adulthood. Theoretically an individual can initially acquire and refine taste desires in any of the following stages: (1) in utero, (2) during breast or bottle feeding, (3) while passively being fed solids, (4) while more actively seeking different nonspecific foods, and (5) while purposely seeking specific foods.[1]

Taste buds are present and functioning before birth, a fact demonstrated by injecting sweetening agents into the amniotic fluid during the fourth month of pregnancy.[2] The sweetened amniotic fluid results in an increased rate of swallowing by the fetus. At birth, infants show a taste preference for sucrose, and their taste cells are more responsive to sucrose than to other sugars. Whether it is simply a pleasurable taste or a true metabolic need is not known.

Taste sensation is initiated by the arrival of a stimulus at the taste buds. Taste recognition occurs when the receptor sites of the cells of the taste buds carry, by cranial nerves, a qualitative and quantitative message to the brain. The message is processed, and the stimulus is recognized as either sweet, sour, salty, or bitter, or some combination of these four.

THE HISTORIC IMPORTANCE OF SWEETENERS

The first recorded evidence of sweeteners dates to 2600 BC. Drawings in Egyptian tombs illustrate beekeeping practices for honey production. The honey was reserved for the rich and powerful.

Cultivating sugarcane began in southeast Asia, India, and China around 100 BC. The earliest known written reference to sugarcane occurs in a scroll dating to AD 375. The Arabs developed the first process for refining sugarcane into sucrose. The cultivation of sugarcane was practiced in southern Europe in the 13th century, and eventually knowledge of it spread to the New World. The cultivation of the root crop called sugar beets started more than 200 years ago.[3]

North American Indians had devised a method of bleeding the sap of the sugar maple tree long before the Pilgrims arrived in Massachusetts. The sugar in the sap of the mature sugar maple is almost exclusively sucrose.

Sweeteners made from corn starch began to appear around 1910. The lesser sweetness of the sugars derived from corn starch, mainly glucose (also referred to as dextrose), was responsible for characterizing them as *substitute* sweeteners. This identity imposed restrictions on their use. Since the last decade, new chemical processes have resulted in the ability to convert the glucose contained in corn starch to a high-fructose corn syrup (HFCS). Because fructose is twice as sweet as glucose, its use has rapidly increased.

The amount of HFCS used as a sweetener surpassed that of sucrose in 1985. Aspartame, which is approximately 180 times sweeter than sucrose, is the most frequently used noncaloric sweetener. From its discovery in 1965, it is now being used by more than 100 million people worldwide.[4]

SUCROSE

Sucrose is the most commonly used sweetener. The use of this natural sweetener in the United States has decreased from the high of 102 lb per person in 1971 to 64 lb per person in 1992 (Fig 14–1).[5] In the past this usage was considered consumption data; however, this is a misnomer. The statistics actually represent the quantity of sweeteners delivered to commercial establishments to be used in various ways. It does not account for any loss, due to waste. It also does not include any additional natural sugars consumed. It has been reported that up to 31% of total sugars consumed by adolescents are hidden sugars in foods, such as in milk and fruit.[6]

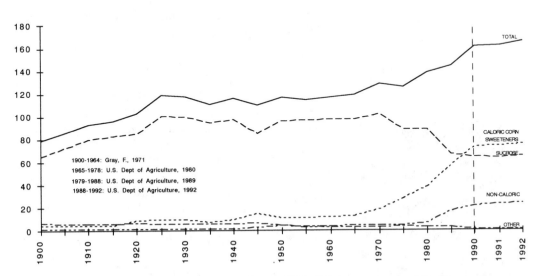

Figure 14–1. Sweetener use in the United States, 1900–1992 in pounds per capita. *(Used with permission of Gray F.[7]; U.S. Department of Agriculture.[8]; U.S. Department of Agriculture.[9]; U.S. Department of Agriculture.[5]*

Individual variation in consumption also occurs. Males generally consume more than females, and teenagers are by far the greatest consumers. Peak consumptions occur among 15- to 18-year old males.[10] A decreased consumption rate occurs among members of large families. The differences in consumption rates in socioeconomic classes do not appear to be as great as in the past when sucrose was a rare commodity and accessible only to the privileged (Fig 14–2).

Uses of Sucrose

Sucrose has several attributes that make it desirable for the food industry. It is ideal in the following roles:

- *Sweetening agent:* The character of the sweet taste can be varied according to pH and temperature used to make a product, as well as by its interaction with other ingredients in the formulation. The level of sweetness is important to the acceptance of certain foods.
- *Flavor blender and modifier:* In some foods such as mayonnaise, sucrose is a flavor blender; in other foods, such as pickles, it reduces the acidic bite and sour taste.

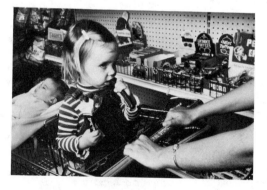

Figure 14–2. I'm not sure if it's genetic or acquired. I just like it.

- *Texture and bodying agent:* Sucrose gives a texture that is highly acceptable to consumers. It provides body and a distinctive "mouth feel" to food products.
- *Dispersing/lubricating agent:* In dry packaged mixes, sucrose is used as an agent to keep other ingredients from packing too closely. This, in turn, permits a better blending of the ingredients during food preparation.
- *Caramelization/color agent:* Caramelization during baking produces a brown color, which increases acceptance. It provides a desirable, characteristic flavor and aroma to the food product.
- *Bulking agent:* When a noncaloric sweetener that may be 200 times sweeter than sugar replaces sucrose, other ingredients must be added to replace the lost sucrose "bulk" to maintain the food's normal appearance and consistency.

Earlier in this century, home canning and baking resulted in a higher per capita consumption of sucrose than for industrially processed foods. Modern-day affluence, the desire to be liberated from the kitchen, and a higher percentage of working women are factors that have helped reverse the trend. Seventy-five percent of the sucrose manufactured between 1910 and 1930 was delivered to households. In 1950, industrial uses of sucrose surpassed that used at home.[3] The food-processing industry has greatly changed the eating habits of the average American by increasing the output of processed foods. No longer are there only three meals during the day; instead, individual food intake patterns have been extended to include a continuous morning-to-night intake of sucrose-containing snacks and beverages.

Sucrose has several disadvantages that restrict its industrial use.

- The high concentration (osmolarity) used in canning often causes shrinkage and wrinkling of canned fruits. Both characteristics detract from the visual appeal of the product.
- It absorbs moisture (hygroscopic) and accordingly makes it difficult to freeze dry food containing high concentrations of sucrose.
- It chars at high temperatures, thus it cannot be used to sweeten items that must be fried—bacon, for instance.
- It supports bacterial growth; hence its use in prepared food increases the potential for bacterial contamination and spoilage.

Evaluation of the Health Aspects of Sucrose

Prior to 1958 few regulatory constraints existed on the introduction of new products into foods. If problems developed, the Food and Drug Administration (FDA) had to prevail on the conscience of the manufacturer to withdraw the product or to prove in court that the product was not safe. Both options were rather daunting because considerable financial interest was usually involved. In 1958, Congress passed the *Foods Additive Amendment* that required *preliminary* marketing clearance. The act required the following information on additives: (1) chemical composition, (2) method of manufacture, (3) analytic method used for the detection of the additive, (4) proof that the additive accomplished its intended effect and that it did not occur in excess of the amount required to achieve that effect, and (5) proof that it was safe.[11] The burden of proof in substantiating any of these factors resided in the petitioner applying for the clearance—and not with the FDA.

The *Foods Additive Amendment* decreed that all components added to processed foodstuffs prior to 1958 were classified as *food ingredients*, whereas those added thereafter were called *food additives*. With this act, Congress authorized a list of food ingredients which it called *generally regarded as safe* (GRAS). Sucrose was listed as a food ingredient and placed on the GRAS list. At that time items on the list were considered as relatively immune from future regulatory action. With the passage of time, however, all the items listed on the original GRAS list of food ingredients have come under review.[12] This action occurred as new information raised questions about their safety.

The FDA in 1986 formed a Sugars Task Force that critically reviewed all of the recent scientific literature addressing potentially adverse health effects associated with sugars consumption. They investigated the cause-and-effect relationship between the use of sugar and diabetes, cardiovascular disease, hypertension, heart disease, and obesity. They concluded that no conclusive body of research links any of the above to sugar consumed in moderation.[10] The concluding summary paragraph of the report entitled "Evaluation of the Health Aspects of Sucrose as a Food Ingredient" states:

1. "Reasonable evidence exists that sucrose is a contributor to the formation of dental caries when used at the levels that are now current and in the manner now practiced.
2. Other than the contribution made to dental caries, there is no clear evidence in the available information on sucrose that demonstrates a hazard to the public when used at the levels that are now current and in the manner now practiced. One of the seven major recommendations of the *Surgeon General's Report on Nutrition and Health* in 1988 was to "Avoid too much sugar."[13]

Role in Caries Formation

Sucrose has been called the "arch criminal of dental caries."[14] Eating large amounts of sucrose can increase the dental caries incidence, but a great deal of epidemiologic evidence indicates that this is not entirely true.[12] Much depends on the physical form in which sucrose is eaten, other ingredients of the food with which it is eaten, the presence of certain acid-producing bacteria in dental plaque, the frequency of ingestion, the time of ingestion such as before bedtime, and undoubtedly on other circumstances not as yet comprehended.[15]

Bowen, from the National Institutes of Health, stated at the National Symposium on Dental Nutrition that "Evidence incriminating sugars has continued to accumulate from the results of epidemiological and animal research and has now reached such proportions that no reasonable person would deny that frequent consumption of sugars by caries susceptible humans will result in the development of dental caries."[16] Two animal studies and four human clinical studies have contributed to the understanding of the importance of sugar in the development of caries.

In 1955, the first animal study[17] was conducted with rodents in a gnotobiotic (germ-free) environment. Two groups of rats were used. The first group was fed a caries-producing diet containing large amounts of sugar. The second group was fed the same diet, but at the same time specific microorganisms were introduced to the otherwise germ-free environment. Those rats receiving the cariogenic diet alone did *not* develop caries; those with the cariogenic diet plus the bacteria *did* develop lesions (Table 14–1). Observations at that time and since have conclusively demonstrated that certain microorganisms and strains of organisms are more caries-productive than others.

In a second rodent study,[18] one group of rats was fed a caries-producing diet by

TABLE 14–1. DENTAL CARIES IN GERM-FREE RATS AND CARIES-FREE RATS INOCULATED WITH KNOWN BACTERIAL CELLS (ENTEROCOCCI PREDOMINATING)

Group	Microbial State	No. of Rats	No. of Rats Developing Molar Caries
A	Germ-free	9	0
B	Inoculated with Enterococci plus others	13	13

(*Copyright by the American Dental Association. Reprinted by permission. From Orland et al., J Am Dent Assoc. 50, 1955.[17]*)

means of a stomach tube, with no food coming in contact with the teeth. No caries resulted. When the same diet was fed orally and allowed to *come in contact* with the teeth, caries *did* occur (Table 14–2).

These two studies conclusively demonstrate that (1) bacteria are essential for caries development, regardless of diet, and (2) the action of the sugar in carious development is *local*, not systemic.

Several human studies have supported and further clarified the animal studies. Two of the most cited occurred at Hopewood House[19] in Australia and at Vipeholm in Sweden.[20]

Hopewood House was an orphanage in Australia that accommodated up to 82 children. From its beginning, sugar and other refined carbohydrates were excluded from the children's diet. Carbohydrates were served in the form of whole meal bread, soy beans, wheat germ, oats, rice, potatoes, and some molasses. Dairy products, fruits, raw vegetables, and nuts were prominently featured in the typical menu. As illustrated in Figure 14–3, dental surveys of these children from the ages of 5 to 11 years revealed a greatly *reduced* caries incidence compared with the state school population in that age group. The children's oral hygiene was poor, with about 75% suffering from

TABLE 14–2. CARIES IN RATS FED A DECAY-PRODUCING DIET VIA NORMAL AND STOMACH TUBE ROUTES

Group	Method of Feeding	No. of Rats	Avg. No. of Carious Molars	Avg. No. of Carious Lesions
A	Normal	13	5.0	6.7
B	Stomach tube	13	0	0

(*From Kite, Shaw, and Sognnaes, J Nutr. 42, 1950.*[18])

gingivitis. When the children became old enough to earn wages in the outside economy, they deviated from the original diet. A steep increase of decayed, missing, and filled teeth (DMFT) after the age of 11 years indicates that the teeth did not acquire any permanent resistance to caries (Fig 14–3).

The Vipeholm study was conducted at a mental institution in that city located in southern Sweden. Adult patients on a nutritionally adequate diet were observed for several years and found to develop caries at a slow rate. Subsequently the patients were divided into seven groups to compare the cariogenicity accompanying various changes in frequency and consistency of carbohydrate intake. Sucrose was included in the diet as toffee, chocolate, caramel, in bread or in liquid form. Caries increased significantly when foods containing sucrose were ingested *between* meals. In addition to the *frequency* of eating, the *consistency* of the sugar-containing food was very important. Sticky or adhesive forms of food that maintained high sugar levels in the mouth for a longer time were much more cariogenic than forms that were rapidly cleared.

The Vipeholm study also demonstrated that it was possible to increase the average consumption of sugar from about 30 to 330 g per day with little increase in caries, *provided* the additional sugar was consumed at mealtime in solution form.[20]

Other less publicized studies have emphasized the close relationship of sucrose exposure to caries production. A Swedish dental scientist, von der Fehr, and colleagues instituted a dental study[21] in which all oral hygiene procedures were discontinued and the subjects rinsed their mouths nine times a day with a 50% sucrose solution. Within 23 days demineralization of the teeth could be demonstrated. This study emphasized the importance of reducing between-meal snacks of sucrose-rich food, especially in people with poor oral hygiene.

Finally, some people suffer from a condition known as hereditary fructose intolerance (HFI). After the intake of fructose, these persons become nauseated, vomit, and sweat excessively; malaise, tremor, coma, and convulsions may develop. As a result,

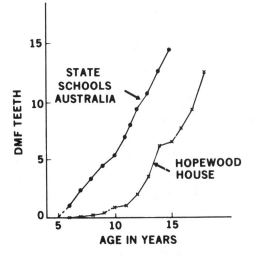

Figure 14–3. Plot of the mean number of DMFT versus chronologic age in state schools of Australia and in Hopewood House. (*Reprinted by permission. Marthaler, Caries Res. 1, 1967.*)[19]

these individuals learn to carefully avoid foods with fructose or sucrose where fructose is one of the metabolic products. Those HFI individuals who have survived this disorder by successfully avoiding fructose or sucrose from any source are either caries-free or have very few caries.[22] The low prevalence of caries in HFI patients indicates that starchy foods alone do not produce decay, whereas sugary foods do (Table 14–3).

What is the threshold level of sugar content above which a food is highly cariogenic? The answer requires some value judgment. Many animal and human studies have followed the drop and recovery of plaque pH following consumption of specific foods. Data tend to indicate that a "safe," or at least an acceptable level of sugar consumption in which the incidence of caries is acceptably low, is 10 kg per person per year. When fluoride is widely available, the acceptable level increases to 15 kg per person per year.[23]

An epidemiologic study of the caries prevalence in 12-year-olds and the per capita sugar use was conducted in 47 countries.[24] The data reveal a statistically significant relationship between the availability of sugar and the number of DMFT. When daily per capita supply of sugar was less than 50 g, the DMFT index was less than 3.0 (Table 14–4). The achievement of this low caries-prevalence rate in 12-year-olds is a goal of the World Health Organization (WHO).

Streptococcus mutans has generally come to be regarded as the microorganism having the greatest cariogenic potential in man. Sucrose enhances the colonization and growth of *S mutans* in dental plaque more than other monosaccharides or disaccharides. These bacteria (1) ferment sucrose rapidly, producing acids; (2) convert sucrose to extracellular polysaccharides that facilitate the adherence of the bacteria to teeth and may function as a reserve of fermentable carbohydrate necessary for the production of acids; and (3) reduce plaque permeability that in turn decreases the rate at which saliva can neutralize or dilute acids formed in the depths of the plaque.[25]

Question 1. Which of the following statements, if any, are correct?

A.   Some sweeteners with a per-gram calorie content equal to sucrose can result in a lesser calorie intake because of their intense sweetness.

TABLE 14–3. HEREDITARY FRUCTOSE INTOLERANT (HFI) SUBJECTS AND CONTROL SUBJECTS COMPARED

	HFI Subjects (*n* = 17)	Control Subjects (*n* = 14)
DMFT score	2.1	14.3
Plaque index	1.2	1.2
Average number sucrose-containing food items per day	0.83	4.32
Average intake of sucrose per day (g)	2.5	48.2
Average intake of carbohydrates per day (g)	163	185
Mean age (years)	29.1	26.5
Percent caries-free	59	0

(*Reprinted by permission. Copyright by the American Dental Association. From Newbrun et al., J Am Dent Assoc. 101, 1980.*[22])

TABLE 14–4. SUGAR SUPPLY AND CARIES PREVELANCE IN 12-YEAR-OLD CHILDREN OF 47 COUNTRIES

DMFT Index	Sugar supply (g/person/day)		
	50	*50–120*	*120*
3.0	21 countries	9 countries	
3.0–5.0		9 countries	1 country
5.0		1 country	6 countries

(Reprinted by permission. From Sreebny LM. Community Dent Oral Epidemiol. 10:1982.[24])

B. The *Foods Additive Amendment of 1958* established the basis for the GRAS list.

C. A *food ingredient* is less subject to FDA study than a *food additive.*

D. Approximately 50% more sugar is required in the diet of gnotobiotic (germ-free) rats to induce caries, than in the diet of control rats.

E. Individuals with hereditary fructose intolerance (HFI) usually have more caries than sugar-tolerant individuals.

CORN SWEETENER USE

The large increase in the cost of sucrose in 1974 prompted a search for a less expensive alternative. The availability of high-fructose corn syrup (HFCS) with 42% fructose provided one alternative. By late 1977 a process to produce 55% fructose was developed. The use of HFCS per capita has jumped from 0.7 lb in 1970 to 51.3 lb in 1992.[5] In early 1980, the whole-sale list price of HFCS was approximately two thirds that of sucrose. The caloric sweetener HFCS seems to be reaching maximum use on a per capita basis, and its production is not expected to continue increasing as rapidly in the future as it did in the 1970s and early 1980s. High-fructose corn syrup use in soft drinks accounted for over 70% of its use in 1992.[26]

A study by Scheinin[27] determined the relative cariogenicity of fructose and sucrose. Fructose was used exclusively by one group who developed 3.8 new carious lesions, whereas the sucrose group developed 7.2 new lesions. The large decrease in caries incidence in the United States may partially be explained by the increased use of HFCS sweeteners with a concurrent decrease in a sweetener that appears to be much more cariogenic—sucrose.

The consumption of glucose and dextrose corn syrup has remained fairly constant over the past 60 years at 3.5 lb. The three leading uses are the brewing industry, confectionary, and cereal products.[9]

Effects of Other Sugars

Fructose, maltose, and lactose are also caloric sugars found in nature. A considerable amount of the first two sugars is contained in fruits and vegetables. Lactose in varying concentrations is present in all mammalian milk. The sweetness of these other sugars ranges from 0.2 to 1.8 times the sweetness of sucrose (Table 14–5).

The subjective evaluation of the sweetness of a substance is usually judged by tasting panels. Several methods are used: (1) having the members of the panel write down in their own words a subjective perception of the sweetness, time of onset, aftertaste, or other descriptive terms; and (2) comparing the test sweetener against a ref-

TABLE 14–5. RELATIVE SWEETNESS* OF SUGAR AND OTHER SWEETENERS

Substances	Sweetness	Substances	Sweetness
Lactose	.2	Naringin dihydrochalcone†	100
Galactose	.3	Mesperidin dihydrochalcone†	100
Maltose	.3	Aspartame	180
Sorbitol	.5	Acesulfame K	200
Mannitol	.6	Stevioside	300
Glucose	.7	Saccharin	300–500
Sucrose	1.0	Sucralose	600
Xylitol	1.0	Neohesperidin dihydrochalcone†	2000
Glycerol	1.0	Thaumatin†	2000
Invert sugar (glucose–fructose)	1.3	Alitame	2000
Fructose	1.7	Monellin†	3000
Cyclamate sodium	30	Sweetener 2000	10,000
Ammoniated glycyrrhizin†	50		

*Sucrose is assigned a value of 1.0. Sweetness depends on concentration, pH, temperature, and sensitivity of taster.
†Sweeteners of natural origin, which are found in various fruits, berries, roots, and leaves of plants.

erence sweetener, possibly sucrose. These two evaluations indicate *quality* but not *intensity* of the test material. For intensity, *threshold detection* and *recognition* levels are noted. For threshold detection testing, extreme dilutions of the sweetener are used. The *threshold level* is the lowest concentration at which sweetness can be *discerned*. Recognition tests are based on the least concentration at which a panel can *recognize the specific sweetener* being tested. Testing is accomplished with the sample solutions at 37°C because temperature does modify taste perception. The threshold level is much lower than the recognition level.

The Polyols as Sweeteners

The most commonly known polyols include sorbitol, mannitol, and xylitol. These polyols are not sugars in the strictest sense. Each molecule resembles a sugar, with the exception that an alcohol grouping is attached to one carbon atom.

The polyols have similar *caloric content* to sucrose. Because sorbitol and mannitol are only half as sweet as sucrose, there

may be a tendency to increase caloric intake with the use of these two polyols. Xylitol has the same sweetness as sucrose. Polyols have similar physical characteristics as sucrose, and their substitution does not change the customary size and weight of a product. Browning or caramelization, however, do not occur with food products that have been sweetened with polyols.

Sorbitol. Sorbitol, first isolated in 1872, is mainly used in chewing gum, toothpaste, and some candy. The dental interest in sorbitol results from its use in so-called sugar-free gum, which has been claimed to be noncariogenic. This claim of noncariogenicity has not been substantiated by clinical trials, but intraoral studies have indicated that the plaque pH seldom drops below 5.7 after chewing sorbitol-sweetened gum.[28] The need for further studies is emphasized by the fact that *S mutans* is known to metabolize sorbitol.

Mannitol. Mannitol, which occurs naturally in seaweed, is also derived from the sugar mannose. This sweetener is metabolized very slowly by oral microorganisms; therefore it is thought to have a low cariogenic potential. Mannitol is used in toothpastes, mouth rinses, and as a dusting agent for chewing gum.

Xylitol. The polyol that has received the greatest amount of attention by the dental profession is xylitol.[29] Xylitol is derived from birch trees, corn cobs, and oats, as well as from bananas and certain mushrooms. As with other polyols, the appearance and texture of xylitol is similar to sucrose. Its cost is about 10 times that of sucrose. Even with a significant expansion in xylitol production, the cost cannot be reduced by much more than half.

It is the best nutritive sucrose substitute with respect to caries prevention. It has been shown to be nonacidogenic and therefore noncariogenic.[a] Microbiologic experiments have shown that xylitol cannot be used by microorganisms to produce tooth-destroying acids.[30] Some have reported this polyol to be anticariogenic.[b][31,32] It is now felt that this property is the result of the (1) increased rate of salivary flow and accompanying rise in pH and (2) the increase in salivary calcium concentration that occurs during chewing gum. These two actions also occur when chewing a sorbitol- or even a sucrose-based gum,[33] however the incidence of caries is decreased only with the xylitol- and sorbitol-based gums, with the xylitol-based gum proving to be the much less cariogenic of the two.[34]

Xylitol has been found to inhibit the growth and metabolism of certain strains of microorganisms, such as *S mutans*,[29] to the same degree as some antimicrobials.[35] The main use of xylitol appears to be where it is used in partial substitution for other sugars. This takes advantage of its microbial action, with the food item still being competitive in price.

Question 2. Which of the following statements, if any, are correct?

    A. Hopewood House in Australia established the fact that *restricting sugar intake* reduces caries incidence, whereas the Vipeholm study in Sweden demonstrated that *frequency of intake* and *consistency* of sugar products are important in evaluating cariogenicity of foods.

    B. A higher concentration of a sweetener is required for recognition than for detection.

    C. It is possible for a noncariogenic substance to be anticariogenic, but not all noncariogenic agents are anticariogenic.

    D. All products with *polyol* sweeteners are considered sugar-free.

    E. Xylitol has the potential of preventing, arresting, and reversing incipient caries.

INTENSE SWEETENERS

The need for intense sweeteners is acute. For primary preventive dentistry practices, a noncarious product that could be used in oral medications, mouth rinses, dentifrices, and all forms of "candy" or between-meal snacks is highly desirable. The American Dental Association (ADA) is encouraging the use of intense, or artificial, sweeteners. It stated "For many years the ADA has encouraged the use of sugar substitutes and therefore it welcomes the development and FDA approval of new artificial sweeteners that are shown to be safe and noncontributary to tooth decay. Studies have shown that

---

[a] Noncariogenic = Does not cause caries.
[b] Anticariogenic = Reverses the caries process prior to cavitation (by enhancing remineralization).

sugar rich snack foods can contribute to tooth decay and that replacing their sugar content with an artificial sweetener results in fewer cavities."[36]

More than 10 million diabetics live in the United States. Until noncaloric sweeteners became available, it was common to tell diabetics that they must forego sweet foods. One of the nation's leading health problems is obesity. An intense sweetener should permit caloric reduction without sacrificing palatability. A sweetener with a low physical weight is also highly desirable for reducing the size of product packages and the shipping cost of goods. Weight and bulk are major considerations in foods being considered for extended space flights.

Very small amounts of intense sweeteners can be used to achieve acceptable levels of sweetness. Even though the cost of these sweeteners may be 100 times greater than an equal amount of sucrose, they are 90% more economical than sucrose because their equivalent sweetness can be 1000 times that of sucrose.

The US Senate Select Committee on Nutrition and Human Needs in 1977 proposed as a dietary goal for the United States that no more than 10% of the total daily calories be from refined sugars and other caloric sweeteners. In 1978, the average daily diet provided 18%[37] of total calories through sugar and caloric sweeteners. In 1986, however, that percentage had dropped to 11%[10] (Fig 14–4). Reaching closer to this goal was made possible by a reduction in sugar intake and an increase in the use of acceptable intense sweeteners.

The three most popular intense sweeteners in the United States are saccharin, aspartame, and acesulfame-K.

Saccharin. Saccharin is considered approximately 300 times sweeter than sucrose. In 1988, approximately 6 lb per person

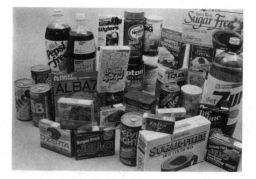

Figure 14–4. Sweeteners are making significant inroads into the sucrose market.

(sugar-sweetness equivalent weight) was delivered for use as a sweetener in the United States, a drop from 10 lb in 1984. Due to its intense sweetness, the use of saccharin is only about 4% as costly as an equivalent sweetness derived from sucrose.[38] Saccharin is compatible with most food and drug ingredients. It is stable in an aqueous solution and can be used in most formulated and processed foods over a considerable pH range. Its major deterrent, its metallic aftertaste, can be recognized by most users.

On April 15, 1977, on the basis of alleged carcinogenicity the revocation of previous approvals for saccharin was proposed by the FDA, with the recommendation that saccharin be classified as a drug, meaning it could only be sold by prescription. This decision set off a consumer furor across the nation, resulting in bills being passed in Congress to postpone the ban on saccharin for 18 months. Congress has reacted with a series of 2-year moratoriums that prohibit the FDA from banning use of saccharin in diet sodas and food while permitting more time for further research. In 1987 and 1992, five-year moratoriums were passed by Congress. The moratorium was to be in effect through May 1, 1997. To everyone's surprise, in 1992, the FDA formally withdrew its 1977 proposal to ban the use of saccharin. The agency did not address the safety of saccharin, but stated it would re-propose the ban later should such action be warranted.[39]

Aspartame. Aspartame, better known by the tradename NutraSweet, is void of an unpleasant aftertaste. It is a dipeptide of two naturally occurring amino acids, phenylalanine and aspartic acid, but it is not found in nature. It was a serendipitous discovery by James Schlatter, a chemist with G. D. Searle & Company, who produced aspartame in 1965 while working on a new antiulcer drug.[4] Aspartame has 4 Cal/g, which is characteristic of proteins; however, because it is 180 times sweeter than sucrose, the caloric intake is insignificant.

Aspartame was originally approved for use in July 1974 by the FDA as an artificial sweetener. During the review period following the initial approval, objections were filed. In December 1975 the FDA retracted its aspartame approval pending a more detailed inspection of the manufacturer's research and public hearings. In July 1981, aspartame was reapproved for use as an artificial sweetener. In 8 years its per capita use increased to 14 lb (sugar-sweetness equivalent weight). More people have voluntarily consumed considerable quantities of aspartame within a few years of its introduction than of any other new chemical entity in history.[40] It was about 30 times more expensive than saccharin; however, in 1992, the Nutrasweet patent expired and the cost of the sweetener decreased substantially. In Canada the expiration of the patent precipitated a 50% drop in cost for the product. Approved uses include free-flowing sugar substitute for table use, and for use by manufacturers in over 100 products, such as cold cereals, drink mixes, instant coffee, instant tea, soft drinks, gelatins, puddings, pie fillings, toppings, dairy products, and multivitamin food supplements.[41] The FDA Commissioner concluded his statement on aspartame before the Committee on Labor and Human Resources of the United States Senate by stating, "in conclusion, we do not have any medical or scientific evidence that undermines our confidence in the safety of aspartame."[42] Aspartame is a flavor enhancer, especially for sweetening acid flavors. It is also a flavor extender, lengthening the period of flavor for chewing gum for five to seven times as long as gums sweetened with sugar. Aspartame appears to be noncariogenic. The ADA has issued a statement supporting the approval of aspartame as a sweetener.[43] *People with phenylketonuria (PKU) should avoid the intake of aspartame* because of its phenylalanine content. Products sweetened with aspartame must be labeled with the statement "Phenylketonurics: Contains Phenylalanine."

Acesulfame K. Acesulfame K is a noncaloric sweetener 200 times sweeter than sucrose, with a pleasant taste. Its sweetness is quickly perceptible and diminishes gradually without any unpleasant aftertaste. It is a derivative of acetoacetic acid. It is marketed under the tradename "Sunette" by the Hoechst Celanese Corporation and is classified as a noncariogenic sweetener.

This sweetener was discovered in 1967; however, it was not approved for use by the FDA in the United States until the summer of 1988. Acesulfame has been tested in more than 90 studies and was in widespread use in 20 countries before it was approved for use in the United States. In approving the sweetener the FDA stated that the studies it has reviewed do "not show any toxic effects that could be attributed to the sweetener."[44] It is approved for use in such items as toothpastes, mouth washes, pharmaceuticals, dry beverage mixes, instant coffee and tea, chewing gum, gelatins, puddings, and as a tabletop sweetener. It has a synergistic action with other low-calorie sweeteners, as do most of the intense sweeteners. This means the combination of ingredients are sweeter than the sum of the individual ingredients in sweetness. It is excreted quickly and totally, unmetabolized by both animals and humans.

Cyclamate. Cyclamate has a pleasant, sweet taste and a relative sweetness approximately 30 times greater than sucrose. It was originally included on the GRAS list. In 1960, the FDA requirements for studies were expanded to include testing for teratology and carcinogenicity. In early October 1969, there were indications of some cases of rodent bladder cancer. The FDA ruled in 1970 that cyclamate would no longer be allowed even if it were classified as a drug. As a result, the sweetener was withdrawn from the marketplace amidst considerable protest. Before cyclamate is returned to the marketplace, the FDA has noted it will conduct an extensive review of the National Academy of Science's exonerating report of the sweetener and resolve other questions that relate primarily to the acceptable daily intake for cyclamate.

Promising New Noncaloric Sweeteners

Many sweeteners have been submitted to the FDA for approval in the United States.

Two of the more promising ones are *Alitame* and *Sucralose*. Another being prepared to be submitted for approval is *Sweetener 2000*.

Alitame is 2000 times sweeter than sucrose. It is composed of two amino acids, L-aspartic acid and D-alanine. It is metabolized in the body; however, due to its concentration, the caloric contribution to the diet is insignificant. It has a synergistic effect with other sweeteners. Alitame has a clean taste and is stable both at high temperatures and broad pH ranges.

Sucralose is a noncaloric sweetener 600 times sweeter than sucrose that is derived from sucrose. It also exhibits synergistic sweetening effects. It will probably be several years before these two sweeteners are introduced in the United States.

Sweetener 2000 is 10,000 times sweeter than sucrose. Originally discovered and patented by researchers at Claude Bernard University in Lyon, France, Sweetener 2000 is exclusively licensed by the NutraSweet Company. It tastes similar to sugar and promises excellent stability in all possible applications. This sweetener will likely be presented to the FDA for its approval in 1996. It could literally change the way the world thinks about sweeteners.[45]

Other sweeteners are being used in other parts of the world (Table 14–6).[46,47] Over 150 plants have been identified as prossessing a sweet taste.[48]

TABLE 14–6. REGULATORY STATUS OF INTENSE SWEETENERS

Sweetener	Relative sweetness (× sugar)	USA	Canada	Europe	Japan
Acesulfame K	200	A	P	A	N
Aspartame	180	A	A	A	A
Cylamate	30	P	A	A	N
Saccharin	300	A	N	A	A
Sucralose	600	P	A	P	P

A = Approved, P = Petition filed, N = Not Approved
(*From U.S. Department of Agriculture, 1991.*[46])

CURRENT LEGISLATION REGARDING SWEETENER USE

In 1960, the FDA required that all petitions for new food additives must include information from studies relating to teratology, mutagenicity, and carcinogenicity.

Many questions have to be answered before a sweetener is advertised and marketed. If a noncaloric sweetener is to be used as a food additive, it must pass the Delaney clause, mandated by Congress in 1958, which states "no additive shall be deemed to be safe if it is found to induce cancer when ingested by man or animal."[49] Congress has excepted saccharin by legislation but is unlikely to exempt any future sweeteners, because sweeteners, such as aspartame and acesulfame-K, are now available that have passed the Delaney clause.

The specific use of a sweetener must be stated before it can be approved for commercial use. Will it be used as flavoring, or will it be as an anticaries agent? Such differences in intended use can greatly affect the cost of getting the product on the market. If it is to be used as a sweetener, then only *safety, teratology, mutagenicity,* and *carcinogenicity* are subjects of investigation. If anticariogenicity is claimed such as is possible in the use of xylitol, a great amount of additional money must be spent in animal and human caries incidence studies before such claims can be advertised. Estimates on the time and expense of marketing an entirely new sweetener range up to 10 years and as high as $20 million. If it is classified as a new drug, it may require a dosage statement and package insert carrying warnings of complications, contraindications, and incompatibility with other drugs.[50]

On the other hand, public safety is paramount. Many of the original food additives were chosen from organic and inorganic compounds that were intended for fabric and paper coloration, with safety being secondary to product appeal. With such teratogenic tragedies as accompanied the use of the tranquilizer thalidomide in the late 1950s the FDA is understandably reluctant to move rapidly in approving new drugs and additives that will be consumed by large segments of the population.

Question 3. Which of the following statements, if any, are correct?

A. The two amino acids in aspartame are phenylalanine and aspartic acid.
B. Sweetener 2000 has equivalent sweetness to saccharin but no reported aftertaste.
C. Sunette, the sweetener, is known as aspartame K.
D. The Delaney clause provides the FDA with the power to *exempt* new products from rigid regulation, provided the risks are low and the cost benefits high.
E. Sweetness is related to cariogenicity.

SUMMARY

There is little doubt that the consumption of sugar is associated with the caries process. Sweetness is such a cultural characteristic, however, that behavior modification to exclude it from the diet is considered an impossibility. It is estimated that carbohydrate sugars are the basis for a $59 billion economy in the United States. Also, the nonsweetening benefits of sucrose in industry would probably guarantee its continued use. In many industrial applications in the preparation and processing of food, other caloric and noncaloric sweeteners are preferable to sucrose. New sweeteners have been recently introduced that are less cariogenic and many hundred or thousand times the sweetness of sucrose. Many of them are nonacidogenic and noncaloric. From a dental standpoint these new sweeteners offer the potential for a considerable decrease in caries incidence.

ANSWERS AND EXPLANATIONS

1. A, B
   C—incorrect. A food additive is considered suspect, whereas the food ingredient has a long-term record of use and apparent safety.
   D—incorrect. Without bacteria, no amount of sugar is going to produce caries in the gnotobiotic rats.
   E—incorrect. People with HFI cannot consume sucrose without adverse systemic problems and hence experience few if any caries.

2. A, C, D, E
   B—incorrect. It requires more sweetener to identify the product, than to identify the sweet taste.

3. A, C
   B—incorrect. Sweetener 2000 is 10,000 times sweeter than sucrose, whereas saccharin is 300 times the sweetness of sugar.
   D—incorrect. The Delaney clause is quite rigid; if there is any evidence of cancer risk, the product is to be kept from the marketplace.
   E—incorrect. Cariogenicity is related to sugar, not sweetness.

SELF-EVALUATION QUESTIONS

1. Two synthetic caloric sweeteners are _____ and _____; two synthetic noncaloric sweeteners are _____ and _____.

2. Peanut brittle made with saccharin would be a very unusual product, mainly because the sweetener lacks the _____ (characteristic) that sucrose imparts to a product. Three other attributes of sucrose that are desirable from a commercial viewpoint are _____, _____, and _____.

3. Four properties of sucrose that make it undesirable for the preparation of some consumer products are _____, _____, _____, and _____.

4. The acronym GRAS refers to _____ _____.

5. The Vipeholm study demonstrated that two key factors relating to cariogenicity of foods were (1) frequency of intake and (2) _____; the lesson learned at Hopewood house was _____.

6. The lowest concentration at which a substance is identified to be sweet is known as the _____ concentration; the tasting of higher concentrations to identify *specific sugars is known as* _____ *testing.*

7. The *sugar alcohols* are more correctly referred to as _____ (name). Three of these compounds are _____, _____, and _____.

8. The *anti*cariogenicity of xylitol is related to its ability to induce _____ of previously diagnosed carious teeth.

9. A sweetener that is much sweeter than sucrose is referred to as an _____ sweetener.

10. The FDA acted to withdraw saccharin from the market because of the _____ clause.

11. Three of the most popular sweeteners are _____, _____, and _____.

12. One sweetener that is on the market today because of Congressional action is _____.

13. A new product to be accepted must include data relating to carcinogenicity, _____, and _____.

14. Aspartic acid and phenylalanine are the two molecules that make up _____ (name of sweetener).

15. The chemical name for Sunette is _____.

REFERENCES

1. Weiffenbach JM. The development of sweet preference. In: Shaw JH, Roussos GG, eds. _Proceeding: Sweeteners and Dental Caries. Special Supplement. Feeding, Weight & Obesity._ Abstract. Washington, DC: Information Retrieval Inc.; 1978:75–91.

2. Mandel ID. Dental caries. _Am Sci._ 1979; 67:680–688.

3. Institute of Food Technologists. _Sugars and nutritive sweeteners in processed foods. A scientific status summary by the I.F.T. expert panel on food safety and nutrition._ Chicago, Ill: Institute of Food Technologists; May 1979.

4. Homler BE, Deis RC, Shazer WH. Aspartame. In: Nabors LO, Gelard RC, eds. _Alternative Sweeteners._ New York, NY. Marcel Dekker, Inc.; 1991:39–63.

5. US Department of Agriculture. _Sugar and sweetener outlook and situation report._ SSRV17N3. Washington, DC; Government Printing Office; September 1992.

6. Rugg-Gunn AJ, Hackett AF, Appleton DR, et al. The dietary intake of added and natural sugars in 405 English adolescents. _Hum Nutr Appl._ 1986; 40A:115–124.

7. Gray F. _Sweeteners consumption, utilization and supply patterns in the United States: Past trends and relationships, and prospects for target years 1980 and 2000._ Dissertation, Baltimore, MD: University of Maryland, Department of Agricultural Economics, 1971.

8. US Department of Agriculture. _Sugar and Sweetener Outlook and Situation Report,_ SSRV5N7. Washington, DC; Government Printing Office; May 1980.

9. U.S. Department of Agriculture. _Sugar and Sweetener Outlook and Situation Report,_ SSRV140N2. Washington, DC; Government Printing Office; June 1989.

10. Glinsmann W, Irausguin H, Park YK. Evaluation of health aspects of sugars contained in carbohydrate sweeteners: Report of Sugars Task Force, 1986, _J Nutr._ 1986; 116(11S): S1–S216.

11. Ronk RJ. Regulatory constraints on sweetener use. In: Shaw JH, Roussos GG, eds. _Proceeding: Sweeteners and Dental Caries. Special Supplement. Feeding, Weight & Obesity._ Abstract. Washington, DC; Information Retrieval Inc, 1978:131–134.

12. US Department of Commerce, Food and Drug Administration. _Evaluation of the Health Aspects of Sucrose as a Food Ingredient._ Washington, DC; Government Printing Office, PB 262–668; 1976.

13. US Department of Health and Human Services. _The Surgeon General's Report on Nutrition and Health._ Washington, DC; Government Printing Office 017-001-00465-1; 1988.

14. Newbrun E. Sucrose, the arch criminal of dental caries. _Odontologisk Revy._ 1967; 18(4):373–386.

15. Marthaler TM. Changes in the prevalence of dental caries: How much can be attributed to changes in diet? _Diet, Nutr Dent Caries Res._ 1990; 24(Suppl 1):3–15.

16. Bowen WH. Role of carbohydrates in dental caries. In: Wei SHY, ed. _Proceedings of the National Symposium on Dental Nutrition._ Iowa City, Ia. University of Iowa Press; 1979:78–86.

17. Orland F, Blayney R, Harrison W, et al. Experimental caries in germ free rats inoculated with enterococci. _J Am Dent Assoc._ 1955; 50:259–272.

18. Kite O, Shaw J, Sognnaes R. The prevention of experimental tooth decay by tube-feeding. _J Nutr._ 1950; 42:89–103.

19. Marthaler TM. Epidemiological and clinical dental findings in relation to intake of carbohydrates. _Caries Res._ 1967; 1:222–238.

20. Gustafsson BE, Quensel CE, Lanke LS, et al. The Vipeholm dental caries study. The

effect of different levels of carbohydrate intake on caries activity in 436 individuals observed for five years. *Acta Odont Scand.* 1954; 11:232–364.

21. von der Fehr FR, Löe H, Theilade E. Experimental caries in man. *Caries Res.* 1970; 4:131–148.

22. Newbrun E, Hoover C, Mattraux G, et al. Comparison of dietary habits and dental health of subjects with hereditary fructose intolerance and control subjects. *J Am Dent Assoc.* 1980; 101:619–626.

23. Sheiham A. Why free sugars consumption should be below 15 kg per person per year in industrialized countries: The dental evidence. *Br Dent J.* 1991; 171(2):63–65.

24. Sreebny LM. Sugar availability, sugar consumption and dental caries. *Community Dent Oral Epidemiol.* 1982; 10:1–17.

25. Sheiham A. Sugars and dental decay. *Lancet.* Feb. 5, 1983:282–284.

26. US Department of Agriculture. *Sugar and Sweetener Outlook and Situation Report,* SSRV17N4. Washington, DC: Government Printing Office; December 1992.

27. Scheinin A. Caries control through the use of sugar substitutes. *Int Dent J.* 1976; 26:4–13.

28. Park KK, Shemehorn BR, Stookey GK. Effect of time and duration of sorbitol gum chewing on plaque acidogenicity. *Pediatr Dent.* 1993; 15:197–202.

29. Bar A. Caries prevention with xylitol. *World Rev Nutr Diet.* 1988; 55:183–209.

30. Bibby BG, Fu J. Changes in plaque pH in vitro by sweeteners. *J Dent Res.* 1985; 64:1130–1133.

31. Scheinin A, Makinen KK, Tammisalo E, et al. Turku sugar studies XVIII. Incidence of dental caries in relation to 1-year consumption of xylitol chewing gum. *Acta Odont Scand.* 1975; 33(suppl 70):269–278.

32. Leach SA, Green RM. Reversal of fissure caries in the Albino rat by sweetening agents. *Caries Res.* 1981; 15:508–511.

33. Jensen M, Wefel J, Sheth J. Plaque pH responses to meals and effects of chewing gums. *J Dent Res.* 1988; 67(SI):279. Abstract 1329.

34. Makinen KK, Bennett CA, Isokangas P, et al. Caries-preventive effect of polyol-containing chewing gums. *J Dent Res.* 1993; 72(SI):346. Abstract 1945.

35. Loesche WJ, Grossman NS, Earnest R, et al. The effect of chewing xylitol gum on the plaque and saliva levels of *Streptococcus mutans. J Am Dent Assoc.* 1984; 108:587–592.

36. American Dental Association. *Statement on Aspartame,* 17 July 1981.

37. Shaw JH. The metabolism of the polyols and their potential for greater use as sweetening agents in foods and confections. In: Shaw JH, Roussos GG, eds. *Proceedings: Sweeteners and Dental Caries. Special supplement. Feeding, Weight & Obesity.* Abstract. Washington, DC: Information Retrieval Inc. 1978:157–176.

38. US Department of Agriculture. *Sugar and Sweetener Outlook and Situation Report,* SSRV17N1. Washington, DC: Government Printing Office; March 1992.

39. Withdrawal of certain Pre-1986 Proposed rules: Final Action. *Federal Register.* 30 Dec 1991; 56:67442.

40. Dews PB. Summary report of an international aspartame workshop. *Fed Chem Toxic.* 1987; 25:549–552.

41. Aspartame, chewable multivitamin food supplement. *Federal Register.* May 30, 1984; 49:22468–22469.

42. Young FE. *Statement by FDA Commissioner before Committee on Labor and Human Resources, United States Senate.* Nov. 3, 1987.

43. American Dental Association. Aspartame important as a sucrose substitute. *ADA News.* July 27, 1981:1.

44. US Food and Drug Administration. Food additives permitted for direct addition for human consumption; acesulfame potassium. *Federal Register.* 1988; 53:28379–28383.

45. Sweetener for the 21st century? *Food Processing.* 1991; 52(6):54.

46. US Department of Agriculture. *Sugar and Sweetener Outlook and Situation Report,* SSRV16N4. Washington, DC: Government Printing Office; Dec 1991.

47. Newbrun E. The potential role of alternative sweeteners in caries prevention. *Isreal J Dent Sci.* 1990; 2(4):200–213.

48. Kinghorn AD, Soejanto DD. Intensely sweet compounds of natural origin. *Med Res Rev.* 1989; 9(1):91–115.

49. Isselbacher, KJ. Saccharin—the bitter taste. *N Eng J Med.* 1977; 296:1348–1350. Editorial.

50. Macay DAM. Sucrose and sucrose substitutes: Industrial considerations. *Pharmacol Ther Dent.* 1979; 3:69–74.

Chapter 15

Nutrition, Diet, and Oral Conditions

Carole A. Palmer

Objectives

At the end of this chapter it will be possible to

1. Explain how dietary standards such as the Recommended Dietary Allowances (RDAs), Reference Daily Intakes (RDIs) and Daily Reference Values (DRVs) are derived and utilized.
2. Discuss why severe malnutrition during organogenesis is more damaging than that occurring later in the development process.
3. Discuss why all foods with equal amounts of sugar are not necessarily equally cariogenic.
4. Describe how dietary patterns and the physical consistency of foods affect cariogenic potential.
5. Discuss the effects of food on buffering capacity and neutralization of plaque acids.
6. Discuss the role of nutrition in periodontal disease.
7. Identify two vitamins critical for the formation of epithelial or connective tissue, respectively, and indicate how their marginal deficiency can affect periodontal disease.
8. Explain why elderly patients are at higher nutritional risk than other age groups.
9. Discuss the relevant nutritional considerations for patients who are diabetic, those who are immunocompromised, and those having head and neck surgery.

Introduction

The relationships between diet, nutrition, and oral health are many. Nutrition is an important factor in the growth and continued integrity of oral tissues. During periods of *rapid* development (such as during gestation and the first few years of life), malnutrition, as well as disease or drugs, can have *irreversible* effects on the developing oral hard and soft tissues. Once the organs have achieved their genetic potential, nutritional deficiencies or toxicities, although reversible, can affect physiologic function, tissue integrity, and resistance and response to irritation and infection.

Prior to tooth eruption, nutritional status can influence *enamel maturation* and chemical composition as well as *tooth morphology* and size.[1,2] After eruption, the effects of diet on the dentition are topical rather than systemic. Diet is essential for the initiation and progression of carious lesions, and dietary factors and patterns can exacerbate or minimize caries status.

Because the oral tissues have a more rapid turnover rate than most other tissues in the body, aberrations in nutrition are often manifest first in the oral cavity. In addition, the patient who often undergoes oral or periodontal surgery or who has dentures or other dental disability may require dietary guidance to ward off deleterious changes in diet. Patients with diabetes mellitus, oral cancer, or acquired immunodeficiency syndrome (AIDS), may all suffer from oral problems that can compromise nutritional status.

Thus, the dental clinician should know not only how diet and nutrition can affect oral health but also how oral conditions can affect diet and ultimate nutritional status. It is the role of the dentist to screen patients for nutritional risk, provide appropriate dietary guidance, and refer patients to nutri-tional professionals for treatment when indicated.[3,4]

ESTABLISHING DIETARY STANDARDS

Daily food intake must be of sufficient quantity and quality to meet metabolic requirements for nutrients and energy. The actual requirements vary among individuals. However, dietary standards have been developed that provide consensus on the nutrient needs for *population groups* categorized by sex, age, and body composition.

In 1940, the National Research Council of the National Academy of Sciences established the *Food and Nutrition Board* with a mandate to establish human nutrition requirements, based upon the best scientific information of the time. The *Recommended Dietary Allowances (RDAs)* are recommendations by that body for the daily consumption of a variety of nutrients for different age and sex groups. The RDAs are reevaluated and revised approximately every 5 years to reflect current knowledge.

The first Recommended Dietary Allowances (RDA) were published in 1941 and included recommendations for calories and nine essential nutrients. The 1989 RDAs include specific recommendations for calories and 19 nutrients, as well as a suggested range of intake for 7 others.

The RDAs are set at a level considered adequate to meet the needs of *most healthy people, with a sufficient margin of safety to allow for individual variation.*[5]

GUIDELINES FOR FOOD CHOICES

Food Labeling
Over the years, the *Food and Drug Administration (FDA)* has developed various

methods for helping consumers evaluate the nutrient content of packaged foods by providing information on food labels. In 1973, under the *Federal Food, Drug, and Cosmetics Act,* the FDA developed a labeling standard *(USRDA),* which was derived from the RDA and which displayed the nutrient content of foods on food labels as a *percentage* of the US RDAs.

In 1990, the *Nutrition Labeling and Education Act (NLEA)* (effective in 1994)[6,7] expanded the number of foods for which nutrition information on labels is mandatory and developed new labeling standards. The term *Reference Daily Intake (RDI) replaces* the USRDA. It is based on an average of the 1989 RDA values for various age and sex groups. For food components, such as fat or fiber, for which the RDA is not defined, a *Daily Reference Value (DRV)* is used. For simplification, all reference values on food labels are referred to as *Daily Values (DVs).*

The standard format for food labels includes

- A standardized portion size
- The amounts of total calories and calories from fat per serving
- The percentage daily value of mandated nutrients based on a 2000-Cal diet (eg, total fat, saturated fat, cholesterol, sodium, total carbohydrates, dietary fiber, sugars, protein, vitamin A, vitamin C, calcium, and iron—in that order)
- Specific daily recommendations of target nutrients for 2000- and 2500-Cal diets
- The number of Calories per gram of fat, carbohydrate, and protein

Other information, such as the amounts of polyunsaturated or monounsaturated fats or other vitamins and minerals, is optional. In addition, descriptors, such as "free," "low," "high," "light," "lite," "lean," or "reduced," may be used on the label *as long as a standard portion meets specified criteria.* For example, to be labeled "low-calorie" a serving must have no more than 40 Cal. To be "low-fat," no more than 3 g of fat must be in a serving. Also, certain health claims are allowed *if* they meet specific requirements. Figure 15–1 shows the new label format.

DIETARY GUIDELINES

In addition to educating consumers via food labels, various food guides have been used over the years to promote a healthy diet.[8] Food guides, such as the "basic seven" and the "basic four" were designed to provide the foundation for a good diet. They used the RDAs as a basis for grouping foods of similar nutrient content, with an emphasis on meeting basic nutritional requirements. These food guides, however, did not address such current issues of nutritional concern as *overconsumption* and diet's relationship to degenerative diseases. Thus, additional recommendations such as the *Dietary Guidelines for Americans* have been developed by government and professional organizations to target the prevention of nutrition-related disease. The recommendations include

- Eat a variety of foods.
- Maintain a healthy weight.
- Choose a diet low in fat, saturated fat, and cholesterol.
- Choose a diet with plenty of vegetables, fruits, and grain products.
- Use sugars only in moderation.
- Use salt and sodium only in moderation.
- If you drink alcoholic beverages, do so in moderation.

Most recently, the U.S. Department of Agriculture retired its familiar *Guide to Good Eating* in favor of the new *Food Guide Pyramid* in order to address these issues of nutritional concern. The pyramid

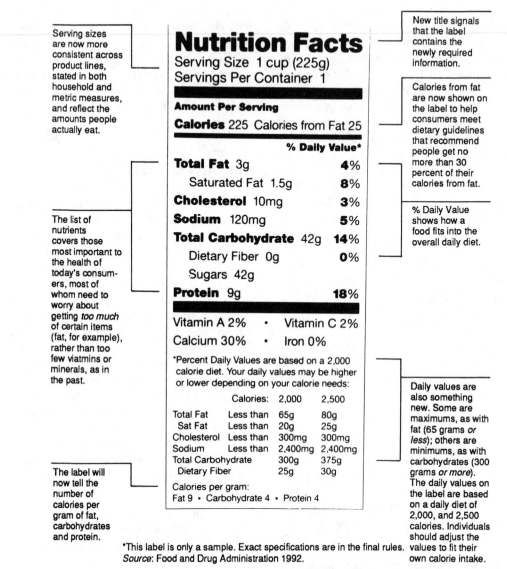

Figure 15–1. The New Food Label at a Glance

design presents the recommended distribution of foods in the diet more graphically and revises the recommended number of servings from various groups (Fig 15–2).[9] The active involvement of government in fostering nutrition's role in health promotion is also evident in major reports such as the *Surgeon General's Report on Nutrition and Health,* which details health-related goals and objectives for the nation, including goals for nutrition and oral health.[10]

In summary, dietary guidelines have been used as tools for teaching good nutrition for many years. Recently, however, the

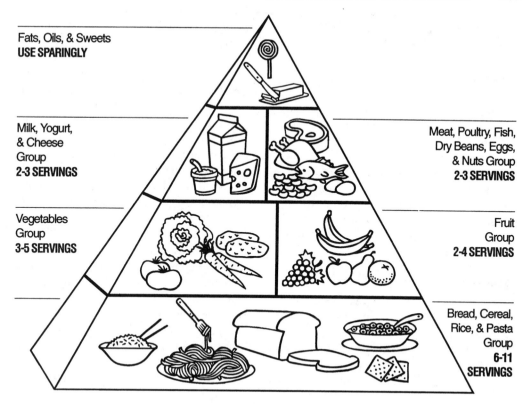

Figure 15–2. The Food Guide Pyramid: A Guide to Daily Food Choices is an outline of what to eat each day. Not a rigid prescription but a general guide that lets each person choose a healthful diet, the Pyramid calls for eating a variety of foods to get the needed nutrients while consuming the right amount of calories to maintain a healthy weight. (*Courtesy U.S. Department of Agriculture, Human Nutrition Information Service*).

goal of these guidelines has moved beyond meeting basic requirements and avoiding deficiency to *promoting health and avoiding nutrition-related disease and disability.*

Question 1. Which of the following statements, if any, are correct?

A. The abbreviation RDA stands for *Recommended Daily Allowances.*

B. The *Nutrition Labeling and Education Act* provides the legal basis for *requiring* nutrition information on packaged goods.

C. The information supplied by the Reference Daily Intake is presented in a standardized format.

D. Descriptors such as "low," "high," and "light," for product content *must* conform to government specifications applying to truth in advertising.

E. The Food Guide Pyramid is a guide to daily food choices, which recommends the same number of servings from the fruit group as from the pasta group.

NUTRITION DURING GROWTH AND DEVELOPMENT

Aberrations that occur during periods of organ formation may have potentially irreversible effects on the developing organism. Such effects can be seen in the tetracycline staining of teeth, fluorosis, and fever-induced enamel hypoplasia seen in the primary teeth. The effects of malnutrition are less well documented in humans but lead to the impression that malnutrition during these "critical periods" of growth can result in a dentition that is more susceptible to dental caries.

The Early Role of Proteins

Impaired protein synthesis has been found if protein malnutrition occurs during the developmental stage. Menaker and Navia[11] demonstrated that the offspring of rats on a protein-deficient diet exhibited a lower salivary flow, an altered protein content, and a greater susceptibility to caries. Marginally and severely malnourished humans had a decreased lysozyme level, as well as lower secretory IgA levels.[12] When young, healthy monkeys were placed on a short-term protein-deficient diet, the output of salivary protein was lower during the period of the deficiency, but it returned to normal levels once the regular diet was resumed.[13] It has been suggested that the linear hypoplasia reported in the enamel of primary teeth of children in underprivileged populations contributes to their high prevalence of dental caries. This type of hypoplasia appears to be related to the severity of malnutrition.[14,15]

Many of the protein molecules secreted by the salivary glands are of extreme importance in protecting the integrity of the teeth and the soft tissues throughout life. The protein molecules forming the pellicle can influence future colonization of the plaque; secretory IgA can likewise be adsorbed to the hydroxyapatite to influence plaque formation or to react directly with oral bacteria. Glycoprotein molecules aggregate bacteria, either for eventual swallowing or for incorporation into the plaque. Salivary peroxidate, lactoferrin, lysozyme, sialin, and statherin are other protein molecules that are part of the defense arsenal secreted by the salivary glands. All of these can be diminished in volume or altered in structure during severe periods of malnutrition.[15,16]

Minerals

Minerals are classified as macrominerals or as microminerals, depending on the amount contained in the body. Calcium, magnesium, phosphorus, sodium, potassium, and sulfur are examples of macrominerals, and chromium, cobalt, copper, fluoride, iodine, molybdenum, selenium, and zinc are microminerals, or trace elements. Iron is sometimes considered a macromineral, and sometimes a micromineral. Forty elements can be quantitated in enamel and can affect the plaque or tooth via contact from food or water, or they can be absorbed in the intestinal tract and later secreted in the saliva.

The effect of most of the trace elements on bacterial metabolism or on hard and soft tissue defense and repair is either unknown or not completely understood. It is known that *small* amounts of strontium can substitute for calcium in the apatite crystal; similarly, fluoride can substitute for the hydroxyl grouping, and carbonate can replace phosphate. Most of the other elements are adsorbed onto the great amount of surface area of the crystals or are found in the matrix.

The function of iron is of interest because iron deficiency is the most common deficiency in this country. Although documenting a role for a preeruptive nutritional iron deficiency in subsequent caries susceptibility has been difficult, it is important to cite the evidence for iron having such a role. Even a marginal deficiency of iron in the rat diet predisposes these rodents to caries. Conversely, supplementation of the caries-promoting diet with iron produced a major reduction in caries, with the greatest effect being shown in the neonatal period.[17]

Part of the difficulty in understanding the role of all trace elements is that they occur in such minute amounts. Feeding experiments are difficult to conduct, because it is nearly impossible to develop a diet free of trace minerals that may be physiologically active in the range of parts per billion.[18]

CARIOGENIC POTENTIAL OF FOODS

Historic Perspective

The introduction of mass methods for the production of sugar ushered in the "great caries era" starting in the 18th century. Before that time, caries was a disease of the affluent who could afford to pay approximately 50 times the cost of a loaf of bread for a pound of sugar.[19] The same trend later occurred in Ghana, where better paid workers developed caries, whereas those who could not afford refined carbohydrates had fewer caries.[20] At the end of the 19th century a second major contribution to the caries epidemic occurred: the introduction of the roller-milling process to refine flour.[21] The baker was now able to combine the sweetness of sugar with the cereal foods to produce appetite-satisfying confections and breads (Fig 15–3). The effect of the availability of sweets is illustrated in one study in which the number of carious lesions found in a children's population varied inversely with the distance they lived from the only

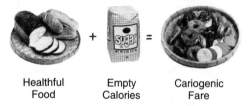

| Healthful Food | Empty Calories | Cariogenic Fare |

Figure 15–3. The addition of sugar, which has no food value other than calories, to healthful cereal grains results in a more cariogenic product.

sweet shop in the area.[22] During World Wars I and II, the incidence of caries in the countries affected by the naval blockades was markedly reduced.[23,24]

Factors Affecting Food Cariogenicity

Type of Carbohydrates. All of the simple carbohydrates—sucrose, fructose, lactose, galactose, and glucose—can be cariogenic. For instance, sucrose is used to aid in the implantation of *Streptococcus mutans* in experimental animals.[25] Several exposures to sucrose are probably necessary before the bacterial populations change from a noncariogenic to a cariogenic plaque. In the study by von der Fehr and associates in which dental students rinsed their mouths nine times daily with sucrose, only 23 days elapsed before incipient lesions (white spots) began to appear.[26] In another study, subjects maintained on a high-sucrose diet for about 2 weeks demonstrated a marked increase in the numbers of *S mutans* and lactobacilli; by 4 weeks the change was even greater.[27,28] Conversely, when patients with a high lactobacilli count were placed on a restricted sucrose diet, approximately the *same* amount of time—2 to 4 weeks—was necessary before the lactobacilli were reduced to baseline levels.[28] Similarly, when subjects were placed on a sucrose-free diet for 17 days, *S mutans* counts fell to near zero. Thus the cariogenic potential of the plaque fluctuates quite rapidly, depending on the frequency of sugar intake.

The use of *honey* as an alleged "safe" sugar substitute has resulted in an even higher caries development than with sucrose. The sap of the *maple* tree which is used to make maple sugar candy is almost exclusively sucrose. *Sugar beets*, a crop that has been cultivated for over 200 years in the United States, produce a major alternative source of sucrose.[29] *Sugar cane* is the world's traditional source of sucrose. All of these different sources of sucrose are cariogenic. If sucrose is baked with starch in the form of cakes and cookies, the products are even more cariogenic because of their slow clearance time from the mouth.[30] Even after the food has been cleared, acid is still produced in the plaque.[31] The cariogenicity of foods incorporating refined carbohydrates depends on such variables as saliva flow, contact time of the product with the plaque, bacterial constituents of the plaque, and individual plaque control measures— all of which help determine *how long and how often the plaque is in a "demineralizing mode."*

Physical Forms of Food and Clearance Time.

Diets that result in the *greatest retention of refined carbohydrates over the longest period are the most cariogenic.* Different foods are cleared from the mouth at different rates. Foods that may not be cariogenic if cleared in a short time can be cariogenic if retained in an area for a longer period. The clearance of refined carbohydrates is not the same at all sites and depends on such factors as alignment of teeth, gingival recession, and proximity to glandular duct openings, as well as on the physical form of the carbohydrate.

Oral glucose clearance times range from approximately 6 to 24 minutes, with the average times being near 15 minutes.[32] Demineralization does not cease, nor does remineralization begin until the carbohydrate substrate has been cleared. With a more frequent intake of refined carbohydrate, damage time is increased and tooth repair time (ie, remineralization) decreased proportionately. Over repeated 24-hour periods, this negative mineral balance can mean the difference between caries and no caries.

In quantitative terms, a demineralizing pH may last for 40 to 60 minutes after a cariogenic meal or for about 10% of the day for three such meals. If a person superimposes four snacks at about 2-hour intervals between meals, each cariogenic snack lowers pH for another 40 to 60 minutes, and demineralizing pH occurs for more than 20% of the day. Loesche made such calculations and then cited data to show that besides increasing demineralization time directly, frequent snacking further prolongs demineralization time by favoring a high population of acidogenic plaque bacteria.[33]

Particle size and fluidity can affect the clearance time for foods. As a practical point, health educators should not imply that sugary solutions are necessarily less cariogenic than sticky snacks. A significant positive association between the frequencies of at- and between-meal consumption of soft drinks and high caries scores has been noted.[34] Another good example of rampant caries caused by fluids is *"baby bottle" caries*.[a] Milk sugar (ie, lactose) can be just as cariogenic as sweetened beverages or fruit juice when allowed to remain in contact with children's teeth over a prolonged period.[35,36]

---

[a] "Baby bottle" caries and "nursing bottle" caries are synonyms for dental decay resulting from bottles filled with milk, formula, or juice remaining in a child's mouth while it sleeps.

Diet Control of Caries in Rats

When two out of four groups of rats were fed either high-cariogenic diets (HCD) or low-cariogenic diets (LCD) on different daily schedules for over 18 days, the rats that were continually on the HCD developed an average of 30.6 lesions, whereas those on the LCD developed only an average of 5.4. Three very important findings emerged from the data concerning the other two groups.

1. The caries scores developed were in *direct proportion* to the number of days out of the 18-day experimental period the HCD was fed.
2. The maximum numbers of caries occurred when sugar was consumed throughout any given 24-hour period.
3. When the HCD was fed only on weekends, only two-sevenths of the number of lesions occurred, as compared with the control group.

These studies suggest that individuals on high-cariogenic diets can reduce caries activity by changing diet patterns, a fact that *if applied to childrens' cafeteria diets during school days, could possibly reduce caries by as much as 70%.*[37] Progress towards this goal only needs the school dietitian to substitute fruit desserts for those with a high sugar content.

Assessing Relative Cariogenicity of Foods

Despite the fact that the relationship between sugar and caries is inescapable,[38,39] the *cariogenicity of food cannot be evaluated simply on the basis of sugar content.* Other physical characteristics of food, such as solubility and retentiveness, the ability to stimulate the flow and chemical changes of

the saliva,[40] and the texture and particle size of food must be considered.[41]

Several methods have been attempted to establish the relative cariogenicity of foods. One of the earliest methods used to observe acid production by food was employed by W. D. Miller in the late 19th century.[42] Bread was placed in a tube with pooled saliva, and the acid production was quantitated. Many studies have since used the same method, or modifications thereof, employing different foods instead of bread. In other studies, pooled saliva is placed in a tube with the test food and a tooth. Variables, such as pH drop, amount of acid formed, and calcium release from teeth, have been studied.

In vitro tests are indirect and cannot consider the dynamic events that characterize plaque metabolism: acidogenicity of the bacteria, changing substrates, neutralizing and buffering capacity of the plaque, and diffusion of acids through the plaque. Such tests cannot consider the various interactions occurring between the foods being tested and the salivary components, nor can they consider the effects of physiologic and pathologic conditions, such as differences in clearance time, hypersalivation, and xerostomia. Finally, they cannot consider the effect of restorations, retention sites, and tongue-and-cheek muscle actions. All these factors can only be considered by going directly to the mouth in which the action is occurring. This can only be done by using living models, both *human and animal.*

The use of both animal and human models is sufficiently advanced to begin to predict food cariogenicity. Both paradigms are used extensively, and both contribute information that leads to a better general understanding of plaque metabolism following ingestion of foods. Human data, of course, have the advantage of being directly applicable to all humans. The disadvantages to the human paradigm are that feeding schedules and diets cannot be artificially manipulated over long periods and that it is unethical to feed humans foods that are known to be cariogenic. Animal models do not have these restrictions, however. Most animal models for testing food cariogenicity use the rat because a cariogenic diet produces results similar to caries in humans.[43] Efforts have been made to standardize protocols used to determine the in vivo potential cariogenicity of food for both animal and human models, which would allow results from different laboratories to be compared.

Probably the most direct animal model was developed by Bowen and colleagues.[44] In their studies, rats were fed a basal diet via stomach tube, and the test foods for intraoral exposure were presented to the rodents by a feeding rack that could be programmed for any desired time schedule. Sucrose acted as the control food. A variety of other food items, such as sugar-coated cereals, potato chips, and chocolate cookies with soft filling, were studied. The resulting caries score for each food item was compared with the sucrose controls to secure a *caries potential index (CPI)*. Later studies by S.A. Mundorff and colleagues provided a similar comparison of the caries potential of various foods (Table 15–1).

Question 2. Which of the following statements, if any, are correct?

A. Severe malnutrition during the teenage period is apt to cause more permanent changes in secretory patterns than severe malnutrition during the first trimester of pregnancy.

B. On a diet very restricted in refined carbohydrates, over a *2-week period* both lactobacilli and streptococci counts can be reduced to near zero.

C. An oral clearance time of 5 minutes is considered excessive.

TABLE 15–1. COMPARISON OF THE CARIES POTENTIAL OF VARIOUS FOODS

Foods	Caries Potential Index	
	Buccal	*Sulcal*
Raisins	1.3	0.95
Bananas	1.2	1.17
French fried (chips)	1.2	0.98
Granola (a breakfast cereal)	1.1	0.64
Sucrose	**1.0**	**1.0**
Bread	0.82	0.90
Grahams (digestive biscuits)	0.66	0.79
Cup cakes	0.62	1.73
Chocolate	0.59	0.81
Cornstarch	0.47	0.76
Sponge cake	0.44	0.95
Rye crackers	0.36	0.86
Saltines (savoury crackers)	0.36	0.69
Peanuts	0.30	0.43
Pretzels	0.21	0.77
Jello (fruit jelly)	0.11	0.43
Yoghurt	0.11	0.65
Corn chips	0.10	0.54

(*Adapted from Mundorff SA, Featherstone JDB, Eisenberg AD, et al. Cariogenicity of foods: Rat study. J Dent Res. 64:(special issue) 1985; 294. Abstract 1071.*)

D. The lactose derived from breast feeding, will *not* cause "baby-bottle" caries.

E. A *caries potential index* permits the cariogenicity of test foods to be compared with that of sucrose.

Measuring Plaque pH Change

It is assumed that if a given food does not cause the pH to drop below the critical demineralization point for enamel over a given period, no caries can occur. The pH at which enamel demineralization begins usually ranges between an upper pH of 5.5 down to 5.0.

Three methods have been considered scientifically valid for measuring the pH changes on the surface of the tooth: (1) *plaque sampling,* (2) *touch electrodes,* and (3) *proximity telemetry.*[45] To determine the pH by plaque sampling, a small sample of plaque is removed from the tooth, placed on a microscope slide, and the pH measured. Determining pH via touch electrodes involves an in situ measurement of the pH of the plaque while still on the tooth. Using either of these two methods, reproducing measurements over time is impossible. Proximity telemetry, however, is the most informative because it permits an automatic, continuous monitoring of a changing pH.

With the proximity method, the pH electrode is part of a miniature high-tech radio transmitter that is built into a bridge or large restoration. As food is chewed, the pH at the site of the electrode is continually transmitted to an extraoral receiver. The rate and extent of the fall and rise of pH can be recorded over the entire time of the experiment. With this method it is possible to state positively that the mastication of a given food results in a pH that is above, or below pH 5.6[46]

At a symposium on food cariogenicity, the consensus was that agreement in results from any two of these methods could be used to assess the safety of food.[46] *Sorbitol* has been selected as the noncariogenic reference food because it is minimally, if not absolutely, noncariogenic.[47]

DIET AND ROOT CARIES

Research has indicated that the dietary factors responsible for root surface caries may be similar to those responsible for coronal caries. The prevalence of root caries is much higher in older than in younger adults and is associated with periodontal disease and gingival recession.[48] Studies of primitive peoples showed an association between the use of complex carbohydrates and root caries.[49] More recent studies of individuals with periodontal disease showed significant correlations between the incidence of root caries and total carbohydrate intake,[50] the frequency of consumption of fermentable carbohydrates,[51] the frequency of use of liquid and solid fermentable carbohydrates, and the use of slowly dissolving fermentable carbohydrates.[51]

CARIES-PROTECTIVE EFFECTS OF FOOD

"Self-Cleansing Foods"

The detergent effect of such foods as carrots,[52] apples,[53] and celery[54] has been studied many times and each time found relatively ineffective in removing plaque (Fig 15–4). Alexander and associates pointed out that if an area of the tooth is to be considered self-cleansing, it implies that under normal circumstances bacterial plaque and food debris are removed from the surface either by the friction of food and the oral tissues, the action of oral fluids, or by means *other* than the deliberate oral hygiene procedures employed by the individual. In their study to determine if self-cleansing

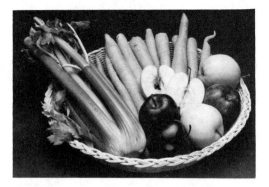

Figure 15–4. Fibrous foods good for the body *but not* good for removing plaque.

areas did exist, a scaling and polishing procedure was completed for 40 male dental students, followed by a recording of their individual plaque accumulations over 5 days. In no instance were there plaque-free areas.[50]

In another study by Arnim,[54] subjects refrained from plaque control procedures for 7 days. Then, over a 3-hour period, they chewed sugar cane, apples, whole carrots, and celery. In comparing before-and-after photographs, it was determined that only 3% to 19% of the plaque had been removed.[54] In another study, the eating of three raw carrots three times a day over an 18-day period had no effect on the amount of plaque that accumulated at the gingiva and interproximally.[52]

Despite the evidence that "detergent" foods do not remove plaque, the clinical fact still remains that when teeth are not used in chewing, as when there are no opposing teeth or when pain occurs because of an exposed pulp, more extensive plaque or calculus formation (or both) results. Probably the fibrous foods serve to *limit* the amount of plaque rather than to prevent its accumulation.

Aside from the function of limiting plaque formation, fibrous foods have other functions that help to prevent caries or periodontal disease or both. For example, flavorful, fibrous, raw, unrefined, or minimally processed vegetables and fruit require chewing and promote salivation. The stimulated salivary flow aids in the removal and dilution of sugars and their fermentation products, which can threaten the teeth and gingiva. The stimulated saliva is of higher pH and buffer capacity and, along with the greater abundance of calcium and phosphate ions due to increased volume, favors remineralization of enamel following an acid attack.

Buffering and Neutralizing

The simple acts of chewing, smelling, looking at, or anticipating good food increase both the flow of saliva and the concentration of bicarbonate. Chewy foods such as meat provide a greater stimulant for flow and buffering action than do soft foods such as mashed potatoes. The buffering capacity of the saliva is greater after eating fruits and vegetables.

Cheese as a Buffering Agent. Cheese has also been found to be a powerful buffer.[56] When a group of foods were tested after rinsing with a 10% sucrose rinse, aged cheddar cheese prevented the pH from dropping below 6.0.[57]

The intraoral cariogenicity test was used to measure tooth indentation hardness differences between a control group using a 10% sucrose rinse only and an experimental group using the rinse plus a 5-g piece of cheese. The Knoop[b] indentation for the control group was 3.79, compared with 1.11 for the cheese group. Concurrently, the minimum pH for the control group was 4.7 and for the experimental group 5.7.[58] In another similar study, in which the cheese was processed with 3% urea, the pH fell to only 6.3.[59]

This desirable effect of eating cheese is probably due to one or more of the following factors:

1. Buffering of the saliva by the cheese
2. Stimulation of saliva flow
3. Fatty acids in the cheese exerting a protective effect

---

[b] The Knoop hardness tester is a device with a small, dull stylus that is forced against the tooth surface. Both the pressure and the depth of penetration can be measured. The depth of penetration is inversely related to the hardness of the specimen being tested, meaning, the harder the tooth surface, the less penetration.

4. Possible presence of peptones acting similar to sialin
5. The calcium and phosphorus product causing an ion supersaturation of the plaque[60]
6. Cheese enhancing remineralization[61]

The apparent noncariogenic or anticariogenic properties of a variety of cheeses,[62,63] as well as peanuts[56] and chewing gum,[64] provide a healthy way of ending a meal. A piece of cheese, some peanuts, or a stick of xylitol chewing gum keeps the salivary defenses high for half an hour while the mouth is being cleared and the plaque pH is returning to normal.[65]

Sugar Alcohols and Noncariogenic Sweeteners

Perhaps one of the most promising of sugars to be studied is xylityol, a sugar alcohol that has been demonstrated to be noncariogenic (does not support bacterial metabolism) as well as anticariogenic (encourages remineralization). One explanation for this dual action is its ability to enhance saliva-buffering capacity. Other polyols and compounds are used as sweeteners that also do not support bacterial metabolism. The substitution of these sweeteners for sucrose in the diet essentially eliminates the cariogenic challenge. The importance of these compounds in dentistry is detailed in Chapter 14.

Minerals and Cariogenic Potential

Studies indicate that other as yet unknown elements or combinations of elements present in food or water protect the teeth. Arnold found that two different municipalities with approximately the same fluoride level could often have different decayed missing, or filled tooth indexes (DMFT).

For instance, Nashville, Tennessee had 0.0 ppm F and a total hardness to the water of 79 ppm, whereas Key West had 0.1 ppm F and only 36 ppm water hardness. Despite the approximate equality of fluoride, Key West had 1071 carious lesions/100 children, and Nashville had 461.[66] On the basis of human and animal studies, Navia has probably best summarized the cariogenic status of many of the minerals in a list compiled to indicate relative cariogenicity.[18]

- Cariostatic elements: F, P
- Mildly cariostatic: Mo, V, Cu, Sr, B, Li, Au
- Doubtful: Be, Co, Mn, Sn, Zn, Br, I
- Caries-inert: Ba, Al, Ni, Fe, Pd, Ti
- Caries-promoting: Se, Mg, Cd, Pt, Pb, Si

Curzon has noted that zinc and calcium may show promise as antiplaque agents, whereas strontium and zinc may enhance remineralization of enamel.[67] There are indications that aluminum salts that do not form complexes can be considered cariostatic. In vitro studies have found aluminum salts equivalent to stannous fluoride in preventing acid dissolution.[68] In combination with iron salts, root resistance is increased more than with fluoride alone.[69]

Question 3. Which of the following statements, if any, are correct?

A. The increasing cariogenic potential of cariogenic foods is directly related to the number of times they must be cleared from the mouth over a given period of time.

B. Touch electrodes provide the most reliable data on the constantly changing pH of plaque.

C. "Self-cleansing" foods with a high fiber content *remove* rather than *limit* plaque buildup.

D. Peanuts, sugarless chewing gum, and cheddar cheese can be used as after dinner items to modify buffering and to increase salivary flow.

E. In general, phosphorus and fluoride are considered cariostatic, whereas magnesium and lead are considered cariogenic.

PERIODONTAL DISEASE AND NUTRITION

Periodontal disease is an infectious disease, and like caries, (1) it is of multifactorial etiology, (2) in health the bacterial challenge factor is matched by a host defense and repair capability, and (3) it has periods of progression and remission. It is often difficult to determine whether the remissions are due to a lessening of the challenge by the subgingival plaque organisms or to a more effective defense and repair due to better body health.

Unlike the close relationship between sugar and the caries process, no food is specifically indicted as triggering the onset and continuation of periodontal disease. The nutritional concepts that apply to preventing infection and enhancing wound healing elsewhere in the body apply also to the prevention and management of the periodontal lesion.[70]

If both the challenge to and the defense and repair capabilities of the periodontal tissues are in balance, nutrition could possibly be the deciding factor in whether health or disease results. Even when the periodontium is healthy, there is continual need for nutrients to maintain the tissues; once inflammation is established, that need for nutrients escalates. The relationship between malnutrition and infection is a close one, with infection aggravating malnutrition and malnutrition abetting infection. The amino acids, ascorbate, riboflavin, folic acid, vitamin A, and zinc are critical to recovery and for maintenance of a healthy periodontium.[71-74] Whenever routine scaling, prophylaxis, and oral plaque control procedures fail to reverse gingivitis and before any treatment for periodontitis is attempted, a thorough nutritional evaluation and patient counseling session(s) should be conducted.

The Defense: Nutrients Affecting the Periodontium

The defenses of the gingival crevice against the bacteria causing periodontal disease are mainly dependent on the secretions of the salivary glands: (1) the flow of saliva aids in the flushing and aggregation of bacteria; (2) the nonimmunologic defenses, such as lysozyme, salivary peroxidase, and lactoferrin, aid in maintaining a bacteriostatic status; and (3) the secretory IgA molecules act against invading bacterial cells. A few antibodies and polymorphonuclear (PMNs) leukocytes and antibodies from the underlying connective tissues filter through the epithelial barrier and enter the oral cavity via the gingival sulcular fluid. If the glands have been compromised in the early stages of fetal development by nutritional deficiencies, any or all of these functions can be affected.[75]

A much more complex defense force exists in the connective tissue, consisting of PMN leukocytes, macrophages, lymphocytes, and plasma cells supplemented by antibodies, complement, and lymphokines. Each of these defense components requires an adequate intake of *all* nutrients to ensure adequate reproduction and function of defense and supporting cells. For example, basal epithelial cells, fibroblasts, and osteoblasts are needed to repair damaged epithelial and connective tissue. Liver cells are needed to synthesize the glycoproteins in immune functions and to remove toxins.

In a healthy periodontium with only a relatively few challenge organisms, the crevicular epithelium is sufficient to maintain both the oral and the tissue defenses on a standby basis. Little gets through to the underlying connective tissue because of the close contact of the epithelial cells and the integrity of the basement membrane. However, if the end products of the bacterial cells in the pocket are sufficiently toxic to overwhelm the oral defenses or in the presence of deficiencies of zinc, folate, and ascorbate, the permeability of the epithelial barrier and the basement membrane are altered. The toxic substances move between the cells and through the basal lamina into the connective tissue. As soon as this occurs, *lymphokines,* which are secreted by lymphocytes in the connective tissue, trigger the inflammatory response. Additional defense cells arrive; more connective tissue fluid enters the pocket as gingival sulcular fluid, often sweeping defense cells and antibodies into the mouth. This is the beginning of gingivitis. Along with the increased metabolic needs of the army of defense cells plus the additional demands by the tissue cells attempting to maintain and to repair the damaged areas, a much greater flow of all nutrients is needed.

Effect of Protein Deficiency

The normal, very rapid turnover of epithelial tissue[76] in the crevice requires a continual supply of nutrients. Every 3 to 6 days the basal epithelium of the gingiva undergoes renewal.[77] Any severe deficiency of protein-calorie intake results in a decrease of mitotic activity of the crevicular epithelium as well as elsewhere in the body.[78] In comparing periodontal involvement in patients with severe malnutrition (kwashiorkor) with that in healthy control individu-

als in South India,[16] fewer caries and more periodontal disease was found among the undernourished group. Because the oral hygiene indexes (OHI) of these groups were similar, it was assumed that the difference was due to nutritional factors. It should be noted that any malnutrition of the severity of kwashiorkor represents a multinutrient deficiency and not merely a protein deprivation.

With the exception of the cleansing and diluting effect of saliva, each of the defense mechanisms depends on an adequate supply of proteins. The glycoproteins that result in aggregation of bacteria arise from the salivary glands. Lysozyme, salivary peroxidase, and lactoferrin are also glycoproteins. Secretory IgA (sIgA) arises mainly from the labial and buccal glands and is an immunoglobulin. Finally, the cell types involved in cellular immunity (ie, the polys and the macrophages and their enzymes used in phagocytosis) also require protein for their production.[79]

Probably one of the most deleterious effects of a protein-calorie deficiency is manifest in a depletion of the cellular and immunocellular defenses of both the oral and the connective sides of the barrier epithelial cells lining the gingival crevice. In general, the severity of the impaired immunologic response parallels the severity of the protein or calorie deficiency. This deficiency is reflected by deficiencies of both sIgA and complement factors.[17]

Vitamin Effects

Vitamin A. Vitamin A is essential for the integrity of *epithelial tissue* throughout the body. It also affects the synthesis of constituents of mucus, such as the mucoproteins and mucopolysaccharides. Deficiencies of vitamin A have not been directly associated with periodontal disease; however, the effects of vitamin A toxicity on the periodontium have been reported.[80] Effects include, proliferation of oral epithelium, reduction of the keratin layer, thickening of the basal membrane, and increase of the granular layer. A patient who took 200,000 IU of vitamin A daily for more than 6 months, presented with painful gingival lesions, along with nausea, vomiting, xerostomia, and headaches. Clinical examination revealed gingival erosions, ulcerations, bleeding, swelling, loss of keratinization, color changes, and desquamation of the lips. With the levels of oral hygiene unchanged, all pathologic manifestations disappeared within 2 months of the elimination of the vitamin A supplements.

Vitamin C and the Connective Tissue.
Normally, turnover of the collagen in connective tissue is continual. Vitamin C is an essential nutrient in *catalyzing this collagen formation. Iron* serves as a cofactor with ascorbic acid in the synthesis of collagen whereas *copper* is needed as part of a metalloenzyme to stabilize the collagen.[81]

A vitamin C deficiency results in a greater permeability of the *capillaries* and of the *basement membrane*. These two conditions accelerate the movement of serum transudate from the vascular system, out into the connective tissue, through the basement membrane, and then between the separated epithelial cells before entering the gingival sulcus.[82] An acute scurvy can be produced by placing monkeys on a vitamin C-deficient diet for 90 days, with a resultant extensive pocket formation and mobility of teeth due to degradation of the collagen making up the periodontal ligament fibers. Subacute conditions are more difficult to produce experimentally. In two studies, however, gingival inflammation

could be produced on suboptimal amounts of vitamin C if the gingival tissue of a guinea pig was initially stressed by painting the gingiva with silver nitrate,[83] or stressed, in the case of a monkey experiment, with the use of a ligature around the teeth. Part of the reaction in the monkey experiment was attributed to a reduction in phagocytic capability (defense) by the leukocytes in the experimental group.[84]

Several human studies have been conducted to determine the effect of vitamin C in existing periodontal disease with equivocal results. The use of ascorbic acid and multivitamin supplementation over a 69-day period for young children in an African village where gingivitis and bleeding gums afflicted 40% of the populace produced no results.[85] Woolfe[86] could see no effect from the use of megadosage of vitamin C. In a major study of over 8000 people as part of the American National Health and Nutrition Examination Survey (HANES), only a weak relationship emerged between vitamin C levels and periodontal disease.[87] This has prompted the plea to treat periodontitis with scaling, root planing, and plaque control programs and not with megadosages of vitamin C.

B Complex Vitamins.
The B complex vitamins are water-soluble vitamins essential in many instances as coenzymes but *not stored by the body*. A deficiency of these vitamins has produced gingival lesions and changes in the periodontal ligament and bone, but the changes are not those of periodontal disease.[88] A deficiency of the B complex does have an adverse effect on antibody formation, which is an essential part of the body defense system.

Individual deficiencies of B vitamins are *rare*.[89] When they do occur, they often first manifest in the oral cavity with signs such as *cheilosis* (cracks in the corners of the mouth), inflamed tongue, and changes in salivary content.

Folate. The use of oral contraceptives and pregnancy have been associated with gingivitis.[90] Both conditions have been attributed to a deficiency of folate, which is an indispensable factor for the normalcy of rapidly regenerating epithelium.[91,92] With contraceptives, gingivitis can take up to a year to develop.[90] In pregnancy the gingivitis peaks at around 8 months, at a time when nutrition is not adequate to match fetal and maternal demands.[90,92]

MINERAL EFFECTS

Zinc

Zinc regulates function in inflammation by *inhibiting the release of lysosomal enzymes and histamines. A deficiency of zinc can inhibit the formation of collagen and reduce cell-mediated immunity.*[93,94] Theoretically, therefore, tissue levels of zinc can modify periodontal defense mechanisms. Such effects have been shown in rabbits,[95] but the results of human studies have been equivocal.[96,97]

Calcium and Phosphate

Studies relating calcium and phosphate intake to periodontal conditions in humans have been equivocal.[98,99] Dietary calcium-to-phosphate ratios were associated with alveolar bone resorption in edentulous individuals when low calcium intake and low dietary calcium-to-phosphate ratios were positively correlated with severe alveolar ridge resorption. Conversely, a high calcium intake and high calcium-to-phosphate ratio was related to a more normal alveolar ridge.[97–102]

Question 4. Which of the following statements, if any, are correct?

A. The defense against the periodontal diseases resides mainly in the saliva on the oral side of the crevicular epithelium and in the body's immunologic response on the connective tissue side.

B. Even if two end organs received the same amount of nutrient supply from the blood, one might be deficient due to higher nutrient requirements.

C. The basal epithelium of the sulcus turns over every *10 to 14* days.

D. In general, the severity of an impaired immunologic response parallels the severity of a protein deficiency and is reflected by deficiencies of both sIgA and complement factors.

E. Vitamin C and folate deficiencies have been linked to gingivitis.

DIET COUNSELING FOR TREATING PLAQUE DISEASE

Diet Counseling for Treating Caries

The *actual* cariogenicity of different foods will probably never be known, because this can only be determined in the mouth on an individual basis. However, with animal and the human studies it is possible to establish a relative ranking of the *potential* cariogenicity of various foods. This array of information is desirable for research purposes; however, for counseling it is problematic although still useful. A prevention counselor can only safely recommend those foods that consistently result in a pH that is *above* the demineralization range of 5.5 to 5.0. He or she can equally advise against consumption of foods that consistently produce a prolonged drop of pH *below* 5.6. It is impossible however, to evaluate the effect on pH of foods that fall between pH 5.5 and 5.0, because the ultimate caries status in this range is determined by the *magnitude of bacterial challenge, adequacy of host defense, and the remineralization potential of each individual*. This principal is recognized in Switzerland, where if the pH of a commercially available food remains above pH 5.7 for over a 30-minute period following ingestion, the product is considered "safe." Manufacturers are permitted to include this fact on the labels of their products after proof of adequate testing.

Table 15–1 contains a summary of the current estimates of relative cariogenicities of foods. How a carbohydrate is used is often more important than its cariogenic rank, because even the lowest rank used in an unhealthful manner can be hazardous. See Chapter 21 for specific counseling procedures.

Dietary Counseling for Treating Periodontal Disease

Due to the complexity of factors that can affect the course of inflammatory periodontitis, it is difficult to isolate those effects attributable solely to nutrition. Research to date suggests important nutrition-related associations, but much more research is needed. Nevertheless, the following recommendations can be made to patients to help ensure optimal nutrition as a defense mechanism against periodontal disease.

- Ensure that the diet is adequate in nutrient quality and quantity.
- Consume a variety of foods.
- Increase the use of saliva-stimulating fibrous foods.
- Minimize the consumption of sweets.

- Avoid fad diets, which could be deficient in nutrients.
- Avoid megadoses (10× the RDA or greater) of vitamins and minerals.
- Avoid single vitamin supplementation.

Other Nutrition Concerns

Today's dental practitioner is not only concerned with educating patients for the prevention of caries and periodontal disease but also plays an important role in *screening* patients for other health risks. Just as medical history and blood pressure evaluation are used to screen for underlying medical conditions, a dietary assessment and screening can help pinpoint potential nutritional problems that can affect or be affected by dental care. Because of the large number of patients seen regularly in dental practice, the dental team is in an excellent position to recognize areas of nutritional risk and provide referral to patients for appropriate care.[3]

Eating Disorders

Eating disorders, especially *bulimia*, are often first diagnosed in the dental office. Patients, usually young females present with *severe erosion* of teeth, especially lingual surfaces, often accompanied by red, sore, inflamed esophagus and swollen salivary glands. Bulimia is characterized by recurrent episodes of binge eating, (involving the consumption of large amounts of food at a sitting), followed by self-induced vomiting. The use of laxatives or diuretics to induce fluid loss and malabsorption is also common. The acid from regurgitation irritates the soft tissues and causes severe tooth erosion.[103]

Although at first patients usually deny having an eating disorder, when confronted with the oral evidence, they often admit to the disorder. At this point the dentist should refer the patient to a clinic that specializes in eating disorders and elicit patient agreement to undergo treatment. Such clinics are available in many medical facilities. The diagnosis of this disorder by the dentist, and the dental destruction wrought by the disorder, often convince patients to agree to treatment. The treatment requires a multidisciplinary team approach, generally including physicians, psychiatrists, psychologists, nutritionists, and social workers. The patient must be cautioned that for dental rehabilitation to be successful, the underlying problem (the eating disorder and its causes) must be resolved.

Elderly Patients

The older patient may be faced with a variety of changes that affect their nutrition and oral health. Compared with younger individuals, elders have a significantly decreased ability to respond to physiologic challenges. The physiologic changes associated with aging can affect the patient's ability to digest, absorb, and utilize food properly. Psychosocial problems, such as loneliness, depression, and lack of money or access to food, can all undermine good eating habits. Functional problems, such as arthritis, or vision difficulties can directly affect the ability to prepare and eat food. In addition, disorders of the oral cavity, such as missing teeth and dentures, have been considered major factors in the poor eating habits of the elderly.[104] For these reasons, elders have been identified as a group especially susceptible to malnutrition.[105]

Diabetic Patients

The diabetic dental patient is at greater risk for developing oral infections and periodontal disease than the nondiabetic.[106] The dental team should be aware of current approaches to diabetes management and carefully monitor the patient's health status prior to initiating dental treatment.

The nutrition care plan generally requires that patients have meals and snacks of specific nutrient composition at *regularly scheduled intervals* to be coordinated with insulin and exercise. Dietary management has progressed from the high-fat, low-carbohydrate diets of past decades to the more liberal use of complex carbohydrates and the reductions in fat recommended today.[103,107] Use of cariogenic fermentable carbohydrates should be infrequent so a diabetic diet should be low in cariogenicity. Frequent use of hard candies or other foods designed to counteract hypoglycemia are signs that the diabetes is not well controlled. Patients with diabetes that is not controlled should be referred for further medical care. In addition, quickly assimilated foods, such as juices, milk, and crackers, should be kept readily available *in the dental office* in case diabetic patients develop symptoms of hypoglycemia. This may happen if they have taken their insulin but delayed eating until after the dental appointment.

Cancer and Immunocompromised Patients

When providing dental services to patients suffering from cancer or AIDS, it is essential that team members understand the nutrition principles underlying the care of such patients, so that the preventive dental services provided can be coordinated effectively with total care. Immunocompromised patients, such as those suffering from cancer or AIDS, often have increased requirements for nutrients in the face of various physiologic and psychosocial impediments to eating. To meet nutrition needs in the face of such obstacles, the nutrition care plan often requires that patients consume frequent small meals, which may be high in sugars and in total calories.[108] In such cases, the dental team should *not* caution patients to reduce the frequency of eating, because this contradicts the nutritional management goals. Rather, thorough cleaning and use of fluoride mouth rinses before bed should be stressed. This approach is standard for immunocompromised patients as part of the usual aggressive preventive program.[109] All cancer patients should be cautioned, however, about the potential oral sequelae of an increased frequency of eating. Patients should also be cautioned to avoid the use of slowly dissolving hard candy to assuage the xerostomia that may result from surgery or radiation therapy.

Oral and Periodontal Surgery and Wired Jaws

The patient who has had oral surgery, whether it be therapeutic or as a result of trauma, is a candidate for special nutrition consideration.[110] An adequate diet *before* surgery is essential to support adequate postsurgical response. The surgery itself can result in an inability to chew, anorexia, and increased metabolic requirements.[111] After surgery, a patient may need a liquid diet for 1 or 2 days but should be graduated as soon as possible to a soft diet of high nutritional quality until normal eating ability is restored. In some cases, nutritionally complete liquid supplements may be appropriate and should be prescribed in consultation with the patient's dietitian and physician.[112,113]

Question 5. Which of the following statements, if any, are correct?

A. Bulimia is strongly associated with the facial erosion on teeth.

B. *Complex carbohydrates* add to the burden of fermentable carbohydrates in diabetes control.

C. A nutritional deficiency *plus* a gingival irritant (calculus) is more damaging to the gingiva than a nutritional deficiency alone.

D. In an epidemiologic study, it is *easy* to identify single-nutrient deficiencies.

E. An oral surgery patient who has extreme difficulty in chewing or swallowing can usually be *started on a soft* diet and then changed to a normal diet in a few days.

SUMMARY

Caries and periodontal disease exist because bacterial challenges can overwhelm the body's defenses. This bacterial attack leads to the incipient lesions for caries and periodontal disease, that is the white spots for caries and gingivitis for periodontal disease.

To cope with these attacks, the body has an arsenal of biologic defenses, including peroxidase, lactoferrin, lysozyme, sialin, and statherin, backed up by the immunologic and humoral defense systems. For the repair systems involving osteocytes, fibroblasts, and epithelial cells to function, all nutrients must be available on demand, otherwise the quality of the replacement tissue is downgraded. To meet these biologic defense requirements, the body stores some nutrients, synthesizes others, and depends on the timely and continuous ingestion of still others.

The best advice for using nutrition as a primary preventive dentistry tool is to consume a daily diet that at all stages of life meets the RDA requirements while adopting dietary patterns that limit cariogenic potential.

Because dental professionals see patients more frequently than other health care providers, they are in an ideal position to screen patients for nutritional risk and refer patients to a physician or dietitian for appropriate care. Patients whose nutrition problems are related to their oral condition should receive appropriate diet counseling from the dentist or hygienist. This may mean recommending changes in the texture or consistency of foods so as to alleviate masticatory difficulties or providing appropriate preventive dietary guidance for caries or periodontal disease. No longer can the dental school nutrition course consist of the single dictum "Sugar is bad, and fluoride is good."

ANSWERS AND EXPLANATIONS

1. B, C, D.
   A—incorrect. Should be Recommended *Dietary* Allowances.
   E—incorrect. The daily consumption of the fruit group (2–4 servings) is considerably less than the 6 to 11 servings of the pasta group.
2. A, B, E
   C—incorrect. Clearance times range from 6 to 24 minutes, with the average near 15 minutes.
   D—incorrect. Frequent breast feeding can cause "baby-bottle" caries.
3. A, D, E
   B—incorrect. Proximity telemetry furnishes the most complete and accurate data.
   C—incorrect. The reverse is true; foods serve to limit rather than prevent plaque buildup.
4. A, B, D, E
   C—incorrect. Very rapid—every 3 to 6 days.
5. C
   A—incorrect. It is the lingual surface that is affected by the vomiting of the acid stomach contents.
   B—incorrect. Complex carbohydrates along with a low-fat intake are currently being advocated in diabetes control.

D—incorrect. Dietary factors are so closely linked that it is very difficult to identify a single-nutrient deficiency.
E—incorrect. The starting diet should be a liquid diet, then a soft, and finally a normal diet.

SELF-EVALUATION QUESTIONS

1. The National Academy of Sciences established the _____ and _____ Board in 1940 in anticipation of possible wartime rationing (The last part is true).
2. All *daily reference values,* for simplicity's sake, are designated as _____.
3. The *Food* _____ (geometric figure) is a diagrammatic means of presenting the diversity of food groups recommended for daily consumption.
4. An example of a macromineral is _____; of a micromineral _____; and a mineral sometimes considered a macro- and at other times a micromineral _____ _____.
5. A severe protein deficiency can lead to a lower level of the salivary immunoglobulin, secretory _____.
6. Two events in history that have contributed to the extensive consumption of sugar are _____ and _____.
7. Caries resulting from the use of sugary solutions in baby bottles is known as _____ _____ caries, or _____ _____ syndrome.
8. In establishing a *caries potential index* the basal diet is fed by _____, whereas the test diet is fed orally. Explain why.
9. Three methods for determining plaque pH are: plaque sampling, _____

_____, and _____
_____.

10. Three items that should be on an after-dinner menu to reduce caries risk are _____, cheddar cheese, and a stick of _____ _____.

11. Two cariogenic minerals are _____ and _____; two cariostatic minerals are _____ and _____.

12. Demineralization of teeth occurs in the range of pH _____ to _____.

13. A vitamin C deficiency leads to a greater permeability of the blood _____ and of the _____ _____.

14. Habitual self-induced vomiting, which erodes the teeth, is termed _____.

REFERENCES

1. Navia JM. Evaluation of nutritional and dietary factors that modify animal caries. *J Den Res.* 1970; 49:1213–1227.

2. Watson RR. Nutrition, disease resistance and age. *Food Nutr News.* 1979; 51:1.

3. Palmer C, Dwyer J, Clark RE. Expert opinions on nutrition in clinical dentistry. *J Dent Educ.* 1991; 23:291–293.

4. Stager S, Levine A. The need for nutritionists: A survey of dental practitioners. *J Am Diet Assoc.* 1990; 1:100–102.

5. *Recommended Dietary Allowances,* 10th ed. Washington, DC. National Academy Press. 1989.

6. Crawford LM. The food label reform initiatives of the U.S. Departments of Agriculture and Health and Human Services. *Nutrition Rev.* 1992; 50:2–3.

7. Mandatory nutrition labeling—FDA's final rule. *Nutr Rev.* 1993; 51(special report): 101–105.

8. Welsch S, Davis C, Shaw A. A brief history of food guides in the United States. *Nutr Today.* Nov/Dec. 1992:6–11.

9. Welsh S, Davis C, Shaw A. Development of the food guide pyramid. *Nutr Today.* Nov/Dec. 1992:12–13.

10. US Department Health and Human Services. *The Surgeon General's Report on Nutrition and Health; Summary and Recommendations.* USPHS. 88-50211; 1988.

11. Menaker L, Navia JM. Effect of undernutrition during the perinatal period on caries development in the rat: V. Changes in whole saliva volume and protein content. *J Dent Res.* 1974; 53:592–597.

12. McMurray DN, Reyes MA, Watson RR. Secretory and cellular immunity in severely malnourished children during nutritional recuperation. *Fed Am Soc Exp Biol.* 1977; 36:1171. Abstract 4758.

13. Alvares, O. The effects of protein malnutrition on monkey parotid saliva. In: Kleinberg I, Ellison SA, Mandel ID, eds. Proceedings on saliva and dental caries. *Microbiol Abstracts.* 1979; (special suppl) 123–126.

14. Pindborg JJ, Bhat M, Roed-Peterson B. Oral changes in South India children with severe protein deficiency. *J Periodont.* 1967; 38:218–221.

15. Alvarez J, Carley K, Caceda J, et al. Infant malnutrition and dental caries: A longitudinal study in Peru. *J Dent Res.* 1992; 71(special issue):749. Abstract 1864.

16. Watson RR, McMurray DN. Effects of malnutrition on secretory and cellular immunity. In: Furia TE, ed. *CRS—Critical Reviews of Food and Nutrition.* Cleveland, OH. CRS Press; 1979.

17. Sintes J, Miller S. Influence of dietary iron on the dental caries experience and growth of rats fed an experimental diet. *Arch Latinoam Nutr.* 1983; 33:322–338.

18. Navia JM. Prevention of dental caries: Agents which increase tooth resistance to dental caries. *Int Dent J.* 1972; 22:427–440.

19. Hardwick JL. The incidence and distribution of caries throughout the ages in relation to the Englishman's diet. *Br Dent J.* 1960; 108:9–17.

20. MacGregor AB. Changing diet and its effect on caries prevalence in Ghana. *J Dent Res.* 1963; 42:1086. Abstract 16.

21. Read TG. Some chemical changes occurring in the mouth during the mastication of food composed of roller flour. *Br Dent J.* 1901; 22:590–595.

22. Mecredy RJR. Some observations on dental caries and allied conditions. *N Zeal Med J.* 1924; 23:324–329.

23. Parfitt GJ. The apparent delay between alteration in diet and change in caries incidence; A note on conditions in Norway reported by Toverud. *Br Dent. J.* 1954; 97:235–237.

24. Takeuchi M. Epidemiological study on relation between dental caries incidence and sugar consumption. *Bull Tokyo Dent Coll.* 1960; 1:58–70.

25. de Jong MH, van den Kieboom CWA, Lukassen JAM, et al. Effects of dietary carbohydrates on the numbers of *Streptococcus mutans* and *Actinomyces viscosis* in dental plaque of mono-infected gnotobiotic rates. *J Dent Res.* 1985; 64:1134–1137.

26. van der Fehr FR, Löe H, Theilade E. Experimental caries in man. *Caries Res.* 1970; 4:131–148.

27. Dennis DA, Gawronsky TH, Sudo SZ, et al. Variations in microbial and biochemical component of four-day plaque during a four-week controlled diet period. *Dent Res.* 1975; 54:716–722.

28. Jay P. Reduction of oral *Lactobacillus acidophilus* counts by the periodic restriction of carbohydrates. *Am J Orthod.* 1947; 33:162–184.

29. Institute of Food Technologists. *Sugars and Nutritive Sweeteners in Processed Foods. A Scientific Status Summary by the I.T.T. Expert Panel on Food Safety and Nutrition.* Chicago, IL; Institute of Food Technologists, May 1979.

30. Bibby BG. Changing perspectives on dental caries. In: Storey E, ed. *Diet and Dental Caries. Changing Perspectives.* Melbourne, Australia. University of Melbourne; 1982:1–17.

31. MacFadyen EE, Campbell MS, Weetman DA. Oral sugar clearance and pH of plaque and saliva. *J Dent. Res.* 1990; 69(special issue):941. Abstract 65.

32. Cox GF, Draus FJ, Entress CP. How long does sugar remain in the mouth? *Dent Prog.* 1963; 3:152–154.

33. Loesche WJ. Role of *Streptococcus mutans* in human dental decay. *Microbiol Rev.* 1986; 50:353–380.

34. Ismail AI, Burt BA, Eklund SA. The cariogenicity of soft drinks in the United States. *J Am Dent Assoc.* 1984; 109:241–245.

35. Johnson D, Nowjack-Raymer R. Baby bottle tooth decay (BBTD): Issues, assessment, and an opportunity for the nutritionist. *J Am Diet Assoc.* 1989; 8:1112–1116.

36. Sclavos S, Porter S, Kim Seow W. Future caries development in children with nursing bottle caries. *J Pedodontics.* 1988; 13:1–10.

37. Madsen KO. Influencing dental caries by daily control of the diet. *J Dent Res.* 1985; 64(special issue):293. Abstract 1070.

38. Newbrun E. Sugar and dental caries. *Clin Prevent Dent.* 1982; 4:11–14.

39. Rugg-Gunn AJ, Edgar WM. Sugar and dental caries: A review of the evidence. *Community Dent Health.* 1984; 1:85–92.

40. De Paola DP, Alfano MC. Diet and oral health. *Nutr Today.* 1977; 12:6–11; 29–32.

41. Navia JM, Lopez II. Rat caries assay of reference foods and sugar-containing snacks. *J Dent Res.* 1983; 62:893–898.

42. Miller WD. The microorganisms of the human mouth. Cited in Noto WA, ed. *Oral Microbiology,* 2nd ed. St Louis, Mo. C.V. Mosby Co.; 1973:251.

43. Tanzer JM. Testing food cariogenicity with experimental animals. *J Dent Res.* 1986; 65(special issue):1491–1497.

44. Bowen WH, Amsbaugh SM, Monell-Torrens S, et al. A method to assess cariogenic potential of food stuffs. *J Am Dent Assoc.* 1980; 100:677–681.

45. Edgar WM, Dodds MWJ, Highham SM. The control of plaque pH and its significance in relation to the evaluation of food

cariogenicity. In: Leach SA, ed. *Factors Relating to Demineralization and Remineralization of the Teeth.* Oxford. IRL Press; 1986:115–126.

46. Proceedings, scientific consensus conference on methods of assessment of the cariogenic potential of foods: Executive summary. *J Dent Res.* November 17–21, 1985; 65(special issue):1540–1543.

47. Slee AM, Tanzer JM. The repressible metabolism of sorbitol (D-glucitol) by intact cells of the oral plaque forming bacterium *Streptococcus mutans. Arch Oral Biol.* 1983; 28:839–845.

48. US Department of Health and Human Services. *Oral Health of U.S. Adults: The National Survey of Oral Health in U.S. Employed Adults and Seniors (1985–1986), National Findings.* NIH Publication No. 87-2868. 1987.

49. Schamschula RG, Keyes PH, Hornabrook RW. Root surface caries in Lufa, New Guinea. I. Clinical observations. *J Am Dent Assoc.* 1972; 85:603–608.

50. Papas A, Palmer C, McGandy R, et al. Dietary and nutritional factors in relation to dental caries in elderly subjects. *Gerodontics.* 1987; 3:30–37.

51. Ravald R, Hamp SE, Birked D. Long term evaluation of root surface caries in periodontally treated patients. *J Clin Periodontol.* 1986; 13:758–767.

52. Lindhe J, Wicen PO. The effects on the gingiva of chewing fibrous foods. *J Periodont Res.* 1969; 4:193–201.

53. Longhurst P, Berman DS. Apples and gingival health. *Br Dent J.* 1973; 134:475–479.

54. Arnim SS. The use of disclosing agents for measuring tooth cleanliness. *J Periodont.* 1963; 34:227–245.

55. Alexander AG, Morganstein SI, Ribbons JW. A study of the growth of plaque and the efficiency of self-cleansing mechanisms. *Dent Pract.* 1969; 19:293–297.

56. Krobicka A, Bowen WH, Espeland MA. The effect of ingestion of cheese and peanuts on composition of saliva from rats. *J Dent Res.* 1985; 64(special issue):188. Abstract 123.

57. Jensen ME, Schachtele CF. The acidogenic potential of reference foods and snacks at interproximal sites in the human dentition. *J Dent Res.* 1983; 62:889–892.

58. Silva MFA, Jenkins GN, Burgess RC, et al. Effects of cheese on experimental caries in man. *J Dent Res.* 1985; 64(special issue): 188. Abstract 124.

59. Jensen ME. Human plaque pH responses to processed cheese food with urea. *J Dent Res.* 1985; 64(special issue):347. Abstract 1554.

60. Rosen S, Min DB, Harper DS, et al. Effect of cheese with and without sucrose, on dental caries and recovery of *Streptococcus mutans* in rats. *J Dent Res.* 1984; 63:894–896.

61. Featherstone JDB, Myers ML, Zero DT, et al. Effects of cheddar and processed cheese on de/remineralization in vivo. *J Dent Res.* 1990; 69(special issue):181. Abstract 584.

62. Harper DS, Osborn JC, Hefferren J, et al. Cariostatic evaluation of cheeses with diverse physical and compositional characteristics. *Car Res.* 1986; 20:123–130.

63. Jensen ME. Responses of interproximal plaque pH to snack foods and effect of chewing sorbitol-containing gum. *J Am Dent Assoc.* 1986; 113:262–266.

64. Hall AF, Crenor WH, Gilmour WH, et al. Effect of a sugar-containing chewing gum on in situ enamel lesion remineralization. *J Dent Res.* 1993; 72(special issue):395. Abstract 2332.

65. Shin C, Hsieh C, Dodds MWJ, et al. Effect of increased mastication on plaque pH and parotid saliva. *J Dent Res.* 1990; 69(special issue):321. Abstract 1699.

66. Arnold FA. Fluorine in drinking water: Its effect on dental caries. *J Am Dent Assoc.* 1948; 36:28–36.

67. Curzon MEJ. Influence on caries of trace metals other than fluoride. In: Guggenheim B, ed. *Cariology Today.* New York. Karger; 1984:125–135.

68. Putt MS, Kleber CJ. Dissolution studies of human enamel treated with aluminum solutions. *J Dent Res.* 1985; 64:437–440.

69. Dérand T, Petersson LG. Inhibiting effect on demineralization of permanent root surfaces after different topical application of fluorides and a solution containing Fe- and Al-ions. *Swed Dent J.* 1982; 6:117–120.

70. Navia JM, Menaker L. Nutritional implications in wound healing. *Dent Clin North Am.* 1976; 20(3):549–567.

71. Alfano MC, Miller SA, Drummond JF. Effect of ascorbic acid deficiency on the permeability and collagen biosynthesis of oral mucosal epithelium. *Ann NY Acad Sci.* 1975; 258:253–263.

72. Alfano MC, Masi CW. Effect of acute folic acid deficiency on the oral mucosal permeability. *J Dent Res.* 1978; 57:312. Abstract 949.

73. Joseph CE, Ashrafi SH, Steinberg AD, et al. Zinc deficiency changes in the permeability of rabbit periodontium to ^{14}C-phenytoin and ^{14}C-albumin. *J Periodont.* 1982; 53:251–256.

74. Alfano MC. Controversies, perspectives and clinical implications of nutrition in periodontal disease. *Dent Clin North Am.* 1976; 20:519–548.

75. DePaola DP, Kuftinec MM. Nutrition in growth and development of oral tissues. *Dent Clin North Am.* 1976; 20:441–459.

76. Beagrie GS, Skougaard MR. Observations on the life cycles of the gingival epithelial cells of mice as revealed by autoradiography. *Acta Odont Scand.* 1962; 20:15–31.

77. Enwonwu CO. Role of biochemistry and nutrition in preventive dentistry. *J Am Soc Prevent Dent* 1974; 4:6–17.

78. Alvares O, Worthington B, Enwonwu CO. Regional differences in the effects of protein-calorie malnutrition (PCM) on oral epithelia. *J Dent Res.* 1976; 55:B173. Abstract 448.

79. Pollack RL, Kravitz E. *Nutrition in Oral Health and Disease.* Philadelphia, Pa. Lee & Febiger; 1985:136–146.

80. de Menezes AC, Costa IM, El-Guindy MM. Clinical manifestations of hypervitaminosis A in human gingiva: A case report. *J Periodontol.* 1984; 8:474–476.

81. Freeland JH, Cousins RJ, Schwartz R. Relationship of mineral status and intake to periodontal disease. *Am J Clin Nutr.* 1976; 29:745–749.

82. Nakamoto T, McCroskey M, Mallek HM. The role of ascorbic acid deficiency in human gingivitis—a new hypothesis. *J Theor Biol.* 1984; 108:163–171.

83. Glickman I. Acute vitamin C deficiency and the periodontal tissues. II. The effect of acute vitamin C deficiency upon the response of the periodontal tissues of the guinea pig to artificially induced inflammation. *J Dent Res.* 1948; 27:201–210.

84. In the JAMA under section entitled From the NIH. Primate studies indicate that subclinical and acute vitamin C deficiency may lead to periodontal disease. *J Am Med Assoc.* 1981; 246:730.

85. Prentice AM, Lamb WH, Bates CJ. A trial of ascorbic acid and of multivitamin supplementation on the oral health of West African children. *Trans Roy Soc Trop Med Hyg.* 1983; 77:792–795.

86. Woolfe SN, Kenney EB, Hume WR, et al. Relationship of ascorbic acid levels of blood and gingival tissue with response to periodontal therapy. *J Clin Periodontol.* 1984; 11:159–165.

87. Ismail AI, Burt BA, Ecklund SE. Relation between ascorbic acid intake and periodontal disease in the United States. *J Am Dent Assoc.* 1983; 107:927–931.

88. Chawla TN, Glickman I. Protein deprivation and the periodontal structures of the albino rat. *Oral Surg Oral Med Oral Pathol.* 1951; 4:578–602.

89. Scrimshaw NS, Suskind RM. Interactions of nutrition and infection. *Dent Clin North Am.* 1976; 20:461–472.

90. Lindhe J, Branemark P. The effects of sex hormones on vascularization of granulation tissue. *J Periodontol Res.* 1968; 3:6–11.

91. Streiff RR. Folate deficiency and oral contraceptives. *J Am Med Assoc.* 1970; 214:105–108.

92. Thomson ME, Pack AR. Effects of extended systemic and topical folate supplementation on gingivitis of pregnancy. *J Clin Periodontol.* 1982; 9:275–280.

93. Solomons NW. Zinc and copper. In: Shills M, Young V, eds. *Modern Nutrition in*

Health and Disease. Philadelphia, Pa. Lea and Febiger; 1988:238–250.

94. Pekarek R, Sandstead H, Jacob R, et al. Abnormal cellular immune responses during acquired zinc deficiency. *Am J Clin Nutr.* 1979; 32:1466–1471.

95. Nizel AE, Papas A. *Nutrition in Clinical Dentistry,* 3rd ed. Philadelphia, Pa. WB Saunders; 1989:201–203.

96. Frithiof L, Lavstedt S, Eklund G, et al. The relationship between bone loss and serum zinc levels. *Acta Med Scand.* 1980; 207: 67–70.

97. Freeland J, Cousins R, Schwartz R. Relationship of mineral status and intake to periodontal disease. *Am J Clin Nutr.* 1976; 29:745–749.

98. Binkley L. *The Relationship of Alveolar Bone Loss to Calcium and Phosphorus Ingestion in Humans.* Columbus, OH: Ohio State University; 1978. Thesis.

99. Sweeney E, Shaw J. Nutrition in relation to dental medicine. In: Shills M, Young V, eds. *Modern Nutrition in Health and Disease,* 7th ed. Philadelphia, Pa. Lea & Febiger; 1988:1069–1098.

100. Wical K, Swoope C. Studies of residual ridge resorption, Part II. The relationship of dietary calcium and phosphorus to residual ridge resorption. *J Prosthet Dent* 1974; 32:13–22.

101. Wical K, Brusse P. Effects of a calcium and vitamin D supplement on alveolar ridge resorption in immediate denture patients. *J Prosthet Dent* 1979; 41:4–11.

102. Sorensen R. *A Study of Dietary Calcium and Phosphorus Intakes in Relation to Residual Ridge Resorption.* Loma Linda, Calif: School of Health, Loma Linda University; 1977. Thesis.

103. Weinsier RL, Morgan SL. *Fundamentals of Clinical Nutrition.* St. Louis. Mosby Year Book; 1993:42–48.

104. Roe D. *Geriatric Nutrition.* Englewood Cliffs, NJ. Prentice Hall, Inc.; 1983:75–77.

105. Palmer CA. Nutrition and oral health of the elderly. In: Papas A, Niessen L, Chauncy H. *Geriatric Dentistry: Aging and Oral Health.* St. Louis. Mosby Year Book; 1991:264–282.

106. Holdren RS, Patton LL. Oral conditions associated with diabetes mellitus. *Diabetes Spectrum.* 1993; 6:11–17.

107. The DCCT Research Group. Nutrition interventions for intensive therapy in the diabetes control and complications trial. *J Am Diet Assoc.* 1993; 93:768–772.

108. Smith TJ, Dwyer JT, LaFrancesca JP. Nutrition and the cancer patient. In: Osteen RT, Cady B, Rosenthal P, eds. *Cancer Manual,* 8th ed. Boston. American Cancer Society; 1990: Chapter 39.

109. Dwyer JT, Efstathion MS, Palmer C, et al. Nutritional support in treatment of oral carcinomas. *Nutr Rev.* 1991; 49:332–337.

110. Sintes JL. Nutrition intervention in general dentistry. *Compend Continuing Educ Dent* 1990; 11:734–739.

111. Soliah L. Clinical effects of jaw surgery and wiring on body composition: A case study. *Diabetic Currents,* volume 14. Columbus, OH. Ross Laboratories; 1987.

112. Kendall BD, Fonseca RJ, Lee M. Postoperative nutritional supplementation for the orthognathic surgery patient. *J Oral Maxillofac Surg.* 1982; 40:205–213.

113. Rugg-Gunn AJ. Current issues concerning the relationship between diet and dental caries. *J Int Assoc Dent Child.* 1990; 20:3–7.

Chapter 16

Understanding Human Motivation

Arden G. Christen
Clifford A. Katz

Objectives

At the end of this chapter it will be possible to

1. Discuss Bloom's hierarchy of educational objectives in relation to patient education.
2. Explain how the learning ladder integrates attainment of educational objectives with patient motivation.
3. Discuss how value systems are developed.
4. Define motivation, and explain the difference between intrinsic and extrinsic motivation.
5. Name the components of the five-tier hierarchy of human needs, as proposed by the humanistic psychologist Abraham Maslow, and explain their relationship to motivation as affluence and learning levels improve.
6. Define adherence, and discuss its importance in the development of a patient home care program.
7. Explain the role of the health provider and the role of the health consumer in accomplishing behavioral changes.

Introduction

Dentists are not people oriented. They are things oriented. They are technique oriented. They don't know enough about people. The only trouble is that they have to work with and on people. Too bad we can't work on typodonts. The first thing we should learn is that, to every tooth there is attached a person.—Charles W. Jarvis, DDS

The Problem

About half of the people in the United States do not see a dentist regularly, and among low-income people, the proportion not receiving care is even higher.[1] Christen's[2] review of the literature revealed a number of stated reasons why people avoid dental treatment (Table 16–1).[3–15] They include

1. Habitual personal neglect
2. A perceived high cost of dental care

3. Pessimism and ignorance concerning dental diseases and dental treatment
4. A questioning of the dentist's motives and reactions to the patient
5. Fear and anxiety of a conscious and unconscious nature
6. Negative feedback or unflattering statements about dentistry received from friends or relatives.

Other factors identified as having helped people lose confidence in dentists include poorly executed or ineffective prior treatment (technical quality of care); work that does not last long enough; lack of access; unnecessary or questionable extractions or other treatments or charging a fee for work that was ineffective or had to be repeated. Previous painful experiences and perceived negative dentist behaviors (as when a dentist was arrogant, sarcastic, inconsiderate, or lost his or her temper) appear to be especially important to the anx-

TABLE 16–1. PERCEIVED ORIGINS OF ADVERSE REACTIONS TO DENTISTRY

Reasons	No. Responses	% Total Participants Giving Responses*
Negative expectations from others	83	16.9
Much painful dental work	67	13.5
Perceived dentist error	45	8.3
Fear of needles (specifically)	41	8.3
Perceived poor management	32	6.8
Dislike of dentist's personality	23	4.7
General fear of dentistry (unspecified)	13	3.0
Fear of drill	10	2.4
Physical abuse by dentist or assistant	8	1.5
Dislike of procedure and setting	8	1.5
Not knowing what to expect	7	1.3
Dislike of doctors in general	3	<1.0
Dislike of other's hands in one's mouth	3	<1.0
Fear of reprimand for poor oral hygiene	1	<1.0
Total negative reasons	344	

*Percentages computed by dividing number of respondents giving a particular response by total number of participants, N = 487. Some gave more than one reason, others did not respond, thus, percentages do not total 100%.
(From Kleinknecht RA, Klepac RK, Alexander LD. Origins and characteristics of fear of dentistry, J Am Dent Assoc. 1973; 86:842–846.)

ious individual who is mentally preparing for dental treatment (Table 16–1). All of these allegations are people-to-people problems and in the majority of cases can be solved by effective educational programs and by an understanding, sensitive, and common-sense interpersonal relationship between the health professional and the patients. This possibility for changing the public's attitude is reinforced by the fact that recent polls indicate that the image of dentistry is very high and improving.[2]

Psychology and Education in Prevention Programs

In previous chapters the point was made that primary preventive dentistry can be effectively implemented by using five actions: (1) plaque control, (2) sugar discipline, (3) fluoride therapy, (4) use of pit-and-fissure sealants, and (5) education. The successful use of any of these measures requires an interaction of health professionals and patients to achieve and maintain a maximum level of oral health. Three major factors are necessary for both parties to achieve this rapport—*information, motivation,* and *psychomotor skills.* The psychomotor factor is thoroughly discussed in Chapter 19, in which physical and neurologic handicaps are considered. In this chapter the interrelationships of education, motivation, human values, socioeconomic needs, and behavioral modification are considered—all with the objective of helping the health professional to become a more understanding, knowledgeable, and effective health educator and health counselor.[15] This task of educating the patient, the health professional, and the community can be greatly simplified by a knowledge of and the application of a few basic precepts of educational psychology and human motivation. These same precepts apply equally to either private or public health practices.

Sources of Information

For any preventive dentistry program to succeed, information must be available to both the health professional and the patient about what *needs* to be done and *how* it is to be accomplished. For the layman this information—and sometimes misinformation—is learned through public school programs; from the dentist, the media, and advertising; and from peers, friends, neighbors, and family. On the other hand, the health professional learns preventive dentistry as part of the undergraduate school curriculum and after graduation by reading dental journals, attending society meetings and major conventions, or by participating in continuing education programs. The void between the information possessed by the lay person and the health professional is great. This gap poses a problem in health education because people tend to seek what they already believe and avoid exposure to anything that mandates change.[2] As a result of the disparity in backgrounds, the task of the health professional is to attempt to "fit" new information into a framework of what is already known to the health consumer.[16] Many clinicians believe that information is the basis for motivational change. Unfortunately, however, the patient's having information does not mean that he or she is actually moved to action.

METHODS FOR FACILITATING LEARNING

The Learning Process

Because information transmittal involves learning, it is desirable to turn to the teaching profession for how information is best imparted to ensure long-term retention. Getting a patient to comply with a home care regimen can be the most difficult part of therapy.[17] According to Bloom's taxonomy of educational objectives, a hierarchy of six levels of learning attainment proceeds from a complete lack of information to goal attainment.[18] These successive levels are *knowledge, comprehension, application, analysis, synthesis,* and *evaluation.* Most teaching today is at the entering-knowledge stage. On mastery of this stage, the learner can *only* define, repeat, or name facts; it is only partial learning at best. Possible verbs used in stating cognitive outcomes of teaching programs starting with the knowledge level up to evaluation are listed in Figure 16–1.

The implication of partial learning is apparent when applied to plaque control methods. The average person *knows* and *comprehends* that brushing and flossing

clean the teeth. They can even *demonstrate* that they can brush their teeth in some fashion. But how many people can *evaluate* the effectiveness of their efforts? How many can *analyze* where problems lie, and how many can *propose* innovations to their personal oral hygiene program that might make it more effective?

At each cognitive level the teaching should feature an *explanation* of the subject, followed in sequence by *demonstration, application, feedback,* and *reinforcement.* The employment of these sequential steps in all teaching helps to ensure a mastery of the subject. In moving from one level of complexity to the next, the learner is exposed to an *organized* continuum of interrelated facts. Even after successfully

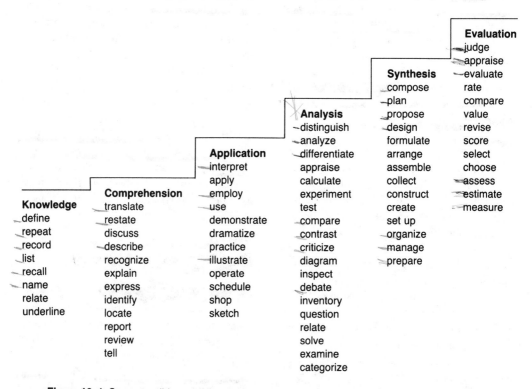

Figure 16–1. Some possible verbs for use in stating cognitive outcomes. (*Courtesy of Marybelle Savage.*)

mastering all levels of Bloom's hierarchy, however, it is very possible that a skill or subject area learned in an academic environment is not applied on a routine basis. The day-to-day application occurs only after the individual has learned sufficient information to determine that a specific benefit accrues to him or her from its use. Education involves learning; practical application involves self-motivation.[19]

Incorporating Knowledge into Value Systems

The mouth represents a body area of special importance and value for children and adults. According to Horowitz and coworkers,[20] the mouth is associated with the development of (1) a healthy personality, (2) perceptions, (3) gross motor skills, and (4) the overall experience of pleasure. Many areas of the mouth, especially the gingival tissues, are easily accessible for self-diagnosis and primary preventive treatment. Gums that are red or bleeding can be easily detected by the patient. The tongue, with its highly developed neurosensory feedback system, can be useful in helping patients to assess their own plaque levels and the resultant need for improved oral hygiene behavior. As a result, dental personnel and school health educators should be able to devise strategies for motivating self-care oral behavior by teaching individuals how to recognize their own signs of dental distress or neglect.

The application of knowledge requires that an individual have enough *facts* to develop *concepts* and then a sufficient number of *concepts* to develop a *value*.[2] Graphically this concept is portrayed in Figure 16–2. The base of the pyramid consists of facts, which are the building blocks of all learning. Sometimes great voids or even misinformation occur in this body of information. Yet, regardless of its completeness or accuracy, this substratum of information is where concepts are formed by use of one's reasoning power. Concepts, less numerous than facts, represent the organization and classification of facts into a meaningful personal pattern. The greater the number of correct facts arising from different inputs, the greater the possibility of developing correct concepts. On top of these supporting facts and concepts rest values—beliefs and bodies of

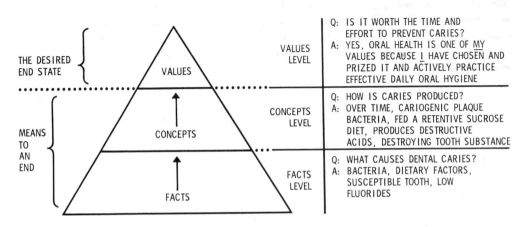

Figure 16–2. The interrelationship between values, concepts, and facts using oral health as a positive end value. Learning on all three levels helps individuals discern facts, make sense of them and, finally, to live by the meanings they perceive.

knowledge important to the individual. These values are only as strong as the supporting information. It should be noted that all dental values are not positive. For individuals living under impoverished conditions who do not appreciate the value of teeth from a health or social viewpoint or where the loss of teeth is considered as normal, the facts, concepts, and values are often negative. These negative perceptions can motivate nonparticipation in dental programs.[9] A health educator must carefully consider the possible myriad facts and concepts that can make up this pyramid when trying to change a patient's value system—a value system that is valid to only the patient.

Values are not neutral but are held with personal feeling.[2] When they are challenged, they frequently generate an emotional, defensive response. Making changes in one's behavior is often very difficult and involves dealing with conflict. Hayakawa expands this idea when he writes, "the process of learning, which is also the process of growth, is essentially a means of resolving conflicts . . . a conflict must always be present before learning can occur . . . conflict then is a necessary accompaniment of personality development, and the progressive assimilation of disturbing stimuli is the only practical means by which a stable organization can be attained. Without conflict, no learning results."[21]

Therefore it is necessary that the health professional understand that because of this value system, resistance is normal and permanent changes in some forms of behavior are difficult to achieve. This same resistance is met from the patient in the dental office, or from many in the community, when new health programs are proposed. For example, sugar discipline is difficult to instill because of concepts and values shaped early in childhood by the media and the candy-laden shelves in the supermarkets; water fluorida-

tion efforts have failed in some areas because of a barrage of misinformation and distorted facts, leading to strongly held values by those voting against fluoridation. Such resistance to change should not prevent the continual education and pressure for more effective oral disease control programs. In this quest, however, we must be careful how we approach the value systems of our patients or of the community. We must respect the fact that others have their own value systems tied to their own set of expectations that may be quite different from ours.

Can human values be changed? The answer is yes, but this statement must be qualified. Values are slow to form and slow to change.[2] Even if the factual information is complete and adequate, *time* is required for concepts to *evolve* and to *mature;* even more time is required before other additional facts and concepts are acquired to support a new value. Stated another way, a health professional should not expect dramatic and immediate changes in patient behavior as a result of only one or two counseling sessions.[a] Thus to attain a behavioral change, a health education program is often confronted with the imposing requirement to modify or reconstruct completely the facts and concepts making up an existing value structure. No wonder so many health education programs fail. A case in point is the American smoker. Virtually all smokers have enough facts necessary to develop the concept that the addiction, cigarette smoking, is harmful. Yet many have not accepted this concept into their own value systems to the point of behavioral change, namely of *not* smoking. It is also seen in caries and pe-

---

[a] Counseling is an interpersonal process that establishes the educational basis and recommended actions for patient motivation and action to accomplish a specific task.

riodontal disease control programs in which patients are unwilling to conduct lifelong programs of plaque control.

Conditions for Value Change

In 1974, Haynes and Matthews[22] presented four rules to consider before attempting to change another person's values. They have been modified to the dental workplace as follows:[2]

- Dental personnel must *be aware of their own values* and how they affect their choices in planning for, and implementing changes in, dental behavior.
- Dental personnel must *understand the needs and values held by the patient* before planning a dental health education program. Values may be inferred from the patient's behavior, active listening, and by careful observation. The prompt fulfillment of immediate needs is often vital. For example, relieving pain or improving the patient's appearance by temporarily restoring a broken anterior tooth helps promote respect and trust between the patient and oral health team members.[17]
- Dental personnel must not impose *their* values or related behaviors on a patient who has a different set of values. Sometimes these patient values can be altered by education and peer pressure.
- The methods used to obtain change and the degree of success is determined in part by the degree of "fit" between the advocated change and the individual's value system.

Bakdash[17] adds two steps to the educational-motivational model.

- Discover what motivates the patient to seek treatment.
- Reinforce prior instruction. It often takes three to five sessions to achieve good plaque control levels.

Merging Motivation and Education

A second popular way of looking at the education process, other than Bloom's hierarchy of learning, is based on communications research indicating that humans learn in a sequential series of steps. This approach is exemplified by the *learning ladder,* a ladder with six rungs, which begins with total *unawareness* of the area to be discussed and extends up to *habit formation* (Fig 16–3).[23–25] Health professionals often mistakenly assume that patients will comply with their wishes and totally revise their oral hygiene habits after only one session on oral health care. In fact, many of our office educational programs are based on the false premise that "knowing *how* to do something" motivates people to do it.

The first task to be resolved in helping to facilitate another person's learning (or our

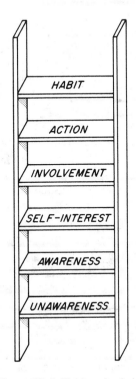

Figure 16–3. The learning ladder.

own) is to determine on what rung of the learning ladder the learner stands. The sequence of progress usually cannot be varied, nor can any steps be eliminated.[26] Attempts to change behavior by "leapfrogging" over one or several steps can result in failure to reach the top of the ladder. In such an event no permanent behavior change occurs.

The lowest level, *unawareness,* is often the current behavior of the patient. The individual simply lacks information or has faulty data concerning the problem. For example, if one does not realize that a relationship exists between oral hygiene and caries, then the person is *unaware.* Likewise, if a person believes that calculus "causes" periodontal disease or that "soft teeth" are inherited, this misinformation also constitutes unawareness. *Awareness* occurs when the correct information is obtained but does not have any *personal* meaning or effect. Stated another way, awareness is a recognition but is not accompanied by any inclination to action.

Even though there is no action, progress has been made, because nothing can happen unless an individual has reached the awareness stage. The real value of reaching the awareness stage is appreciated when an individual—for some conscious or subconscious reason—realizes that the information applies personally; at this time the knowledge has become personalized. The person then enters the *self-interest stage,* which is characterized by a recognition of a prospective objective and a mild inclination to action. If action does occur, the *involvement* stage has been reached. If action does not occur, regression to the awareness stage usually occurs. At this stage of involvement on the learning ladder, most teaching efforts fail. At this time personal attitude is affected, with a feeling component being activated. It becomes important to act on the situation. A desire for knowledge is accelerated; this, in turn, hastens the entry into the next *action stage.* This is a movement phase in which new concepts and practices are tested. True learning is manifest by changes in behavior and results. For instance, after 2 weeks of brushing and flossing as part of the testing, the patient notices that both the swelling and the redness of the gingiva have stopped. Self-satisfaction can directly result from the new practice of brushing and flossing. With this self-satisfaction, the final stage, *habit (commitment),* is reached and practiced over a longer period. The new behavior becomes a part of the individual's lifestyle. At this point, the top of the learning ladder and the top of the pyramid of higher human needs (self-actualization) and of human values (health) come together.

The progress from awareness to habit may be intermittent. Conceivably many years could elapse from the stage of awareness until some triggering event personalizes the information to make upward progress possible.

Note that the sequence of events seen in Bloom's hierarchy and in the learning ladder are somewhat parallel. The main difference is that Bloom's hierarchy emphasizes the learning process per se, whereas the learning ladder focuses on how *motivation* must be considered along with learning in skills development to facilitate and accelerate attainment of the top rung. Once that top rung has been reached with habit formation, the learner has a new value. In other words, the facts are gained at the bottom of the ladder, the concepts acquired as the learner progresses, and a full value emerges at the top.

Question 1. Which of the following statements, if any, are correct?

doesn't accept lots persuasion

A. The layman who is undereducated in dental health readily accepts suggested changes in preventive programs that are directed to better oral health.

1st occurs at limited level — the facts — 2nd at evaluation level

B. Most education results in the learner being able to attain the cognitive level of evaluation on Bloom's hierarchy.

C. Different groups of individuals presented with the *same* facts can develop *different* concepts.

D. Once facts and concepts are a part of an individual's life, values automatically fall in place.

two (reception)

E. The learning ladder approach to goal attainment discourages a too rapid progression from unawareness to habit.

MOTIVATION

What is motivation? Everyone is motivated to action or to inaction. Not to be motivated is to be dead. Some argue that what humans do is primarily *instinctual* in nature. This concept is difficult to accept because of the varied nature of human behavior. If the "instinct theory" were valid, all personalities would show a uniformity of behavior across all cultures.[24] This, of course, is not the case. Others believe that behavior is learned and that environment determines actions. No one should downplay the importance of environmental forces on human behavior; however, humans do initiate their own activities and often appear to act without regard to external forces. Furthermore, these actions seem to fit into a sort of coordinated pattern that reflects a composite of the educational background, socioeconomic status, and cultural mores of the individuals. Despite the fact that human behavior is highly

variable and at times unpredictable, one thing is certain: *Individuals' performances or outputs are based on the degree to which they are motivated.* Motivation makes the difference.

Motivation can be best defined as *the internal knowledge and will of the entire individual to act*. It is an *inner* drive *pushing* an individual to satisfy a need.[27] It is not something that one can produce in someone else; it can only be reinforced and supported by others. When individuals have found a motive to spur them to action, we say that they are motivated.[28] Motivation is not achieved by using certain "tools" or methods but rather is a distinct property of life itself. The "push process" usually seems to occur naturally and gradually without any specific effort on the part of the individual. When we *want* to do something, we motivate ourselves internally by means of innate forces. Only *we* can motivate ourselves by using our own generator and self-starter. Others can fuel the generator with encouragement, ideas, and actions, but only we have the key to start the generator. Motivation is that "something" that moves patients to take the action necessary to prevent dental disease.[14]

Human motivation is complex. It is based on a blending of expectations, ideas, feeling, desires, hopes, attitudes, values, and other factors that initiate, maintain, and regulate behavior toward achieving a given goal or outcome. Other factors, such as previous adverse experiences, educational insufficiency, nonacceptance by peers, a poor self-image, and impoverished socioeconomic circumstances can cause negative behaviors. Some of these positive or negative "motivators" are operating at a subconscious level. Motivation factors can change with the passage of time. Humans are strongly goal-oriented and can demonstrate a tremendous drive to achieve their personal ambitions. For some, however, a significant part of the pleasure is derived from working toward a goal; after they have "arrived," their pleasure is somewhat diminished. For these individuals, getting there is not only half the fun, it is possibly all the fun. For example, some individuals periodically become intensely motivated to upgrade their oral health status. Appointments are made with the dentist, all restorative work is completed, preventive programs are developed with a great amount of patient participation until all dental care has been completed, at which time the individual appears to lose interest until another sudden flurry of interest may occur at a later date.

Intrinsic and Extrinsic Motivation

Intrinsic motivation results from an internal decision; it is truly self-generated. Basically people are strongly driven to make their own decisions and do what they wish. In most cases these decisions are made on the basis of facts, concepts, and values held by the individual. Nearly everyone's behavior is self-justified. A naturally developing intrinsic motivation that is based on an individual's own desires usually produces *long-lasting* learning or action. The health educator should provide the information and establish an environment that allows an individual to make an informed decision freely.

In contrast to intrinsic motivation, the primary source of influence in *extrinsic motivation* resides outside the individual. *Persuasion* can be regarded as an example. Persuasion can be defined as the attempt to influence through appeal to reason or to a personal relationship. These are powerful methods to influence behavior, especially when the health educator and patient have developed a relationship of trust or when the patient is seeking logical answers to a problem. Often simple persuasion becomes, in reality, *manipulative persuasion*, which consists of more overt external reinforcement designed more to meet the needs of the educator than the patient. In this case results are achieved by giving or removing rewards, approval, or encouragement or by employing punishment, fear tactics, biased presentations, or threats from the outside source. Sometimes the difference between persuasion and subtle manipulative persuasion is rather indistinct.

Because only the individual concerned can be motivated, when we as health educators speak of "motivating people to do something," we are technically in error. All that the health professional does is to establish the proper learning environment, deliver accurate and timely information, and persuade and facilitate an individual's desire for behavioral change.

SOCIOECONOMIC NEEDS AND PREVENTIVE MOTIVATION

Maslow's Hierarchy of Human Needs

Abraham Maslow, the late humanistic psychologist, viewed the human organism as an integrated, organized whole and not as a collection of separate organs and functions.[29] The inner forces that drive a person to action were referred to by Maslow as *needs*. He believed that an individual takes action to satisfy these needs, and he conceptualized *five levels of basic human needs*.[29] These five levels can be arranged in a pyramid form (Fig 16–4), with the highest priority needs being at the base.

In this pyramid two *lower order needs* and three *higher order needs* occur. The two basic lower order needs are (1) *physiologic* needs, which include those necessary to maintain body homeostasis, such as the need for food, water, oxygen, proper tem-

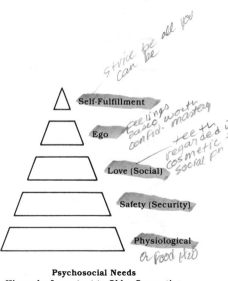

Strive be all you can be

Feelings basic worth confid. mastery

teeth regarded w cosmetic social fn

Self-Fulfillment

Ego

Love (Social)

Safety (Security)

Physiological

or food h2O

**Psychosocial Needs
Hierarchy Important to Older Generation**

Figure 16–4. Maslow's hierarchy of needs is presented in a pyramidal graphic format. The size of each level represents its relative importance to the other needs in the hierarchy.

perature, sleep, and other functions necessary for human survival; and (2) *safety* and *security* needs, which control the number of hazards that can cause physical and mental damage as well as guaranteeing a stable and predictable environment. For example, Burdette and Gale[30] believe that people who have been suffering chronic toothache pain may have great difficulty dealing with anything other than seeking relief from that discomfort. Patients with chronic pain do not become accustomed to it, but rather seem to become more sensitive and to suffer more with the passing of time.[30] Once the majority of physiologic and safety needs have been met, the sociopsychologic needs then become the prime motivating force. These higher order needs have been learned or acquired as a part of the developing individual's socialization process. They are more cognitive than physiologic and more concerned with the individual's sense of *self* and uniqueness. These needs are not easily and permanently satisfied.[29] The higher need for *love and social belongingness* implies group acceptance, social ac-

ceptability, and opportunity to give and to receive friendship and love. This is the point at which teeth are regarded as having important cosmetic and social functions.[10,29,32] The *ego* (self-esteem) needs involve our feelings of basic worth, including achievement, confidence, mastery, competence, prestige, and status. Finally, the highest need for *self-actualization* is based on a positive tendency for development, growth, and self-enhancement. At this level the individual strives to become the person one has the potential to be.

To Maslow, as long as individuals are subjected to lower need bondage, they cannot concentrate on satisfying the higher needs.[33] To put it simply, if a person is worried about where the next meal is coming from (physiologic), he or she will probably have little concern about upper level needs such as the kind of toothbrush and toothpaste available for dental health care. Similarly, an infantryman who worries about surviving in the heat of battle has little interest in oral health care. Concerns about love, ego, and self-actualization all take a back seat in these circumstances. These examples also underline a very important point about education and motivation. It is futile to attempt to educate an individual during an emergency, when he or she is in pain, or when the patient's life is severely disrupted.

Maslow's Concepts Brought Up to Date

In an important, provocative paper, Drumm updated Maslow's concepts to reflect more closely the age in which we live.[34] He pointed out that the older generation (over 35 years of age) had values based on the conventional work ethic: "To work is good, and to work even harder is better." These traditional, achievement-oriented concepts, developed during the era of scarce commodities and scattered population, accentuated the omnipresence of Maslow's lower order needs (Fig 16–4). As the older generation made gains toward the "good life," enjoying the greater abundance of commodities and sociologic advances, and as society took collective steps to decrease personal concerns about meeting physiologic or safety needs, individual *need systems* changed. The reduced emphasis on physiologic and, to a lesser extent, on security needs changed the pyramidal configuration to that of a diamond (Fig 16–5). When overwhelming emphasis was subsequently placed on the higher needs, the emerging younger generation devoted more and more energy to ego satisfaction and self-fulfillment; a further metamorphosis of the pyramid occurred, and an inverted pyramid emerged (Fig 16–6). This gap between today's older and younger generations often makes it difficult for one group to understand the other. Stated differently, many of

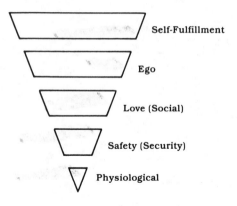

Emerging Generation Needs
(lower needs satisfaction guaranteed)

Figure 16–6. Inverted pyramidal shape of Maslow's hierarchy resulting from a much higher emphasis being placed on the fulfillment of higher order needs in the emerging generation.

the older generation see the need for behavioral patterns that ensure a continuance of emphasis on lower order needs, whereas the younger generation that did not experience the Great Depression can focus only on behavior that is oriented toward self-actualization. To summarize, *assessing need patterns of the potential audience is vital for any person who seeks to communicate effectively with others.* Also, as the lower order needs diminish and the higher needs begin to dominate, individuals are more likely to consider oral health programs, especially prevention, as one of their values associated with self-fulfillment.

Alternative Preventive Approaches for Different Levels of Patient Motivation

Medical science can deal with many acute and infectious diseases. Coping with diseases that can be prevented, arrested, or ameliorated with *behavioral change,* as is the case with smoking-induced disease and periodontal disease and caries has not been

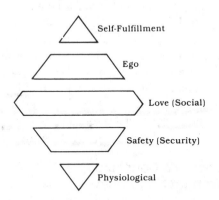

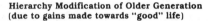

Hierarchy Modification of Older Generation
(due to gains made towards "good" life)

Figure 16–5. A diamond-shaped modification of Maslow's hierarchy of needs is illustrated for the traditionalists who have their safety and physiologic needs largely met. The love and belongingness (social) needs emerge as the most important in motivating behavior. (*From Drumm RH. The Air Force Man and the Cultural Value Gap. Air Univ. Rev. 1968; 19:20–24.*)

as successful.[35] The only barrier to preventing the ravages of these chronic diseases is behavioral change, a change that can range from either a minimally motivated person passively accepting continual preventive care provided by health professionals to active participation by the patient, or both.

Surgeon General C. Everett Koop stated that the combined use of sealants and fluorides should essentially eliminate dental caries.[36,37] There is also evidence that a thorough prophylaxis at 2- to 4-month intervals plus a high level of daily oral hygiene maintains good periodontal health.[1,38] With an appropriate recall interval, use of pit-and-fissure sealants, topical applications, and prophylaxes, a relatively high level of oral health can be maintained with little motivation of the patients to develop their own self-care programs. The *only* motivation requirement is that the patient respond to a mailed or telephone recall appointment. This passive method of plaque disease control is expensive,[39] and if more than a quarterly recall appointment is necessary, it is not practical on a mass population basis.

The other two approaches to plaque disease control, sugar discipline and plaque control, do require behavioral changes and self-discipline. Theoretically, if an individual were to use self-discipline to minimize sugar intake, coupled with meticulous brushing and flossing techniques, a high level of oral health could be maintained. Unfortunately both of these approaches require a continuous, lifelong motivation to achieve.

Self-motivation to accept sugar discipline is not easy to achieve because sugar is an integral part of our culture—a reward in the form of pastries and candy. It is available in most prepared foods.[40] Any change in eating patterns represents a major shift in attitude. Eating practices are deeply ingrained and can be influenced by one's upbringing, lifestyle, socioeconomic status,

religion, emotional status, interest in personal health and appearance, outside commercial pressures, and availability of different types of food.[38] Probably the simplest way to change sucrose consumption patterns is to *persuade* dietitians and mothers to restrict the availability of sweets in institutions and in the home environment. Appeals can also be made to patients to reduce the frequency of eating sweets to permit a longer time for saliva-induced remineralization, of applying effective plaque control procedures to minimize the effect of acidogenic episodes, and, finally, to increase the use of fluoride preparations to reduce demineralization and to enhance remineralization. Such actions require a knowledgeable and concerned (motivated) public.

Plaque control measures are difficult to accomplish and require considerable time, skill, and perseverance. In fact, current measures of oral hygiene requiring fastidious removal of all supragingival plaque may be beyond the average individual.[41,42] Thus a blend of education, motivation, and psychomotor skills are necessary to ensure good personal oral hygiene measures. There is *no* good evidence to support the fact that mass education alters individual behavior. Instead, individualized approaches are usually necessary, and even these are not always successful.

For a dentist entrusted with the preventive care of a moderately motivated individual, the recall program should be at sufficiently frequent intervals to compensate for lapses in patient self-care routines. At the same time, the educational and motivation phases of patient education should be emphasized to improve the participation and effectiveness in self-care programs. In this way the health professional assumes the task of caring for the patient to the extent that compensates for the shortcomings of the patient while preparing the patient to assume a greater role in maintaining personal oral health status. Ultimately it is the patient who must assume as much responsibility for self-care as possible and to seek out the health professional for evaluation (examination) and reinforcement when deficiencies are noted or suspected.

Adherence

The term *motivation* applies to the enthusiasm and desire of an individual to achieve a given objective. *Adherence* is the term used to indicate the actual cooperation of a patient in carrying out recommended directions and actions for the prevention or treatment of a disease. It is used interchangeably with the term *compliance*. Compliance is a problem for all the health professions.[43] A counseling session is of little use if the patient does not choose to secure the necessary drugs or follow the recommended actions for self-care. Even when serious medical problems are present, it is estimated that 30% to 70% of the recommended regimens are not followed.[44] Adherence is greatest when the recommended act is simple, of short duration, and produces immediate results; conversely, it is least effective when the task is complex, of long duration, or does not produce dramatic results.[45] Preventive procedures usually fall in the latter category because they only produce a lifelong continuum of good health.

Despite the fact that adherence is critically important for self-care programs, relatively little is known about how to identify the patient who demonstrates adherence. Common sense dictates that the patient must know exactly what is expected. Thus the education program should be directed to achieving *both* patient motivation and adherence. Patients with a good record of participating in preventive recall visits and with a higher occupational status, educational level, and income tend to demonstrate more adherence to recommended self-care programs. The greatest success in adherence is attained with a patient who

- Believes that he or she is susceptible to the disease;
- Is convinced that the disease can be prevented;
- Understands that prevention is preferable to disease; and
- Knows that he or she can modify the course of the disease.[46,47]

To illustrate this point, in a retrospective factory study in which free dental care was available, 80% of those who had made a preventive visit over the past 3 years subscribed to these beliefs. To the contrary, no visits were made by individuals believing the contrary.[47]

When all is said and done, probably the maximum success in attaining adherence depends on the personality, persuasiveness, and interest of the practitioner, the health professional–patient rapport, and the enthusiasm and motivation of the patient to cooperate in recommended self-care programs.

Question 2. Which of the following statements, if any, are correct?

A. Intrinsic motivation, rather than extrinsic motivation, produces the longest lived learning or action.

B. An individual usually gives a higher priority to physiologic needs than to security needs and to both of these higher priority than to oral health needs.

C. Ideally a primary preventive care program is designed to permit the dentist to compensate for small or large discrepancies in a patient's self-care regimen.

D. In considering a patient's motivation potential, a greater amount of self-motivation is required for plaque control and sugar discipline than for primary prevention using fluoride therapy and sealants.

E. Adherence—or compliance—implies motivation plus a directed action to accomplish a recommended objective.

SELECTING METHODS OF INFLUENCING BEHAVIOR ALTERATION

The Health Professional's Role

It is tempting for the health professional to try to impose his or her views on the patient without explanation because he or she knows that the principles of health care are well founded and applicable in general.[28,48,49] Most patients, however, are willing to cooperate in employing health care procedures *if they understand the reasons behind the rec-ommended treatment.* Health professionals must make their own interests clear-cut and known to the patient to ensure that the patient does not feel manipulated by an omniscient and socially distant expert.[24] The approach used to influence or to inform the patient should be guided by the individual's needs, motives, and self-established values.[25] In dental practices, or in any business or personal relationship, failure to show sensitivity to the feelings of others destroys the foundation of mutual trust and cooperation. The option of selecting different styles of participation or methods of influence to affect either lower or higher order needs is shown in Figure 16–7. When dealing with higher order needs, the use of authority, bargaining, coercion, and fear arousal should be avoided. These manipulative methods may produce *short-term success* but are unlikely to result in a long-term behavior change.

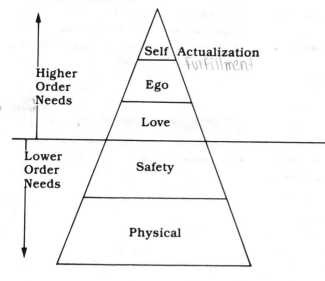

Higher Order Needs

Self Actualization
Fulfillment

Ego

Love

1. Acceptance
2. Intellectualization
3. Persuasion
4. Reward

Lower Order Needs

Safety

Physical

1. Authority
2. Bargaining
3. Coercion
4. Fear Arousal

Figure 16–7. Methods of influencing higher and lower order needs. It is prudent to avoid dealing with lower order needs because the methods of influence are geared toward manipulative nonproductive methods.

Authoritarian or Nonauthoritarian Styles

The health professional has the choice of two ways to relate to a patient, either as an *authoritarian* or as a *nonauthoritarian*. According to Barkley,[15] most dentists and other health professionals are practicing authoritarians and are adept at applying external pressures on people. For the health professional in command, authority provides a means of achieving quick, efficient, and gratifying results.[25] Many individuals are not even aware of their authoritarian image because it is so ingrained in their daily patterns of dealing with others.

The authoritarian is forceful, doing most of the talking and advice giving, with the patient expected to listen and to obey.[50] Sometimes there is a tradeoff, with the health professional giving praise *if* the patient has cooperated and relinquished his or her right to make decisions regarding his or her involvement in the diagnostic and treatment processes. It should be mentioned, however, that some patients welcome the authoritarian approach, because it frees them from the responsibility of decision making; in this scenario the responsibility for initiating, altering, or maintaining the desired behavior remains in the hands of the authoritarian—not in the hands of the patient.

Some other serious problems are associated with the authoritarian style. Authority often generates resentment and *temporary*, grudging compliance, as long as the external pressure is being applied. Exercising authoritarian influence is tyrannical, because people are not achieving *their* own goals. They are not doing the things they want to do, and eventually they rebel. The specter of an authoritarian menacingly pointing a forefinger and stating, "You really should *want* to keep a clean mouth," does not qualify as a universal incentive to action.[50–51] Generally, excessive fear arousal

leads to unpredictable behavior and the blocking out of other important information.[23] Also, direct frontal attacks on personal value systems are often counterproductive. The confronted person may avoid the professional in the future or may even retaliate.

On the other hand, sometimes the authoritarian approach is absolutely necessary. In times of emergency, when correct decisions must be made quickly to avoid life-threatening events, the authoritarian should take command. Also, the same authoritarian approach is justified in dealing with individuals not capable of decision making, such as the young and the mentally retarded. Whenever possible, such decisions should be made in concert with parents or guardians.

The nonauthoritarian approach seeks to develop the potential of the patient's desire to satisfy his or her needs. The health professional and the patient conjointly explore the various preventive options and planning objectives. The nonauthoritarian appeals to higher order means of acceptance, including reasoning, nonthreatening persuasion, and rewards. He or she talks less, listens more, questions, reacts, clarifies, or synthesizes when necessary.[41] This nonauthoritarian approach is based on Carl Rogers' paradoxic self theory, which states that learning and change best take place when a person is free to reject change. According to Rogers,[26] this freedom of choice allows the patient to be his or her true self, thus increasing the possibility of learning new behavior.

Accurate Empathy: Emotional Understanding

According to Mittelman,[21] our professional background has taught us some faulty assumptions. For example, we incorrectly assume that those "correct and good" things that *we* want for our patients are desired by our patients as well. It is humanly difficult to keep from projecting our standards and values onto our patients and to accept their present motives, desires, and emotions. This is exactly the true nature of empathy and rapport, however. Mittelman[21] had rightly concluded that "human communication is essentially an exchange of feelings, not information. . . . People seldom think. They always feel."[21]

Our task, therefore, is to seek out and to understand our patient's real, current desires and motives. To accomplish this we need to become involved in what Rogers terms "accurate empathy" (ie, nonpossessive warmth).[26] The patients' experiences and verbalizations are accepted without imposing preconditions. Patients are allowed to have their own feelings and are appreciated for being themselves, regardless of their behavior. Even though we have great difficulty in sharing our patients' emotions, we should appreciate and be aware of those feelings.

To summarize, humans are born with a drive to maximize their potential as human beings (eg, to learn all they can, to master challenge, and to develop fully and use their talents).[29] One of our most important tasks as professionals and as employers is to provide a growth-enhancing environment. If we create a repressive, inhibiting, or punitive environment, those around us will fail to self-actualize (eg, their natural growth processes will become distorted or diminished).

Modeling or Vicarious Learning

One of the most important ways that people learn new behaviors and are motivated to maintain such behaviors is by observing others, or what psychologists often refer to as *modeling*, or *vicarious learning*. Psychologic research has shown that certain characteristics of given individuals make them more important as models than others, with status or prestige being an extremely important

variable. To us as health professionals this means that our patients are going to look at us as being important models, especially in the area of health behavior.

How many of us have heard our parents say, "Do as I say, not as I do"? Which part of our parents' message was really the most influential? Most likely their actions were more important than their words when it came to the way we actually responded. When the words and the actions are too incongruent or discrepant, we become faced with a *credibility gap*. This gap often results in distrust or cynicism on the part of those exposed to such situations. To illustrate the point, take a few moments to imagine the following scenes.

First Scene

You're going to your physician for a checkup and in the reception room are several attractive posters dealing with the health dangers of cigarette smoking. You are impressed with the physician's concern for your good health and well-being. Then, as you are ushered into the private office, the physician exhales a large cloud of smoke, puts the cigarette down in an ashtray full of butts, and stands up to greet you.

Second Scene

You're going to attend a public lecture on the importance of good nutrition on health and longevity. The speaker is supposed to be an expert on the benefits of nutrition and nutritional research. As the speaker approaches the podium, you see that the expert is extremely obese and seems to have difficulty just walking up the three or four steps to the stage.

Third Scene

You are going to your dentist to have your teeth cleaned and checked. While performing the prophylaxis, the dentist talks to you about the importance of regular prophylaxis, oral hygiene, and reduction of sweets. At one point the dentist grins broadly and you notice that his or her teeth are stained, there are obvious calculus deposits at the gingival margins of the lower anterior teeth, and the gingival tissues are inflamed in several areas. As you leave, the receptionist gives a lollipop to each of your children.

What reaction did you have to these scenes? How much confidence would you place in what these professionals had to say about various health practices? Are these scenes far-fetched? Variations of these scenes do occur continuously in health care settings; often the professionals involved are frustrated that their patients just do not seem to follow their directions or suggestions. Sadly, there is some evidence that physicians who smoke or do not exercise are less likely to be concerned about such practices among their own patients; this is also true of a dentist who does not floss and who indiscriminately consumes refined carbohydrates. We tend often to be blind to the practices of others when we ourselves have not managed to overcome them. These practices, whether deliberate or not, tend to undermine seriously the effect of our message. In one way or another we present our patients with a credibility gap that renders us less effective in influencing their behavior. It is not that we do not believe what we are saying, it is that the belief lacks conviction or commitment without which behavior does not change.

As health professionals we can more effectively get ourselves to do what we know *we* should do in order that we might not only help ourselves but also be more effective models for our families, friends, staffs, and patients. This should not imply that if a dentist or auxiliary serves as a perfect role model concerning preventive health practices, patients will do likewise. Rather, sound practices on our part help re-move an important block to behavior change by our patients (the credibility gap) and furnish positive, successful, motivating models for them to attempt to emulate.

Behavioral Change Strategies for the Patient

Sometimes the motivation is strong to accomplish a behavioral change; however, a strong habit may already exist that interferes with attainment of the desired objective. This dilemma is well illustrated by the obese individual who desires to reduce, by the individual with an insatiable craving for sweets, and by the individual who is a chain smoker. The question is, "What strategies are available to eliminate the old behavior to substitute the new?" Two general approaches are *positive thinking*, which implies one decision to get rid of the old habits and to bring in the new simultaneously, through simple determination; and *behavioral self-control*, which involves a planned process to permit coping with the interfering habit.

Positive Thinking. Anyone visiting the psychology section of almost any bookstore will realize that books on self-improvement, self-understanding, and self-motivation are abundant. Many of the popular books are based more or less on the concept of "*positive thinking*." Basically this approach states that "you can, if you think you can"—and then concentrates on developing a positive attitude about succeeding at any given task and of developing a positive self-image. *The Power of Positive Thinking*[52] by Norman Vincent Peale and *Psychocybernetics*[53] by Maxwell Maltz are two popular examples of this approach to self-motivation.

The fundamental quality that an individual must possess to engage in such an approach is *will power*. Will power is a concept with which we are all familiar, but it is not easily defined nor understood. What is it? From where does it come? Often will power is likened to an almost supernatural inner force or an inherent personality trait that only some people have. How many times have we tried to modify some behavior of our own—such as overeating, exercising, flossing, or smoking—only to find that we did not have sufficient will power to accomplish our goal? We almost feel at times as though we were not blessed with sufficient "will power genes" and are therefore doomed to failure.

Behavioral Self-Control. An alternative approach to changing one's own behavior has developed in the field of behavior therapy and might best be labeled *behavioral self-control,* as opposed to positive thinking. Psychologists Michael Mahoney and Carl Thoresen in their book *Self-Control: Power to the Person*[54] state that behavior and attitudes are learned and then are maintained or altered by both environmental influences (cues) and the resultant consequences of that behavior. The key to effective self-regulation, they feel, is clearly understanding the person–environment relationship rather than focusing strictly on personality traits. Simply stated, the important factors are *cues and consequences;* self-control depends on the individual's ability to recognize and change these two factors. Mahoney and Thoresen[54] refer to the ABCs of human behavior—antecedents, behavior, and consequences—that help us understand what is controlling the behavior to be changed.[16] Actually three processes are involved in successful self-control: (1) specification of the behavior to be changed, (2) identification of the behavior's antecedent environmental cues, and (3) implementation of a plan to alter the cues or consequences or both as needed. What are the necessary steps to accomplish these goals?

Self-Observation. The first step involves careful *self-observation,* by which is meant both paying attention to the behavior of interest and, very importantly, recording the level of occurrences of the behavior. Several benefits arise from careful monitoring of one's own behavior: (1) increased self-awareness, (2) immediate quantitative feedback on what we are doing or not doing, and (3) information about the environmental cues and subsequent consequences. Keeping weight charts; food intake diaries; accounts of where, when, and how many cigarettes smoked; frequencies and duration of jogging or cycling excursions, and so on provide an excellent record and incentive by helping us to visualize our behavior patterns. Do we snack mostly while watching television? Do we smoke more when drinking alcoholic beverages or coffee? Do we exercise more faithfully when someone else is with us than when alone? This type of information is invaluable in helping us to understand what maintains or hinders our behaviors.

Interestingly, research has demonstrated that keeping careful records of behaviors alone can alter their frequency. Recognizing what one is doing may be sufficient enough motivation to stimulate change. A common example in preventive dentistry is the reduction in sugar intake by patients once they have maintained a food diary and become aware of the surprisingly high frequency of their carbohydrate consumption.

Environmental Planning. The next self-control strategy has been labeled *environmental planning* by Mahoney and Thoresen.[54] This involves changing the environment so as to change the cues preceding a behavior. Often this requires the elimination or avoidance of situations that trigger the undesired behavior. Examples might be not eating and watching television at the same time or in the same room, limiting all sugar intake to meal times, arranging to exercise daily with another person, arranging a specific time and distraction-free location for studying, or linking oral hygiene procedures to some regularly occurring event like watching the 10 o'clock news.

Behavioral Management. The third self-control strategy, *behavioral management*, deals with changing the consequences of a behavior rather than the triggering event or situation. Several approaches can be used to accomplish this task, including various forms of self-reward or self-punishment. One approach commonly used is the "when–then" principle, by which is meant engaging in some highly desirable behavior contingent on completion of the behavior to be initiated. For instance, one cannot watch a favorite television program such as the "Tonight Show" until brushing and flossing have been completed or the evening paper cannot be read until one has exercised or jogged. A basic principle of behavior management is that desired behavior must be rewarded to enhance the probability of its being repeated.[55] *Positive reinforcement* is the term for following a desirable behavior with an appropriate reward. In general it is usually better to set some realistically obtainable goal, such as flossing every day for a week, after which you reward yourself and then set a new goal, rather than to set goals so high that you have little chance of success and a high probability for failure and discouragement of future efforts.

Social reward or punishment can be utilized by means of public self-monitoring. Openly displaying the charts or graphs of an individual's progress enlists the aid and encouragement of others in helping achieve goals of specified behavioral change. In addition, we can use internal reinforcement in terms of self-praise and feelings of accomplishment as means of motivating the maintenance of our new behavior. Whereas Maxwell Maltz's[53] *Psychocybernetics* discusses changing one's self-image to effect behavioral change, more recent research has demonstrated that self-image is changed as a result of successful involvement in a behavioral change program. Discovering, perhaps for the first time, that we can quit smoking, begin flossing regularly, lose weight, and so forth can in itself be very satisfying and bolstering to one's self-esteem.

Learning and successfully applying the methods of behavioral self-control provide an individual with a sense of personal accomplishment and fulfillment that derives from *knowing*, not just thinking, that behaviors can be changed to more desirable directions. The difficulty does not lie in a lack of will power but rather in acceptance of responsibility for unwanted behaviors. *If we as health professionals refuse to accept the same responsibility, the probability of our patients doing any better is severely diminished.*

BASIC PHILOSOPHY

A basic philosophy of prevention is itself a value. One basic philosophy concerning preventive dentistry is that *patients deserve to know the cause of their dental diseases and how they can prevent them.* This is a responsibility for the health educator. *Once armed with the knowledge, however, the patient reserves the right to remain sick.* This is a problem of self-motivation. Patients are ultimately responsible for their own dental health. In the final analysis, prevention is a shared responsibility between the practitioner and the patient.

Question 3. Which of the following statements, if any, are correct?

A. The advantages and disadvantages of an authoritarian approach to patient care are reversed in times of crisis.

B. *Vicarious learning* is a negative implication of *modeling*. are synonyms

C. Will power is the method of choice in attempting to change the behavior of large numbers of people.

D. Keeping a record of undesired events is often accompanied by a behavior change without the need for environmental planning or behavioral programming.

E. Primary preventive dentistry receives equal emphasis with secondary and tertiary prevention, mainly because of the motivation of most dentists.

SUMMARY

The maintenance of good oral health requires a partnership between the health professional and the patient. No preventive program can be a success unless the patient participates in a home self-care program to supplement office care programs, with the level of success being proportionate to the amount of participation. Maximum participation can be expected when the patient knows *what* to do, *how* to do it, and above all has the *motivation* to adhere to recommended procedures. Educational strategies can be used to teach facts and skills, but these are useless without motivation. Motivation can be initiated by an individual based on some need or desire, or it can be stimulated by persuasion from external sources. With or without motivation, learning is best achieved in sequential steps, as seen with Bloom's hierarchy of cognitive levels and similarly with the ascending rungs of the learning ladder. As an individual accumulates facts, the facts merge into concepts and ultimately into values, which in turn engender motivation. Motivation can be either positive or negative, depending on environmental or cultural factors. According to Maslow, environmental factors that threaten physiologic and security needs can often redirect all motivation to survival and away from the more personal, higher level needs associated with acceptance by society and good health. At times motivation provides the drive to alter lifestyle to attain habit patterns necessary to maintain good oral health. The health professional can exert a direct or indirect influence on such a change by assuming a passive modeling role, by taking a more active role as an authoritarian, or by participating as a nonauthoritarian in developing a program of planned change by the patient. Such behavioral changes by the patient may involve positive thinking or, more often, strategies that include self-observation, environmental planning, or behavioral planning. All health education requires learning, but the successful application of all health knowledge requires motivation.

ANSWERS AND EXPLANATIONS

1. C, E
   A—incorrect. The average layman does not accept change without considerable persuasion.
   B—incorrect. Most education is directed to the initial level—facts; very little learning ends up at the evaluation level.
   D—incorrect. Facts and concepts represent unorganized and organized thoughts, respectively; values represent the acceptance and personal application of facts and concepts.
2. A, B, C, D, E
3. A, D

B—incorrect. Modeling and vicarious learning are synonyms.

C—incorrect. For only relatively few individuals is positive thinking an adequate source of self-motivation; for the average individual the behavioral self-control provides the best results.

E—incorrect. More rhetoric exists about prevention than action.

SELF-EVALUATION QUESTIONS

1. To be taught a skill, three major factors are necessary: _Informat^n_, _motivat^n_, and _psychomotor. skill_

2. The six cognitive levels of Bloom's hierarchy of learning are knowledge, _Comprehension_, _Applicat^n_, _Analysis_, _Synthesis_, and _Evaluat^n_.
At each level, to ensure mastery learning, the teaching should include in sequence *explanation,* _demonstration_, _applicat^n_, _feedback_, and _reinforcement_.

3. An individual, through reasoning, organizes facts into _concepts_; which in turn are the basis for a _value_.

4. With the learning ladder, the stage between *awareness* and *involvement* is the _self Interest_ stage. The stage at which most teaching failures occur is the _Involvement_ stage.

5. The self-motivation that occurs as a result of persuasion is called _extrinsic_ motivation.

6. In sequence, from the base to the point of the pyramid, the five levels of needs as conceptualized by Maslow are _Physiological_, _Safety Security_, _Love (social)_, _Ego_, and _Self Fulfillment_. It is probably correct to say that more motivation for health

programs can be elicited at the (top) (bottom) of the pyramid. An older person, remembering the Great Depression, would probably be more cognizant of the (lower) (upper) level needs than the present generation. The (classical) (inverted) pyramid is probably more associated with an affluent society than the diamond-shaped characterization of human needs.

7. In the dentist–patient partnership, it is the _patient_ who must assume responsibility for home care programs, whereas the _HCW_ must assume responsibility of identifying and correcting deficiencies that occur in a home care program.

8. The greatest possibility for securing adherence to recommended regimens is with a patient who believes the following about the possibility of contracting disease: _Susceptible to, Can be prevented, prevent prefered Disease,_ and _modify course disease_ The dentist who *dictates* recommended changes is called an _authoritarian_, and the dentist who participates in a health professional–patient agreed-on program is known as a _non authoritarion_.

9. When others learn by emulating the actions of individuals considered as outstanding in their estimation, the type of learning is termed _vicarious_ or _modeling_. When that individual deviates from accepted norms, a _credibility_ gap is created.

10. A synonym for *positive thinking* in bringing about behavior change is _willpower_. Usually, changes in behavior require a longer process involving *behavior,* which can involve three steps: _Self Obs._, _Env. Planning_, and _Bx Mng_.

11. Two reasons that might explain a reluctance of dentists to embrace primary

preventive dentistry are _____
and _____.

REFERENCES

1. U.S. Department of Health and Human Services. *Healthy People 2000: National Health Promotion and Disease Objectives.* DHHS Publication No. (PHS) 91-50213. Washington, DC. Public Health Service; 1991.

2. Christen AG. The development of positive health values. *Health Values.* 1984; 8:5–12.

3. Bernstein DA, Kleinknecht RA, Alexander LD. Antecedents of dental fear. *J Public Health Dent.* 1979; 39:113–124.

4. Christen AG. Improving the child's dental behavior through mental rehearsal. In: Van Zoost B, ed. *Psychological Readings for the Dental Profession.* Chicago, Ill. Nelson-Hall; 1975:91–96.

5. Coombs JA. Application of behavioral science research to the dental office setting. *Int Dent J.* 1980; 30:240–248.

6. Friedson E, Feldman JM. The public looks at dental care. *J Am Dent Assoc.* 1958; 57: 325–335.

7. Gale EN, Ayer WA. Treatment of dental phobias. In: Van Zoost B, ed. *Psychological Readings for the Dental Profession.* Chicago, Ill. Nelson-Hall; 1975:97–106.

8. Haefner DP. Principles and problems of communicating with patients. *National Conference on Patient Education.* Las Vegas, Nev. American Dental Association; 1965: 1–32.

9. Kleinknecht RA, Klepac RK, Alexander LD. Origins and characteristics of fear of dentistry. *J Am Dent Assoc.* 1973; 86:842–846.

10. Linn EL. Social meanings of dental appearance. *J Health Hum Behav.* 1966; 7:289–295.

11. Milgrom P, Weinstein P, Kleinknecht R, et al. *Treating Fearful Dental Patients.* Reston, VA. Reston Publishing Co. 1980.

12. Sosnow I. The emotional significance of the loss of teeth. *Dent Clin North Am.* 1962; 6:637–650.

13. Reisine S, Weber J. Motivations for Treatment and Outcomes of Care. *J Am Coll Dent.* 1989; 56:19–25.

14. O'Hehir TE. Motivation is our never-ending goal. *RDH.* 1991; 11:29, 44.

15. Barkley RF. A rational basis for a behaviorally sound dental practice. *Successful Preventive Dental Practices.* Macomb, Ill. Preventive Dentistry Press; 1972.

16. Weinstein P, Getz T. *Changing Human Behavior: Strategies for Preventive Dentistry.* Chicago, Ill. Science Research Associates, Inc; 1978.

17. Van Houten P. Motivating patients to self-care takes the staff's personal involvement. *Dent Off.* 1989; 1:8–9.

18. Bloom BS, Engelhart MD, Furst EJ, et al. *Taxonomy of Educational Objectives. Handbook I: Cognitive Domain.* New York, NY. David McKay Company; 1975.

19. Savage MB, Johnson RB, Johnson SR, eds. *Assuring Learning with Self-Instructional Packages, or . . . Up the up staircase,* Chapel Hill NC. Self-Instructional Packages, Inc; 1971:141.

20. Horowitz LG, Dillenberg J, Rattray J. Self-care motivation: A model for primary preventive oral health behavior change. *J Sch Health.* 1987; 57:114–118.

21. Mittelman JS. Getting through to your patients: Psychologic motivation. *Dent Clin North Am.* 1988; 32:29–33.

22. Haynes J, Matthews B. Human values: Implications for health education practice. *Int J Health Educ.* 1974; 57:266–273.

23. Corn H, Marks MH, Corn B. Philosophy and psychology of preventive care. Clinical dentistry. In: Clark JW, ed. *Preventive Dentistry.* Hagerstown, Md. Harper and Row Publishers; 1979; Vol. 2:1–30.

24. Hutchins DW. Motivation in preventive dentistry. *Report on the Proceedings of the Fourth Annual Preventive Dentistry Workshop.* Washington, DC, July 25–26, 1967.

Columbia, Mo. The Curators, University of Missouri; 1968.

25. Moss SJ, ed. *Contemporary Dentistry: Persuasive Prevention.* Cincinnati, Ohio. The Crest Professional Services, Procter and Gamble Co, Medcom, Inc; 1975.

26. Rogers CR. *Carl Rogers on Encounter Groups.* New York, NY. Harper and Row; 1979.

27. Shulman J. Current concepts of patient motivation toward long-term oral hygiene: A literature review. *J Am Soc Prev Dent.* 1974; 4: 7–15.

28. Katz S, McDonald JL, Stookey GK. Understanding the patient as a human being: A must for success in any preventive dentistry program. *Preventive Dentistry in Action.* 3rd ed. Upper Montclair, NJ. D.C.P. Publishing; 1979.

29. Maslow AH. *Motivation and Personality,* 2nd ed. New York, NY. Harper and Row Publishers; 1970.

30. Burdette BH, Gale EN. Pain as a learned response: A review of behavioral factors in chronic pain. *J Am Dent Assoc.* 1988; 116: 881–885.

31. Katz CA. Motivation and actualization in the workplace: Cornerstone of a team-based practice. *Mod Dent Pract.* 1988; 1:19–24.

32. Martin RT. *An Exploratory Investigation of the Dentist/Patient Relation.* Australia. The Dental Health Education and Research Foundation, University of Sydney; 1965: 1–29.

33. Frick WB. *Humanistic Psychology: Interviews with Maslow, Murphy and Rogers.* Columbus, Ohio. Charles E. Merrill Publishing; 1971.

34. Drumm RH. The Air Force man and the clinical value gap. *Air Univ Rev.* 1968; 19: 20–24.

35. Glazier WH. The task of medicine. *Sci Am.* 1973; 228:13–17.

36. American Dental Association. US surgeon general urges greater use of pit and fissure sealants. *Am Dent Assoc News.* June 18, 1984:16.

37. National Institute of Dental Research, RFP No. NIH-NIDR-5-82, IR, National Institutes of Health, May 1982.

38. Federation Dentaire Internationale. The prevention of dental caries and periodontal disease. Report #22. *Int Dent J.* 1984; 34: 141–158.

39. Burt BA, Warner KE. Prevention of oral diseases: Its potential for containing the cost of dental care. In: Kudrle RT, Meskin LD, eds. *Opportunities for Cost-Containment in Dentistry.* Minneapolis, MN. University of Minnesota Press; 1981.

40. Shannon IL. Sucrose—the tooth's mortal enemy; fluoride—the tooth's best friend. *J Dent Child.* 1977; 44:429–437.

41. Brady WF. Periodontal disease awareness. *J Am Dent Assoc.* 1984; 109:706–710.

42. Iwata BA, Becksfort CM. Behavioral research in preventive dentistry: Educational and contingency management approaches to the problem of patient compliance. *Appl Behav Anal.* 1981; 14:111–120.

43. DiMatteo MR, DiNicola DD. *Achieving Patient Compliance.* New York. Pergamon Press; 1982.

44. Sackett DL. The magnitude of compliance and noncompliance. In: Sackett DL, Haynes RB, eds. *Compliance with Therapeutic Regimens.* Baltimore, Md. Johns Hopkins University Press; 1976.

45. Geboy MJ, Ingersoll B. Patient adherence to dental regimens. *Compendium Contin Educ.* 1983; 4:185–190.

46. Kegeles SS. Some motives for seeking preventive dental care. *J Am Dent Assoc.* 1963; 67:90–98.

47. Kegeles SS. Why people seek dental care: A test of a conceptual formation. *J Health Hum Behav.* 1963; 4:166–173.

48. Wright R, LeBloch DS, Lapin L. *Winning Communications for the Successful Practice.* Chicago, Ill. American Dental Association; 1986.

49. Wright R, LeBloch DS. *Interpersonal Skills for the Dental Team.* Chicago, Ill. American Dental Association; 1986.

50. Gold SL. Establishing motivating relations in preventive dentistry. *J Am Soc Prev Dent.* 1974; 4:17–25.

51. Mager RF, Pipe P. Analyzing performance problems or you really oughta wanna. Belmont, Calif. Fearon Publishers; 1970.

52. Peale NV. *The Power of Positive Thinking.* Englewood Cliffs, NJ. Prentice-Hall Inc. 1964.

53. Maltz M. Psychocybernetics: The new way to a successful life. Englewood Cliffs, NJ. Prentice-Hall Publishers; 1960.

54. Mahoney MJ, Thoresen CE. *Self-Control: Power to the Person.* Monterey, Calif. Brooks-Cole Publishers; 1974.

55. Sapp RM, Sapp GL. Patient motivation: a challenge for preventive dentistry. *Dent Assist.* 1987; 56:15–18.

Chapter 17

Dental Public Health Programs

Leonard A. Cohen
Harold S. Goodman

Objectives

At the end of this chapter it will be possible to

1. Define dental public health, and cite the criteria necessary to develop successful dental public health programs.
2. List the various political levels that maintain and support public health departments.
3. Compare the methods involved in public health practice with those of private practice.
4. Outline the scope of traditional dental public health programs.
5. Describe recent changes in the United States that are relevant to the practice of dental public health.
6. Discuss the cooperative liaisons between public health personnel and other people and organizations necessary for developing effective programs.

Introduction

By definition, *dental public health programs are organized efforts to improve the oral health of the public.* These programs vary considerably, and may include activities on a wide spectrum, from small-scale local projects to broad-based national and international programs. Dental public health programs must satisfy the criteria of practicality, feasibility, acceptability, safety, effectiveness, and relatively low cost.[1-2] Public health dentistry has a rich tradition of improving the oral health status of the U.S. population. All segments of the dental profession, public and private, including those whose activities involve efforts in education, research, public programs, and private practice, have made significant contributions to the oral health of the public.

HISTORIC PERSPECTIVE

Dental disease has been a significant problem for Americans since our early history.[3] From 1862 to 1864, tooth loss was the fourth most frequent cause for rejection of young men for draft into the Union Army during the Civil War.[4] In 1918, military draftees for World War I were rejected for defective and deficient teeth at a rate that exceeded 10% in some states.[5] Prior to World War II, the *U.S. War Department Mobilization Regulation* required that to be acceptable for military service a man must have a minimum of both three serviceable natural anterior and posterior teeth in opposition in each arch. Fifteen percent of the men could not pass these rather liberal criteria and were rejected.[3]

One of the earliest studies of the dental condition of a large, heterogeneous adult civilian population was conducted by the Metropolitan Life Insurance Company in the 1920s.[6] Dental examinations of more than 12,000 adults revealed that among 20- to 24-year-olds, more than half the teeth had been affected by caries, and this proportion increased steadily in older age groups. The classic rule of thumb established by Knutson[7] states that for every year beyond age 6 years, another tooth became decayed, missing, or filled.

Following World War II, the number of civilian dental surveys increased dra-

matically.[8-13] These studies confirmed the high caries prevalence noted in the military studies. Not only has dental caries caused a high tooth loss and a serious oral health problem in young adults in the past, but the disease also initiates early and affects young children.

A study sponsored by the U.S. Public Health Service (USPHS) of thousands of 6- to 14 year-old children in 26 states across the country between 1933 and 1934 revealed high caries levels in these children.[14] In the classic Hagerstown, Maryland, study of 1937,[15] which introduced the decayed, missing, and filled tooth and surface index (DMFT, DMFS), moderately high caries prevalence was observed among the children examined. Furthermore, the 20% of children with the highest DMFT scores received only 2% of the treatment time rendered by the dentists. The early caries experience of children and the continuing progression of decay to serious levels in most adults provided the rationale for the application of dental public health methods to address the problem. The efforts, cooperation, and interactions of a number of individuals and agencies led to one such method, the implementation of fluoridation.

Fluoridation—A Monumental Public Health Success Story

Fluoridation is the principal dental public health preventive program available in the control of dental caries in the population. Former U.S. Surgeon General Dr. Luther L. Terry stated at a national health meeting in 1966, "Controlled fluoridation is one of the four great mass preventive health measures of all time. The four horsemen of health are the pasteurization of milk, the purification of water, immunization against disease, and controlled fluoridation of water."[16]

The historic development of fluoridation in the United States is an example of the contributions of individuals of varied backgrounds representing public and private segments of the profession. For example, Dr. H. Trendley Dean, considered the "father of fluoridation," had a prominent role in the early developing story of the importance of fluoride to tooth enamel.[17] Dean was an officer in the USPHS who led extensive studies that later established that 1 ppm of fluoride in a community water supply greatly reduced caries prevalence.[18] But, as important as the contributions of Dean and the USPHS were to the subsequent implementation of community fluoridation, we should not lose sight of the importance of the curiosity of Dr Fredrick McKay, a private practitioner in Colorado Springs. McKay and Dr G. V. Black, another practitioner and prominent dental educator, conducted extensive investigations prior to Dean's work into the reason for the "Colorado brown stain," the term applied to teeth exposed to excessive levels of natural fluoride but in which caries was arrested.[19]

In addition, we need to consider the influence of the industrial chemist, H. V. Churchill, who developed the analytic method that enabled detection of minute quantities of fluoride in water, a critical step necessary to establishing the link between the level of fluoride ions in water and the caries experience of the population consuming the water.[20] At the same time, Smith and Smith,[21] agricultural researchers, also linked mottled enamel with water fluoride concentrations. Following these and other studies,[22] independent researchers conducted controlled trials in 1945 and 1946 to test the caries experience of four communities (Grand Rapids, Michigan; Newburgh, New York; Evanston, Illinois; and Brantford, Ontario) where the fluoride concentrations were adjusted to higher (1.0–1.2 ppm) levels.[23–26] These studies successfully demonstrated the caries reduction capability of fluoridation.

Currently, approximately 250 million people in 34 countries receive the benefits of water that has been adjusted to an optimal fluoride concentration.[27] Over 135 million people in the United States, or approximately *65 percent* of the total population, drink adjusted or naturally occurring fluoridated water.[28] Efforts to increase the proportion of the world population drinking fluoridated water have been thwarted, however, in part, because of the continuing political activities of the antifluoridationist movement. This group continues to oppose fluoridation for many reasons, the vast majority of which have no scientific basis.[29]

Despite the efforts of antifluoridationists, community water fluoridation continues to receive widespread support from both the private and public health care sectors. Numerous dental and non-dental health care, consumer, and advocacy groups, as well as the surgeon general, have endorsed community water fluoridation.[30] Most recently, a comprehensive review by the USPHS of the benefits and risks of fluoridation again reaffirmed the value of water fluoridation.[31] The essence of successful dental public health programs is people working together effectively to reduce oral disease in the population.

CURRENT PROBLEM

A public health problem has been defined as (1) a condition or situation that is a widespread actual or potential cause of morbidity or mortality; and (2) an existing perception that the condition is a public health problem on the part of the public, government, or public health authorities.[32] Oral diseases constitute a public health problem for certain subgroups in this country and are among the more prevalent chronic diseases that plague Americans.[33] Yet, the attention given to oral diseases typically has not been appropriate considering their magnitude. Currently, considerable concern has arisen over the future of dental public health programs and funding levels to support them.[34] Total U.S. expenditures for dental care in 1992 were $38.7 billion constituting 5.3% of total health care, an approximate 3% decline since 1960.[35] In comparison, physician services constitute more than 20% of total health expenditures.[35] Less than 5% of the dental care budget, or about $1 billion, supports dental public health programs, and many of these have experienced serious cutbacks in recent years.[36] What is particularly disappointing is that more money is spent annually on both cosmetics and tobacco products than on dental care.

Here are some pertinent dental statistics for the U.S. population:

- The average adult has 23 decayed or filled tooth surfaces.[37]
- Only 42% of adults 65 years and older visit a dentist during a year.[38]
- Of all 17-year-olds, 84% have experienced tooth decay.[39]
- The average 17-year-old has eight decayed or filled tooth surfaces.[39]
- Twenty-five percent of the children have 60% of the caries prevalence in their age group.[40]
- Over 41 million days of restricted activity are caused by dental diseases or visits.[41]
- 7.05 million days of work loss are attributed to dental conditions.[42]
- Only 10.6% of those below the poverty level have dental insurance.[43]
- Utilization of dental services is 10 times lower for minority and poor children compared with the national average.[43]

- Nearly 80% of all Americans have some form of periodontal disease.[37]
- Forty-one percent of older Americans have lost all of their teeth.[37]

These are the principal concerns that need to be addressed in both private practice and the public health sector to improve the oral health of the population.

DENTAL PUBLIC HEALTH METHODS

Private practitioners necessarily treat individual patients for their specific oral disease, and collectively these treatments certainly improve the oral health of the public. Public health dentistry is a discipline that considers the *total community* as the patient and thus is concerned with the oral health of all members of society. When a fluoridation program is successfully implemented in a community, all gain the protective benefit against dental caries. The methods employed by the two modes of practice have been contrasted by Knutson,[44] formerly chief of the dental division of the USPHS. Each consists of six sequential steps that permit a logical progression from the time of identifying a problem to its solution (Table 17–1).

TABLE 17–1. METHODS OF PRIVATE AND PUBLIC HEALTH PRACTICE

Private Practice	Public Health Practice
Examination	Survey
Diagnosis	Analysis
Treatment planning	Program planning
Treatment	Program operation
Payment for services	Financing
Evaluation	Appraisal

(From Knutson JW. In: Pelton WJ, Wisan JM, eds. Dentistry in Public Health. 1955.[44] Reprinted with permission.)

For the individual patient, a private practitioner initiates the treatment process by performing a careful examination and taking a history to provide an accurate diagnosis of the problem. Then a course of treatment is planned to address any problems. Once the services have been provided and paid for, subsequent visits provide for evaluation of the treatment.

The methods employed in public health practice parallel those of the private practitioner but involve the total community instead of an individual. The methods, which are broad in scope, will now be discussed in greater detail.

Survey

Both the nature and extent of a dental problem must be determined. The level of dental caries in a subgroup of children in a community may be considered for study (Fig 17–1). Perhaps children are complaining of toothaches to teachers or missing school to visit dental offices for care. The magnitude of the difficulty can best be assessed by screening examinations of the children in the target population. Epidemiologic methods of study come into play requiring that conditions be measured and quantified accurately based on sound scientific principles. Results obtained through the examinations must be accurate, consistent, valid, and reliable. Rigid standards backed by stated criteria must be adhered to during the conduct of examinations.

Surveys that ascertain the oral health of children, adults, and senior citizens have also been conducted at the national level by the National Institute of Dental Research (NIDR).[37,45] Other surveys conducted by the National Center for Health Statistics (NCHS) in coordination with the NIDR, including the National Health and Nutrition Examination Surveys (NHANES) I (1971–

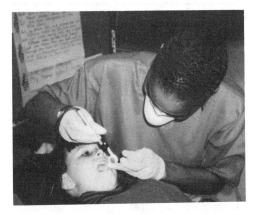

Figure 17–1. Surveys designed to establish the oral health needs of children most often take place in the school setting. (*Courtesy of Dr. Arthur Bonito, Research Triangle Institute, North Carolina.*)

1974) and III (1988–1994) and the National Health Interview Survey (NHIS) series, have also evaluated a variety of oral health care indicators as part of an overall assessment of the health and behavioral status of the public. These surveys carefully chose random statistical samples that validly reflects the experience of the U.S. population as a whole.

Dental Indices

An important tool used in examinations of a population group, the *dental index*, is a numeric score that quantifies the magnitude of the disease measured. A number of indices have been developed for the purpose of providing the objective measurement of the oral health status of a population group. The number of *teeth* that are decayed, missing, or filled, the DMFT index,[15] is a total score of all affected teeth and provides a caries experience score for an individual. A count of tooth *surfaces* that are decayed, missing, or filled is a DMFS index and provides greater precision about the caries history of an individual or a population group when mean scores are derived. The mean DMFT score for a population group is the total average caries experience at a particular time. Caries experience in the primary dentition is denoted by the use of *lowercase letters* to represent the number of decayed, extracted, or filled primary *teeth* or surfaces, deft or defs.[46] This index has recently been modified to dft or dfs because of the difficulty in distinguishing a primary tooth that has been extracted from one that has naturally been exfoliated.

The status of *periodontal tissues* have been evaluated using several alternative indices. The Gingival Index (GI) of Löe and Silness[47] is particularly suited to assessing changes in *gingival* health that might be observed during an evaluation period of an oral hygiene program. The Periodontal Index (PI) of Russell[48] and the Periodontal Disease Index (PDI) of Ramfjord[49] were once used for the assessment of severity of *periodontitis* in adult population groups. They have been *replaced* however, by a simple measurement of the loss of periodontal attachment in the same six teeth used by Ramfjord for the PDI. The Community Periodontal Index of Treatment Need (CPITN) is still used to assess bleeding, calculus, and pocket depth.[50] The CPITN has been widely adopted by World Health Organization (WHO) countries and is employed by the Indian Health Service of the USPHS.

Several plaque indices have also been developed to assess the status of oral hygiene in population groups. The Plaque Index (PLI) of Silness and Löe[51] quantifies the extent of plaque on specified areas of specific tooth surfaces. The Oral Hygiene Index—Simplified (OHI-S) of Greene and Vermillion[52] measures oral debris and calculus on specific tooth surfaces.

These indices can be useful in evaluating the prevalence of a condition or in assessing the extent of a favorable reduction in a reversible condition such as gingivitis or the comparable increments of dental caries in alternative preventive procedures. These indices have specific performance criteria so that the assigned numeric values provide specific information desired in a screening program or an epidemiologic study and are key elements in dental public health practice. In applying these indices to assessing dental diseases or oral status it is important to consider certain *demographic* factors, such as age, sex, socioeconomic status, and ethnic background, that may influence the condition being evaluated. For example, DMFS scores obtained for the purpose of comparing the prevalence of dental caries in two population subgroups have little meaning if the groups have different mean ages because DMFS scores increase with increasing age.

The accumulation of data in the survey process requires the recording of information concerning the status of teeth or the soft tissues of the mouth in a manner dictated by the pertinent *dental index* or indices selected for a study. The need to ensure that all examiners are calibrated is paramount (Fig 17–2). Often mark sense forms (machine-readable) were used to make these appropriate guided entries at the time of the oral examination. Eventually the mark sense forms were read by a machine such as an optical scanner, to provide a summation of the desired data. These data were, in turn, fed into a computer for statistical analysis and eventual presentation in table or graphic form. The mark sense forms are rapidly being superseded by the field use of small, portable, laptop computers that permit the *direct* entry of examination findings. This recent method of data collection bypasses the need for processing hun-

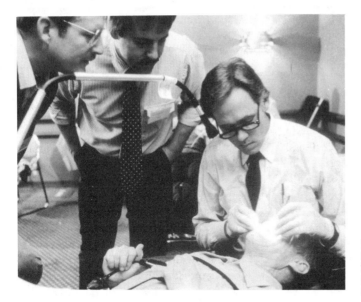

Figure 17–2. Calibration of dental examiners is required to ensure that the data collected are reliable. (*Courtesy of the National Institute of Dental Research.*)

dreds or even thousands of mark sense forms through an optical scanner. The use of the computer, aside from greatly reducing the time, effort, and cost of data processing, also reduces the possibility of errors because programs can be written to block or at least to question the entry of inappropriate data.

Analysis

Once the information has been collected through a survey, analysis of the data is done to answer certain questions. Is there a dental health problem? What is the extent of the problem? Are there appropriate solutions available to solve the problem? Statistical treatment of the data is usually necessary to compile the information into a useful form. For example, children enrolled in a Head Start program may be examined using the dfs index to determine the mean group score for all children surveyed. In addition, it may be desirable to know what portion of their decay has been treated. A ratio of the mean filled surface score (fs) to the total mean decayed-and-filled surface score (dfs) provides the relative amount of restorative care that has been completed in the children. Thus if the group mean fs score is 1.5 and the group mean dfs score is 4.5, only 33% (1.5/4.5) of their treatment needs have been met, or, conversely, two thirds of their restorative needs have not been met. How this problem can best be solved is an appropriate question for the analysis step.

Program Planning

Through the survey and analysis process the problem is identified and its scope defined. Program planning includes the consideration of all aspects of the program to ensure its success. Alternative plans must be considered to avoid loss of a program because contingencies were not anticipated. Communication is made with all concerned individuals and organizations. For example, to provide dental care to Head Start children, it is necessary to contact the parents of the children, to arrange transportation to dental offices or clinics where the care is provided, to obtain agreements from practitioners to provide care to the children, and to schedule appointments. More programs probably fail for lack of careful planning than any other single factor.

Program Operation

Once carefully planned, program operation can be implemented. Program operation usually includes three features: (1) dental health *education,* (2) disease *prevention,* and (3) *clinical services.*[36] Even well-planned programs, however, do not continue to function smoothly indefinitely; problems tend to occur, and continuous surveillance is necessary. Administrative skills are tested in the day-to-day operation of any program. In the Head Start example, it was necessary to determine if dental care was being provided satisfactorily, if transportation was a problem, and if patients were arriving on time and were keeping appointments.

Finance

Operational funding is usually provided by appropriate governmental agencies. Public dental programs are generally supported by local public health departments, which operate and administer local programs. The Head Start, a national program, is supported by federal funds. Allocated amounts of money, usually based on program enrollment, are specifically designated for the dental component of the program.

Evaluation

All programs must be continually evaluated to assess their effect, to measure their success or lack of it, and to consider modifications that might improve the program. In the Head Start dental program, children can be screened following their dental care to evaluate the ratio of fs to dfs to measure the degree to which the ratio has improved since the beginning of treatment. Thus, if

the score improves from the beginning 33% to 83%, additional treatment has been attained to the point where only 17% of the need for care remains, indicating a high degree of success for the program.

Additional Methods

Striffler[53] has suggested a modification to the traditional six sequential steps in public health practice, so that financing, evaluation, and education extend throughout all of the steps. Certainly it is necessary to consider costs and the methods of program financing during all phases of a program. Each step should be evaluated to assess success and to consider alternative approaches that may provide improvement. In addition, education is a critical component of public health practice and should be a part of all other phases. The education of authorities in city or county government, health boards, school boards, school administrators, parents, taxpayers, and the children themselves is necessary and effective in maintaining community understanding and support. To conduct successful health programs it is usually necessary to influence attitudes and to alter behavior in positive directions. A first and most important step in this process is education. To be effective the desired educational outcome and the methods of communication must be relevant to the target population.

Question 1. Which of the following statements, if any, are correct?

A. Approximately 80% of the people in the United States have some form of periodontal disease.

B. About one quarter of children have more than 50% of the decay.

C. The DMFT stands for decayed, missing, and filled tooth *surfaces.*

D. *Examination* is comparable to *analysis* in a public health setting, whereas *treatment* is equivalent to *program operation*.

E. The purpose of an epidemiologic survey is to determine the magnitude of the problem or the success of a program.

An Example Program

A dental public health program illustrating the sequential steps necessary in the development of any public health program is the Columbus, Ohio, Dental Sealant Program begun in 1986[54,55] (Fig 17–3).

Pit-and-fissure sealants can be used in innovative ways in public health programs. They have been found to offer a highly effective means of protecting occlusal fissured tooth surfaces[56] that have been found in recent surveys to be the most susceptible tooth surface attacked by dental caries in children. Sealants have also been used as a primary preventive means of preventing the need for restorative care, in conjunction with minimal restorations, or over incipient lesions where complete sealing is ensured to avoid the loss of tooth tissue.[57] Commu-

nity public health programs administered by the New Mexico[58] and Tennessee[59] Departments of Public Health have effectively used sealants with high success and low cost. By using auxiliary dental personnel to apply sealants whenever possible, allotted funds can be spread over a larger population.[60] Presently, 29 states have functioning community-based sealant programs.[61] Unfortunately, only 10.9 percent of American children have dental sealants, and less usage of sealants is found in lower socioeconomic and minority groups[43] (Fig 17–4).

Survey. It was known from the available national data at that time that various special population groups were at especially high risk for dental caries.[62] The development of an effective and relevant program to address this need however, demanded that local data be generated to confirm the national findings as well as better reflect the changing oral disease patterns of the community. A survey was developed and conducted through a collaborative effort of the Columbus Health Department, Ohio De-

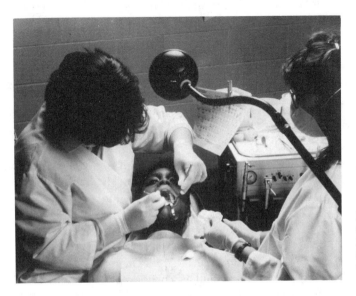

Figure 17–3. School-based sealant treatment programs have been found to be an effective approach to reducing occlusal caries. (*Courtesy of Ohio Division of Dental Health.*)

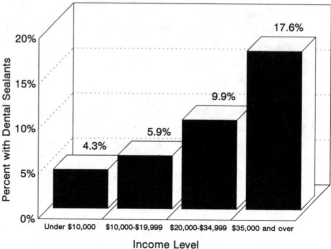

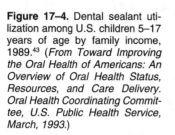

Figure 17–4. Dental sealant utilization among U.S. children 5–17 years of age by family income, 1989.[43] (*From Toward Improving the Oral Health of Americans: An Overview of Oral Health Status, Resources, and Care Delivery. Oral Health Coordinating Committee, U.S. Public Health Service, March, 1993.*)

partment of Health, the Ohio State University College of Dentistry, and the University of Michigan School of Public Health. Among the many age groups identified by the WHO Pathfinder method,[a] school children in grades 1 and 2 and 6 and 7 were screened for their baseline dental caries prevalence using the DMF index and the number of "targeted" permanent molars available for dental sealants. The WHO Pathfinder method is used in developing countries with limited resources and has been adapted in local dental programs in the United States with similar fiscal constraints.[63] Portable microcomputers were used on site for data recording and analysis.

Analysis. A high proportion of children were found to have at least one carious permanent tooth. The caries experience of the children was found to be most prevalent on tooth surfaces with pits and fissures. Only a small proportion of children had received dental sealants.

---

[a] The WHO Pathfinder survey is a simple, inexpensive screening instrument designed to establish the oral health status of a population.

Program Planning. Cooperation between public and private sectors was necessary to design effectively a specific caries-preventive strategy: a school-based dental sealant program. Agencies and organizations involved included those from the city and state health departments, school administrators and educators, as well as the local dental society, community leaders, and private foundations. Planning the dental sealant programs required a knowledge of resources available or needed to provide services. Time, supplies and equipment, facilities, and personnel represented the principal resource requirements. Promotion of the dental sealant program first required marketing to procure resources, build needed public and private constituencies, and educate community leaders and organizations. Survey data were released in a variety of formats to the public through establishment of a local network of interested advocacy groups. A report of the survey's findings was also presented to the local board of health.

Finance. Consideration of finance, education, and evaluation were inherent in all steps of the dental sealant program. Start-up costs for this program were funded by grants from a local foundation, the United Way, and the state health department. The educational and marketing effort helped to convince local policymakers to continue funding for the program by increasing the dental program's general fund appropriation. This commitment was concomitant with the local board of health approving a long-range programmatic plan to utilize survey data. Salaried dental health care providers in the Columbus Department of Health were involved in developing the dental sealant strategy.

Education. Education was also an important step throughout the project. An educational campaign was conducted to ensure communication with all elements in the identified population. Communication was initiated and maintained with parents, school boards, teachers, administrators, school health nurses, health educators, and state and local societies. Parents and school personnel particularly needed to be well informed concerning the purpose, importance, and guidelines for the program. It was important that teachers appreciate the need for children to have their attendance disrupted for time to participate in the program and be made aware that these interruptions would avoid future acute conditions and toothaches that could cause serious problems and greater time lost from school. Cooperation among all the people involved in the project achieved a common goal—the improved oral health of a population in need.

Program Operation. After thorough consideration of the problem, analysis of its severity, careful planning, and procurement of funding, the program was put into operation. In preparation for the initiation of the program, in-service training programs were conducted for all participants to affirm goals

and methods of operation. The actual provision of dental sealants to a large number of school children progressed smoothly because the previous stages had been so well planned.

Evaluation. The program was evaluated by subsequent reviews of school health records and the number of toothaches reported by the participating children. An increase in the number of teeth with dental sealants was evidence of improved protection from future oral health problems. The results of ongoing cost-effectiveness analyses found that the program reflected an effective use of funds for reducing the future costs of dental care to the public. Results from this survey and program eventually served as the basis for a comprehensive, statewide initiative.[64]

LEVELS OF PUBLIC HEALTH OPERATION

All countries have a department or ministry responsible for the public health of the nation. The World Health Organization (WHO) has accepted the responsibility of coordinating the efforts of all member organizations in developing and improving dental and medical health programs throughout the world. In this endeavor they are aided by governmental, international, and private organizations. For instance, the USPHS, the health arm of the Department of Health and Human Services (DHHS); the Federation Dentaire Internationale (FDI), a prestigious organization of outstanding dentists from many nations; and national organizations such as the American Dental Association (ADA) from the United States cooperate in exchanging information and developing dental health programs that will benefit all nations.

In the United States, DHHS is responsible for the planning and implementation of health programs. The USPHS is the operational arm of this department in carrying out health policies mandated and financed by congressional legislation. To accomplish this task, administrative, clinical, and research divisions were created. Planning begins in Washington, D.C., with objectives changing as health needs shift. For example, at one time the need was financing new dental and medical schools to increase the output of health professionals; more recently the need has been for specifically focused programs to accelerate development for either caries or periodontal disease control measures, and continually efforts are being made to refine programs so as to offer better access to, or less cost for, medical or dental care.

To facilitate administration, the United States has been divided into *10 USPHS geographic regions*, each with a central office. These offices provide consulting and monitoring expertise for health programs involving federal funds. From an operational viewpoint, the USPHS provides dental care to the federal prison systems, drug rehabilitation services, and the Coast Guard, as well as care through the Indian Health Service (IHS) to Native Americans. Their research commitment is conducted through NIDR, which is the oral health branch of the National Institutes of Health (NIH), which accomplishes both intramural and extramural research. This last agency (NIH) is the major funding source for all dental research in the United States and at times for outstanding foreign scientists, including grants to universities and nonprofit organizations, financing of international and national symposia to coalesce bodies of research knowledge, and underwriting clinical demonstration programs that aid in translating laboratory accomplishments into better patient care.

Each state has a health department that may or may not include a dental division. Of those states with a dental division, many divide their jurisdictional operation into regions to better administer and monitor state-conducted oral health programs. The regional programs include operation of clinics for needy populations, state prison systems, and in some cases, school systems. Consultations with communities desiring to establish or to improve community oral health, public health education programs, and fluoride initiatives receive major emphasis.

Within each state many of the more populous counties or cities maintain their own clinic facilities under a locally financed health department. These agencies operate clinical facilities in economically underprivileged areas, in schools, or in populations that do not have access to routine dental care. Federal, state, and local tax funds are intermixed in the delivery of care at all levels.

TRADITIONAL DENTAL PUBLIC HEALTH PROGRAMS

Special Population Groups

Although dental public health is the specialty in dentistry that concerns itself with the oral health of the total population, traditional dental public health programs also have consisted of a number of projects designed for special subgroups in the population. Certain groups, because of their occupation, position, or location, do not have ready access to private practitioners and must be cared for in special clinics supported by public or private funds. The oral health needs of these groups, which includes Native Americans, long-term care populations (nursing home and homebound geriatric groups), migrant groups, medically compromised individuals, Department of Veterans Affairs (DVA) hospital patients, the developmentally disabled, homeless individuals, the elderly, and poor or minority children and adults are significantly more severe than the average for the total population.[37,45,65–77] These problems are generally a result of lack of treatment in the past, poor education, neglect of oral hygiene practices, medical complications, and attitudinal barriers.

Native American and Head Start children, for example, experience a disproportionate amount of *baby bottle tooth decay* and other oral health problems because they do not have ready access to educational and behavioral modifications designed to counteract such conditions.[78–80] In addition, both young and old individuals from the general population place themselves at higher risk for developing *oral cancer* because of their use of alcohol, smokeless tobacco, and other tobacco products.[81,82]

Other examples include oral conditions such as *xerostomia* (dry mouth), which are often a consequence of the numerous medications taken by the elderly for various medical and psychological problems.[83,84] Xerostomia is a major risk factor for coronal and root caries as well as periodontal disease in these individuals.[76] Many populations suffering from specific diseases such as Sjögren's syndrome also experience disabling oral manifestations as a direct result of these systemic medical disorders.[85] Medically compromised individuals with diabetes or acquired immunodeficiency syndrome (AIDS) are often predisposed to rapidly progressing periodontal disease and other oral problems.[86,87] Alzheimer's disease and other dementias psychologically and physically compromise the ability of many elderly persons to take care of their mouths.[88,89] Finally, poor attitude and beliefs on the part of dental professionals and

patients alike further preclude the promise of improving oral health status in these special populations.[90–92]

The provision of restorative and preventive care to many of these groups requires special training and particular skills. As a specific example, routine treatment in a dental office is inaccessible to homebound patients. Dentists and auxiliary personnel trained in the use of mobile dental equipment and treatment of the disabled patient, are needed to provide care delivery to the homebound.[93] Removal of the barriers to care and the subsequent improvement in oral health is an example of an effective dental public health program.

Dental public health personnel in public health agencies, local or state health departments, or dental schools are often called on to provide consultation to or to initiate projects that are concerned with particular diseases or conditions. Projects in this category may include a baby bottle tooth decay education program for young mothers, a mouth-guard fabrication program for high school football players, a denture adequacy assessment program for a geriatric population, a fluoride therapy program for cancer patients undergoing head and neck radiation, implementation of a screening program for the Head Start children in the community, an oral cancer prevention and education program, or a workplace treatment or health education and promotion program.

Primary and Secondary Prevention: A Sample Screening Program for Oral Cancer

Primary or secondary prevention programs designed to avert disease incidence or deter further progression, respectively, are additional examples of dental public health practice. Probably the prevention program in which most health professionals participate as a public service is the oral cancer-screening program. Oral cancer accounts for approximately 4% of all cancers.[82] Approximately 30,500 persons develop oral cancers annually in the United States and more than 8000 die.[82] Oral cancer is found more frequently in persons older than 65 years of age, in heavy smokers, or in alcoholics. In addition, the rate of new oral cancer cases is increasing in minority groups, including older women and African Americans.[82]

If detected early, death from oral cancer is one of the most preventable types of cancer mortality. Yet, the majority of diagnosed oral cancer lesions are well advanced when first detected, with at least 50% showing lymphadenopathy.[94] This delayed diagnosis is perhaps attributable to infrequent routine examinations of the mouth for oral cancer. Surveys have reported that the groups at high risk for oral cancer annually visit physicians and other nondental health professionals more frequently than they do dentists.[38,95]

The University of Maryland dental and medical schools and the Department of Veterans Affairs in Perry Point, Maryland, designed an educational and oral cancer-screening and mortality prevention program in a region with a high reported oral cancer mortality rate.[96] Data were initially collected using a written survey questionnaire that assessed physicians' and dentists' knowledge of and behaviors concerning oral cancer. The unique aspect of the program was its attempt to encourage physicians to inspect the oral cavity more routinely. The ultimate goal of the program was to increase the proportion of dentists and physicians who routinely perform oral cancer screening or examinations and referrals.

Prior to conducting the study, communication was begun with the target population, educators, and health professional peers. Lay individuals were interviewed to discern their knowledge of oral cancer, as well as their receptivity to an oral cancer prevention program. A collaborative relationship with an influential local health education consortium, the Western Area Health Education Center (AHEC), was established and support from the American Cancer Society was enlisted. Finally, professional societies and organizations with a prime interest in the program were consulted.

The study was designed to address the following essential questions:

- What is the age makeup of the population?
- What is the populations' use of dental and medical services? Are they being examined more frequently on an annual basis by nondental professionals?
- What are the mortality, morbidity, incidence, and prevalence of oral cancer in this population? The best source of this information is a central tumor registry or a national agency, such as the Centers for Disease Control and Prevention (CDC). If none is available, hospitals in the area need to be canvassed to develop a presumptive evidence of need.
- What is the level of knowledge and behaviors concerning oral cancer among the physicians and dentists practicing in the district? Are continuing education (CE) programs necessary to increase the number and skill level of practitioners, especially nondental professionals, who routinely examine or refer patients at high risk for oral cancer.
- Can the information from these CE programs be used to implement relevant community oral cancer-screening programs that enlist the assistance of dental and nondental professionals alike?
- What existing resources are available for CE and screening programs? Help in this area can be secured

from the Western AHEC, American Cancer Society, dental and medical schools, local health departments, local dental and medical societies, and other advocacy groups.

Planning for the program in Western Maryland began with documentation of need, expected benefits, and methods for accomplishing program objectives. Separate surveys of local physicians and dentists were conducted to assess practitioner character-istics and demographic background; profes-sional education and training; knowledge, attitudes, and behaviors related to oral can-cer prevention, detection, and referral; and characteristics of the patient populations. These results were used to determine the need for and content of subsequent CE ses-sions and community screening programs, as well as to establish a basis for program evaluation. Continuing education programs funded by the University of Maryland and indirectly supported by Western AHEC were conducted in the region. These pro-grams featured nationally recognized ex-perts in the diagnosis of oral cancer. The data generated by this study will be used to secure further funding from governmental, academic, and private sources to conduct community oral cancer-screening programs.

The short-range goal of oral cancer-screening programs is to induce as many people as possible to enter the program; the longer term goal is to reduce the number of deaths resulting from undetected oral can-cer. To achieve the first, which is a prerequi-site for the second, a strong public educa-tion component must exist. It is essential that the target population be convinced that they will benefit from a head-and-neck ex-amination that is short, painless, and effec-tive in identifying possible malignant and benign neoplasia. To accomplish this objec-tive, newspapers, radio, television, hand-outs, posters, and word of mouth should be used. Participants who have been through

similar programs previously can become the best source of public relations once a pro-gram is being planned.

Once the screening phase is com-pleted, it is then necessary to ensure that all referred persons have been seen for a defin-itive diagnosis and that confirmed neoplas-tic lesions are treated. Often the American Cancer Society assumes these important obligations.

It is worth noting that in addition to playing an important role in the detection of oral cancer, dentists are increasingly being asked to participate in its prevention as well. The NCI's Community Intervention Trial for Smoking Cessation (COMMIT) involves dentists and community organizations in joint efforts aimed at implementing tobacco use interventions.[97] Dentists have also been called on to participate in a large demon-stration project (ASSIST—America Stop Smoking Intervention Study) involving 50 million Americans.

Dental Health Promotion and Prevention

Dental health education, promotion, and prevention programs have traditionally constituted a significant portion of dental public health activities. *Health promotion* provides the education, access, and avail-ability of a known preventive method to the population[98] (Fig 17–5). Programs devoted to school children, such as fluoride mouth rinse and tablet programs and dental sealant applications, have been particularly popular because children have been highly suscepti-ble to dental caries. In addition, many chil-dren, especially those with the highest dis-ease levels whose families may not be able to provide for their oral health needs, do not visit dental offices. Yet, virtually all of them attend school and, therefore, are exposed to a school-based program. Many educational and prevention programs for school chil-dren have not, however, demonstrated the

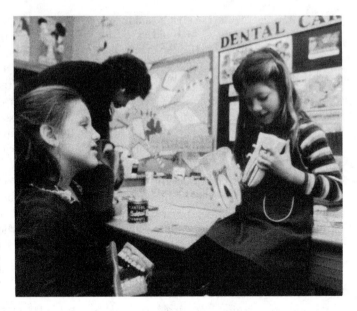

Figure 17–5. Classroom dental health education programs are important, but it is critical to evaluate their effect. (*Courtesy of the National Institute of Dental Research.*)

degree of success that theoretically might be anticipated.[99–101] Enthusiasm for dental health education in many school programs needs tempering because it promotes unrealistic expectations in caries control that are often not realized when programs are carefully evaluated.[1] When expectations are not realized, disappointment may be created, as well as the attitude that all school-based preventive programs are not successful.

School-based preventive services, discussed thoroughly in the following chapter, are seen by dental public health professionals and, hopefully, by most educators as consistent with American educational philosophy and goals that are supportive of improved health.[102] School-based preventive programs should be more effective than private practice-based services because of the large number of children whose parents cannot or will not take them to private offices. Those children of lowest socioeconomic status, who often belong to minority groups, are least likely to have access to private preventive services and are the ones most susceptible to higher levels of dental caries (Fig 17–6). The glaring need in the conduct of these programs, as in dental health education, is that the cost-effectiveness of these preventive services be carefully evaluated.

Rather than eliminating school-based preventive programs that some might think are ineffective, it is important that they be maintained but that they employ careful evaluation methods designed to determine the effect of the program on the oral health of the target population in terms of reduced disease.[103] In the past, many programs were content merely to report the number of children engaged in mouth rinse or dental health education programs with the assumption that such programs are beneficial. A program that has been determined ineffective by evaluation should be replaced by one expected to do better; the replacement program will, in turn, be evaluated. Even when preventive programs appear to be in

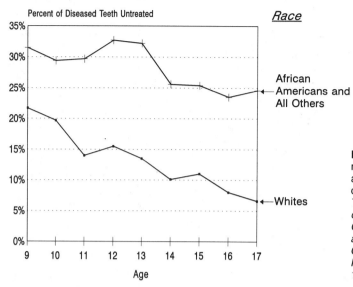

Percent of Diseased Teeth Untreated

Figure 17–6. Percent of permanent teeth with dental caries that are untreated among U.S. children by race, 1986–1987.[45] (*From Toward Improving the Oral Health of Americans: An Overview of Oral Health Status, Resources, and Care Delivery. Oral Health Coordinating Committee, U.S. Public Health Service, March, 1993.*)

place and thought to be functioning effectively, evaluation and monitoring are important aspects that cannot be neglected in dental public health activities. For example, due to the widespread use of fluorides in many modalities, several states are shifting resources from school-based fluoride mouth rinse programs to sealant treatment programs.

Community Water Fluoridation

The fluoridation of community water supplies is an activity that still warrants considerable attention by the dental profession. Fluoridation campaigns have been actively waged by dental public health professionals since fluoridation was first introduced into municipal water supplies. To conduct fluoridation campaigns successfully, it is important to understand the political realities and to recognize all the community resources that can be used to assist in securing a favorable outcome.[104] Successful campaigns require dedicated and enthusiastic people who are coordinated by an individual with

good political skills. Support from all segments of the population, not just health professionals, is crucial. The best method for achieving fluoridation in a small community is through city council action if state laws do not require a referendum. Endorsements are required by strategic role models, such as the mayor, city council members, and community opinion leaders.

Often surveillance of fluoridation of a municipal water system is neglected after a short time. Several states conducted studies that revealed 50% or more of distribution centers contained fluoride lower than recommended levels.[105] Authority should rest with the dental director of the local department of public health rather than with water department personnel who may not assign a high priority to fluoride level monitoring. Periodic meetings should be held between dental and water department personnel to discuss the results of water analyses. Optimum results from fluoridation can be achieved only if proper fluoride levels are continuously maintained.

Question 2. Which of the following statements, if any, are correct?

A. A ratio of 0.5 for the mean fs score to the total mean dms score indicates *more* restorative work *present* than does a 0.78 ratio.

B. An evaluation of program operation usually is made only after completion of the program.

C. Survival rates for oral cancer are greatly improved with early detection.

D. Most public-school-based education programs produce marked reductions in oral disease.

E. The best approach to implementing community water fluoridation is through city council action, not by public referendum.

NEW STRATEGIES NEEDED

Changing Disease Patterns

In the early 1900s, various infectious diseases were so devastating in their mortality and morbidity toll of the population that the entire health profession concentrated its treatment and prevention efforts on these diseases. With the relative control of infectious diseases by the 1950s, the medical and public health community shifted their strategies to addressing the chronic diseases that plagued the population—heart disease, cancer, stroke, diabetes. The principal dental diseases—caries and periodontal disease—are both infectious but are also chronic and deserve their share of prevention attention. Just as attention has shifted with changes in general disease prevalence in medicine, the dental profession should be receptive to new strategies that reflect altered disease patterns.

One of the truly significant developments in the field of dental public health has been the well-documented decline in dental caries during the past 15 years.[39,45,106-114] The reduced susceptibility to dental caries, particularly among children and young adults, is altering the oral health status of the population. The NIH has estimated that the United States saved approximately $100 billion in dental expenditures during the 1980s as a result of this improvement in oral health.[115] The changed caries picture represents a major success for organized dentistry while presenting new challenges to the dental profession.

In the past it was not considered practical to provide the needed care for everyone because dental caries was so highly prevalent in children.[116] Now with caries reduced by about one third and significant numbers of children remaining caries-free, it may be practical to attempt to control the disease in the subset of children who have the most serious problems. The challenge to public health practitioners is not to do less because less dental caries exists, but to exert new efforts to identify high-risk individuals and to expand services for those who have not had access to care. The current trend to decrease spending for public programs as well as to reduce health care costs generally may at least favor *preventive programs that are targeted to smaller numbers of people who have high unmet levels of oral disease.*[117,118]

Limited attention has been given in the past to public health periodontal programs. Now the emerging consensus is that periodontal disease, like caries, can involve children as well as adults, and either can be acute or chronic.[37,45,119] As caries control measures are increasing in effectiveness, emphasis has shifted to developing a nationwide periodontal disease control initiative. Future efforts should be devoted to bringing periodontal disease to the attention of the public and to assessing the extent of the disease through community screening and detection clinics in which hygienists can be used to refer patients to practitioners' offices or clinics for definitive care.[120]

Changing Public Health Practices

As in the case of periodontal disease, dental public health programs should be organized to meet the needs of the population. As these needs change, dental public health efforts should be devoted to current and emerging problems and conditions rather than to expending resources on traditional programs that may be rooted in the past.[121] One accepted characteristic of a profession is that it should be willing in the public interest to respond to changing needs as a result of its own successful preventive and treatment measures.[122] Concern over the ability of the public health profession to adapt to change is addressed in an Institutes of Medicine report on *The Future of Public Health*.[123] The report contends that public health in the United States is disorganized, splintered, and unprepared to accommodate and address future challenges. The means to maintaining and expanding public health programs to meet the demands of a changing environment is through surveillance and assessment, policy development, and assurance including a legal guarantee of services.[123]

Unfortunately, the political and economic mood of the country in the 1990s is not to expand dental public health programs, but rather to curtail or discontinue many of them. *The Future of Dental Public Health* report asserts that the decline of dental public health programs at the national, state, and local levels is, in part, a result of the perception that oral health is not a major concern.[124] Between 1981 and 1988, local dental public health programs suffered losses in personnel and averaged a 10% reduction in funds.[33,36] Neighborhood health centers, as well as centers treating rural, migrant, and homeless populations, have suffered severe cutbacks in federal outlays for dental services, personnel, and scope of services.[124] Public health dentistry curricula in many schools of public health are experiencing major reductions or outright dissolution. Many community dentistry programs in dental schools are only modest in scope relative to the concentration of resources devoted to these programs when first initiated.[124]

Why has the downsizing of dental public health programs progressed with relatively few challenges? One answer may be the lack of an organized constituency or advocacy group for dental public health issues. A partnership between the public and private dental sectors is essential if oral health concerns are to be effectively promoted. Often the aims of professional groups within dentistry tend to be compartmentalized and narrowly defined. Public dental programs may also be seen as competitive with private practitioners. Preventive approaches are apt to be erroneously classified as public sector or private sector programs. Yet the efforts of both should reinforce common goals. Fluoridation, for example, may be seen as an effective public health measure, but the promotion of fluoride dentifrices may not be. Yet they complement each other, and both are public health measures.[125]

Cooperation between dental public health organizations, such as the American Association of Public Health Dentistry (AAPHD), the American Public Health Association (APHA) Oral Health Section, and the ADA can help resolve the differing perspectives of the private and public sectors. Cooperation can also foster an influential alliance in local and national campaigns addressing dental public health issues. Collaboration with a multitude of national and local voluntary nondental health and educational organizations, such as the Children's Defense Fund, American Association of Retired Persons, or the National Health Education Coalition, is equally important in promoting oral health as essential to overall health and in integrating oral health issues within the health, educational, and policy directives of these organizations. By working together on certain broad-based popular issues (ie, access to health services), these separate partnerships can evolve into a coalition, such as the National Oral Health Alliance, that can be recruited to support specific oral health issues actively.

With reductions in funds to support public health programs, administrators must become more opportunistic and adaptive in order to conduct effective programs. An innovative prototype that embraces this notion is the New Jersey Statewide Network for Community Oral Health Care.[126] This program establishes a network of oral health care facilities through a collaborative and proactive effort of the New Jersey Dental School, USPHS, Bureau of Health Manpower, New Jersey State Dental Association, and the New Jersey State Department of Health. These clinics serve underserved, low socioeconomic, and other special population groups in the State.

Other advocacy measures that can be pursued in support of dental public health programs may be advanced through regulatory and legislative routes. An area of activity often entered with some reluctance is the political arena. Those in dental public health programs characteristically go about their duties quietly, content to live within the constraints imposed by citizens who, for example, vote against fluoridation. Niessen believes that community regulatory roles exist for dental public health regarding compliance with fluoridation and infection control standards.[127] If successful, efforts to educate and persuade others of the impor-

tance of these issues can pay big dividends. The preventive benefit provided to a community by initiating and monitoring fluoridation or a practice act that addresses infection control may be greater than the benefit attained from a lifetime of practice by a dozen dentists.

Successful public health workers need to be opinion leaders and community decision makers regarding oral health programs and services. Gaupp expands this notion when stating that, ". . . it is opportune for the oral health interest groups to strike out on their own by working toward a national, comprehensive, oral health bill."[128] Resource development can also be expedited if dental public health programs attained influence in the regulatory and legislative arenas.

National Oral Health Objectives

An effective means of expanding on advocacy and regulatory activities in generating support for oral health programs is through the setting of measurable health objectives. In 1980, the federal government established a program entitled *Promoting Health/Preventing Disease: Objectives for the Nation*[129] to identify and monitor specific health objectives, including 12 that addressed dental health and fluoridation. Although this program was an early opportunity to promote oral health alongside other national health priorities, it did not adequately address the means by which states and localities could achieve these objectives. A subsequent program, *The National Health Objectives for the Year 2000*,[130] builds on the previous framework by recognizing both the relationship of oral health and total health and the strategies required to achieve these oral health objectives by dental and nondental professionals alike. This program addresses 16 oral health objectives constituting a wide array of oral diseases.[130]

Model standards have been established that provide guidance for community attainment of the year 2000 national health objectives. Twenty-nine measurable oral health objectives and indicators are outlined in *Healthy Communities 2000: Model Standards*.[131] In addition, periodic reports identifying and monitoring specific activities directed toward achieving the year 2000 health objectives at the federal, state, and consortium levels have been mandated.[132–134] Finally, an enterprising voluntary initiative with an array of nondental professional, advocacy, and corporate entities in the private sector—the Oral Health 2000 National Consortium—has been established to promote and attain the year 2000 oral health objectives for the nation.[135]

Special Population Needs

Insomuch as recent budget restrictions and the changing epidemiology in caries prevalence have either curtailed or changed public dental programs, other issues and trends also affect the ability of these programs to successfully achieve the year 2000 oral health objectives for the nation. For example, the United States has experienced in recent years an increase in special population groups, such as long-term care patients,[66] medically compromised individuals, patients with AIDS,[70] and the homeless,[73,74] whose high unmet oral health needs clearly affect already depleted financial resources. A proportional decrease has also occurred in the number of children relative to older population groups in the United States.[136] This growth in the aging population create substantial numbers of older members of society who have periodontal disease and root surface caries.[2,137–139] Despite recent upward trends in the use and demand for dental services, the elderly overall still have the poorest utilization rates of any age group over 4 years of age.[37] This is likely to

change as the rate of edentulism continues to drop among aging cohorts.[37]

Access to dental services for special population groups as well as the growing number of the working poor compromises the ability of dental public health programs to attain oral health objectives. Only a small proportion of these groups have private dental insurance coverage, and dental benefits through federal or state entitlement programs for the poor such as Medicaid are rapidly dwindling[43,140,141] (Fig 17–7). The Medicaid outlay for dental services has decreased by almost 30% since 1987, far more than any other health service. Only 15% of all dental service expenditures among the poor in 1987 was paid by Medicaid, with 56% paid out-of-pocket.[142]

Other Trends Affecting Oral Health

Other recent trends that influence the attainment of oral health objectives include new technologic advances and dental education and personnel requirements. New advances in dental implants, restorative methods, chemotherapeutic agents, and diagnostic hardware will clearly affect future disease treatment modalities and costs. Advanced computer skills should also lead to new research developments in periodontology, salivary gland dysfunction, and the provision of health services. Going hand in hand with these advances is the realization of the need to pay greater attention to *risk assessment* and the identification of *risk factors* for oral diseases.[143] The potential for advances in the dental health care delivery system to improve oral health for all citizens is muted, however, by poor access to dental services and personal oral health behaviors and attitudes.

The level of dental personnel required to meet the need or demand of the public for care is also a crucial factor affecting the success of oral health programs. Unfortu-

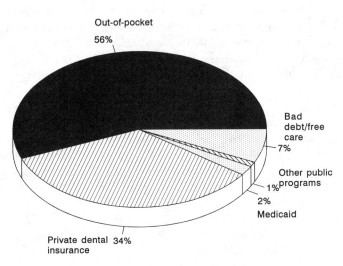

Figure 17-7. Source of payment for dental services, 1987.[142] (*From Toward Improving the Oral Health of Americans: An Overview of Oral Health Status, Resources, and Care Delivery. Oral Health Coordinating Committee, U.S. Public Health Service, March, 1993.*)

nately, the predictor models used to ascertain an "appropriate" measure of required level of dental staffing suffer from a lack of critical data and are generally unable to account for epidemiologic, social, economic, and political change.[144] The traditional model used in dental personnel planning, the dentist-to-population ratio, projected a high number of dentists per population, indicating an oversupply of dentists. This staffing prediction has been complicated by a decrease in dental school applications and enrollment with the accompanying closure of five dental schools.[145] The most recent federal report, *Health Personnel in the United States: Eighth Report to Congress, 1991,* projected that the actual number of dentists will peak between 1997 and 2005, and then decline for 15 to 20 years.[146] Whether an oversupply or undersupply of dentists occurs, maldistribution of dental personnel still exists in the United States as embodied by over 1000 federally designated "dental health manpower shortage areas."[147]

The dental educational curriculum may be evolving as a result of funding and budgetary pressures arising from changes in student enrollment, oral epidemiology, changes in health delivery systems, information transfer, and population makeup. Reforms, if enacted, will almost certainly affect the year 2000 oral health objectives. Recommended changes generally underscore the need for more interdisciplinary research, preventive modalities, and community-based initiatives to better complement the current clinical curriculum.[148]

Emerging Public Concerns

Public and professional reactions to perceived risks in the oral health care delivery system affect treatment modalities, service utilization, and, ultimately, oral health status. Well-publicized reports of individuals contracting a number of conditions from fluoride and amalgam restorations have prompted the dental research community to review the risks associated with the use of these fundamental components of dental prevention and treatment.[31,149] Of even greater threat to the practice of dentistry and the recruitment of future dental personnel is the fear, by both health care providers and patients, of contracting AIDS in the dental office.[150,151] Although dental public health professionals have been at the forefront in ensuring access for patients infected with the AIDS virus, many dental practitioners are still reluctant to treat known AIDS patients. On the other hand, the revelation of the probable occupational transmission of the AIDS virus from a dentist to five of his patients has generated a high level of concern and anxiety among the public about receiving dental care.[151–153] Dental public health activities have been directed at preventing transmission of infectious diseases in the dental office by assisting dentists to comply with recommended ADA and CDC infection control guidelines and the Occupational Safety and Health Administration's bloodborne pathogens standard. Implementation of these edicts, however, is already dramatically changing the scope and cost of delivering dental services.[154–156]

Health Care Reform

Infection control is only a small element of the potential changes facing the U.S. dental delivery system. The current debate over health care reform presents enormous implications and opportunities for future dental delivery systems. A U.S. Health Care Reform Commission has been established by President Clinton to study measures for reducing the current high cost of health services while providing *universal* and *uniform* health care access. Recommendations to reform the U.S. health care system have ranged from emulating a *single-payer governmental model* like that employed in Canada, Sweden, and the United Kingdom to a *government–private industry partnership* as practiced in Germany, Japan, and the Netherlands.

Dentistry may be at a momentous juncture concerning its participation and inclusion in a health care reform package. The debate over health care reform could

provide dentistry with unique opportunities to promote oral health as an essential primary health care component of total health as well as to define its inclusion within a comprehensive health benefits package. Although health care reform will most likely connote change for the dental delivery model, the greater risk to the oral health of U.S. citizens would be the failure to consider oral health at all within health care reform.

To prevent such an occurrence, a USPHS Oral Health Coordinating Committee was commissioned by the Chief Dental Officer to formulate an oral health benefits package under health care reform.[157] Although the submission of this package and related activities make it likely that public health dentistry will be heard in the debate, inclusion of an oral health benefits package within health care reform would benefit from the tacit support of the private dental sector as represented by the ADA. If the ADA chooses *not* to participate, as appears likely at this time,[158] oral health services may once more be accorded ancillary and discretionary status as in past programs and continue to fail to meet the burgeoning oral health needs and demands of the country's more unfortunate citizens.

Insomuch as dentistry's future may be, in part, determined by the direction and content of health care reform, mutually supportive research agendas, interdisciplinary workshops, innovative policies, and creative administrative programs are needed to secure dentistry's position. Recent examples abound. The NIDR, DVA, APHA and AAPHD, and surgeon general have drafted comprehensive research agendas related to issues of oral health status, behaviors, attitudes, utilization, and disease sequelae.[159–162] The Health Resources and Services Administration (HRSA) in coordination with the Maternal and Child Health

Bureau (MCHB) established regional interdisciplinary workshops that addressed the oral health issues of women and children.[163] Finally, HRSA's Bureau of Health Professions is planning a conference to redefine primary oral health care and its role in a changing health care system.

Although funding for more oral health projects is needed, MCHB and HRSA recently developed special projects of regional and national significance (SPRANS) grants to state and local MCH agencies to integrate oral health into their range of primary care services. In addition, MCHB's block grant review policy now includes a specific consideration for oral health programs, including the completion of an oral needs assessment. The MCHB is also working with the Association of State and Territorial Dental Directors to develop and test a model statewide oral health survey protocol. The Bureau of Health Professions is developing policies and programs regarding dental, allied dental health, and dental public health education; dental treatment and management of HIV-positive and AIDS patients; and grant-training programs related to the oral health care of underserved populations such as geriatric patients. In addition, the National Health Service Corps (NHSC) is once again placing dentists alongside other health professionals in underserved urban and rural areas in the United States.[164] The NHSC provides scholarships and loan repayments in return for a minimum period of paid service. This progress can continue if dentistry accepts new challenges that require altered approaches to conducting dental public health programs that are effective in preventing dental diseases.

Question 3. Which of the following statements, if any, are correct?

A. Public health dentistry programs are *expanding* rapidly because of their need and effectiveness.

B. The prevalence of both root and coronal caries is decreasing while the prevalence of periodontal disease is increasing.

C. To ensure their success, dental public health programs must have strong constituency support.

D. The need to *target* public health services to susceptible populations is important to make the most effective use of scarce resources.

E. Over the last 5 years, the Medicaid outlay for dental services has *decreased* more than any other health service.

SUMMARY

Dental public health programs are organized efforts to improve the oral health of the public. The most outstanding dental public health success story is water fluoridation, which is one of the great mass disease-preventive measures of all times. Yet, there is much that needs to be done for a large percentage of the population that either does not seek or does not have geographic or economic access to timely preventive or treatment services. One approach is to set measurable objectives, such as the oral health objectives for the year 2000, that identify a number of oral health issues and, in the process, help develop and coordinate strategies for addressing them. The dental problems of a population are determined by epidemiologic surveys that quantify levels of disease, using either caries, periodontal, or other dental indices. Once a problem is tentatively identified, it is addressed through use of six sequential steps: survey, analysis, program planning, program operation, financing, and evaluation. Public health programs are usually identified with subsets of the population other than the affluent. When traditional programs prove ineffective, they should be replaced by more cost-effective approaches. The need is great for methods that permit better targeting of individuals at high risk for oral disease. The combination of less disease, more effective use of professional personnel, and improved technology and better preventive methods, particularly sealants, provides opportunities to target community-based oral health programs to subgroups who have been traditionally neglected. To do this, a constituency of public and private, dental and nondental advocacy groups is needed. Ultimately, however, dentistry's position in health care reform may be the most important factor determining the success of these efforts in improving the overall oral health status of the nation.

ANSWERS AND EXPLANATIONS

1. A, B, E
   C—incorrect. The DMFT stands for decayed, missing, filled *teeth,* not *surfaces.*
   D—incorrect. Examination is equivalent to *survey,* not *analysis.*
2. C, E
   A—incorrect. A higher ratio indicates the presence of *more* restorations.
   B—incorrect. Evaluation of a program should be an ongoing process.
   D—incorrect. Most school education programs produce disappointing results.
3. C, D, E
   A—incorrect. Money for dental public health is always sparse.
   B—incorrect. The prevalence of root caries is increasing because people are living longer and retaining more teeth.

SELF-EVALUATION QUESTIONS

1. By definition, public health programs are _____.
2. The four great public health measures of all time have been _____, _____, _____, and _____.
3. Approximately $_____ (amount) is spent annually in the United States for dental care.
4. DMFS stands for decayed, missing, and filled surfaces, whereas, _____is used to designate the same index for primary teeth.
5. The World Health Organization is the health organization coordinating international health efforts; in the United States, the cabinet-level department of government responsible for national health is the department of _____; the service within that department responsible for implementing department and congressional mandates is the _____ (Service). At state level there is a _____ to accept responsibility for planning and implementation of health programs to meet the oral health needs of the state.
6. The following are comparative methods used in private and public health practice:
   1. Examination   1. _____
   2. _____ 2. Analysis
   3. Treatment   3. _____
      planning
   4. _____ 4. Program operation
   5. Payment for   5. _____
      services
   6. _____ 6. Appraisal
7. Two indices for assessing gingival health are _____ and _____; two for assess-

ing severity of periodontal disease are _____ and _____; and two for assessing oral hygiene (plaque indices) are _____ and _____.

8. Program operation usually involves three basic elements: _____, _____, and _____.

9. _____ is essential to maintaining community understanding and support.

10. Three (of several) outreach type programs in which public health departments or dental schools often participate are _____, _____, and _____.

11. The two most cost effective means of reducing caries are _____ and _____.

REFERENCES

1. Cons NC. Using effective strategies to implement a program administrator's goal. *J Public Health Dent.* 1979; 39:279–285.

2. Graves RC. Aspects of the practical significance of current public health methods for the prevention of caries and periodontal disease. *J Public Health Dent.* 1982; 42: 179–189.

3. Klein H. The dental status and dental needs of young adult males, rejectable or acceptable for military service, according to selective service dental requirements. *Public Health Rep.* 1941; 56:1369–1387.

4. Lewis JR. Exemptions from military service on account of loss of teeth. *Dent Cosmos.* 1865; 7:240–242.

5. Britton RH, Perrott GJ. Summary of physical findings on men drafted in World War I. *Public Health Rep.* 1941; 56:41–62.

6. Hollander F, Dunning JM. A study by age and sex of the incidence of dental caries in over 12,000 persons.*J Dent Res.* 1939; 18: 43–60.

7. Knutson JW. Epidemiological trend patterns of dental caries prevalence data. *J Am Dent Assoc.* 1958; 57:821–829.

8. Fulton JT, Hughes JT, Mercer CV. *The Natural History of Dental Diseases.* Chapel Hill, NC. University of North Carolina School of Public Health; 1965:80.

9. Moen BD. Survey of needs for dental care II: Dental needs according to age and sex of patients. *J Am Dent Assoc.* 1953; 46: 200–211.

10. Pelton WJ, Pennell EH, Druzina A. Tooth morbidity experience of adults. *J Am Dent Assoc.* 1954; 49:439–445.

11. National Center for Health Statistics. *Basic Data on Dental Examination Findings of Persons 1–74 Years: United States, 1971–1974.* Department of Health, Education and Welfare, Public Health Service. DHEW Pub. No. (PHS) 79-1662, Series 11, No. 214. Washington, DC. U.S. Government Printing Office; 1979.

12. National Center for Health Statistics. *Decayed, Missing, and Filled Teeth among Children, United States.* Department of Health, Education and Welfare, Public Health Service. DHEW Pub. No. (HSM) 72-1003, Series 11, No. 106. Washington, DC. U.S. Government Printing Office; 1971.

13. National Center for Health Statistics. *Decayed, Missing, and Filled Teeth among Youths 12–17 Years, United States.* Department of Health, Education and Welfare, Public Health Service. Pub. No. (HRA) 75-1626, Series 11, No. 144. Washington, DC. U.S. Government Printing Office; 1974.

14. Messner CT, Gafafer WM, Cady FC, et al. Dental survey of school children, ages six to fourteen years, made in 1933–1934 in twenty-six states. *Public Health Bull.* 1936:226.

15. Klein H, Palmer CE, Knutson JW. Studies on dental caries. I. Dental status and dental needs of elementary school children. *Public Health Rep.* 1938; 53:751–765.

16. Ast DB. Response to receiving the John W. Knutson distinguished service award in dental public health. *J Public Health Dent.* 1983; 43:101–105.

17. Russell AL. Epidemiology and the rational bases of dental public health and dental

practice. In: Young WO, Striffler DF. *The Dentist, His Practice and His Community.* Philadelphia, Pa. WB Saunders Co.; 1969: 35–62.

18. Dean HT. Endemic fluorosis and its relation to dental caries. *Public Health Rep.* 1938; 53:1443–1452.

19. McKay FS, Black GV. An investigation of mottled teeth. *Dent Cosmos.* 1916; 58:477–484.

20. Churchill HV. The occurrence of fluorides in some waters of the United States. *J Dent Res.* 1932; 12:141–159.

21. Smith H, Smith MC. *Mottled Enamel in Arizona and Its Correlation with the Concentrations of Fluorides in Water Supplies.* University of Arizona, College of Agriculture Experimental Station, Tech Bull 43; July 1932.

22. Dean HT, Arnold FA Jr, Elvove E. Domestic water and dental caries. V. Additional studies of the relation of fluoride domestic waters to dental caries experience in 4,425 white children aged 12–14 years of 13 cities in 4 states. *Public Health Rep.* 1942; 57: 1155–1179.

23. Dean HT, Arnold FA Jr, Jay P, et al. Studies on mass control of dental caries through fluoridation of the public water supply. *Public Health Rep.* 1950; 65:1403–1408.

24. Ast DB, Finn SB, McCaffrey I. The Newburgh-Kingston caries-fluorine study. I. Dental findings after three years of water fluoridation. *Am J Public Health.* 1950; 40: 716–724.

25. Blayney JR, Tucker WH. The Evanston dental caries study. *J Dent Res.* 1948; 27: 279–286.

26. Hutton WL, Linscott BW, Williams DB. The Brantford fluorine experiment. Interim report after five years of water fluoridation. *Can J Public Health.* 1951; 42:81–87.

27. Federation Dentaire Internationale. *Basic Fact Sheets.* London. The Federation; 1987.

28. Department of Health and Human Services, USPHS. Letter: FL-139, May 1992. Atlanta, Ga. Centers for Disease Control; 1992.

29. Easley MW. The new antifluoridationists: Who are they and how do they operate. *J Public Health Dent.* 1985; 45:133–141.

30. American Dental Association. Fluoridation facts: Answers to questions about fluoridation. Chicago, Ill. American Dental Association; 1980.

31. U.S. Department of Health and Human Services. *Review of Fluoride Benefits and Risks.* Public Health Service. Washington, DC. Department of Health and Human Services; 1991.

32. Burt BA, Eklund SA. The practice of dental public health. In: Burt BA, Eklund SA. *Dentistry, Dental Practice, and the Community,* 4th ed. Philadelphia, Pa. WB Saunders Co.; 1992.

33. Graves RC. Dental health needs and demands in American society: Current methods. *Health Values.* 1984; 8:13–20.

34. Symposium on the future of public health and public health dentistry. *J Public Health Dent.* 1989; 49:93–98.

35. Health Care Financing Administration. Office of National Cost Estimates, Office of the Actuary. Washington, DC. Health Care Financing Administration, U.S. Department of Health and Human Services; 1992.

36. Kuthy RA, Odom JG. Local dental programs: A descriptive assessment of funding and activities. *J Public Health Dent.* 1988; 48:36–42.

37. National Institute of Dental Research. *The Oral Health of United States Adults: The National Survey of Oral Health in U.S. Employed Adults and Seniors, 1986–1987.* US Department of Health and Human Services, National Institutes of Health. DHHS Pub. No. (NIH) 87-2868. Bethesda, Md. U.S. Government Printing Office; 1987.

38. Jack S, Bloom B. *Use of Dental Services and Dental Health, 1986.* Vital and Health Statistics, National Center for Health Statistics, Public Health Service, Department of Health and Human Services, DHHS Pub. No. (PHS) 88-1593, Series 10, No. 165. Washington, DC. U.S. Government Printing Office; 1988.

39. Brunelle JA, Carlos JP. *Recent Trends in Dental Caries in U.S. Children and the Effect of Water Fluoridation.* International Fluoride Symposium; March 1989; Pine Mountain, Georgia.

40. Graves RC, Bohannan HM, Abernthy JR, et al. Contrasts in dental caries in US children by risk groups. *IADR Prog Abst.* 1985; 64(456):225.

41. Gift HC, Reisine ST, Larach DC. The social impact of dental problems and visits. *Am J Public Health.* 1992; 82:1663–1668.

42. Reisine ST. Dental health and public policy: The social impact of dental disease. *Am J Public Health.* 1985; 75:27–30.

43. Bloom B, Gift HC, Jack SS. *Dental Services and Oral Health: United States, 1989.* Vital and Health Statistics, National Center for Health Statistics, Public Health Service, Department of Health and Human Services, DHHS Pub. No. (PHS) 93-1511, Series 10, No. 183. Washington, DC. U.S. Government Printing Office; 1992.

44. Knutson JW. What is public health? In: Pelton WJ, Wisan JM, eds. *Dentistry in Public Health,* 2nd ed. Philadelphia, Pa. WB Saunders Co.; 1955:20–29.

45. National Institute of Dental Research. *Oral Health of United States Children: The National Survey of Dental Caries in U.S. School Children, 1986–1987.* Department of Health and Human Services, National Institutes of Health. DHHS Pub. No. (NIH) 89-2247. Bethesda, Md. U.S. Government Printing Office; 1989.

46. Gruebbel AO. A measurement of dental caries prevalence and treatment service for deciduous teeth. *J Dent Res.* 1944; 23:163–168.

47. Löe H, Silness J. Periodontal disease in pregnancy. I. Prevalence and severity. *Acta Odont Scand.* 1963; 21:533–551.

48. Russell AL. A system of classification and scoring for prevalence surveys of periodontal disease. *J Dent Res.* 1956; 35:350–359.

49. Ramfjord SP. Indices for prevalence and incidence of periodontal disease. *J Periodont.* 1959; 30:51–59.

50. World Health Organization. *Community Periodontal Index of Treatment Needs, Development, Field Testing, and Statistical Evaluation.* Geneva, Switzerland: Oral Health Unit, World Health Organization; 1984.

51. Silness J, Löe H. Periodontal disease in pregnancy. II. Correlation between oral hygiene and periodontal condition. *Acta Odont Scand.* 1964; 22:112–135.

52. Greene JC, Vermillion JR. The simplified oral hygiene index. *J Am Dent Assoc.* 1964; 68:25–31.

53. Striffler DF. What is public health? In: Striffler DF, Young WO, Burt BA, eds. *Dentistry, Dental Practice and the Community,* 3rd ed. Philadelphia, Pa. WB Saunders Co.; 1983:58–72.

54. Siegal MD, Martin B, Kuthy RA. Usefulness of a local oral health survey in program development. *J Public Health Dent.* 1988; 48:121–124.

55. Kuthy RA, Martin BW, Siegal MD, et al. Development of an oral health survey: Columbus, Ohio. *J Public Health Dent.* 1988; 48:116–120.

56. Massachusetts Department of Public Health. *Preventing Pit and Fissure Caries: A Guide to Sealant Use.* Boston, Mass. Massachusetts Department of Public Health; 1986.

57. Simonsen RJ. Potential uses of pit-and-fissure sealants in innovative ways: a review. *J Public Health Dent.* 1982; 42:305–311.

58. Calderone JJ, Mueller LA. The cost of sealant application in a state dental disease prevention program. *J Public Health Dent.* 1983; 43:249–254.

59. Hardison JR. The use of pit-and-fissure sealants in community public health programs in Tennessee. *J Public Health Dent.* 1983; 43:233–239.

60. Horowitz AM, Frazier PJ. Issues in the widespread adoption of pit-and-fissure sealants. *J Public Health Dent.* 1982; 42:312–323.

61. Cohen LA, Horowitz AM. Community-based sealant programs in the United

States: Results of a survey. *J Public Health Dent.* 1993; 53:241–245.

62. US Department of Health and Human Services. *The Prevalence of Dental Caries in United States Children: the National Dental Caries Prevalence Study 1979–80.* National Institutes of Health. NIH Pub. No. 82-2245. Washington, DC. U.S. Government Printing Office; 1981.

63. World Health Organization. *Oral Health Surveys: Basic Methods*, 3rd ed. Geneva. World Health Organization; 1987.

64. Siegal MD, Carnahan BW. Oral health of Ohio school children, 1987–88: findings of a statewide survey and implications for caries prevention strategies. In: Pit and fissure sealants (monograph). *The Ohio Dental Journal: Special Emphasis.* 1989:3–7.

65. Kaste LM, Marianos D, Chang R, et al. The assessment of nursing caries and its relationship to high caries in the permanent dentition. *J Public Health Dent.* 1992; 52: 64–68.

66. American Dental Association. Oral health status of Vermont nursing home residents. Council on Dental Health and Health Planning, Bureau of Economic and Behavioral Research. *J Am Dent Assoc.* 1982; 104:68–69.

67. Marcus P, Kaste L, Monopoli M, et al. Barriers to dental care for homebound elders in Boston. *J Dent Res.* 1989; 68(special issue):238. Abstract.

68. Woolfolk M, Hamard M, Bagramian RA. Oral health of children of migrant farm workers in northwest Michigan. *J Pub Health Dent.* 1984; 44:101–105.

69. Entwistle BA, Swanson TM. Dental needs and perceptions of adult Hispanic migrant farmworkers in Colorado. *J Dent Hyg.* 1989; 63:286–289.

70. Little JW, Falace DA. *Dental Management of the Medically Compromised Patient.* St. Louis, Mo. CV Mosby; 1988.

71. Niessen L, Dunleavy HA. Meeting the oral health needs of the aging veteran. In: Wetle T, Rowe JW, eds. *Older Veterans: Linking VA and Community Resources.*

Cambridge, Mass. Harvard University Press; 1984:369–407.

72. U.S. Public Health Service. *Special Report: Dental Care for Handicapped People.* U.S. Department of Health and Human Services. DHHS Pub. No.(PHS) 81-50154. Washington, DC. U.S. Government Printing Office; 1980.

73. Gelberg L, Linn LS, Rosenberg DJ. Dental health of homeless adults. *Spec Care Dent.* 1988; 8:167–172.

74. Jago JD, Sternberg GS, Westerman B. Oral health status of homeless men in Brisbane. *Aust Dent J.* 1984; 29:184–188.

75. Beck JD. Trends in oral disease and health. *Gerondontology.* 1988; 7:21–25.

76. Beck JD, Hunt RJ. Oral health status in the United States: Problems of special patients. *J Dent Educ.* 1985; 49:407–425.

77. Klein SP, Bohannon HM, Bell RM, et al. The cost and effectiveness of school-based preventive dental care. *Am J Public Health.* 1985; 75:382–391.

78. Broderick E, Mabry J, Robertson D, et al. Baby bottle tooth decay in Native American children. *Pub Health Rep.* 1989; 104: 50–54.

79. Louie R, Brunelle JA, Maggiore ED, et al. Caries prevalence in Head Start children, 1986–87. *J Pub Health Dent.* 1990; 50:299–305.

80. Jones DB, Schlife CM, Phipps KR. An oral health survey of Head Start children in Alaska: Oral health status, treatment needs, and cost of treatment. *J Pub Health Dent.* 1992; 52:86–93.

81. Little SJ, Stevens VJ, LaChance PA, et al. Smokeless tobacco habits and oral mucosal lesions in dental patients. *J Public Health Dent.* 1992; 52:269–276.

82. National Cancer Institute. *Cancer Statistics Review, 1973–1987.* NIH Pub. No. (NIH) 88-2789. U.S. Department of Health and Human Services. Bethesda, Md. Government Printing Office; 1989.

83. Levy SM, Baker KA, Semia TP, et al. Use of medications with dental significance by a non-institutionalized elderly population. *Gerodontics.* 1988; 4:119–125.

84. Navazesh M. Xerostomia in the aged. *Dent Clin North Am.* 1989; 33:75–80.

85. Atkinson JC, Fox PC. Sjögren's syndrome: Oral and dental considerations. *J Am Dent Assoc.* 1993; 124:74–86.

86. National Institutes of Health. *Detection and Prevention of Periodontal Disease in Diabetes.* U.S. Department of Health and Human Services, Public Health Service. NIH Pub. No. 86-1148. Bethesda, Md. U.S. Government Printing Office; 1986.

87. Silverman S. AIDS update: Oral findings, diagnosis, and precautions. *J Am Dent Assoc.* 1987; 115:559–563.

88. Niessen LC, Jones JA. Alzheimer's disease: A guide for dental professionals. *Spec Care Dent.* 1986; 6:6–12.

89. Ship JA. Oral health of patients with Alzheimer's disease. *J Am Dent Assoc.* 1992; 123:53–58.

90. Antczak AA, Branch LG. Perceived barriers to the use of dental services by the elderly. *Gerodontics.* 1985; 1:194–198.

91. Gilbert GH. "Ageism" in dental care delivery. *J Am Dent Assoc.* 1989; 118:545–548.

92. Cohen LA, Grace EG. Infection control practices related to treatment of AIDS patients. *J Dent Pract Admin.* 1990; 7:108–115.

93. Steifel DJ, Lubin JH, Truelove EL. A survey of perceived oral health needs of homebound patients. *J Public Health Dent.* 1979; 39:7–15.

94. Mashberg A, Samit AM. Early detection, diagnosis, and management of oral and oralpharyngeal cancer. *CA.* 1989; 39:67–88.

95. National Center for Health Statistics. *Physician Contacts by Sociodemographic and Health Characteristics, 1982–83.* Vital and Health Statistics, Department of Health and Human Services, DHHS Pub. No. 87-1589, Series 10, no. 161. Washington, DC. U.S. Government Printing Office; 1987.

96. Yellowitz JA, Goodman HS, Wertheimer DA. Physicians' and dentists' oral cancer knowledge and practices. *J Public Health Dent.* 1994; 54:115. Abstract.

97. Mecklenburg RE. Managing hard-core smokers: oral health team challenges and opportunities. *Health Values.* 1994; 18:6–16.

98. Frazier PJ. Public health education and promotion for caries prevention the role of dental schools. *J Public Health Dent.* 1983; 43:28–42.

99. Graves RC, McNeal DR, Haemer DP, et al. A comparison of the effectiveness of the "Toothkeeper" and a traditional dental health education program. *J Public Health Dent.* 1975; 35:85–90.

100. Smith LW, Evans RI, Suomi JD, et al. Teachers as models in programs for school dental health: An evaluation of the "Toothkeeper." *J Public Health Dent.* 1975; 35:75–80.

101. Stamm JW, Kuo HC, Nail DR. An evaluation of the "Toothkeeper" program in Vermont. *J Public Health Dent.* 1975; 35:81–84.

102. Kenney JB. The role and responsibility of schools in affecting dental health status—a potential yet unrealized. *J Public Health Dent.* 1979; 39:262–267.

103. Johnson BG. Introduction: Establishing a conceptual framework for the critical analysis and planning of school dental programs. *J Public Health Dent.* 1979; 39:259–261.

104. Faine RC, Collins JJ, Daniel J, et al. The 1980 fluoridation campaigns: A discussion of results. *J Public Health Dent.* 1981; 41:138–142.

105. Bronstein E. Letters to the editor: Fluoridation monitoring. *J Public Health Dent.* 1979; 39:248.

106. Bell RM, Klein SP, Bohannan HB, et al. *Treatment Effects in the National Preventive Dentistry Demonstration Program.* Santa Monica, Calif. Rand; R-3072-RWJ; 1984.

107. Bohannnon HM, Bader JD. Future impact of public health and preventive methods on the incidence of dental caries. *J Can Dent Assoc.* 1984; 50:229–233.

108. Brunelle JA, Carlos JP. Changes in the prevalence of dental caries in US school-

children: 1961–1980. *J Dent Res.* 1982; 61:1346–1351.

109. Bryan ET, Collier DR, Howard WR, et al. Dental health status of school children in Tennessee—a 5-year comparison. *J Tenn State Dent Assoc.* 1982; 62:31–33.

110. DePaola PF, Soparker PM, Tavares M, et al. A dental survey of Massachusetts schoolchildren. *J Dent Res.* 1982; 61:1356–1360.

111. Glass RL. Secular changes in caries prevalence in two Massachusetts towns. *Caries Res.* 1981; 15:445–450.

112. Hughes JT, Rozier RG, Ramsey DL. *The Natural History of Dental Disease in North Carolina, 1976–77.* Durham, NC. Academic Press; 1980.

113. Zacherl WA, Long DM. Reduction in caries attack rate—non-fluoridated community. *J Dent Res.* 1979; 58:227. Abstract.

114. Burt BA. The future of the caries decline. *J Public Health Dent.* 1985; 45:261–269.

115. Beazoglou T, Brown LJ, Heffley D. Dental care utilization over time. *Soc Sci Med.* 1993; 37:1461–1472.

116. Friedman JW. A consumer advocate's view of community dentistry. *J Dent Educ.* 1977; 41:656–659.

117. Federation Dentaire Internationale. Technical Report No. 31. Review of methods of identification of high caries risk groups and individuals. *Int Dent J.* 1988; 38:177–189.

118. Stamm JS, Disney JA, Graves RC, et al. The University of North Carolina caries risk assessment study. I. Rationale and content. *J Public Health Dent.* 1988; 48:225–232.

119. Page RC. Oral health status in the United States: Prevalence of inflammatory periodontal disease. *J Dent Educ.* 1985; 49:354–367.

120. Catherman JL. Role of the dental hygienist in public health periodontal programs. *J Public Health Dent.* 1983; 43:135–138.

121. Galagan DJ. Some comments on the future of dental public health. *J Public Health Dent.* 1976; 36:96–102.

122. Dunning JM. Guest editorial: The stone wall. *J Public Health Dent.* 1979; 39:175–176.

123. Institutes of Medicine. *The Future of Public Health.* Washington, DC. National Academy Press; 1988.

124. Corbin SB, Martin RF, eds. *The Future of Dental Public Health Report.* American Public Health Association Dental Health Section, American Association of Public Health Dentistry. *J Public Health Dent.* 1994; 54:80–91.

125. Glass RL. The use of fluoride dentifrices: A public health measure. *Community Dent Oral Epidemiol.* 1980; 8:278–282.

126. Harmon RG. Oral health care for the underserved in the 1990's: The HRSA perspective. *J Public Health Dent.* 1993; 53: 46–49.

127. Niessen LC. New directions-constituencies and responsibilities. *J Public Health Dent.* 1990; 50(special issue):133–138.

128. Gaupp PG. New initiatives for advocacy in national maternal and child oral health. *J Public Health Dent.* 1990; 50(special issue): 396–401.

129. United States Department of Health and Human Services. *Promoting Health/Preventing Disease: Objectives for the Nation.* Washington, DC. Public Health Service; 1980:54.

130. U.S. Department of Health and Human Services. *Healthy People 2000: National Health Promotion and Disease Prevention objectives.* Public Health Service. DHHS Pub. No.(PHS)91-50212. Washington, DC. U.S. Government Printing Office; 1990.

131. American Public Health Association. *Healthy Communities 2000: Model Standards.* Washington, DC. American Public Health Association; 1991.

132. U.S. Department of Health and Human Services. *Healthy People 2000: Public Health Service Action.* Public Health Service. Washington, DC. Government Printing Office; 1992.

133. U.S. Department of Health and Human Services. *Healthy People 2000: State Action.* Public Health Service. Washington, DC. Government Printing Office; 1992.

134. U.S. Department of Health and Human Services. *Healthy People 2000: Consortium Action.* Public Health Service. Washington, DC. Government Printing Office; 1992.

135. American Fund for Dental Health. *Proceeding of the National Consortium Meeting: Oral Health 2000.* Chicago, Ill. American Fund for Dental Health; 1992.

136. American Association of Retired Persons. *A Profile of Older Americans: 1990.* Administration on Aging, U.S. Department of Health and Human Services; 1990.

137. Burt BA. New priorities in prevention of oral disease. *J Public Health Dent.* 1982; 42:170–179.

138. Hand JS, Hunt RJ, Beck JD. Incidence of coronal and root caries in an older adult population. *J Public Health Dent.* 1988; 48: 14–19.

139. Stamm JW, Banting DW, Imrey PB. Adult root caries survey of two similar communities with contrasting natural water fluoride levels. *J Am Dent Assoc.* 1990; 120:143–149.

140. American Dental Association. *Dental Programs in Medicaid: The 1989 Survey.* Council on Dental Care Programs. Chicago, Ill. American Dental Association; 1990.

141. Office of Technology Assessment. *Children's Dental Services under the Medicaid Program.* Congress of the United States; 1990.

142. Agency for Health Care Policy and Research. *National Medical Expenditure Survey: Annual Expenses and Sources of Payment for Health Care Services.* Center for General Health Services Intramural Research. Rockville, Md; 1992.

143. Bader JD, ed. *Risk Assessment in Dentistry.* Chapel Hill. University of North Carolina Dental Ecology; 1990.

144. Goodman HS, Weyant RJ. Dental health personnel planning: A review of the literature. *J Public Health Dent.* 1990; 50:48–63.

145. American Association of Dental Schools. *Manpower Project Report No. 2.* Washington, DC. American Association of Dental Schools; 1989.

146. U.S. Department of Health and Human Services. *Health Personnel in the United States: Eighth Report to Congress, 1991.* Public Health Service, Health Resources and Services Administration, Bureau of Health Professions. DHHS Pub. No. HRS-P-OD-92-1, Sept. 1992.

147. Interim Study Group on Dental Activities. *Improving the Oral Health of the American People: Opportunity for Action.* Washington, DC. US Department of Health and Human Services; 1989.

148. Machen JB. Education and dental environment: The future for dental schools. *J Am Coll Dent.* 1989; 56:33, 42–44.

149. National Institutes of Health. *Technology Assessment Conference Statement: Effects and Side Effects of Dental Restorative Materials.* Department of Health and Human Services, August 26–28, 1991.

150. Cohen LA, Grace EG, Ward MA. Maryland residents' attitudes towards AIDS and the use of dental services. *J Public Health Dent.* 1992; 52:81–85.

151. Verrusio AC, Neidle EA, Nash KD, et al. The dentist and infectious diseases: A national survey of attitudes and behaviors. *J Am Dent Assoc.* 1989; 118:553–562.

152. Ciesielski C, Marianos D, Ou C-Y et al. Transmission of human immunodeficiency virus in a dental practice. *Ann Int Med.* 1992; 116:798–805.

153. Cohen LA, Grace EG, Ward MA. Changes in public concern about transmission of AIDS from dentist to patient after CDC report. *Clin Prev Dent.* 1992; 14:6–9.

154. American Dental Association. Infection control recommendations for the dental office and the dental laboratory. Council on Dental Materials, Instruments, and Equipment; Council on Dental Therapeutics; Council on Dental Research; Council on Dental Practice. *J Am Dent Assoc.* 1992; 123(suppl):1–8.

155. Centers for Disease Control. Recommended infection control practices for dentistry. *MMWR* 1986; 35:237–242.

156. U.S. Department of Labor, Occupational Safety and Health Administration. Occupa-

tional exposure to bloodborne pathogens (29 CFR 1910.1030). *Federal Register*. December 6, 1991; 56:64004–64182.

157. U.S. Public Health Service, Oral Health Coordinating Committee. *An Essential Oral Health Benefits Package: Working Draft*. Department of Health and Human Services, 1993.

158. ADA Task Force on Access, Health Care Financing, and Reform. *Change and Continuity in Health Care in the United States: A Position Paper on Access, Health Care Financing, and Reform*. American Dental Association; 1993.

159. National Institute of Dental Research. *Broadening the Scope, Long-Range Research Plan for the Nineties*. Department of Health and Human Services. NIH Pub. No. 90-1188. Bethesda, Md. U.S. Government Printing Office; 1990.

160. Veterans Administration. *A Research Agenda on Oral Health in the Elderly: A Collaborative Research Project of the National Institute on Aging, the National Institute of Dental Research, and the Veterans Administration*. Washington, DC. Veterans Administration; 1986.

161. American Public Health Association, Oral Health Section; and the American Association of Public Health Dentistry. A research agenda for dental public health. *J Public Health Dent*. 1992; 52(special issue): 1–39.

162. Department of Health and Human Services. *The Health Consequences of Using Smokeless Tobacco: A Report of the Advisory Committee to the Surgeon General*. Bethesda, Md. Department of Health and Human Services, NIH Pub. No. 86-2874; 1986.

163. Department of Health and Human Services. *Equity and Access for Mothers and Children: Strategies from the Public Health Service Workshop on Oral Health of Mothers and Children*. Public Health Service, Health Resources and Services Administration, Maternal and Child Health Bureau. Washington, DC. National Maternal and Child Health Clearinghouse; Sept. 1989.

164. Department of Health and Human Services. *National Health Service Corps: Fact Sheet*. Public Health Service, Health Resources and Services Administration. Washington, DC. Department of Health and Human Services; 1992.

Chapter 18

School-Based
Oral Health Programs

Norman O. Harris
Jacquelyn L. Fried

Objectives

At the end of this chapter it will be possible to

1. Explain why some teachers are concerned about teaching oral health, and discuss how these concerns can be partially or completely allayed.
2. Explain why oral health teaching presentations that impart facts only are not as satisfactory as those involving students in combined education–prevention programs.
3. Name at least four different school and classroom preventive actions that can accompany educational presentations to produce *rapid, predictable,* and *significant reductions in DMFS.*
4. Describe a preventive dentistry program that can be easily accomplished by teachers and a school nurse; and by teachers, a school nurse, and a dental hygienist.
5. Explain why school-based sealant programs should be target-specific, that is, directed to the "high-risk" children, not to all children.
6. State five sports for which helmet protection and mouth-guards are mandated to prevent orofacial injuries and three other sports for which mandated protection is desirable.
7. Justify the need for school intervention programs to prevent children from smoking and using smokeless tobacco.

Introduction

School-based oral health programs give children a chance to experience optimal oral health, but developing relevant programs that address the needs of today's children is a complex task. Our increasingly heterogeneous society poses challenges to the school health program planner. Shifting demographics and attendant cultural diversity present a patchwork of societal and psychosocial variables that influence planning decisions. Trends in children's caries patterns and the overwhelming prevalence of gingivitis and periodontitis also shape the objectives of today's school-based programs. In addition to caries and periodontal disease, timely programs must address accident prevention, mouth protection, malocclusion, tobacco use interventions, nutrition, fluorides, and pit-and-fissure sealants.

Several changes in caries incidence and patterns affect the planning of school-based programs. In general, in the United States caries has declined among children.[1,2] Approximately 50% of children aged 6 to 8, however, still experience dental caries in their permanent dentition.[2,3] The highest caries rates are associated with lower socioeconomic status.[4,5] As children reach the age of 15 to 17 years, about 90% of all caries are found in occlusal, buccal, and lingual pits. With the widespread use of fluorides, including water fluoridation, the "halo effect" of water fluoridation, fluoride supplements, fluoride mouth rinses, and fluoride dentifrices, the incidence of smooth-surface caries has declined.

The presence of gingivitis and periodontal disease among children is ubiquitous. It has been reported that 92% of school children have mild or moderate gingivitis.[6] Current research also reveals that children are experimenting extensively with cigarette smoking and smokeless tobacco

(ST) use.[7] In 1989, more than 30% of male teenagers reported current or previous use of smokeless tobacco.[7]

School-based oral health programs that are designed to help children must be relevant and offer interventions based on current research findings.[8] Different target populations present with different needs, and the astute planner must address these. For example, children at high risk for caries may require different program strategies from children at less risk who live in fluoridated communities. No one standardized program completely meets the needs of all children. Economic constraints also affect the scope of many school-based programs.

Despite the challenges posed by overwhelming need and limited resources, children deserve to receive information that allows them to make informed choices. They also deserve the chance to learn skills and develop attitudes that permit them to practice desirable behaviors that enhance their oral and overall health. Finally, they deserve to receive services that prevent and treat oral disease. The knowledge, the methodologies, and the techniques that allow children to be free of oral disease are *now* available. Less obvious are the political and administrative means needed to make these cost-efficient measures available to the children. School administrators, legislators, oral health professionals, and parents must all work together to ensure that children eventually are afforded the opportunity to achieve optimal oral health.

Treatment is not the answer to solving children's oral health problems; instead, *prevention* is the key. Schools have been and will continue to be important environments for the dissemination of disease preventive information.[8] Because the classroom maximizes the numbers of children reached simultaneously, school-based education, health promotion, and preventive efforts are efficient. Schools serve as institutions that support the adoption and practice of behaviors deemed desirable by society. In the school setting, students also are prepared to assume responsible roles as future parents and community leaders.

The year 2000 objectives[3] help provide a focus for relevant and comprehensive school-based oral health programs. Appendix 18–1 provides a listing of the health status, risk reduction, and services and protection *objectives* that specifically relate to children and school-based programs. As services and protection objective 8.4 indicates, schools have an obligation to plan and provide quality school health education from kindergarten through 12th grade.[9]

In this chapter we suggests ways to create and implement successful school-based oral health programs. The following is a comprehensive overview of the essential elements and strategies that ensure success.

CHALLENGES AND SOLUTIONS

To involve communities, families, or individuals in assuming responsibility for *their own* dental health, two main ingredients are necessary: *knowledge* and *motivation.* Approximately 56 active dentists serve every 100,000 people in the United States.[10] In addition a total of 81,000 active dental hygienists serve the same population.[11] It is impossible for these dental professionals to assume the tremendous task of imparting oral health facts to the public and encouraging the behaviors that are requisite to oral health care. Such mass education can only be accomplished through the *public school systems.*[12]

Considerable debate rages about what should be taught by the public schools. Reading, writing, arithmetic, history, and geography are examples of traditional subjects. Yet, along with these, there are continual demands for curriculum time to teach about other urgent concerns of our society. Cultural sensitivity, drugs, AIDS, economic, social, physical and psychologic issues are but a few of the topics relevant to a school-aged population. Despite the great competition for the little time available in the curriculum, it should be stressed that the end purpose of education is to (1) provide the information and experience for people to *earn a living* and (2) *make life more worthwhile.* Optimal oral health contributes to the latter objective.

Public schools have traditionally accepted the responsibility of teaching dental health as a part of general health. Often times, however, programs are episodic and lack depth. Many erroneously consider education like an inoculation—once an individual is exposed, results are permanent.[13] A school-based oral health curriculum should include education and health promotion, along with primary preventive and treatment services. The core components of a school oral health program are shown in Table 18–1.[8]

TABLE 18–1. COMPONENTS OF A SCHOOL ORAL HEALTH PROGRAM

Services
Appropriate regimens to prevent dental caries, gingivitis, and oral cancer. Assurance of periodic oral examination and treatment. Effective referral and follow-up procedures for children in need of treatment. Emergency first aid for accidental oral injuries at school.

Instruction
A comprehensive educational curriculum for all grade levels, including both personal and community health topics.

Environment
An environment consistent with what is taught; that is, healthy for both students and school personnel. Incorporation of safety measures in the school building and in sports.

In today's fast-paced society, in which children often live in single-parent or dual-career families, the school can become a reliable bastion of constancy. Messages in school can be reinforced readily. Oral health education and promotion should begin in the early school years but should extend into adulthood, then parenthood, and finally into community wellness initiatives as a public service responsibility.

CREATING EFFECTIVE SCHOOL-BASED PROGRAMS

To maximize program success, a school-based oral health program should include all the elements contained in the mnemonic, CAPITE,[14] that is,

- **C**   **Compatible** with the needs of the nation and of the population served.
- **A**   **Administratively sound,** requiring political, professional, educational, and community planning to ensure a source of oral health and teaching personnel, money, materials, and facilities necessary to support the objectives of the school oral health program.
- **P**   Incorporate effective **Preventive** and **Promotive** regimens into school and classroom activities as part of the oral health curriculum.
- **I**   Periodic oral screening inspections to **Identify** impending or actual pathology implying the need for preventive, screening, and referral programs requisite for optimal student oral health.
- **T**   Provisions for screening and **Treatment** referral programs requisite for optimal student oral health.

- **E**   **Education** that supports the acquisition of knowledge and develops the attitudes for self-care.

Planning a School-based Program

A successful school-based program does not just happen. *Planning* is the key to success. A diverse and involved work group ensures a greater variety of input, a representative commited audience, and a broad-based sense of ownership. It is important that cooperative working relationships be established in the initial planning stages among parents, community leaders, teachers, school administrators, and oral health professionals. Planning procedures must include collecting and analyzing needs-assessment data; establishing priorities; setting goals that include monitoring oral health status changes; establishing objectives; planning activities geared toward these objectives; identifying resources; developing a budget; and implementing, monitoring, and evaluating program objectives.[15] *An integrated plan of action spanning kindergarten through 12th grade is essential, as is a clear delineation of program responsibilities.*[8] Judicious planning ultimately can result in meaningful, target-specific programs that are integrated throughout the school years. With this strong academic base, positive attitudes and behaviors can be developed regarding oral health that will accompany children into adulthood.

Before implementing a school-based oral health curriculum, it is necessary to consider that

- People interpret health messages through the "filter" of their own values and attitudes. This needs to be understood, if the educational process is to have any chance of success.
- The most successful education maximizes self-involvement of the participants.

- Health professionals must accept that not all people share their values about the importance of physical health. An acceptance of all components of wellness helps in dealing with the infinite variety of human beliefs on health.[16]

DENTAL HEALTH TEACHING CONSIDERATIONS

Commited, knowledgeable *teachers* are the cornerstone of all effective school-based oral health programs. Yet, they have concerns about teaching oral health. Unfortunately, teachers receive little dental information in undergraduate training to prepare them to teach the subject. Usually the dental subject matter contained in undergraduate texts used in teacher's colleges and education curricula relates to the physiology and anatomy of the teeth, the supporting tissues, and the salivary glands. Such a grounding enables the school teacher to communicate basic information about oral physiology. Teachers cannot, however, be expected to possess expertise in a constantly changing pool of scientific knowledge about primary preventive procedures, health promotion, and dental treatment options. Also, few sources are *accessible* for periodic updates of dental information that allow teachers to remain current on dental education objectives. Hence, teachers are reluctant to teach what could be incorrect or obsolete information.[17] Kay and Baba suggest that this problem might be addressed by involving the teachers in the formative evaluation of teaching materials. This involvement, they suggest, would promote teacher confidence and foster individualized, experiential, and participatory student learning.[18]

The priority given to school oral health education programs has been questioned by teachers and the dental profession alike. Sometimes the questions are asked by the educators because the time taken for dental education competes with the time needed for other subjects.[19] Is oral health instruction more important than, for instance, mathematics or vocational training? Health professionals also question the time devoted to school programs that feature mainly information transmittal, rather than a combination of education and active preventive programs. One of the findings of the National Preventive Dentistry Program was that the teaching of dental information was the *least expensive* and the *least effective* way of bettering oral health status.[20] This is partially due to the fact that it is possible to transmit information without immediately improving the aptitudes and attitudes necessary for long-term self-care, especially if the need for behavioral change is not emphasized. On the other hand, it is always possible that knowledge acquired in public school will become meaningful in adult life when the importance of good health becomes more apparent. Although the results of teaching information alone are equivocal in evaluating attitudes, beliefs, and even actual health status, Flanders concludes that such efforts should be continued.[21] This conclusion is based primarily on the fact that children are fast learners, and that learning started at an early age can be reinforced with a variety of teaching techniques that enhance absorption and retention.[8,15,21] It also is posited that without having appropriate information, behavior change cannot occur.

The amount of dental health taught in school is often too little to be assimilated by students, and not long term enough to be amenable to good evaluation. A school health education evaluation, developed by the U.S. Public Health Service (USPHS), also sheds light on the needs of school health education.[22] A key finding from this national evaluation revealed that changes in health-related knowledge, practices, and attitudes increase with the amount of instruction; therefore greater integration of oral health education into the curriculum should be a goal of a school-based program. Inservice training conducted by oral health educators also helps faculty develop greater competencies and aids them in their classroom endeavors.

Question 1. Which of the following statements, if any, are correct?

   A.   Today, educators are required to teach subjects, such as cultural sensitivity, sexual orientation, and health; each new subject taught reduces the time needed for teaching reading, writing, and arithmetic.

   B.   The teacher can effectively disseminate integrated oral health information developed by parents, community leaders, other teachers, school administrators, and health professionals.

   C.   The "E" in the mnemonic CAPITE is to emphasize the role of *education* in implementing oral health programs.

   D.   Teaching oral health self-care is one of the most *effective* means for reducing oral disease.

   E.   Teachers are well prepared academically to teach current concepts of oral health care and disease prevention.

Dental Teaching—Teacher or Parent Responsibility

School-aged children are almost totally dependent on parent or school-based interest for exposure to and inclusion in preventive dentistry or dental treatment programs (Fig 18–1). Many teachers believe that oral health awareness should be the responsibility of parents and dental health professionals—not teachers.[23] This belief might be legitimate if, universally, parents were able to care for their children's teeth. As recently as 1986 through 1987,[2] however, almost three fourths of 14-year-olds had caries in their permanent teeth. In addition, the continued growth in numbers of children living in poverty coupled with cuts in public health programs may not bode well for this underserved population's access to dental services. A child raised in a home where the parents are subject to cultural, ethnic, economic, and educational disadvantages often can be dentally neglected. In these homes, parental intercession in the oral health care of a child frequently begins with seeking help to relieve pain. Too many working mothers and single parents cannot participate in or are apathetic about involvement in school activities and tend to relinquish responsibility to the school authorities. Even with highly motivated parents, knowledge about dental health is often minimal. In addition, behavioral change can be more

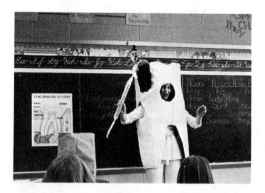

Figure 18–1. Teaching about teeth can be fun; all that is needed in this case is a homemade instructional aid. (*Courtesy of Learning Resource Center, Indiana University—Purdue University at Fort Wayne, Indiana.*)

difficult to influence at home under parental guidance than under the tutelage of the teacher. In other words, the parents themselves do not know how to help their children help themselves and need the support of a school oral health program.

Parent Participation

Whenever possible, the parent[a] must be included in a school-based oral health program.[24] One or both of the parents can provide strong positive reinforcement, either through role modeling or verbal messages, that supports the attitudinal and behavioral changes promulgated in the school setting.[24,25] Ideally, parent education should parallel child education; in this way, parents can learn to better their own oral health as well as have the guidelines to aid their children.[26] This educational process of parents is often needed to overcome the barriers raised by *their* past adverse experiences with dental disease and its financial hardship. As an example of the need to surmount barriers, in a recent study in England, a dental hygienist volunteered to visit some of the homes of school children to instruct their parents. Much to the chagrin of the study directors, some parents resented the intrusion into their homes, whereas others stated they were satisfied with their own level of dental knowledge.[27]

Professional Involvement

In addition to parental support, professional involvement in the school program is desirable. The luxury of having salaried dentists or dental hygienists (or both) employed by school systems, however, is rare. Therefore, opportunities for dentist and dental hygienist volunteerism in school-based programs abound. The involvement of oral health professionals is important to the success of local school efforts.[8] Representatives from local professional societies should be included in the oral health curriculum-planning phases. Professional input is valuable for identifying teaching–learning resources; for speaking to students, faculty, and parent groups; for in-service teaching of faculty and administrators; and for aiding the schools on special occasions, such as "career day." The support of the professional community enhances a program's credibility, improves the image of the oral health professions, and is a practice builder for the participating dentists. A more consistent presence of the oral health professions throughout the academic year is needed to help strengthen school–community relationships.

CHILDREN'S AND ORAL HEALTH PROGRAMS

The Preschooler

In 1965, Head Start, a national preschool program that provides early learning experiences to poor and underprivileged children, was initiated under the *Economic Opportunity Act of 1964.* Health care and health education, including a dental component, have been a continual part of this program.[28] The dental care component includes annual examinations, preventive services, follow-up care, and classroom instruction. Yet after about four decades of existence, there is evidence that many Head Start centers do not comply uniformly with U.S. Public Health Service standards. As it now functions, Head Start is meeting the needs of only a fraction of the eligible population.[29,30]

Today many other private and public preschool programs exist, with the number expected to increase dramatically if a national day care policy is established. The

---

[a] Guardians are included in this use of the word *parent.*

great majority of preschool programs will be under the auspices of private individuals or organizations with possibly limited expertise in health education, specifically in oral health objectives and preventive practices. Levy[31] in a review of preschool programs, found that the dental teaching components were generally flawed in design and lacked proper methodologies for evaluation.

Academically, preschool programs must include objectives, lesson plans, and the evaluation instruments needed to measure if objectives have been attained. Even at preschool age, the important preventive dentistry related words *fluoride* and *sealants* can be introduced into a child's vocabulary to be reinforced later in higher grades. At preschool age, children are willing to learn if it is enjoyable, but appropriate training aids and teaching programs are needed to meet this specification (Fig 18–2).

Parents and infant caregivers should be encouraged to participate in preschool programs because they are influential role models. Through preschool programs, parents and caregivers can learn how to care for their children's teeth, including the prevention of baby bottle caries.

Student Participation. Philosophically, *all* children should be entitled to receive maximum information and primary preventive dental care. Delivering maximum oral health treatment to *all* children, however, is not feasible. Following completion of the National Preventive Dentistry Demonstration Program, it was found that 60% of the carious lesions occurred in only 20% of the school children.[32] These statistics parallel a Finnish report in which a 50% commitment of dental personnel was required for 20% of high-risk children.[33] Thus, any school-based primary and secondary preventive dentistry program, other than classroom education, mouth rinse, or tablet programs, should be

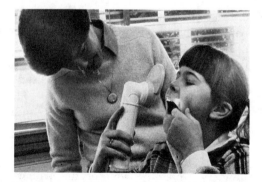

Figure 18–2. Encouraging a child to become familiar with the oral structures raises dental health awareness. *(Courtesy of Learning Resource Center, Indiana University—Purdue University at Fort Wayne, Indiana.)*

selective in *targeting the children most at risk* for a higher level of care. Once criteria are established defining "high risk," however, *all* students meeting the *high-risk* criteria should be eligible for the same preventive and treatment benefits. The economic status of individual students should not be a consideration, because poor dental health occurs among the affluent as well as among the poor. Interestingly in one study, it was found that following a few years of participation in an intensive caries prevention program, individuals were transformed from high risk to low risk.[34]

The extent of student involvement in program activities is an important issue. As previously indicated, the most highly successful programs include considerable student involvement and participation.[4] Personal involvement tends to have a greater effect on behavior, attitudes, and beliefs. Active participation enhances instruction about oral disease prevention measures, such as appropriate fluoride use and the employment of methods for the mechanical disruption or removal of plaque.

One of the few opportunities for innovative student participatory learning comes during Children's Dental Health Month (February). This American Dental Association (ADA) and American Dental Hygienists' Association (ADHA) sponsored program was initiated in 1941 and was intended to provide an annual forum for dental health. Historically, both the dental and dental hygiene associations have participated in this program. Children's Dental Health Month has developed into the professions' most widely supported and publicly recognized oral health event. It is a time when schools, in cooperation with dental manufacturers, local dental and dental hygiene societies, and other sponsors, develop dental health fairs for the public and for students. As a part of these health fairs, students engage in entertainment events, undergo screening examinations, watch demonstrations related to seat belt and air bag protection of the face and body, hear discussions about the deadly effects of cigarette smoking, and learn about health-promoting behaviors.[35] During this time, the students develop group posters and exhibits, discuss nutritional information with their peers, and learn that dentistry is not a profession to be feared. The informality of the occasion can enhance student learning and development of desirable attitudes towards self-care and self-image.

HELPING THE TEACHER TO TEACH

In a school curriculum, the teaching of mathematics becomes more sophisticated as a child progresses from grade to grade. In first grade the child is taught to add 1 and 1; yet at the high school level the young adult is able to perform problems of calculus. In many courses, such as chemistry, the didactic information is reinforced by laboratory programs; the combination of information

and experience helps develop student attitudes and motor skills. This same approach should be used to teach oral health. Also, oral health programs should be planned so that each grade level receives a greater diversity and complexity of subject matter and practical experience. For example, elementary school children have less dexterity than junior high students. Flossing therefore is more easily taught and comprehended in the upper grades.

At the high school level, students should have an advanced lay knowledge of the terminology, anatomy, and functions of the oral cavity and the etiology and consequences of oral disease. They should also have a knowledge of what to do to accept responsibility for (1) preventing oral disease, (2) identifying the presence of their own oral diseases at an early stage, and (3) seeking treatment once oral disease is suspected or identified. In other words, students should be taught to open their eyes when they open their mouths in front of a mirror.

The Tattletooth II Integrated Program

To construct an integrated curriculum for oral health that is applicable to a continuum of grade levels, it is first necessary to consider what information is relevant for each grade level. One such comprehensive grade-to-grade program developed for teaching dental health is exemplified by *Tattletooth II, A New Generation* program, developed by the Texas Department of Health (Fig 18–3).[36]

This comprehensive dental health curriculum targets students from prekindergarten through grade 6. In 1993, with funds appropriated by the state legislature, the Texas Bureau of Dental Health Services employed approximately 20 dental hygienists and dental assistants to implement the program statewide.[36]

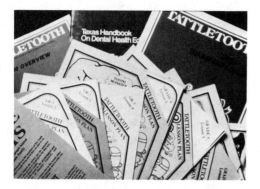

Figure 18–3. *Tattletooth* provides the public school teacher with integrated lesson plans for each grade; both the teacher and the students learn.

Each grade level has five core lessons and two enrichment lessons. Background information *for the teacher* is provided at the beginning of each lesson. Educational strategies are described for integrating dental topics into discussions involving other subjects, such as language, arts, mathematics, and science activities. To facilitate bilingual education, the program is being translated into Spanish for prekindergarten through third grade.

In addition, the curriculum includes scope and sequence charts, a unit test, bulletin board suggestions, audio–visuals lists, and suggested parent letters. A videotape illustrating the appropriate techniques of brushing and flossing is available on loan to schools. The curriculum and training materials were designed, tested, evaluated, retested, reevaluated, and again revised. Finally, the curriculum was reviewed by health and education specialists throughout the state.

To obtain the program for their classroom, teachers *must* attend in-service training provided by the state's regional dental hygiene staff. The staff uses a multimedia approach in their training. The program is copyrighted; however, out-of-state educa-

tors may secure it on loan and reproduce it at their own expense.[b] Other states, such as Connecticut,[37] Ohio,[38] and North Carolina,[15] have developed similar, large-scale teaching programs that can act as models for other state educational agencies.

Question 2. Which of the following statements, if any, are correct?

   A. Most parents are well prepared to teach oral health to their children.

   B. Head Start dental programs were designed to include annual examinations, preventive services, follow-up care, and classroom instruction.

   C. Approximately 20% of school children can be classified as high risk for dental caries.

   D. Once a child is categorized as high risk, he or she can be expected to always remain at high risk.

   E. Grade-integrated oral health teaching programs provide a means of helping teachers better teach the children.

ACTIVE PREVENTIVE DENTISTRY PROGRAMS

School Water Fluoridation

In 1992, schools in North Carolina, Indiana, Kentucky, Wisconsin, and Vermont constituted 332 of the total 351 schools in the United States using their own adjusted fluoridated water supply (Table 18–2).[39] School fluoridation can be used only if all the surrounding areas in which the students live have a low fluoride content. Consolidated rural schools are ideal for this approach, because all grades from kindergarten to senior

---

[b] For information on the *Tattletooth II* program, contact Ms. Cheryl Aiello, Texas Department of Health, Bureau of Dental Health, 1100 W. 49th Street, Austin Texas 78756.

TABLE 18–2. PROGRAMS FOR FLUORIDATION OF SCHOOL WATER SUPPLIES, BY STATE, 1989.

State	Number of Schools (Enrollment)
North Carolina	103 (41,658)
Indiana	85 (35,899)
Kentucky	78 (24,933)
Wisconsin	43 (7,261)
Vermont	23 (5,630)
Total	332 (115,381)
Total in U.S.	351 (122,458)

States with the largest number of schools using adjusted water fluoridation, and number of children deriving benefits.
(*From Department of Health and Human Resources. Fluoridation Census, 1989–Summary.*[39])

high school are usually housed in the same building complex.

Installation costs are relatively high, but the cost-effectiveness of the program increases as the program continues. The cost of preventing each carious lesion has been estimated at $1.90.[40] Unfortunately, the fluoridation of school water supplies can encounter resistance. Any effort to fluoridate the school system is subject to possible confrontation by antifluoridation groups, with the attendant possibility of legal or political challenges. The cost of the installation, supplies, and maintenance competes with other budgetary needs. In addition, some custodial and backup personnel must be trained for the continual operation, maintenance, and monitoring of the fluoridation unit.

The recommended concentration of fluoride for school programs is 4.5 ppm, mainly because students receive only a very

small amount of their daily fluid while at school.[41] An approximate 40% reduction in caries and only a few cases of mild fluorosis were experienced after 12 years of study using this concentration.[42] With the increasing number of communities instituting water fluoridation, interest in school fluoridation has gradually waned.

Diet and Prevention

Basic information on diet and nutrition[c] should be a part of all health education. Children need to understand that sugar consumption is a key component of the dental decay process and that sugar must be present for caries to occur. At the same time, instruction on sugar restriction alone is insufficient if a program's aim is caries prevention.[8] Ideally, dietary information should be mixed with the preventive benefits of appropriate fluoride regimens, oral hygiene measures, and pit-and-fissure sealants.

Often, once the teacher has reinforced the message that sugar causes tooth decay and suggests that the child *avoid* excessive and frequent ingestion of refined carbohydrates, the child then goes to the cafeteria. In the cafeteria, the child is confronted with attractive, sugar-laden desserts. The question then is, What message do the children really get—the message they hear in the classroom or the message that they see, smell, and taste in the cafeteria?

Schools need to provide an environment that allows children to refrain from excessive sugar consumption. One important method of meeting this specification is for the *school dietitian* gradually to reduce the number of days a week in which the confections are available. Instead, desserts can be selected that are nutritionally sound and yet

---

[c] Diet = The total oral intake of food items.
Nutrition = The study of the metabolism that occurs following the ingestion of a food item(s).

limit the amount of sucrose. Thus, in the same way that a water engineer *adds* fluoride to reduce dental decay in a community, so can the dietitian *limit* sugar consumption to reduce dental decay for an entire school population.

A second strategy for reducing student sucrose intake is for the *school principal* or *superintendent* to remove all vending machines that dispense candy and junk foods.[43] Essentially, the income from these machines uses the teeth of the children to subsidize nonbudgeted school expenses. Many schools have removed the machines or have substituted more nutritious snacks, including milk, fruit, and juices.

Classroom Toothbrushing

The *daily* brushing of teeth in the classroom may be an *ideal objective* but is often *impractical*. Despite the need for emphasis on toothbrushing, some basic problems arise. Many teachers are willing to teach the *mechanical* art of toothbrushing so long as they do not have to demonstrate the unfamiliar details of plaque control. Very few are willing to incorporate daily toothbrushing in their classroom teaching schedule because it infringes on essential teaching time for other subjects. The daily hygienic storage and continual replacement of worn-out and lost brushes poses major problems for a teacher. Unless toothbrushes are continually made available to the children without cost, dedicating classroom time for activities in which several students may not benefit due to economic or other factors may be resisted. Finally, few classrooms have the water supply and the sinks necessary for conveniently scheduling daily brushing as a classroom activity.

Despite these problems, many classroom brushing programs have been a success.[44] (See Appendix 18–2 for a suggested method of teaching toothbrushing.) Although little evidence indicates that tooth-

brushing alone reduces caries incidence, *overwhelming* evidence supports the fact that toothbrushing with a fluoride dentifrice is beneficial; consequently, the use of a fluoride dentifrice should be emphasized. Other studies show that there is only questionable support that school toothbrushing programs have any *long-term* effect on gingival status, although it is known that plaque control through toothbrushing can be effective in helping to control gingivitis (Fig 18–4). Thus the teacher should endeavor to habituate correct daily use of the Bass technique to help control gingivitis, and the use of a fluoride dentifrice to help control caries. The ultimate objective of toothbrushing instruction is *prevention*, not toothbrushing as an *exercise*. Reinforcement of the therapeutic benefits of toothbrushing coupled with the use of fluoride dentifrices is required, because even in well-directed programs in which improvement is noted, a relapse can be expected during summer vacations.[45]

Putting it All Together—Education and Active Prevention

At present, the national debate about how best to ensure universal health care is intense. Preventive care for children is one of

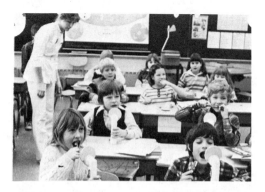

Figure 18–4. A dental hygienist assists children in identifying and removing plaque. *(Courtesy of Learning Resource Center, Indiana University— Purdue University at Fort Wayne, Indiana.)*

the most important objectives of the effort. It is critical that the dental profession, health educators, and public health departments take the steps necessary to ensure that dentistry is represented in the planning and implementation of such a national effort. Salient to the success of such a dental program is that it be *acceptable, equitable, affordable,* and *accessible to all—with a priority on treatment for high-risk students.* There is no better location than a *school system* to implement dental health education, prevention, and care systems that meet these essential criteria.

Dunning and Dunning[46] pointed out the several advantages to a school-based program: (1) The children are available for preventive or treatment procedures, (2) school clinics are less threatening than private offices, (3) school dental programs facilitate and increase the effectiveness of teaching dental subjects, and (4) the dental services supplement the school nursing services by helping to provide total health care for school children. In New Zealand, 96% of all school children are enrolled in a nationwide school dental program featuring both preventive and treatment care,[47] and in Sweden the number of children so cared for approaches 100%.

The initiation of combined education *and* active preventive programs in U.S. schools would reduce the amount of learning time lost in going and coming from a treatment facility. School programs would also obviate the loss of studying time due to pain and apprehension before and after treatment. This lost time can be considerable; for example, children missed more than 51 million hours of school in 1989 because of *acute* dental problems.[48] Combined school dental education and active preventive dentistry programs for all schools should be feasible and cost-effective in terms of staffing, money, and material. Most importantly, with school programs the DMFT of

students should demonstrate a substantial and steady decrease over the years. Such active prevention programs can be established at one or more of three levels.

Level 1. Level 1 includes the following activities:

- Use of a comprehensive teaching curriculum such as the *Tattletooth II* program
- Routine classroom fluoride mouth rinse or tablet regimens in water fluoride-*deficient* areas

The first level program involves only classroom participation by the *existing* school staff and superimposes little additional time commitment, other than that expected within the present school curriculum. To implement the program, both the teacher and the school nurse should be trained to use pretested curricular material, such as that incorporated into the *Tattletooth II* program. This minimizes the need for teachers to search out and organize lessons in an unfamiliar field. In addition, the teacher with the help of the school nurse can conduct weekly fluoride mouth rinses or daily fluoride tablet programs. The nurse is responsible for preparing the mouth rinses or making the tablets available on a schedule approved by the teachers. In one review of mouth rinse effectiveness, caries reductions ranged from 17% to 47%, with an average of 27%.[49] Thus even at this low level of classroom preventive dentistry activity, *major oral health benefits can be realized.* The types of fluoride programs used in level 1 preventive activities are described later on.

Classroom-based Fluoride Programs

The use of fluoride mouth rinses and tablets provide caries-preventive options that are effective and easy to implement (Figs 18–5

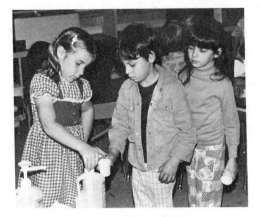

Figure 18–5. Everyone wants to make sure that there is 10 mL of fluoride rinse in the cup.

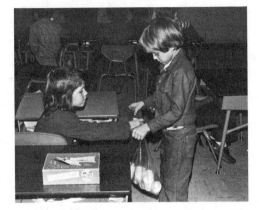

Figure 18–6. Being the trash person is an honorable job.

and 18–6). Horowitz and Frazier[8] provide complete descriptions of logical fluoride combinations and appropriate self-applied fluoride regimens for use in kindergarten through grade 12. In addition, the National Institute of Dental Research offers a free document entitled *Preventing Tooth Decay: A Guide for Implementing Self-Applied Fluorides in School Settings,* which addresses all aspects of fluoride program planning, implementation, and continuation.[50]

The supplies needed for a 32-week school year mouth rinse program consist of a fluoride solution pump dispenser, cups, napkins, and plastic disposal bags. These supplies are available in a commercial kit for approximately a dollar per child per 32-week school year.[d] The dispenser consists of a container with a plastic pump. It is graduated so that a 2.0-g package of sodium fluoride powder can be placed in the jug and water added to the 1000-mL mark. The sodium fluoride, which is in a tearproof package, is nonflavored and nonsweetened

to discourage swallowing.[51] Rinsing programs are advised for grades 1 through 12 but not below. Many younger children cannot master the technique of swishing without swallowing. If desired, the use of a plain-water rinse provides a good preparatory educational experience for kindergarten children. (See Appendix 18–3 for details on conducting a mouth rinse program.)

Fluoride mouth-rinsing programs received official recognition of safety from the Food and Drug Administration (FDA) in 1974 and by the ADA Council on Dental Therapeutics in 1975.[52] The estimates for the number of children enrolled in fluoride mouth rinse programs in the United States vary from 3 million[53] to 8 to 12 million.[54] The state of Kentucky targets their programs to the 10% of the school population that is not receiving community water fluoridation.[55] Aside from the United States, seven other nations—Denmark, Finland, New Zealand, Netherlands, Norway, Thailand, and Sweden—support major mouth rinse programs. In comparison with the estimated 6% of U.S. children involved in school mouth rinse programs, Finland has 80%, Norway 90%, and Sweden 100%.[56]

---

[d] Medical Products Laboratories, 9990 Global Road, Philadelphia, PA 19115

The fluoride tablet program is easier to accomplish than the mouth rinse regimen. One tablet is given to each student. The tablets contain either 1.0 or 0.5 mg of fluoride, with the choice depending on the level of fluoride in the local water supply. The students then chew and swish the sodium fluoride around the mouth for a minute and then swallow. The swish-and-swallow technique provides the benefits of a topical application—as with the mouth rinse; it also provides the optimal systemic benefits of fluoride ingestion that occur during the period of development and maturation of the remaining teeth. The daily tablet appears to be more effective than the weekly mouth rinse, as well as being preferred by the teachers.[57]

It is important to note that the effects of school fluoride programs are not permanent. After an 11-year follow-up study in Norway it was concluded that the residual benefits of school-based fluoride programs decrease as the length of time between previous participation and follow-up increase. This information underlines the need for the *continued use* of fluoride supplements, fluoride mouth rinses, and fluoride dentifrices throughout life in nonfluoridated areas.[58]

Level 2. Level 2 consists of

- Level 1 requirements, plus
- The addition of a dental hygienist to the school health staff

The inclusion of a dental hygienist on the school health staff involved in a comprehensive education–prevention program is salient. A dental hygienist is educated to *plan and participate* in programs that include topical fluoride applications, oral prophylaxes, the teaching of toothbrushing and flossing, counseling on diet, placement of pit-and-fissure sealants, and screening and referral of suspected oral pathology for definitive diagnosis and treatment. The dental hygienist also acts as a program resource person.

Many school districts or public health agencies have dental trailers that are used for prophylaxis and screening programs for children. Students with gingivitis and calculus are seen in increasing numbers as they progress towards senior high school.[19] A periodic prophylaxis with its removal of calculus by a dental hygienist during the school years can help delay the onset of an irreversible stage of gingival damage. Input from the hygienist can also help the teenager develop satisfactory plaque control techniques and to learn to seek professional care when needed.

The same trailer used for the prophylaxis program may be used by the dental hygienist for placement of sealants with little extra cost for supplies. The placement procedure for the sealants is rapid and painless; once placed, the sealants are *highly effective* in protecting the occlusal, lingual, and buccal pits and fissures—sites where up to 90% of all carious lesions occur.[2] In 1988 in the United States, only 6.4% of children age 5 to 8, and 11.5% of those age 9 to 11 years had sealants placed.[59] In contrast, in Finland so many of the occlusal surfaces are covered with sealant that these surfaces are often excluded in DMFS studies.[60]

The great effect of sealant placement in rapidly reducing caries incidence was reported by Sterritt and Frew in a study conducted in Guam.[61] Seventy-five thousand teeth of 15,000 children in grades 1 through 8 were sealed by 17 preventive dentistry technicians. In a period of *2 years the average number of carious lesions per child dropped from 5.35 to 2.92.* The first year retention rate for the self-curing sealant was 94% for first molars, 97% for premolars, and 75% for second molars. Sealant placement, when coupled with a follow-up gel application of fluoride helps provide protection to the *whole* tooth.[62]

The state of New Mexico also has a major sealant program, with up to 22,180 participating school children. Sealants are placed at second and sixth grade levels. To measure the effect of the program, 6447 *previously sealed* occlusal surfaces of first permanent molars were compared with 3060 cohort sixth graders who had *never* had sealants. Over the 4-year interval separating second from sixth grade, the previously sealed cohort group had developed 37 decayed surfaces, compared with 193 for the never-sealed group over an equivalent time. Only 171 of the previously sealed surfaces had fillings, compared with 669 of the never-sealed group. After adjusting for cohort size differences, the sealed group had 208 DF occlusal surfaces, whereas the never-filled had 1818 DF—an 8.74 times greater occlusal involvement for the never-sealed children.[63]

It has been correctly pointed out by Ripa and colleagues that the combined use of sealants and exposure to classroom fluoride programs can result in a *virtual elimination of dental decay in elementary school children*.[64] The importance of this statement is further emphasized by the realization that neither sealants nor fluoride programs require compliance or behavior changes for a successful outcome. Reports of the actual cost per child for sealant placement vary.[20,65-67] Minimal costs rest on the utilization of dental hygienists or dental assistants.[67] For example, the cost of sealing a tooth in two different studies has been as low as $1.37[68] and $1.20[69] per tooth, respectively. On the other hand, restoration of a neglected occlusal lesion averages about $51.00.[70]

Question 3. Which of the following statements, if any, are correct?

A. The United States lags *far behind* New Zealand and Nordic countries in providing preventive and treatment services to school children.

B. Classroom-based fluoride tablet programs require *additional* school personnel and about *30 minutes per day* for efficient implementation.

C. Daily fluoride tablet programs tend to be *more* effective in lowering the caries increment than do weekly rinsing programs.

D. Fluoride protection gained in school programs eliminates the need for future fluoride protection.

E. Usually a decade must pass before the effectiveness of sealants as a caries-preventive measure can be assessed.

Level 3. Level 3 consists of

- Level 1 and 2 requirements, plus
- The addition of a treatment delivery option

The third and final level of preventive dentistry sophistication in a school program involves the identification and referral for early treatment of children with oral pathology. To attain this objective, *an annual screening should be performed for all children and at least a semiannual screening done for children classified as high risk* (Fig 18–7).

State practice acts permitting, triage with possible referral to a treatment facility can be efficiently accomplished by a hygienist.[71] During routine prophylaxis procedures and sealant placement, the hygienist has an opportunity to identify early pathology and to refer the child for expeditious definitive diagnosis and treatment.

The present method of managing school children with oral problems is to send home a note indicating the need for treatment and suggest that the child be

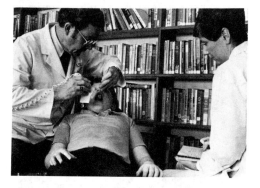

Figure 18–7. Dental screening examinations take place in the most interesting places. *(Courtesy of Dr R. Schimmele, Indiana University School of Dentistry.)*

taken to the dentist. This approach assumes that the parent immediately seeks a private dentist. In turn, it is assumed that when the dentist has completed treatment, a postcard is returned to the school hygienist or nurse, indicating that the referred pathology has been treated. This referral system has the advantage that it uses the professional delivery systems existing in the child's neighborhood. It does not always work, however. Not all parents respond willingly, if at all, to suggestions for child treatment. The nonresponse may be due to apathy, educational level, or economics. Equally troubling is that all dentists do not complete and return forms. In summary, follow-up methods for ensuring that a child was treated are often nonexistent.

A second option for referral involves contracting with local practitioners to offer specific procedures for predetermined fees. In this case, the referral can be a direct transaction between the school system and the dentist(s). The bill submitted by the dentist for completed work constitutes a verification that the child received treatment.

Other possible models include the dental care delivery system used in the Nordic countries, where the public health

services are utilized for school education, prevention, and treatment programs. In Australia and New Zealand, the dental therapists who constitute the backbone of the New Zealand School Dental Program provide the education, preventive, and many of the treatment services. In New Zealand, the average DMF of 12- to 14-year-old students fell from 10.7 in 1973 to 1.88 in 1991.[72] (See Chapter 22, New Zealand National School Dental Health Service.)

To ensure coordination of preventive and treatment scheduling plus follow-up, centralized planning is necessary.[73] The financing and administration of a total school oral health delivery system requires especial consideration. School educators should not be asked to have important educational needs compete for time and money with vital health needs. *If schools are to be made an important vehicle for addressing societal health problems, then additional school time in the form of a longer school year and a separate health budget must be considered.* The objective of whatever option is selected, is that all referrals are expeditiously seen, necessary treatment delivered, and follow-up actions taken to ensure completion of referred oral health needs. *Once the primary preventive dentistry procedures have reduced the incidence of oral disease to that of the annual workload treatment capability, the number of extractions for a school population should approach zero.*

Within the three levels of preventive dentistry programs, various health education and promotion topics should be included. Two of the more current topics are addressed in the following sections.

Preventive Dentistry in Sports

Sports are an important morale ingredient for both student athletes and the student body. During the 1989–1990 school year, in only grades 9 through 11, the Ohio High

School Athletic Association, which is the governing body for high school athletes in the state, listed 167,000 boys and 92,000 girls as competing in organized athletics with tournament play.[74] In many of the sports, the facial structures are highly vulnerable to damage. The causative agents might be a hockey puck or a baseball speeding at 70 to 90 mph; a bone-crunching tackle or a thrown baseball bat; or an elbow following a spectacular basketball slam dunk.

In each session of athletic competition, athletes face a 10% chance of orofacial injury, and a 33% to 56% possibility over a playing career. Protective equipment, rules, and regulations have been developed to reduce this toll. For instance, prototype leather football helmets with padding came into general use at the turn of the century but were not required until 1939. By the 1950s, the leather helmet had been replaced by a more protective hard plastic. The helmet protected the cranium and the ears more than the lower face and mouth (Fig 18–8).

In 1960, the ADA, along with the American Association of Physical Education, issued a report that highlighted the fact that when high school players did not wear *mouth guards,* 50% of all football injuries occurred in and around the mouth.[75] The ADA House of Delegates soon passed a resolution urging that all athletes participating in contact sports wear intraoral mouth guards. This objective came to fruition in 1962 when several sports organizations mandated the wearing of the mouth guard. *It is estimated that as a result of that action, from 100,000 to 200,000 oral injuries to football players are prevented annually.*[75]

Football is not the only school sport for which orofacial protection of the athletes is needed. At the amateur level, five sports now mandate the use of mouth guards dur-

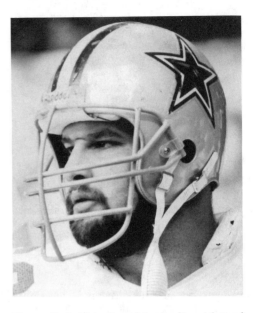

Figure 18–8. Protection of the head and face of Crawford Kerr, offensive lineman. Note how the hard plastic helmet protects the cranium and the ears, whereas the cage protects the orofacial structures. The National Football League does not require players to use a mouth guard to protect the teeth. (*Courtesy of Dallas Cowboys.*)

ing practice sessions and in games: boxing, football, ice hockey, lacrosse, and women's field hockey. It is interesting that the Academy of Sports Dentistry[e] has listed 40 different sports, including soccer, bicycling, skate boarding, and basketball, in which cranial or orofacial protection should be considered.[74]

The mouth guard is constructed of soft plastic which is interposed between the maxillary and mandibular dentition. As such, it helps to prevent violent contact between the lips, cheeks, and teeth, and be-

---

[e] The Academy of Sports Dentistry was formed in 1983, with the objective of preventing oral and facial injuries. The academy is open to all dentists, athletic trainers, physicians, coaches, and players with an interest in learning from or contributing to the latest techniques and treatment of sports-related injuries.

tween the upper and lower teeth. It reduces the possibility of fractured jaws as well as lessening the likelihood of neck injuries, concussion, cerebral hemorrhage, unconsciousness, serious central nerve damage and death.[75]

Prior to a game, it is the responsibility of the game officials to check with the coaches to ensure that the players are provided with the required protective equipment.[76] When mouth guards and other protective equipment are not worn in football, for instance, penalties are levied, ranging from a reduction in the number of time outs to 5 yard penalties. In the past decade, the thrust for protective equipment has been emphasized in an effort to reduce the possibility of bleeding injuries. In some states, any bleeding injuries are cause for the game officials to eject a player from the game due to the increased possibility of transmitting AIDS.[77]

In many locales, dentists are volunteering to assist home teams in the fabrication of mouth guards for all sports. In states where licensure permits, hygienists also can perform this service. By their involvement, dental professionals are extending the concept of primary prevention from an understanding of bacterial disease alone to prevention of orofacial damage by trauma.

Question 4. Which of the following statements, if any, are correct?

A. The placing of a sealant requires long-term student compliance and possible behavioral changes before caries reductions can be identified.

B. In a school treatment program, triage is necessary to ensure diagnosis and treatment priority for the students at highest risk.

C. Fluoride best protects the smooth surfaces of the teeth, whereas sealants best protect the pits and fis-

sures; between the two, the virtual elimination of caries is possible.

D. Protective equipment is optional for all *high school sports* except football.

E. Sports protective equipment is mainly directed towards preventing *major* injuries.

Tobacco Avoidance and Cessation

Tobacco use interventions (both avoidance and cessation) must be included in the curriculum of any comprehensive school-based oral health program. Experimentation with smoking is occurring at earlier ages than ever before; most users starting to smoke or use smokeless tobacco begin in adolescence.[78] Thirty thousand new cases of oral cancer are reported each year, with 8000 people dying annually from this disease.[79] Users of cigarettes and smokeless tobacco are at several times greater risk for oral cancer than are nonusers.[80]

The year 2000 objectives 3.5, 3.9, and 3.10 (Appendix 18–1) directly address children and tobacco.[78] To respond to these objectives, school-based programs in elementary, middle, and secondary schools must include smoking and smokeless tobacco use interventions and provide students with tobacco-free environments.

A recent national survey reveals that an estimated 16% of U.S. teenagers currently smoke, and an additional 29% has experimented with cigarettes.[81] In the 16- to 18-year-old response group, 60% reported either experimenting with or currently using cigarettes.[81] Growing trends for smokeless tobacco use among teenagers also have been reported.[82] To date, approximately 20% to 30% of U.S. teenage males are using smokeless tobacco products.[82]

It appears that school smoking-prevention programs can delay the onset of tobacco use.[83] This is particularly important given the current decreasing age of smoking initiation, especially among young girls.[84] By delaying the onset of smoking, school programs have the potential to (1) prevent some students from ever starting; (2) reduce the possibility that young students will become regular adult users; and (3) make it easier for those who do start tobacco use to stop.[83] These same principles also can be applied to smokeless tobacco use intervention programs.

The National Cancer Institute has provided a list of strategies that help ensure successful school-based tobacco use intervention programs.[83] First, curriculum content must receive significant attention. Ideally, the topics of smoking and use of smokeless tobacco should be introduced in *primary school,* with continuing reenforcement through middle school and junior high and booster sessions in senior high school. Tobacco subject matter may be integrated into preexisting curriculum units on drug abuse prevention or incorporated into health or physical education classes.

Another important ingredient for success is inclusion of content on *refusal skills*.[83,84] Children must be taught how to resist peer and media pressure by developing decision-making and problem-solving skills that facilitate refusal of undesirable habits and influences. Children must also be taught to realize that tobacco use is *not the norm* and has immediate and long-range adverse physical and esthetic effects.

A strong supportive network among students, parents, and teachers promotes program success. Student involvement is paramount. Although sessions should be teacher-led, students can assist in program delivery. Student role-playing and modeling exercises enhance student participation.[85] Parental support is another critical component; the parental values opposing tobacco use and favoring antiuse programs enhance

program credibility. Finally, teachers must be well trained and commited.

Examples of successful programs are mentioned briefly to provide guidance to future program planners. A joint project of the American Cancer Society, The Heart Association, and the American Lung Association, called the "Smoke-Free Class of 2000 Project" addresses the need to reach out to young children.[86] This 12-year education and awareness campaign focuses on children who entered first grade in 1988 and who will graduate in the year 2000. The program is designed to help children (1) understand that health is related to personal choices based on sound decision-making skills; (2) become more aware of factors that influence personal choice; (3) realize that tobacco use is not compatible with a positive image; and, (4) express increased support for a tobacco-free environment. Teachers' guides, posters, and numerous classroom activities are included in the program package.

The Ohio Division of the American Cancer Society designed an education program specifically geared to decreasing use of smokeless tobacco.[87] The program packet includes a teacher's guide with lesson plans, suggested classroom activities and discussion questions, pamphlets, pretests and posttests, and posters. Content areas include facts about smokeless tobacco; its history, ingredients, usage, and health risks; social drawbacks to its use; federal law; and advertising. The Centers for Disease Control has also developed a smokeless tobacco curriculum specifically for grades K through 2 entitled, "I Don't, I Won't."[88] This education activity is designed to educate teachers, students, and their parents about the health risks associated with using smokeless tobacco. Included are a teacher's manual, a flip chart, comic books, stickers, and slides.

Frequently, smokeless tobacco use is related in a positive way to sports achievements and is linked to star athletes who often serve as role models to adolescent males.[89] Appropriately, on June 16, 1993, major-league baseball's executive council, the governing body of the sport, announced an on-the-field ban of all tobacco products for every uniformed employee of minor-league baseball. Under the policy, use of tobacco products of any kind is not permitted in any team area. Violators are subject to fines ranging from $100 to $300 and face game ejections.[89] Unfortunately, this ban does not extend to major-league baseball.

The urgent need for establishing effective tobacco avoidance and cessation programs early is starkly iterated by Glynn: "Today, as in every other day of the year, more than 3000 adolescents will smoke their first cigarette on the way to regular smoking. During their lifetime, it can be expected that of these 3000 children, about 23 will be murdered, 30 will die in traffic accidents, and nearly 750 will be killed by smoking-related diseases."[90]

Question 5. Which of the following statements, if any, are correct?

A. Approximately 15% (±5%) of 16- to 18-year-old U.S. teenagers either have experimented with or now smoke cigarettes.

B. The use of tobacco products by minor-league baseball players on the playing field continues to prompt teenagers to imitate their heroes.

C. The ideal grade level in school for introducing tobacco prevention teaching is at sixth grade.

D. Tobacco *refusal skills* are especially important in the presence of peer student smokers.

E. More people die from tobacco-associated diseases each year than from violent crime and traffic accidents combined.

SUMMARY

School systems need to provide, to the extent possible, a disease-free, safe environment. This goal is challenged by the fact that during the 12-year period that a child attends school, dental caries, plaque, calculus, and periodontal pathology are continuing problems that jeopardize the health of the teeth and their supporting structures. During the same period, the students' orofacial structures are subject to accidents and injuries in routine play and sports activities. Finally, the addiction of students to cigarette smoking and use of smokeless tobacco during the school years needs to be strongly addressed in tobacco avoidance and cessation programs.

Although no consensus has arisen about what the objectives of a school oral health program should be, all the elements of the mnemonic CAPITE must be present. Many school health curriculum planners need help in designing and evaluating textual materials and training aids. Teachers also may need assistance in developing lesson plans that are relevant to the age and social needs of the student. The centralized development of grade-integrated teaching plans for teacher use is a plausible solution. These plans impart oral health information to help children develop an appreciation of good oral health and teach the means of achieving it.

Opinions conflict about the effectiveness of present school teaching programs in reducing the incidence and severity of the plaque diseases. The major successes of school-based dental health programs have been achieved when education has been *combined with active prevention, or active prevention and treatment programs.* Unfortunately, too few schools have routinely included active preventive dentistry regimens—fluoride mouth rinse and tablet programs, sealant applications, and strong emphasis on the use of fluoride dentifrices while brushing—all of which can *rapidly* and *predictably* reduce the DMFS of a school population, with only minimal change in self-behavior or compliance required of the student. Highly effective primary preventive dentistry techniques can be easily introduced into present school routines with only a relatively small additional requirement for time, staffing, money, and material.

A few school systems have employed dental hygienists as resource personnel to aid in the teaching programs or to provide primary preventive services or both. The availability of a dental hygienist provides an effective and economic means for schools to plan and participate in higher level preventive programs, inasmuch as the hygienist can teach and participate in preventive programs, accomplish triage, and arrange for referral and follow-up to ensure completeness of treatment. The ubiquitous availability of sucrose-laden desserts and snacks can be best controlled by the school dietitian reducing the availability and frequency of desserts with high sucrose content and by the school administrator prohibiting the on-campus placement of vending machines that dispense high-sucrose snacks.

The combination of education, active prevention programs, and appropriately trained personnel has the potential of greatly reducing the dental treatment workload of a school system. *Once the incidence of the plaque diseases equals that of the workload output over a similar period, a zero or near-zero extraction incidence is possible.* This is an objective worth working for. Protecting the oral health of future generations is a commitment that must be shared by parents, teachers, school administrators, legislators, and oral health profes-

sionals. This is especially apropos now when national health objectives for total child health care are being debated. Possibly the time *is* propitious to think in terms of a *national school oral health policy*—one that endorses universal access to oral health education, health promotion, preventive regimens, triage, and treatment referral capabilities for discerned pathology.

ANSWERS AND EXPLANATIONS

1. A, B, C

   D—incorrect. Teaching self-care is an *inexpensive* but *not* the most *efficient* means of reducing oral disease.

   E—incorrect. Courses in teachers' colleges do not provide in-depth education relating to oral health care.

2. B, C, E

   A—incorrect. Most parents are not well prepared to teach their children oral hygiene because in all probability many may not have been taught themselves.

   D—incorrect. Children in intensive preventive programs often acquire behaviors and attitudes leading to healthy self-care programs.

3. A, C

   B—incorrect. Only about 5 to 10 minutes of the teachers' time is required daily.

   D—incorrect. As time passes, some of the fluoride protection is lost; for this reason, the daily home use of commercial fluoride rinses and dentifrices is indicated after leaving a school fluoride program.

   E—incorrect. In the study cited in the book, a reduction in the incidence of pit-and-fissure caries as a result of sealant usage was detected at the end of

2 years; often no more than one year is necessary.

4. B, C

A—incorrect. The sealant placement usually occurs with no student dissent; after the placement, compliance is of no concern.

D—incorrect. At the high school level, mouth guards are *required* for all participants in boxing, football, ice hockey, lacrosse, and women's field hockey.

E—incorrect. Emphasis is placed on preventing *all* injuries—major, minor, and bleeding.

5. D, E

A—incorrect. Sixty percent is more accurate.

B—incorrect. Although major-league baseball has banned *minor*-league athletes from using tobacco products when the teams are in the ball park, major-league players have no such prohibition.

C—incorrect. The teaching of tobacco use prevention should begin as early as possible in primary school.

SELF-EVALUATION QUESTIONS

1. The two major objectives of education are (1) to make a living, and (2) _____.

2. The elements of a successful school oral health program as embodied in the mnemonic CAPITE are _____, _____, _____, _____, _____, and Education.

3. The (least)(most) expensive and the (least)(most) effective way of bettering oral health is by use of education—compared with sealant placement, fluoride product use, and oral hygiene.

4. Some Head Start centers (are)(are not) uniformly in compliance with U.S. Public Health Service standards.

5. The 1 month out of the year used by the ADA and the American Dental Hygienists Association to concentrate on a national health promotion crusade is called _____ _____ _____ Month.

6. The concentration of fluoride in the water of a school fluoridation system is _____ ppm.

7. Two people on the school staff who can aid in greatly reducing the sugar consumption by the children are the principal (or superintendent) and the _____.

8. To make a toothbrush effective in combating caries, it is necessary to add a _____ dentifrice.

9. A level 1 classroom prevention program in a fluoride-deficient area requires only (1) a prepared, integrated teaching program, and (2) the classroom use of either a fluoride _____ or a fluoride _____.

10. A level 2 school program is an escalation of the level 1 plan; the additional dental professional needed for sealant placement in this program is the _____ _____.

11. A level 3 program is an extension of a level 2 program, inasmuch as it provides a means to prevent and to _____ the oral pathology of high-risk students.

12. The football helmet best protects the cranium and ears; the mouth guard and cage best protects the _____ structures.

13. Approximately one out of every _____ (number) teenagers uses either cigarettes or smokeless tobacco.

14. (More) (fewer) of the high school students who start smoking *today* will eventually die from tobacco related diseases than by homicides and traffic accidents.

REFERENCES

1. Brunelle JA, Carlos JP. Recent trends in dental caries in U.S. children and the effect of water fluoridation. *J Dent Res.* 1990; 69 (special issue):723–727.
2. U.S. Department of Health and Human Services. U.S. Public Health Service, National Institute of Dental Research. *Oral Health of United States Children. The National Survey of Dental Caries in U.S. School Children: 1986–87. National and Regional Findings.* NIH Pub. No. 89-2247. Washington, DC. Government Printing Office; 1989.
3. U.S. Public Health Service. *Healthy People 2000: National Health Promotion and Disease Prevention Objectives.* DHHS Pub. No. (PHS) 91-50213. Washington, DC. Government Printing Office: 1991;352.
4. Carmichael CL, Rugg-Gunn AJ, Farrell RS. The relationship between fluoridation, social class, caries experience in 5-year-old children in Newcastle and Northumberland. *Dent J.* 1989; 167:51–57.
5. Pinkham JR, Casamassimo PR, Levey SM. Dentistry and the children of poverty. *J Dent Child.* 1988; 55:17–24.
6. National Institute of Dental Research. *Dental Needs of United States Children: 1979–1980.* NIH Pub. No. 83-2246. Bethesda, Md. National Institutes of Health; 1982.
7. Connolly GN, Winn DM, Hecht SS, et al. The reemergence of smokeless tobacco. In: Halleb AI, ed. *Smokeless Tobacco. Professional Education Publication* (booklet). New York, NY. American Cancer Society; 1988.
8. Horowitz AM, Frazier PJ. Effective oral health programs in school settings. In: Clark J., Ed. *Clinical Dentistry,* Vol. 2. Philadelphia, Pa. Harper and Row; 1986 1–17
9. U.S. Public Health Service. *Healthy People 2000: National Health Promotion and Disease Prevention Objectives.* DHHS Pub. No. (PHS) 91-50213. Washington, DC. National Academy Press; 1990;349.
10. Solomon ES. Errors in federal report on dental health personnel presents problems. *J Dent Educ.* 1990; 54:499–501.
11. U.S. Department of Health and Human Services, Public Health Service, Health Resources and Services Administration, Bureau of Health Professions. Eighth report to the President and Congress on the status of health personnel in the United States. *Dentistry.* September 1992:112, 271.
12. Kenney JB. The role and responsibility of schools in affecting dental health status—a potential yet unrealized. *J Public Health Dent.* 1979; 39:262–267.
13. Horowitz AM, Frazier PJ. Effective public health education: Family and community health. *J Health Educ.* 1980; 3:91–101.
14. Harris NO. Elements of an Organized Delivery System for Prevention: Manpower Considerations. In: JP Carlos, ed. *Prevention and Oral Health.* DHEW Pub. No. (NIH) 74-707. Bethesda, Md. National Institutes of Health; 1974.
15. Jong AW. *Community Dental Health,* 3rd ed. St Louis, Mosby. 1993:1–17.
16. Burt BA, Eklund SA. *Dentistry, Dental Practice and the Community,* 4th ed. Philadelphia, Pa. WB Saunders Co.; 1992.
17. Bouchard JM, Farquhar CL, Carnahan BW, et al. Oral health instructional needs of Ohio elementary educators. *J School Health.* 1990; 60:511–513.
18. Kay EJ, Baba SP. Designing dental health education materials for school teachers: Formative evaluation research. *J Clin Pediatr Dent.* 1991; 15:195–198.
19. Cons NC. Using effective strategies to implement a program administrator's goal. *J Public Health Dent.* 1979; 39:279–285.
20. Klein SP, Bohannan HM, Bell RM, et al. The cost and effectiveness of school based preventive dentistry care. *Am J Public Health.* 1985; 75:75–82.
21. Flanders RA. Effectiveness of dental health educational programs in schools. *J Am Dent Assoc.* 1987; 114:239–242.
22. U.S. Department of Health and Human Services. US Public Health Service, Centers for Disease Control. Current trends: The effectiveness of school health education. *MMWR.* 1986; 35:593.

23. Boyer EM. Classroom teachers' perceived role in dental health education. *J Public Health Dent.* 1976; 36:237–243.

24. Lee AJ. Parental attendance at a school dental program: Its impact upon the dental behavior of the children. *J School Health.* 1978; 48:423–427.

25. Rubison L. Evaluating school dental health education programs. *J School Health.* 1982; 52:26–28.

26. Rayner JF, Cohen LK. A position on school dental health education. *J Prev Dent.* 1974; 1:11–23.

27. Rayner JA. A dental health education programme, including home visits, for nursery school children. *Br Dent J.* 1992; 172:57–62.

28. Klass M, Rhoden C. Aspects of dental health education for preschool children and their parents. *J Dent. Child.* 1981; 48:357–363.

29. Nowjack-Rayner R, Gift HC. Contributing factors to maternal and child oral health. *J Public Health Dent.* 1990; 50(special issue): 370–378.

30. Parker WA, Fultz RP. Dentistry's commitment to Head Start: An evaluation of selected programs. *J Am Dent. Assoc.* 1986; 113:654–658.

31. Levy GE. A survey of preschool oral health education programs. *J Public Health Dent.* 1984; 44:10–18.

32. Miller AJ, Brunelle JA. A summary of the NIDR Community Caries Prevention Demonstration Program. *J Am Dent. Assoc.* 1983; 107:265–269.

33. Seppa L, Hausen H, Pollanen L. et al. Effect of intensified caries prevention on approximal caries in adolescents with high caries risk. *Caries Res.* 1991; 25:392–395.

34. Tönisson C, Barenthin T, Sporre D-M. Three-year follow-up study of teenagers with high risk for caries. *J Dent. Res.* 1992; 71(divisional Abstract: 1093. Abstract) 57.

35. Horn SD, Kaster CO. A model for a children's dental health carnival. *J Dent. Child.* 1991; 58:320–327.

36. Aiello C. Personal communication. Director, *Tattletooth II Program.* Texas Department of Health, Bureau of Dental Health, Austin, TX, 1993.

37. Roberto MV. Personal communication. Chief, Office of Health Policy Development. Department of Health Services, State of Connecticut, 1993.

38. Carnahan BW. Personal communication. Assistant Chief, Ohio Department of Health, 1993.

39. Department of Health and Human Services, Public Health Service, Centers for Disease Control, *Fluoridation Census 1989—Summary.*

40. Newbrun E. Cost-effectiveness and practicality features in the systematic use of fluorides. In: Burt BA, ed. *The Relative Efficiency of Methods of Caries Prevention in Dental Public Health.* Ann Arbor, Mich. University of Michigan; 1978:27–48.

41. U.S. Department of Health and Human Services, Public Health Service, Centers for Disease Control. *Water Fluoridation. A Manual for Engineers and Technicians.* Atlanta, Centers for Disease Control; September 1986, reprinted May 1991.

42. Horowitz HS, Heifetz SB, Law FE, et al. Effect of school water fluoridation on dental caries: Final results in Elk Lake, Pa. after 12 years. *J Am Dent Assoc.* 1972; 84:832–838.

43. Crawford L. Junk foods in our schools? A look at student spending in school vending machines and concessions. *J Can Diet Assoc.* 1977; 38:193.

44. Khanna SL. A new approach to dental health care: The classroom teacher as a dental health educator. *Can J Public Health.* 1978; 69:371–374.

45. Kerebel LM, Le Cabellec MD, Kerebel B, et al. Effect of motivation on the oral health of French schoolchildren. *J Dent Child.* 1985; 52:287–292.

46. Dunning JM, Dunning N. An international look at school-based children's dental services. *Am J Public Health.* 1978; 68:664–668.

47. Peterson M. Personal communication. Dental Therapist. Community Health Services, Otago Area Health Board, Dunedin, New Zealand.

tor-, and self-applied gels) in an era of decreased caries and increased fluorosis prevalence. *J Public Health Dent*. 1991; 51: 23–40.

50. Horowitz AM. *Preventing Tooth Decay: A Guide for Implementing Self-Applied Fluorides in School Settings*. Washington, DC. U.S. Department of Health and Human Services; 1981.

51. Horowitz HS. Safety first. *J Public Health*. 1983; 43:194–195. Editorial.

52. American Dental Association. Council on Dental Therapeutics. Council classifies fluoride mouth rinses. *J Am Dent Assoc*. 1975; 91:1250–1251.

53. Connolly GN, Bednarsh H. *Preliminary Report on Fluoride Mouth Rinse Programs of State and Local Health Departments*. Massachusetts Department of Health, Boston, Massachusetts. 1984. Mimeographed handout.

54. Miller AJ, Brunelle JA. A summary of the NIDR Community Caries Prevention Demonstration Program. *J Am Dent Assoc*. 1983; 107:265–269.

55. Fowler R, Jr. Personal communication. Dental Program Administrator, Cabinet of Human Resources, Commonwealth of Kentucky. Frankfort, KY. 1993.

56. Changing patterns of oral health and implications for oral health manpower: Part I. Working group Federation Dentaire Internationale and the World Health Organization. *Int Dent J*. 1985; 35:235–251.

57. Driscoll WS, Nowjack-Raymer R, Selwitz RH, et al. A comparison of the caries-preventive effects of fluoride mouthrinsing, fluoride tablets, and both procedures combined: Final results after eight years. *J Public Health Dent*. 1992; 52:111–116.

58. Haugejorden O, Lervik T, Birkeland JM, et al. An eleven-year follow-up study of dental caries after discontinuation of school-based fluoride programs. *Acta Odontol Scand*. 1990; 48:257–263.

59. Ripa LW. A half-century of community water fluoridation in the United States: Review and commentary. *J Public Health Dent*. 1993; 53:17–44.

60. Sepp AL, Hausen H, Pollanen L, et al. Effect of intensified caries prevention on approximal caries in adolescents with high caries risk. *Caries Res*. 1991; 25:392–395.

61. Sterritt GR, Frew RA. Evaluation of a clinic-based sealant program. *J Public Health Dent*. 1988; 48:220–224.

62. Calderone JJ, Davis JM. The New Mexico sealant program: A progress report. *J Public Health Dent*. 1987; 48:220–224.

63. Calderone J. Personal communication. Dental Director, State of New Mexico Department of Health, Santa Fe, New Mexico. 1993.

64. Ripa LW, Leske BS, Sposata A. The surface specific caries pattern of participants in a school-based fluoride mouth rinsing program with implications for the use of sealants. *J Public Health Dent*. 1989; 48:39–43.

65. Rebick T. School-based preventive dental care: A different view. *Am J Public Health*. 1985; 75:392–394.

66. Garcia AL. Caries incidence and costs of prevention programs. *J Public Health Dent*. 1989; 49(special issue):259–271.

67. Burt BA. Fissure sealants: Clinical and economic factors. *J Dent Educ*. 1984; 48:96–102.

68. Calderone JJ, Mueller LA. The cost of sealant application in a state dental disease prevention program. *J Public Health Dent*. 1983; 43:249–254.

69. Hardison JR. The use of pit and fissure sealants in public health programs in Tennessee. *J Public Health Dent*. 1983:43:233–239.

70. Blair KP. Fluoridation in the 1990's. *J Am Coll Dent*. 1992; 59:3.

71. Wang N. Substitution of dentists by dental hygienists in child dental care. *J Dent Res*. 1993; 72(special issue):172. Abstract 551.

72. MacKenzie FM. Personal communication. Principal Dental Officer. Community Health Services, Otago Area Health Board, Dunedin, New Zealand. 1993.

73. O'Riley M, Gavin O. Planning primary care dental services for schoolchildren. *J Dent Res*. 1992; 71(divisional abstract):1025. Abstract 2269.

74. Ranalli DM. Prevention of craniofacial injuries in football. *Dent Clin North Am.* 1991; 35:627–645.

75. Johnsen DC, Winters JE. Prevention of intra oral trauma in sports. *Dent Clin North Am.* 1991; 35(4):657–666.

76. Ranalli DN, Lancaster DM. Attitudes of college football officials regarding NCAA mouthguard regulations and player compliance. *J Public Health Dent.* 1993; 53:96–100.

77. Morrow, R. Personal communication. University of Texas Dental School at San Antonio, TX. 78284. 1993.

78. U.S. Public Health Service. *Healthy People 2000: National Health Promotion and Disease Prevention Activities.* DHHS Pub. No. (PHS) 91-50213. Washington, DC. Government Printing Office; 1991:143.

79. Crossett L. Oral cancer: Community-based programs. *Dent Hygien News.* 1992; 5:1–3.

80. Winn D. Smokeless Tobacco and Cancer: The Epidemiologic Evidence. In: *Health Effects of Smokeless Tobacco.* Proceedings of a Symposium Booklet published by American Cancer Society. Atlanta, Georgia. 1988.

81. Moss AJ, Allen KF, Giovino GA. Recent trends in adolescent smoking, smoking-uptake correlates and expectations about the future. *Advanced Data from Vital and Health Statistics.* No. 22. Hyattsville, Md. National Center for Health Statistics; 1992.

82. U.S. Department of Health and Human Services. *Spit Tobacco and Youth,* DHHS, Office of the Inspector General. USDHHS Pub. (DEI) 06-92-00500. Washington, DC. 1992.

83. Glynn TJ. School programs to prevent smoking: *The National Cancer Institute Guide to Strategies That Succeed.* Smoking Tobacco and Control Program, NCI, USDHHS. NIH Pub. No. 90-500. Washington, DC. 1990.

84. Centers for Disease Control. *Reducing the Health Consequences of Smoking: 25 years of Progress, a Report of the Surgeon General.* Public Health Service. DHHS Pub. No. (CDS) 89-8411. Washington, DC. 1989.

85. Botvin GJ, Tortu S. Preventing adolescent substance abuse through life skills training. In: Price RH, Cown EL, Lorian RP, Ramos-McKay J, eds. *Fourteen Ounces of Prevention.* Washington, DC. American Psychological Association; 1988.

86. *Smoke-Free Class of 2000.* Atlanta, Ga. American Cancer Society.

87. *With Smokeless Tobacco, You're Out.* Dublin, Ohio. American Cancer Society, Ohio Division, Inc.

88. *I Don't, I Won't.* Centers for Disease Control. Atlanta, Ga. U.S. Department of Health and Human Services.

89. O'Keefe K. Baseball snuffs tobacco in minors. *San Antonio Express-News.* June 14, 1993; 1B, San Antonio, Texas.

90. Glynn TJ. Essential elements of school-based smoking prevention programs. *School Health.* 1989; 59:181–187.

Appendix 18–1. Health Objectives for the Year 2000 Related to School-based Programs

HEALTH STATUS OBJECTIVES

13.1 Reduce dental caries (cavities) so that the proportion of children with one or more caries (in permanent or primary teeth) is no more than 35% among children age 6 through 8 and no more than 60% among adolescents age 15.

13.2 Reduce untreated dental caries so that the proportion of children with untreated caries (in permanent or primary teeth) is no more than 20% among children age 6 through 8 and no more than 15% among adolescents age 15.

RISK REDUCTION OBJECTIVES

13.5 Reduce the initiation of cigarette smoking by children and youth so that no more than 15% have become regular users by age 20.

13.9 Reduce smokeless tobacco use by males aged 12 through 24 to a prevalence of no more than 4%.

13.8 Increase to at least 50% the proportion of children who have received protective sealants on the occlusal (chewing) surfaces of permanent molar teeth.

13.10 Increase use of professionally or self-administered topical or systemic (dietary) fluorides to at least 85% of people not receiving optimally fluoridated public water.

13.11 Increase to at least 75% the proportion of parents and caregivers who use feeding practices that prevent baby bottle tooth decay.

SERVICES AND PROTECTION OBJECTIVES

2.19 Increase to at least 75% the proportion of the nation's schools that provide nutrition education from preschool through 12th grade, preferably as part of quality school health education.

3.10 Establish tobacco-free environments and include tobacco use prevention in the curricula of all elementary, middle, and secondary schools, preferably as part of quality school health education.

8.4 Increase to at least 75% the proportion of the nation's elementary and secondary schools that provide planned and sequential kindergarten through 12th grade quality school health education.

13.12 Increase to at least 90% the proportion of all children entering school programs for the first time who have received an oral health screening referral and follow-up for necessary diagnostic, preventive, and treatment services.

Appendix 18–2. Small-Group Toothbrushing Instruction

PREREQUISITE
Secure written permission from parents to participate.

SUPPLIES NEEDED
Toothbrush (in cellophane wrapper)
Staining tablet
Paper cup
Paper napkin
Magnifying hand mirror
Oversized dentoform model and large toothbrush
Waste basket
Dentifrice (for taking home)

ROUTINE
1. Six to eight students sitting at a table can be taught as a manageable group.
2. Without removing the toothbrush from the cellophane wrapper, the students are asked to demonstrate how to remove some imaginary (and some not so imaginary) dirt from the cuticle of the thumb nail. (Most place the brush at a 45° angle and use short vibratory strokes similar to those used in the mouth in performing the Bass technique.)
3. Reinforce the 45° concept on an oversized dentoform model, letting each child use the large toothbrush to demonstrate understanding and prowess.
4. Give each child a disclosing tablet to chew and swish around the mouth, expectorating the excess saliva into the cup. Wipe the face with a napkin and force napkin into cup to avoid any spillage.
5. Encourage the children to look at the red-stained teeth of their neighbors. (They enjoy it.) Point out that all people have plaque.
6. Pass around the magnifying mirror to allow the students to look at their own teeth, explaining that where the red occurs bacteria live that cause decay and gum disease.
7. Begin dry toothbrushing (without dentifrice), emphasizing the need to brush the teeth in a definite sequence. (During the entire process, appropriate corrections and reinforcements should be made as soon as identified.)
8. Pass around magnifying mirror to demonstrate the success in removing the red plaque.
9. Place all cups and debris in waste basket.

Appendix 18–3. Conducting a Fluoride Mouth Rinse Program

PREREQUISITE   Secure written permission from parents for child to participate.

SUPPLIES

1000-mL fluoride mouth rinse dispenser°
Paper cups
Paper napkins
Large plastic disposal bag

ROUTINE

1. Send a student to the school nurse's office to pick up supplies.
2. Teacher selects four children to pass out supplies: (1) a *pump–pusher* to dispense the fluoride; (2) a *host* or *hostess* to pass out the napkins; (3) a *cup-passer* to distribute the cups; and (4) a *trashperson* to collect the cups at the end of the mouth rinsing.
3. All students pass the table supporting the fluoride solution dispenser and receive a 10-mL aliquot of mouth rinse before returning to their seats to await instructions.
4. After cautioning against swallowing, the teacher tells the students to begin rinsing for 1 minute.
5. After the rinse is placed in the mouth the teacher keeps up a steady chatter—"the girls are doing better than the boys," "Freddie is the best rinser in the class," etc.
6. At the end of the minute, the students are advised to carefully spit the rinse into the empty cup, then wipe their mouths with the napkin before forcing it into the cup to absorb the liquid.
7. The trashperson goes around the classroom to collect the cups and finally ties the plastic bag before placing it in the trash.
8. Students are instructed not to eat or drink for ½ hour.
9. Return all excess supplies to the school nurse's office.

°Medical Products Laboratories, 9990 Global Road, Philadelphia Pa. 19115

Chapter 19

Preventive Oral Health Care for Compromised Individuals

Roseann Mulligan
Stephen Sobel

Objectives

At the end of this chapter it will be possible to

1. Explain why patients with the same handicaps can respond differently, based on communication and patient treatment techniques used by the dentist.
2. Discuss how visual, auditory, speech, and cognitive deficiencies can be identified and at least partially compensated for in preventive dentistry planning and implementation.
3. Illustrate how some functional deficiencies can be identified that require consideration in prescribing preventive dentistry techniques and devices.
4. Name and describe how new or modified devices or aids can be used to stabilize or aid patients with neurologic or physical disorders.
5. Help the poorly ambulatory or wheelchair patients gain access to the dental office, operator, or dental chair.
6. Cite at least three examples of how fluorides, pit-and-fissure sealants, and sugar discipline can be integrated into the preventive dental program for compromised individuals; also list possible exceptions.
7. Discuss the need to educate dental students, dentists, and lay personnel to aid special patients in the home, in the office, and in institutional settings.

Introduction

A compromised individual is a person who has one or more physical, medical, mental, or emotional problems that result in a limitation of that person's ability to function normally in fulfilling the activities of daily living. It has been estimated that more than 36 million individuals in the United States are compromised.[1]

Although some of the causative factors for these compromised conditions, such as trauma, birth defects, or adult-onset diseases, allow impairment patterns to appear along age stratification lines, the age of the individual per se must not be the main determining factor in deciding the quality and quantity of preventive dental instruction provided for that person. Instead, this decision should be made after consideration of a number of other factors, including the individual's *cognitive abilities, sensory perception, functional expertise,* and *oral hygiene condition.*

When a patient presents for care, the clinician's judgment of the patient's capabilities may be biased. Unrealistic expectations of the ravages of a specific disease may have been formed in advance through the reading of the scientific literature or from firsthand treatment of another patient similarly afflicted. These experiences often cause the practitioner to unconsciously form inaccurate generalizations about a person's capabilities. Such labeling can undermine a patient's preventive oral hygiene program, because it does not take into consideration the individual's actual capabilities.

In the manifestation of any disease, the range of functional, sensory, intellectual, and cognitive capabilities must be assessed prior to initiating a preventive oral health care program. The use of rigid disease or age-oriented models discourages the effective application of current preventive dentistry methods and materials to all patients who would benefit from them. To avoid categorizing persons by age and disease, this chapter presents information on how to assess the capabilities of a patient of *any age* within *any* disease category and offers suggestions on the development of individualized oral disease prevention programs. Oral hygiene aids and techniques applicable to a preventive program for the compromised patient, as well as special management techniques, are included.

SENSORY CAPABILITIES

To communicate ideas and instructions successfully, the patient and the practitioner must first be able to see or hear each other. Communication channels are impeded if the patient's hearing or vision is significantly impaired, in which case a modification in communication modalities must be made. Otherwise recommendations for an oral health home care program will not be understood, much less carried out.

Visual Deficits
A number of factors, from harmful prenatal and perinatal environments to the normal aging process can alter visual acuity.[2,3] These changes may range from correctable deficiencies to total blindness. Other common visual deficits include a loss of peripheral vision as occurs with glaucoma or visual field cuts resulting from a cerebrovascular accident.[2] Often a staff member sensitized in the skills of observation can easily identify visual impairment before the patient reaches the operatory. For example, a staff member may observe that the patient is unable to read and respond to the medical history questionnaire without assistance. This is not an unusual occurrence, because most

commercially produced medical history questionnaires are printed in type so small it is difficult for the visually impaired to read. A patient may need aid from the office staff to complete the form.[4] Also, observing how a patient is occupied in the reception area provides additional clues. Is he or she intently reading, flipping through magazines without reading them, involved in a handcraft such as crocheting or knitting, or being totally inactive? When the patient proceeds to the treatment room, the staff member should be aware if the individual's hands, feet, or a cane are extended in a searching manner to feel for environmental cues.

A patient with a significant visual disability may be carrying a white-tipped cane or may arrive with an escort. If the individual requests, the nondental staff escort—whether human or seeing-eye dog—should be allowed to usher the patient into the treatment room.[3] The escort may then be permitted to stay if space is available in the treatment area and if the presence of the escort contributes to the patient's comfort. If the human escort also functions as an attendant for the patient, he or she should be involved in any oral hygiene instructions and demonstrations. Such involvement often proves to be the crucial element necessary to a successful home care program.

Instructional materials to be used with patients who have decreased visual acuity could include selective use of commercial products that have been developed for pediatric dentistry programs. Routinely, such products have large pictures. Other commercially prepared pamphlets for self-instruction and information have limited value because the size of the print used in such pamphlets is too small for the visually impaired to see comfortably. Custom-made instructional sheets may be produced by the dental office using large black letters of at least 12-point type on off-white or white

paper.[5] Cassette tapes for recording personalized hygiene instructions are also recommended. Chairside instructions of toothbrushing and flossing should be demonstrated on oversized models of the dentition with a giant-sized toothbrush (Fig 19–1). These large models allow the patient with limited visual acuity to see and to understand some of the more subtle aspects of toothbrushing, such as the correct angulation of the bristles into the gingival crevice. A green-colored floss can help when demonstrating flossing to those with visual impairment who have difficulty seeing the conventional white floss. Red floss is also available and can be used; in fact, red is easier for the aging eye to see than green.[6] Although colored floss is useful for demonstrations, once the flossing technique is understood and visual acuity permits, the patient may switch to white floss for regular home use. This change allows the patient to check the color of the floss for possible gingival bleeding.

To demonstrate brushing and flossing techniques in the office, an inexpensive magnifying mirror should be employed to assist the patient in observing his or her own performance. A similar mirror should be

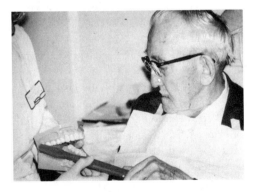

Figure 19–1. Large dental models and a helping hand are needed to perfect toothbrushing habits in the visually impaired.

recommended for the patient's use at home. These mirrors frequently come with attachments that can be hung around the neck, affixed to the wall, or placed on a countertop. Such accessories allow patients to keep their hands free for performing oral hygiene and still use the magnifying mirror to enhance vision. Many patients who have experienced cerebrovascular accident or neuromuscular impairment, however, lack the spatial–perceptual skills necessary to use a mirror. For these people using a mirror causes confusion and therefore is contraindicated. If a patient has visual problems so significant that a mirror cannot be used, he or she must be sensitized instead to the "feeling" and "smell" of a clean mouth to attest to the success of oral hygiene measures.[7]

For individuals with visual field cuts in which random visual fields may be lost[8] or decreases in peripheral vision occur, care should be taken to ensure that all demonstrations take place within the patient's visual field. To check the limits of a patient's vision, the clinician should perform a visual assessment by positioning his or her hand in various locations around the patient's face holding up one or more fingers. Each time this is done the patient should be asked how many fingers can be seen. It is important to notice whether patients move their head rather than just their eyes to see the fingers. Agreed, it would be simpler to ask the patient if he or she can see the demonstrations; however, such a question is frequently answered in the affirmative by visually impaired patients. Asking the patient to respond to the number of fingers displayed confirms if the clinician's face or the object to be used for demonstration is within the patient's peripheral vision or in a visual field cut.

Many patients with visual problems experience an increased sensitivity to light or glare. Indiscriminate positioning of the dental light so that it shines in the eyes of a patient can result in significant discomfort for such a patient. This can be avoided by careful focusing and positioning the operatory light.

Due to the anatomic position of the eye in the socket, the range of upward gaze diminishes with age.[9] A compensatory elevation of the head is not possible in many individuals, due to arthritic changes of the cervical spine.[10] Thus to enhance communication with all patients, it is best to converse from a sitting position rather than towering above the dental chair or wheelchair, requiring the patient to look up.

Hearing Disabilities

Hearing problems occur in all age groups, which can disrupt communication in the dental setting. The sound of dental equipment operating in another room, background music, or street noises can hinder communication with the hearing impaired as these sounds often mask the sound of speech. The commonest problem in communicating with the hearing disabled, however, is that the speaker does not sit directly in front of the patient, at the same eye level, and speak face to face.[2]

Most patients with hearing disabilities do some lip reading to augment their hearing, but even the best lip reader is able to decipher only 26% of a message conveyed entirely through this method.[3] The hearing-disabled patient relies heavily on the communicator's facial expression and body language to understand the message.[11] Therefore speaking distinctly and slightly slower without over exaggeration and in a well-modulated voice, facilitates communication.[12] The progressive loss of hearing of high-frequency tones that commonly occurs among the elderly requires the clinician to lower the pitch of his or her own voice while speaking to be better heard.[2] Avoid back lighting that places the speaker's face in a shadow. Never shout at a hearing-disabled patient because very loud sounds are actually more difficult for the impaired ear to understand.[11] Do not speak to the patient with any equipment running. Similarly, it is not desirable to speak while performing other functions, such as writing with your head down, looking at radiographs with your face turned from the patient, or while entering or exiting the room.

Pantomime and demonstration may be necessary when working with the hearing disabled. When writing information, use a clipboard and a red felt-tipped pen available in the operatory. Specifically designed *assistive listening devices* have been developed for practitioners who routinely deal with the hearing impaired.[13] For instance, in an office setting the patient can be given a pocket-sized FM receiver with a lightweight pair of earphones. The therapist is equipped with a small clip-on microphone transmitter that can transmit an FM voice message to the patient's receiver. This method of communication is good from up to 300 to 600 ft. Or, in a longer education session, a desk microphone wired directly into an amplifier can be used to feed the patient's earphones. In either of these methods (and others) there is no doubt that the entire transmission reaches the patient's ears at a comfortable amplitude, regardless of the speaker's location, voice volume, or lip action, or of extraneous office noises. Even with these aids, however, once the message is transmitted, it is expedient to have the patient demonstrate the suggested oral hygiene skills on models followed by demonstration in his or her own mouth. In this way the therapist can assess how well the message was comprehended.

Hearing aids may be difficult to detect, especially in women whose longer hair covers the ears. Therefore a conscious effort

should be made to look for such aids (Fig 19–2). If preventive instructions are to be given to a patient with a hearing aid, be sure the patient's aid is in place and turned on. Often patients turn off or remove their hearing aids in anticipation of dental treatment, because the proximity of the speaker's body to the aid may cause it to emit high-pitched squeals called *feedback*. Providing dental care with the clinician seated in the 12 o'clock position causes the operator's arm to be nearly in contact with the patient's ear, and it is easy for the cuff of the clinicians's sleeve to accidentally dislodge the hearing aid. Handpieces can also cause hearing aids to produce feedback. Suggest to the patient that the aid be removed or turned off prior to treatment and replaced or turned back on prior to receiving instructions.[3]

Hearing aids are expensive devices, and individuals who wear them usually prefer to remove them themselves. Once removed the aids should be placed in a secure spot, such as the patient's pocket or purse, rather than on the bracket table where they could be forgotten or gathered up and discarded.

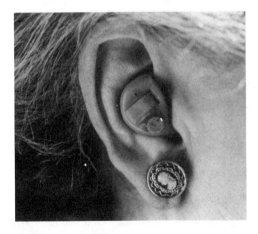

Figure 19–2. When longer hair is combed over the ear, this hearing device can be very inconspicuous—and vulnerable to handpiece noise.

Individuals who have both hearing and visual deficiencies may have their hearing devices constructed as part of the frame of their glasses. The removal of the glasses with the incorporated hearing aid significantly decreases the patient's ability to relate to the environment. In such cases it is recommended that the glasses be left in place but with the hearing device turned off.

For patients with visual or hearing deficiencies, keep distractions to a minimum (It is advisable to have office background music turned off at this time).[7] This includes any interruption of the clinician at chairside as well as the distraction created by auxiliary personnel entering and leaving the room.

Speech and Language Disorders

One cannot discuss the role of communication between the patient and the dental care provider without considering speech and language. Several conditions affect the motor or the cognitive components of speech or both. The patient with cerebral palsy may have speech impairment due to problems in the central nervous system that affect the muscular movements needed for speech.[14] With practice, a clinician who listens carefully and patiently to such speech can become adept at understanding much of it. This is the same sort of technique many dental providers have already achieved in learning to understand patients who attempt to speak with a rubber dam in place. Individuals, such as those who are mentally retarded, even though physiologically capable, may not use language because of their level of intellectual or emotional functioning. Those with neuromuscular diseases may have a weakness so severe that the muscles necessary to articulate sounds are unable to function.[15] Deterioration of speech that once was normal may be due to progressive hearing loss.[15] Individuals who are unable to hear the range of frequencies of the speech spectrum may develop a monotone voice. In addition, such a person often loses the ability to recognize how loudly he or she is speaking.

The patient who has suffered a stroke is particularly prone to language disorders. One type of disorder common to stroke patients is *aphasia*. In aphasia, the reception, integration, and expression of language are impaired.[15] The aphasic patient therefore has difficulty finding the right words to communicate, and this inability may be so pronounced that the patient may become very frustrated. This is particularly true for those individuals who are otherwise cognitively intact. When dealing with these individuals, frame questions so they can be answered with yes or no, or even just a shake of the head.

The aphasic individual may also omit or substitute sounds in words. The words then may be meaningless by themselves but convey intent by the way in which they are expressed. The speech may consist only of nouns, verbs, or a few adjectives. An extreme example of an aphasic patient was a woman who suffered a stroke so severe that her verbal communication was reduced to two exclamatory words that were always said together. With the help of her facial expression, body language, and the force and intonation used in saying these words, dental appointments were completed to the satisfaction of the patient and the provider.

Dysarthria is a speech disorder resulting from a motor dysfunction of the speech-producing elements.[15] This dysfunction may be caused by lesions in the central nervous system, the peripheral nervous system, or in muscles themselves. The symbolic language is intact; however, the coordination necessary to produce speech is impaired. This type of disturbance occurs in patients with

Parkinson's disease, myasthenia gravis, multiple sclerosis, and muscular dystrophy, as well as stroke.[16]

The substitution of written for verbal communication is a possible option for individuals in whom the recognition of language is still intact. Unfortunately, many of the causes of speech disorders result in slight or pronounced paralysis, or tremors that prevent the patient from writing legibly. One solution is to provide the patient with a lap board containing preprinted letters, common words, or pictures. Individuals with a knowledge of language but an inability to speak or to have their speech or writing understood, can point to the letters or words or pictures to communicate. Another method is a sophisticated, small typewriterlike device in which a keyboard is used to type out a tickertape message. Quadriplegic patients may be outfitted with a tongue control that permits very subtle movements of the tongue against a toggle switch. This action causes letters to be printed on a television monitor mounted to a wheelchair or bed.

Today's society places great importance on verbal communication; therefore, an individual with poor verbal skills is perceived as having poor cognitive and intellectual abilities.[11]

Although nonverbal communication, such as smiling, hand holding, and shoulder touching, plays a role in the clinician–patient interaction, it becomes extremely significant when there is no alternative. In such a case the clinician needs to enlist either the patient's attendant or a family member who has become attuned to "reading" the patient's needs. Usually these constant companions can help interpret the underlying message of such nonverbal actions as a rolling of the eyeballs or a fixed stare.

In summary, both verbal and nonverbal techniques play roles in the communication process between a dental care provider and a compromised dental patient. Speaking directly to the patient from a sitting position in front of the patient in a well-modulated, well-articulated voice and reinforcing each step of the communication with nonverbal cues are all techniques that should be used to produce a successful relationship with a patient who has impaired communication skills.

Question 1. Which of the following statements, if any, are correct?

A. Many specialized preventive techniques applicable to one handicapping condition are applicable to other handicapping conditions.

B. The dental personnel in *most* practices have the expertise and experience to successfully identify and instruct visually impaired patients entering primary preventive dentistry programs.

C. During periods of patient–dentist communications, it is better that the dentist be able to clearly see the patient's face than vice versa.

D. An *aphasic* patient is one who has difficulty in articulating personal thoughts and observations.

E. When a patient is unable to form words because of a motor dysfunction problem, the condition is known as *dysarthria*.

COGNITIVE CAPACITIES

The functional capacity of a patient is of far greater importance than that person's intelligence quotient (IQ) test results in determining his or her capacity to benefit from preventive dentistry instructions. For example, a patient who is mentally retarded is expected to have a low IQ, short attention span, and difficulties in understanding oral hygiene instructions. Yet many of these patients, when properly taught and motivated, can successfully perform oral hygiene procedures. To attain this success the dental care provider must first determine the patient's level of cognitive ability and then direct all instruction to that level. Rather than attempting to analyze intelligence test scores, the dental clinician should ask the patient a few simple questions to determine her or his functioning level. Questions of the type that might be asked of the patient, *not* the family member or attendant, could pertain to such everyday conversational topics as (1) What do you do in school, at work, or in retirement? (2) What hobbies do you like? (3) Why do you like a favorite television show, or (4) What has been the most difficult task you performed lately? One mentally retarded patient who responded to such a series of questions confided that he really did enjoy his job as a file clerk in a sheltered workshop environment; however, he did get confused sometimes trying to remember the order of letters in the alphabet. Furthermore, he stated that the most difficult job he faced was paying the rent at the first of each month. Even though he knew he had sufficient money, the responsibility of ensuring that the funds reached his landlord in time caused him a great deal of anxiety.

Such information from the patient offers insights into levels of responsibility, understanding, attention span, usual level of dexterity, and memory for details. These facts greatly assist the dental care provider in selecting the appropriate vocabulary, level of complexity of instruction, and special reward system for adherence to a customized preventive dentistry program. If it

is determined that the patient is intellectually or cognitively impaired, the traditional educational program used to convey preventive oral hygiene techniques must be modified. A problem-oriented approach is one way to ensure that all risk factors specific to an individual patient are considered.[17] For example, it should be recognized that brushing the teeth is a complex task that needs to be broken down into very simple, discrete steps. This allows the impaired patient to follow the instructions and to succeed at every step of the way toward the final goal, thereby integrating the simple tasks into a final complex task.[3] At the first appointment it may be possible to address only the brushing of the occlusal surfaces of the teeth to achieve satisfactory compliance and to reinforce only this activity until it becomes a natural part of the patient's daily routine. Often clinicians in their diligence to get their message across to the cognitively or intellectually impaired patient tend to *do and to say too much*. It is important to keep these instructional periods short with frequent repetition of the information. Use a level of language that is readily comprehended by the patient without being insulting. Written or tape-recorded reminders can be given for homework. At each appointment the individual should be requested to state or show what he or she has been doing since the last visit. This provides feedback about the effectiveness of the previous instructional period and the patient's memory and mastery of the technique.[3]

Demonstrations of appropriate behavior by *any* dental patient, *especially* those with decreased cognitive functioning should always be followed by immediate and positive feedback.[18] Reinforcement throughout the learning period should be supplemented with both verbal and nonverbal rewards; for example, a smile or a gift of a new toothbrush are often motivating techniques. This rapport aids in reducing stress, which can be detrimental to an individual's ability to learn. For this reason all learning should occur in an environment in which the dental staff can reflect warmth and friendliness.

Family members or guardians, teachers, or other caregivers must assume responsibility for oral health care programs of patients with little cognitive ability.[19] The selected individuals should be thoroughly instructed by the dental staff in the proper techniques for that patient's oral health.

FUNCTIONAL PERFORMANCE

To perform preventive dentistry procedures, a person must be able to receive information from the sensory organs, transmit this information through the nervous system to the brain for decision making, and then send it to the muscular and glandular system for action. All of these processes must work in harmony to accomplish a physical task. For instance, toothbrushing and flossing require not only the fine motor skills or dexterity of the small muscles of the fingers and hands but also the gross motor skills of the larger muscle groups in the upper extremities.[20] Numerous muscles and nerves of the head, neck, and upper extremities are all involved, as is the range-of-motion capability of the joints, especially the shoulders and elbows. In many disabilities one or more of these elements may be adversely affected or limited. Arthritis, for example, is a disease of primarily the joints and therefore often restricts the joint range of motion. Cerebral palsy is a central nervous system disorder. Because of aberrant neural signals transmitted to the muscle fibers, fine motor skills are impaired. Muscle contractures also characteristically affect both the range and motion of the joints. A

neuromuscular disease such as myasthenia gravis affects the nerve transmission process itself, resulting in musculature so weak that dexterity, gross motor skills, and range of motion may all be affected.

An accurate assessment of a patient's expected functional performance depends on evaluation of each task necessary to perform the oral hygiene. Once a difficulty has been identified, either a *device* or a person is needed to compensate for the patient's inadequacy. Gross motor skills such as grasping a toothbrush handle can often be improved by *orthotic[a]* appliances (Fig 19–3). Range-of-motion limitations may be altered by exercise, especially in the early stages of injury or disease, or in some cases by surgery. Dexterity such as is necessary for the production of the small vibratory strokes recommended in toothbrushing usually cannot be enhanced through medical or orthotic techniques, although for certain patients, appliances, specifically the electric toothbrush may serve as a highly effective substitute for this lack of dexterity.

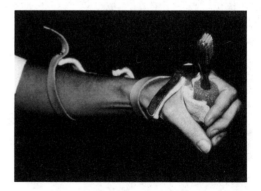

Figure 19–3. An orthotic device that permits a firmer grasp on a modified toothbrush.

---

[a] Orthotic appliances are devices, such as splints and braces, that are used to provide support to deformed or weakened limbs.

Assessment

Specific hand function tests developed for use by occupational therapists to evaluate a patient's ability to use his or her hands can be used by dental clinicians to assess a patient's potential ability to accomplish oral hygiene techniques. As the patient is first greeted, the practitioner should pay attention to the strength of the patient's hand clasp. Those individuals who seem to have a weak grasp should be asked to firmly grip the index finger of the clinician's hand. If the grip is weak, the patient should again be asked to grip the finger "as hard as you can." Repeating this procedure several times using two, three, and four fingers in place of the one finger enables the practitioner to decide at what diameter the patient has the strongest grip[21] (Fig 19–4). Keep this information in mind as you complete the rest of the assessment. If it is determined that the patient would benefit from a manual toothbrush, the handle will need to be increased in diameter to match the number of fingers at which the patient had the strongest grasp.

The range of motion of the elbow and shoulder can be determined by asking the patient to extend and flex the lower arm, or to rotate that arm about the shoulder, but

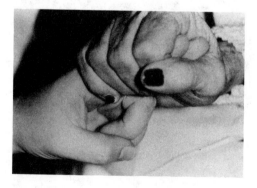

Figure 19–4. The muscular strength of a patient's hand can be assessed by handshake or by a grasp of the clinician's fingers.

this information may be more quickly obtained by asking the patient if he or she is able to feed himself or herself. Individuals who are able to do so, even if they use orthotic splints or other adaptive aids, are probably able to perform oral hygiene procedures. Patients who use special devices to aid in self-feeding should bring these devices to the dental office so that toothbrushes and other oral hygiene aids can be modified to fit their appliances.

The best way to assess whether a patient has sufficient dexterity and cognition to perform adequate oral hygiene is to offer the patient a toothbrush and to directly observe his or her success at actual intraoral plaque removal. Two objectives are accomplished by a patient demonstrating brushing technique before any instruction is given.

1. The clinician can assess the patient's current level of ability and understanding. Noticing the ease or difficulty with which each separate movement is accomplished (grasping the brush, angling and moving it) and the care needed to synchronize these actions into a whole purposeful motion gives the dental professional insight into the capabilities, training, and education of the patient to date.

2. This demonstration establishes a baseline level of achievement against which future improvements or modifications can be measured. A thorough understanding of the patient's current abilities enables the health care provider to determine the type and number of educational interventions to be introduced. Patients with compromised motor skills often compensate for their deficiencies in ingenious ways. Therefore their ability to handle

their own oral hygiene should not be prejudged, but they should be given opportunities to demonstrate their proficiency. Many patients who appear unable to handle a toothbrush or floss, due to deformed fingers or decreased motor functions, compensate and can function reasonably well.

Question 2. Which of the following statements, if any, are correct?

A. It is an *inviolable rule* that as the IQ decreases, so does the possibility of attaining cooperation from a mentally handicapped patient.

B. As an individual's disability increases, the need becomes greater for support from other individuals.

C. Explanations on primary preventive dentistry given to handicapped individuals should be *detailed.*

D. The hand strength and ability of a patient to use a toothbrush can often be determined by a handshake.

E. The best way to find out what a handicapped patient can do is to ask the person to accomplish a stated task.

ATTENDANT CARE

To ensure dental care and compliance with home self-care preventive programs, complete cooperation must be established among the family or caregivers, the health provider, and, to the extent possible, the patient.[22,23] Many compromised individuals are unable to handle their own hygiene due to *sensory, cognitive,* or *physical* deficits. For these individuals an attendant or family member should be instructed in the proper oral health care for the patient.[24] If long-term compliance with instructions is the goal, the comfort of both the caregiver and the patient in performing the oral hygiene program is paramount. For this reason a number of positions have been recommended for the caregiver to assume when providing oral hygiene care to the patient.[25] Facts to be considered include the patient's size and strength, the attendant's size and strength, and the amount of control that needs to be exerted over the *intentional* or *unintentional* movements of the patient. One position that has proven to be successful is for the attendant to stand behind the patient, who is seated in a straight-backed chair or a wheelchair. In this position it is easy to stabilize the patient's head by resting it against the body of the attendant. Brushing then proceeds with the attendant using the same kind of arm and brush positioning as he or she does when cleaning his or her own teeth. Performing this operation in front of a mirror takes further advantage of the attendant's own brushing habits, although a mirror is not a necessity. Other recommended positions include having the patient lie on a sofa or bed with his or her head in the caregiver's lap or sit on the floor in front of a chair in which the caregiver is seated (Fig 19–5).

Caregivers and patients should both be advised that the bathroom is not the only location in which to brush teeth.[25] In fact, it is often the least convenient room in the house due to its space limitations and the need to share its use with other members of the family. Water is not always necessary for toothbrushing, as salivary flow is stimulated by brushing and thus provides moisture. If a patient has tender, friable gingival tissue that can easily become damaged by an initially dry toothbrush, the brush can be moistened beforehand to soften it. When no toothpaste is used, the need for running water and the bathroom lavatory is greatly

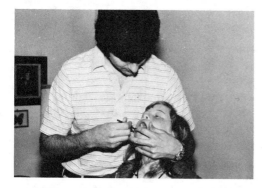
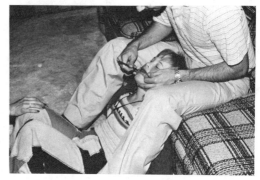
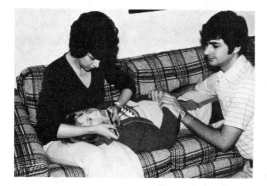
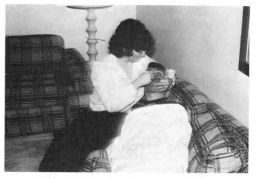
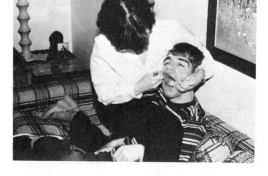

Figure 19–5. Several different positions for a caregiver to use in aiding toothbrushing. (*Courtesy of Tonya Smith Ray and Gayla Hill Taylor.*)

diminished. The elimination of the toothpaste increases visibility and decreases the possibility of gagging. In many cases it has been found that when water and toothpaste brushing were required, many attendants or family members discontinued or decreased the number of toothbrushing sessions. Normally a fluoride toothpaste is an important component of an oral hygiene program in an uncompromised population. In compromised patients, however, if one must omit fluoride toothpaste from the routine, it can be compensated for by using fluorides in other forms.[25]

Those patients who enjoy the taste or appreciate the esthetic value of toothpaste can use a nonfoaming ingestible toothpaste developed for the astronauts. Because this toothpaste does not foam and can be swallowed, it is not necessary for the patient to be near a basin to expectorate.

If a patient likes to rinse with water or a mouthwash after brushing, a two–paper-cup technique can be used. One paper cup holds the rinse; the other is for the expectorate after the patient rinses. Because the cups are lightweight, patients can often hold both, bringing each of the cups up to their lips as needed. This two-cup technique provides a means of controlling dribbling or drooling. This technique is valuable for an individual who is unable to lean over the basin such as an arthritic patient or for an individual who cannot purse the lips to expel the fluid as is the case with muscular dystrophy.

SPECIALIZED EQUIPMENT FOR PATIENT MANAGEMENT

Mouth Props

Several types of mouth props can be used to assist in opening and holding open the patient's mouth for oral hygiene procedures (Fig 19–6). A simple, effective mouth prop can be easily fabricated with two or three tongue blades wrapped together, padded on one end with 2 × 2 gauze squares, and secured in place with adhesive tape.[26] This prop can be used with patients who are unable to understand or to cooperate due to decreased *cognitive functioning,* as seen in mental retardation, mental deficiency, senile dementia, or in patients exhibiting *neuromuscular dysfunction,* such as occurs in cerebral palsy or muscular dystrophy. The mouth prop is first placed in the buccal vestibule and then slid to the posterior part of

the vestible until it reaches the anterior border of the ascending ramus. Pressure applied against this anatomic area with the padded end of the prop causes a reflexive opening of the mouth. When this occurs the mouth prop is immediately flipped over onto the occlusal surfaces of the teeth to maintain the opening. This prop may be used for the duration of the hygiene procedure, or it can be replaced by a commercially manufactured prop, which is placed on the opposite side of the arch. The original mouth prop is then removed with the new prop holding the mouth open.

The two types of mouth props most commonly used are made of rubber or metal.

Rubber Mouth Props. Two rubber, intraoral mouth props are commercially available. One (the McKesson) offers different sizes for adults and pediatric patients, whereas the other (the Pulpdent) is designed to accommodate a variety of individual mouth sizes. When using the McKesson prop, the correct size must be chosen and placed far enough back in the oral cavity to be held in place by the force of the jaws attempting to close. Otherwise, on closure, the prop slides forward along the occlusal surfaces of the teeth. It is not as likely that this will occur with the Pulpdent prop because the serrations and graduated size over the length of the prop resist slippage better. When using either of these props, a piece of floss should be threaded through the hole in the prop and allowed to extend from the patient's mouth. If inadvertent swallowing of the prop occurs, an occluded airway results. In such an event the prop can be retrieved by means of the floss ligature.

It is possible to hyperextend the mandibular muscles with either an oversized mouth prop or an overzealous placement of one. This can cause a muscle

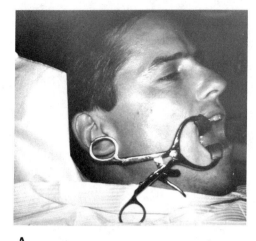

A

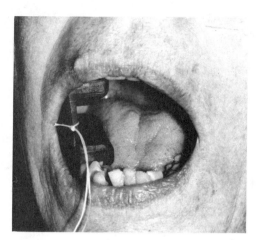

B

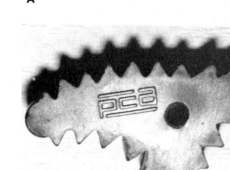

C

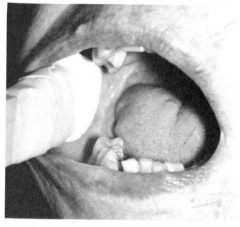

D

Figure 19–6. Several types of mouth props. **A.** Molt device maintaining access to mouth. **B.** McKesson rubber mouth prop. **C.** Close-up view of Pulpdent mouth prop showing serrated edge and graduated size along its length. **D.** Gauze-wrapped tongue-blade mouth prop.

spasm, resulting in considerable discomfort to the patient. When it is necessary to reposition this type of prop, the practitioner's fingers are placed both intraorally and extraorally. Because the patient's jaw might snap shut during the removal of the prop, use the gauze-wrapped tongue blades to assist in the removal of the rubber mouth prop.

Mouth Prop with an Extraoral Attachment. The Molt mouth prop is a commercially available device that is quite commonly found in the dental office. Because of the extraoral ratchet mechanism of the Molt prop it is easy to overextend the patient's mouth opening, which can lead to joint and muscle damage or even to outright dislocation of the temporomandibular joint. The

Molt mouth prop is not recommended for use by inexperienced persons in home care programs. An advantage to the extraoral attachment is that the width of the opening of the jaws can be changed without jeopardizing the caregiver's fingers. It also allows the practitioner to close the patient's mouth easily when desired to allow the patient to relax and rest. A major disadvantage is that once the prop is placed between the upper and lower teeth and activated to separate the jaws, it may tend to slide forward. This often occurs in patients who have one or more severely constricted arches, as is commonly seen in the hypoplastic maxilla of the adult Down syndrome patient, or in either arch of the cerebral palsy individual.

Headrests

There are numerous ways of supporting and stabilizing the head and neck of compromised dental patients. For those individuals who remain in their conventional wheelchairs throughout treatment, a commercially available wheelchair headrest may be purchased and kept in the dental office. This headrest attaches to the hand grips of the wheelchair and adjusts to compensate for different chair widths and sitting heights of the patients.[27] Other types of head stabilizers can be attached to the headrest of the dental chair with velcro straps, which extend around the back of the chair to secure the stabilizing device. The *cervical pillow* is a welcome addition for patients who have cervical spine deformities, such as those present in severely involved arthritic patients. The cerebral palsy head support consists of a block of foam with a depression built in the center to stabilize the patient's head.[4]

Soft Ties

Soft ties, which are cloth or soft leather straps, may be used to support and stabilize

any part of the body, including the head.[28] Most commonly, soft ties are used to secure the upper and lower limbs to an appropriate arm or leg rest. This prevents the limb from spasming, flailing, or hanging off the edge of the rest, a position that can compress nerves and lead to neural damage. Soft ties are *not* meant to be punitive restraining devices but to provide positive support, stability, and security to the patient.

Body Wraps

Full body wraps, such as pedi-wraps and papoose boards, are often used to immobilize smaller patients during dental treatment.[28] These devices have limited usefulness in preventive programs where purposeful attempts are being made to actively involve the patient in his or her own oral hygiene. Body wraps should be considered only when an intraoral procedure needs to be accomplished and the patient is unable to cooperate. For some compromised patients unfamiliar with the dental environment, these full body wraps are welcomed as a source of security and comfort[29] (Fig 19–7). The provider who decides to use a body wrap should be aware that some communities frown on the use of restraints for any purpose. Informed consent in writing outlining the risks and benefits should be obtained from the guardian if restraints are to be used.

ORAL HYGIENE DEVICES

Modifying Toothbrush Handles

In general the principles and techniques of toothbrushing used for a compromised population are the same as for anyone else. In compromised individuals, however, good oral hygiene is much more difficult to achieve and maintain.[17] If it has been determined that the patient has adequate dexter-

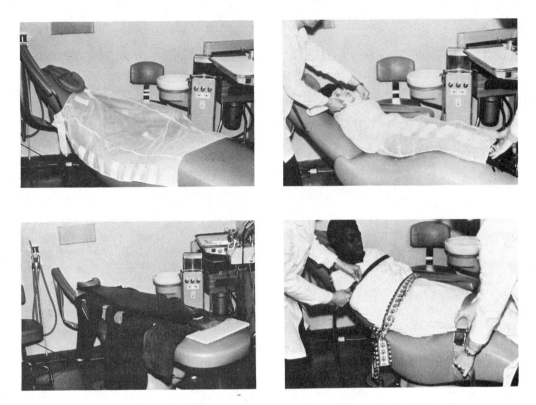

Figure 19–7. Restraining devices. (*Courtesy of Tonya Smith Ray and Gayla Hill Taylor.*)

ity to produce the small strokes needed to brush properly, a manual toothbrush may produce satisfactory results. Even if the patient has a weakened hand grasp or uses orthotic splints or other adaptive appliances, a manual toothbrush can be modified to facilitate usage.[25,30–32] In a well-controlled study of children with cerebral palsy who received modified toothbrushes, plaque removal was increased by 28% to 35% over that achieved when conventional toothbrushes were used.[33] Figure 19–8 illustrates several different methods of quickly augmenting toothbrush handles from materials commonly found around the dental office or home. These include foam wrappings from packing materials, acrylic tray or bite regis-

tration material, the center foam piece from a hair curler, a bicycle grip with plaster anchoring the toothbrush inside, or a juice can with a slotted ball inside to hold the toothbrush.[21] Inexpensive, cylindrical, closed-cell foam can be obtained from orthotic or medical supply stores. This foam cylinder has significant advantages over other types of foam materials because it is composed of closed plastic cells that shed water. This eliminates the increase in weight and the need to squeeze out absorbed water on completion of a hygiene procedure.

Handles augmented with foam can be used by a wide range of compromised individuals. They can be easily adapted to orthotic appliances such as splints. Handles

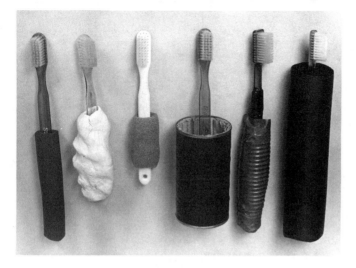

Figure 19–8. Readily available foam tubes, bicycle handles, cans, or dental tray material can be used to modify the size of toothbrush handles.

modified with heavier materials, however, such as a bicycle grip and the juice can, should not be used with arthritics or those with neuromuscular weaknesses. These latter two types of modifications are more appropriately used with mentally retarded individuals, including those with Down syndrome, and with cerebral palsy patients, who usually have strong grips (Fig 19–8).

Patients who are unable to flex their elbows due to joint involvement can be given a toothbrush with an extended handle. This can be fabricated by inserting a bicycle or wheelchair spoke into the original toothbrush handle and fabricating a new acrylic handle out of orthodontic resin or a similar material. Such a handle may be further modified if the patient has grasp difficulties. Other simple modifications include reshaping the plastic handle of the toothbrush by heating it in warm water and bending to the desired configuration or gluing the handle of a nail brush to the toothbrush handle.

Several devices have been developed to assist individuals with limited function to achieve independence. Often, products used to assist in feeding can be adapted for use in brushing the teeth, such as *palmar cuffs* or *activities of daily living* (ADL) *cuffs.*[b]

Question 3. Which of the following statements, if any, are correct?

A. Dentifrices are essential to maintaining good oral hygiene care among the handicapped.

B. *Both* mentally handicapped and individuals with neuromuscular dysfunction may need mouth props.

C. When it is necessary to constrain a neuromuscularly handicapped patient, it should be a nonpunitive action.

D. Body wraps and pedi-wraps are excellent restraint devices for *adults.*

E. A Bunsen burner flame is needed to modify a toothbrush handle.

---

[b] An ADL cuff is a generic term for any kind of appliance adapted to the upper extremity to which various implements can be added, as, for example, a toothbrush, so that the patient might perform his or her own daily living tasks without assistance.

Electric Toothbrushes

Electric toothbrushes are valuable aids in assisting compromised patients.[34] They are especially useful when the patient has the strength to grasp the handle and place the brush in the mouth but does not have the manual dexterity needed to perform the fine movements for the scrubbing function. The length and diameter of the handle of an electric toothbrush approximates those of manual toothbrushes that have been modified for individuals with compromised hand function. These devices cannot, however, be universally recommended for two reasons: (1) their increased weight, and (2) the difficulties in using their on off switch.[35] An electric toothbrush weighs from 25 to 30 times more than a manual toothbrush. This marked increase in weight can present a significant difficulty for people with weakness in their hands or arms. Because switches must be grasped between the thumb and forefinger, many of the on–off switching mechanisms of electric toothbrushes present difficulties for people with dexterity problems. The simple tripping of the switch is a formidable task for most compromised patients, particularly those with incomplete upper spinal cord injuries, cerebral palsy, arthritis, and neuromuscular disorders. Although sliding types of switches on some electric toothbrushes do not require as fine a muscle control to engage, they are frequently stiff and unyielding even for the normal hand. Within the last few years one electric toothbrush model has reached the market that has remedied the switch problem.[c] This device offers a depressible button as its mechanism, or, more importantly, the brushing action can be started simply by exerting pressure against the toothbrush bristles. This revolutionary advance allows people who have never before been able to perform any personal oral hygiene tasks by themselves to brush their own teeth (Fig 19–9). The weight of the electric toothbrush, however, still continues to be a problem. The patient's brushing technique may have to be modified to adjust for this factor. For example, the patient can be shown how to brush seated at a table using the elbows as supports to compensate for the increased weight. If the patient is in a wheelchair, a countertop can be used upon which to rest the bottom of the toothbrush handle while activating the brush in the mouth (Fig 19–9A). In using this method the patient only needs his or her weakened hands to direct the location of the brush while it is activated in the mouth. One particular muscular dystrophy patient, aged 25 years, who had never been able to brush his teeth was successfully introduced to this method. The plaque scores improved dramatically and immediately, as did his mental outlook when he found that he could successfully perform his toothbrushing independent of others.

A newer oral hygiene device has been manufactured that provides the user with all the items needed for oral hygiene. This system, manufactured by Sunbeam (Fig 19–9B), was originally developed at the University of Mississippi. It is an automatic toothbrushing apparatus that allows persons with restricted hand and arm movement to dispense toothpaste and water, brush their teeth, and clean their mouths. The system is set up so that it can be operated by someone who has only head and neck function; that is, the controls can be operated by mouth. Thus the system can be used by patients with quadriplegia, arthritis, a history of stroke, or other conditions that compromise arm and hand function. Its cost, however, is significant.[36,37]

Even though electric toothbrushes seem to be indicated for use in a mentally

---

[c] Teledyne Water Pik, Fort Collins, CO 80525.

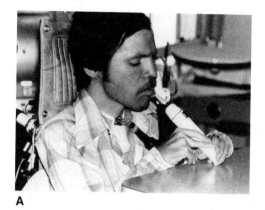

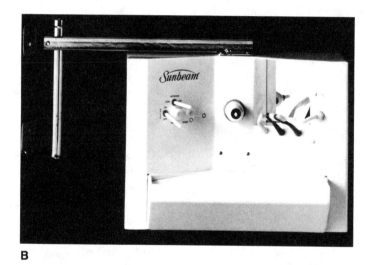

Figure 19–9. A. A pressure-activated toothbrush being used by a severely disabled individual. (Brand name is Water-Pik.) **B.** Dental care system for the disabled with limited upper-extremity capacity. (Brand name is Sunbeam.)

handicapped population, Bratel and coworkers[38] were unable to demonstrate clearly the superiority of electric over conventional toothbrushes whether used independently or aided. In fact, in an aided situation the plaque indices often deteriorated, because the patients appeared to tense up when such devices were used in their mouths.

One additional note of caution should be considered before recommending an electric toothbrush for a compromised patient. An overzealously used electric toothbrush can cause considerable damage to the hard and soft tissues in a short time.

Floss-Holding Devices

Dental flossing is not recommended for all compromised patients. Unless the task of toothbrushing can be learned, it is useless to superimpose the more complex task of flossing. To do so can be so discouraging that all attempts at oral hygiene are abandoned. This is true whether the patient or the attendant is performing the program. Therefore flossing should be introduced on a selective basis for those patients or attendants who have mastered toothbrushing and consistently show low plaque levels on tooth surfaces.

For many able-bodied people, flossing is a difficult task, and therefore it is even more challenging for a compromised individual. Again, an adequate assessment of the patient's ability to understand the technique and the dexterity to achieve the goal must be determined before flossing is introduced.

For some compromised patients, flossing can be performed regularly if a floss-holding device is used. In a recent study, eight such devices were evaluated by people with upper-extremity limitations.[20] This group rated one device significantly higher for its handle dimensions, ease of threading, and ability to keep the floss taut.[d] Although some compromised patients have learned to use parts of their bodies to assist in threading a flossholder, the majority of compromised patients have great difficulty in accomplishing this procedure. One patient with very limited use of his hands described how his wife kept five floss-holding devices threaded on the kitchen counter for use as he needed them. If one became unthreaded during a flossing routine, he simply obtained another. An alternative to multiple floss holders is to create a plaster of Paris base for the floss-holding device, so that it can be stabilized by one compromised hand while the other completes the threading. The holder can then be used with or without the base, depending on the patient's strength and desires.

---

[d] Floss-Aid Co, Santa Clara, California.

Interproximal Brushing

In older patients, gingival recession is a common experience. Often the recession is so pronounced that the use of regular dental floss is not effective in cleaning the long expanse of exposed root structure. In this situation some recommend Super Floss, as it is considerably thicker at one end. If the gingival recession has occurred to such an extent that the papilla no longer fills the interdental space, the use of an interproximal brush is often beneficial.[39] Individuals who have never used floss or who have difficulty manipulating the dental floss or threading a floss holder seem to adapt readily to the interproximal brush. The interproximal brush is also indicated for use in spaces where adjacent teeth are missing.

Interproximal brushing may be introduced near the beginning of the preventive program. Because handles of interproximal brushes are long and sturdy, they can easily be modified in the same manner as the toothbrush. Many interproximal brushes require the assembly of the proper brush head to the handle. This is an intricate task and requires fine motor skills. Therefore preassembled interproximal brushes for compromised patients are advisable. Demonstrations of the use of this brush should be accomplished before the patient leaves the office.

Other Types of Oral Hygiene Aids

From time to time other oral hygiene aids are promoted for use with patients who are in some manner compromised. Frequently these devices have not undergone any testing prior to their marketing but are promoted on the basis of potential worth. When or if such testing is accomplished, claims are not always upheld. An example of such a product is the "foam on a stick" device. In a study by Addems and colleagues[40] able-bodied subjects showed marked increases in plaque and gingival index scores during the week when the foam sticks were used (compared with a week when conventional brushing was performed).

In another study by Kambhu and Levy,[41] four devices were compared for efficacy when used on a simulated dependent care population by a nonprofessional caregiver. An unusual toothbrush with curved bristles,[e] as well as an electric toothbrush with 10 different rotating tufts of bristles,[f] were more effective at removing plaque than a conventional toothbrush. A foam stick device came in a distant fourth in the study. The subjects rated the curved-bristle toothbrush as the most comfortable, and the caregiver rated it as the easiest to use.

A clamping device has been designed to allow a toothbrush to be positioned on a wheelchair so that a patient, specifically a quadriplegic patient, could brush independently.[42]

Other devices can be used independently by compromised patients for plaque removal. These devices are easy to use because the patient simply chews on the device, and features incorporated into its shape disrupt the plaque. One is a soft plastic device with triangular projections; another is a device with filamentlike projections.[43]

Disclosing Techniques

Whatever the patient's age, disclosing products should be suggested to visualize plaque when a patient has difficulty in plaque removal. Although disclosing solutions are readily available over the counter, the price is often prohibitive for daily oral health care. The cost factor can be minimized by purchasing *commercial food coloring*, usually available in the bakery section of any grocery store. The food coloring can then be used in place of the disclosing solution to stain dental plaque. The color should be chosen on the basis of which is easiest to see in the mouth. For example, yellow is difficult to detect on teeth because the color is too close to that of natural tooth color. Blue and green colors, although suitable for teaching plaque control to children, are more difficult for the aging eye to visualize. Red food coloring is the easiest to visualize for all age groups. Because it is a popular color, it can be found packaged in a number of different containers, including individualized plastic bottles that are much easier to use. Two drops of food coloring should be placed on the tongue and the tongue used to wipe the food coloring around all the surfaces of the teeth prior to brushing. The plaque is well stained with this technique, and because the volume of the liquid used is minimal, little drooling or subsequent staining of the individual's clothes occurs. Food coloring can also be used when an attendant is caring for the patient, in which event the dye is applied to all surfaces with a cotton-tipped applicator.

MEETING THE DENTAL PATIENT

Escorting

At times a compromised patient requires an escort.[11] The most comfortable escorting technique is to have the escort at the patient's side, facing in the same direction as the patient. The patient's hand is then guided to the escort's arm just above the elbow.[12] It is best for the escort to precede the patient by a half step, trying to match the size of his or her own stride to that of the patient's. Staying close to the patient provides directional clues and makes it easier to lead. For those individuals who are visually impaired, it is desirable to describe

---

[e] Collis-curve, Inc., Minneapolis, MN 55409.
[f] Interplak, Bausch & Lomb Oral Care Division, Inc., Tucher, GA 30084.

obstacles as they are being approached, using the face of a clock to describe their locations. The escort should lead the person through all doorways into adjacent rooms and hallways, including the dental operatory. It is important for the escort to start and stop smoothly and to avoid any unnecessary or extraneous movements. Once the dental chair has been reached, one hand of the patient should be placed on the seat of the chair. The patient may then feel the configuration of the chair and the direction of the back and arm rests. With this information he or she can become oriented before attempting to sit down (Fig 19–10). Do not leave the side of the patient until he or she is securely in the dental chair and the armrest of the chair has been replaced.

Wheelchair Transfer Considerations

Many compromised individuals arrive at the dental office in wheelchairs. Those persons who spend a great deal of time in their wheelchairs usually have one that is customized to their hip width, sitting height, and leg length. Adjustable seat backs, head rests, leg supports, and seat cushions provide support to vulnerable areas. It is often most comfortable for an individual with a custom-made chair to be treated in it.[29] This is especially true for those individuals with such severe physical handicaps that they are unable to be transferred from their wheelchairs without a mechanized lift.

Normally preventive appointments can be conducted with the patient in the wheelchair. If the office preventive care plan represents only a part of a total treatment, consideration should be given to transferring the patient to the dental chair.

It is best to check with the patients themselves or their attendants about the best transfer techniques. Those individuals who accompany patients for dental treat-

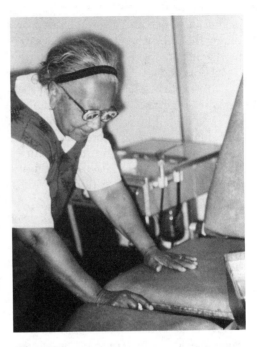

Figure 19–10. Some infirm patients prefer to "feel out" the dental chair before being seated.

ment are usually well versed in the care, transferability, and mobility of the patient and are often adept at transferring him or her. At times patients can transfer from the wheelchair to the dental chair with the use of sliding boards, which they often bring. Other patients have difficulty walking, and they use a wheelchair to improve their mobility. These patients can stand with a little support and are able to move themselves from the wheelchair to the dental chair. The wheelchair should be placed as close as possible to the dental chair before the transfer.

Question 4. Which of the following statements, if any, are correct?

A. When electric toothbrushes are used by handicapped patients, it is often necessary to modify a toothbrush stabilizing device rather then the toothbrush itself.

B. It is easier for the average compromised patient to use finger-directed dental floss than to use a floss holder.

C. Green *food coloring* can be used by the Irish for disclosing plaque on St. Patrick's Day.

D. Wheelchair patients should usually be transferred to the dental chair to benefit from the maximum comfort and back support of the fixed equipment.

E. Intraoffice escort service should be *considered* with *every* compromised patient.

PREVENTIVE THERAPIES

Dietary Considerations and Alternative Reward Systems

For many compromised patients, foods high in sugar are distributed throughout the day as a reward to individuals who have been compliant. Such a reward system encourages between-meal snacking and increases the consumption of highly cariogenic foods.[17] With patients who have a decreased neuromuscular coordination or decreased salivary flow, it is not possible to adequately clear the mouth.[19] Food remains impacted in the buccal vestibule and between the teeth until the next time the patient brushes or is brushed. To reduce the cariogenic potential, it is necessary (1) to restrict between-meal snacking and (2) to limit the use of highly cariogenic foods.[19] If sweets are to be consumed at all, they should be presented at mealtime and the teeth brushed immediately after eating. Bedtime snacks should be discouraged.

An alternative to a reward system based on sugary treats[19] is to present tokens for later redemption for prizes, such as toys, noncarious food, or outings.

Sealants and Fluorides

In spite of the normalization of handicapped individuals into the mainstream of society, it appears that the noninstitutionalized handicapped do not have as high a level of oral health as the rest of the population. The F (filled) value for the DMF (decayed, missing, or filled) scores is often lower in the compromised population, whereas the D and M values are higher.[44,45] Although becoming commoner, preventive strategies that would really benefit this population group are often not available on a regular basis. The use of sealants and fluorides should be considered important preventive techniques to assist in caries control for compromised patients.[45]

Sealant application may be more difficult in some compromised patients, because it may be more difficult to control intraoral moisture contamination. Salivary pooling is often seen in cerebral palsy and muscular dystrophy patients, because they have swallowing difficulties. For the short time needed to apply sealants, antisialogogue medications are usually *not* indicated. Instead, the sealant may be applied in the conventional manner using the techniques to control saliva flow indicated in Chapter 10. To aid in moisture control the patient should be seated upright rather than in a reclining position.

Regular topical fluoride applications by the dental staff are highly important for the compromised dental patient. For the younger patient water fluoridation or tablets are essential.[46] Equally important for this population is a home self-applied fluoride program. Several effective techniques are now available for home fluoride application, ranging from mouth rinses to fluoride gels applied with custom-made trays. Rinses are contraindicated for compromised patients who cannot effectively swish the solution around their mouths. Some individuals with muscular dystrophy and some poststroke patients have an incompetent or hypotonic lip seal and cannot keep the solutions in their mouth for the required period. For fluoride applied in a tray, the patient must keep the tray in place for a minimum of 4 minutes. It is difficult for many compromised patients to cooperate for this long a period, particularly if they have an active gag reflex. A gel-filled tray also stimulates the flow of saliva, which is often difficult to confine. Neither the patient nor the caregiver likes the drooling that occurs. The new brush-on fluoride gels, are therefore often indicated for this population, especially because their application takes advantage of an already learned tooth-brushing behavior.

Fluorides have also been shown to effectively reduce demineralization and to enhance remineralization.[47] Therefore brush-on gel fluorides should be considered for use by elderly compromised patients, particularly those with gingival recession. Fluorides should not, however, be indiscriminantly given to patients for unsupervised use if some question exists as to the patient's ability to understand and follow instructions. This is necessary to prevent accidental ingestion or misuse.[3]

Chemical Plaque Control

When a patient has difficulty removing plaque, even with a conscientiously applied toothbrushing program, a chemical plaque control agent may be introduced. The use of a 0.12% chlorhexidine gluconate (CHX) mouth rinse, twice daily, has been found to reduce plaque and gingivitis in handicapped patients, and CHX has been shown to be more effective than quaternary ammonium compounds, phenolic compounds, and plant alkaloids. Some patients object to the taste, and the major side effect associated with CHX is staining. Consumption of sub-stances containing tannin (tea, red wine, and port wine) increase the level of CHX discoloration. Stain can be minimized with toothbrushing, and when long-term treatment with CHX is indicated, stain may be managed by periodic prophylaxis.[48–51]

Desquamation and painful lesions were found in some subjects in a study using a 0.2% CHX solution; however, no such lesions occurred in studies using concentrations less than 0.2%.[49] The 0.2% concentration is widely used in Europe; the CHX solutions available in the United States are 0.12%.

Chlorhexidine gluconate may be used as a mouthwash, a spray, or a gel. The gel, which has been shown to be the most effective, requires a tray. For handicapped patients, especially those needing assistance with oral hygiene activities, this method may be difficult or impossible. For compliance, the form that is accepted by the user is best.[52]

A study of older subjects showed that rinsing weekly with a 0.12% CHX solution was as effective as rinsing daily.[53]

As mentioned above, CHX is more effective than plant alkaloids; however, in a study done at a psychiatric hospital, sanguinarine was shown to reduce plaque and gingival index scores, and it is generally considered to be better tasting than CHX.[54]

RECALL

Many compromised individuals have a higher incidence of caries and periodontal problems than routine patients, and therefore they should be seen more frequently.[55] The timing of recall appointments should be individualized and should reflect the patient's or caregiver's ability to perform oral hygiene procedures. Often compromised patients are either on fixed incomes or have limited resources available to finance their dental care. Others who are enrolled in government or private insurance plans may have more flexibility in procuring dental care on a regular basis. Documentation by the dentist of the patient's disability and the subsequent oral problems often assists the patient in obtaining a more generous interpretation of the services covered by the third-party provider. This is particularly true for government plans. For some, the cost of dental care is assumed by the patient's family, who realize the importance of preventive oral care and are eager to see the patient benefit from such treatment. In general, the compromised patient has limited resources to expend on dental care. For these patients the dental clinician may wish to consider some innovative financial arrangements to pay for preventive procedures. For example, it might be desirable if a contract could be established whereby the patient is brought in on a regular quarterly schedule for prophylaxis. Each appointment after the first one is performed for a reduced fee if the patient completes the entire series of scheduled visits. Concurrent treatment contracts should also be negotiated for restorative care.

PROVIDER AVAILABILITY

Although compromised children are usually welcomed in most pedodontic practices, it is often difficult for the similarly afflicted adult patient to find dental personnel with the training, empathy, and patience needed to deal with the patient's disabilities. In recognition of this problem, many dental schools are now providing training in special patient care to current students as well as to practicing dentists in continuing education courses.[56] Similarly, geriatric dentistry-training programs are being incorporated into an increasing number of institutional training programs throughout the United States.[57,58] These actions should increase the number of dental clinicians with the expertise and willingness to render special care.

DENTAL CARE IN AN INSTITUTIONAL SETTING

The commonest role for the dental provider in an institutional setting is that of consultant. In this capacity he or she advises the administration about the dental needs of the residents of the facility and recommends the type and frequency of oral hygiene care that should be delivered to the residents.[59,60] The dental clinician should expect to provide in-service prevention-oriented educational training programs for the nursing staff. The administration and the staff must be kept aware of the importance of routine oral health care. The administrator of a facility may agree to a routine dental care program, provided that the dentist trains the staff. This requires a continuous training program because of continual turnover of nurses' aides in such facilities. Training programs can be facilitated by the use of training aids such as videotape recordings of the important aspects of preventive care. The dentist should then participate in staff meetings when needed. A periodic evaluation of the oral hygiene of the residents by the dentist using an established oral hygiene index demonstrates if additional in-service training programs should be scheduled with the nursing staff.

When appropriate, the residents of the various institutions should be encouraged to participate in their own oral hygiene efforts. Instruction in oral hygiene methods, followed by staff supervision and encouragement, can result in improvements in various periodontal indices.[61]

Even the totally disabled or comatose patient who is no longer taking food by mouth but is being nourished via a gastric tube or intravenous line is subject to intra-oral plaque and calculus accumulation and should have daily oral hygiene procedures performed. Ironically, it has been shown that, although plaque accumulates at about the same rate in tube-fed and normally fed patients, calculus accumulates faster in tube-fed patients.[62] The objectives for oral hygiene procedures for these patients are basically the same as for all patients except that more care must be taken, including such steps as lubricating the lips of the patient prior to the hygiene treatment. Petroleum jelly is a fine, inexpensive lubricant that keeps desiccated lips from being injured by mouth props.

The teeth of these comatose patients should be brushed in the conventional manner with a soft-bristled toothbrush. Any edentulous areas should be wiped gently with a gauze square or a disposable foam sponge on a stick, both of which can be lightly moistened. If a mobile or central aspirating system is available, a toothbrush can be used that has been manufactured with an aspirating tube as a part of the brush head.[26] Such a device is an aid to controlling the salivary secretions in the totally debilitated or comatose patient.

Oral hygiene care by nurses' aides in institutional settings should include removal of all full or partial dentures and scrubbing and soaking of these appliances as well as the care of the soft tissue and teeth. A great number of dentures are lost or permanently misplaced in institutions by the staff as well as by the patients themselves. This results in residents with digestive complaints, inadequate nutrition, and speech difficulties, all of which can contribute to a poor self-image. Therefore it is important for the dental consultant to set up denture identifi-cation programs to mark prostheses with the patient's name, social security number, or other means of identification. Then any misplaced appliances can be readily returned to their owner.

Question 5. Which of the following statements, if any, are correct?

A. Often the intake of cariogenic foods can be better controlled by a guardian through judicious cooking than by a compromised patient.

B. Dry-field operation and patient co-operation are the two salient requirements for sealant placement.

C. Fluoride dentifrices should be utilized by *all* compromised patients.

D. Preventive care, even though more economic, usually has a lower priority than treatment.

E. The nurses' aides in institutions for compromised patients are usually well trained to take care of oral health needs.

SUMMARY

Individuals with physical, medical, mental, or emotional problems often have a *greater* need for dental care than their healthy counterparts. This may be because the disability itself has oral manifestations, but more commonly, it is due to (1) the limited capabilities of the individual or the family members to understand and to perform important oral hygiene tasks, (2) a lack of understanding of the importance of preventive dental care, and (3) a lack of ability to finance dental care. When a compromised patient does present to a dental office, the clinician should develop a treatment plan that emphasizes prevention. Assessments should be made of the patient's sensory, cognitive, and functional abilities and be used to customize a preventive plan. When the patient is unable to provide his or her own care, the family or an attendant needs to be taught the appropriate techniques.

Specialized equipment and easy-to-accomplish modifications of conventional oral hygiene devices may be employed to provide oral hygiene care. Strategies such as substituting a noncariogenic reward system to decrease caries incidence are often successful. Dental preventive procedures, such as sealants, fluorides, and chemical plaque control, should be considered for each patient as part of any treatment plan.

The rapport of the compromised patient and his or her family with the dental health provider and the entire office staff is critical to the comfort and compliance of the patient. All of the members of the office staff need to convey a warm receptive attitude to these special patients, assisting them in filling out their medical history forms, and offering their services as escorts when the need arises.

Most institutionalized individuals have great dental needs. The dentist can play a significant role in assessing those needs by communicating recommendations for a daily dental care program to the institutional administrator and offering training to the nursing aids to provide that day-to-day care.

For many compromised individuals, the retention of teeth in a healthy mouth improves mastication and digestion, as well as helps maintain an adequate nutritional status. In addition, the pleasing esthetics afforded by good oral health helps people with disabilities to be more welcomed by others. Good preventive care enhances one's self-esteem. For some patients who are severely compromised, specially adapted appliances may be required to maintain a high level of oral health and may be the only way to keep the mouth intact and free of dental disease. Many individuals, due to neuromuscular problems, have difficulty functioning with any type of oral prosthesis. Because the natural dentition assumes such an important role in the total living environment of the compromised patient, it is of utmost importance that the patient, caregivers, and the dental clinician work together to achieve an effective preventive oral hygiene program for such an individual.

ANSWERS AND EXPLANATIONS

1. A, D, E

    B—incorrect. Most practices serve patients with minimum disability and do not have the expertise to recognize mental and physical handicaps.

    C—incorrect. The patient should be able to see the dentist's face to better understand and to note the dentist's body language.

2. B, E

    A—incorrect. Remember, do not generalize on what a patient might do because of a handicapping condition; there are always exceptions to the rule.

    C—incorrect. Directions given to the handicapped, especially mentally handicapped, should be as simple as possible to get the job done.

    D—incorrect. The cerebral palsy patient has unexpected muscle contractions, whereas the myasthenia gravis patient has muscle weakness.

3. B, C, D

    A—incorrect. It is the brush bristles that disturb the plaque—not the dentifrice.

    E—incorrect. Very hot water is sufficient to soften a toothbrush handle prior to modification.

4. A, C, E

B—incorrect. It is the floss holder that is easier for a compromised patient to manipulate.

D—incorrect. If the care is a short session, the wheelchair often is more comfortable and supportive of the back than is the dental chair.

5. A, B, D

C—incorrect. Fluoride dentifrices are desirable for those who have control of their oral musculature; otherwise undesirable drooling or swallowing of the dentifrice occurs. Other methods of application of fluoride should *always* be considered, however.

E—incorrect. The high turnover of nurses' aides does not permit the development of a good teaching program.

SELF-EVALUATION QUESTIONS

1. A definition of compromised individual is _____. Before initiating any preventive program, it is necessary to evaluate a range of functional, _____, intellectual, and _____ capabilities.

2. A patient may have a simple decrease in visual acuity, which can be noted when the patient begins to _____. If a human guide or guide dog accompanies the patient, they (should) (should not) be allowed in the operatory. Other visual problems are _____ and _____.

3. Three precautions that should be taken to ensure that instructions are presented with maximum effectiveness to a person with loss of hearing are _____, _____, and _____. When a high-speed handpiece is turned on next to a hearing aid, it is uncomfortable for the patient because _____.

4. Patients with a history of previous _____ often have difficulty in speaking. In Parkinson's disease, multiple sclerosis, and muscular dystrophy, there is often an impairment of speech, called _____. A severe impairment in the word sequence in speaking is termed _____. When speech impairment and body paralysis occur, communication can sometimes be accomplished by use of _____ (device).

5. The best way to determine the IQ of a patient is to _____. If the homebound patient cannot complete a task, the _____ (person) should be given the responsibility of helping.

6. A simple test to determine hand muscle strength is _____. To determine whether a patient has the cognitive and psychomotor ability to use a toothbrush, the easiest method is to _____.

7. One position that a caregiver might take in brushing the teeth of a compromised individual is _____. Two disadvantages of using toothpaste are _____ and _____.

8. Two mouth props are the _____ and the _____. Of these, the _____ needs to be secured with a piece of dental floss to prevent its being swallowed, while the second, the _____ prop, can cause an overopening of the mouth.

9. When routinely using a wheelchair in the office, the following two items are convenient for stabilizing the head and extremities, as well as supporting the cervical spine: _____ and _____.

10. At least three modifications of a toothbrush are _____, _____, and _____. Electric toothbrushes can be used by severely weakened patients

by _____. One problem that might be experienced after compromised patients begin using an electric brush is _____. The _____ brush is often convenient for cleaning the interproximal embrasures.

11. A good substitute for commercially available disclosants is _____.

12. Patients with trouble in walking either need another person as an _____ to help or a wheelchair.

13. Reward systems should *not* include _____. In placing sealants, the two key factors to success are _____ and _____. In a nursing home, it is the _____ or the _____ who normally conducts in-service training for nurses' aides. To avoid the loss of dentures in a nursing home, it is desirable to _____ (action).

REFERENCES

1. Meskin L, Berkey D. The next step: A commitment to focus. *Special Care Dent.* 1989; 9(4):98–102.

2. Deckert J, Ham RJ, Smith MR, et al. Some common problems of the elderly. In: Ham RJ, Holtzman JM, Marcy ML, et al., eds. *Primary Care Geriatrics: A Case-based Learning Program.* Boston, Mass. John Wright/PSG Inc.; 1983:279–299.

3. Lange BM, Entwistle BM, Lipson LF. *Dental Management of the Handicapped: Approaches for Dental Auxiliaries.* Philadelphia, Pa. Lee & Febiger; 1983.

4. Sinykin S. The dental assistant and the special patient. *Dent Assist.* Jan–Feb 1984:24–26.

5. Boyce MR. *Guidelines for Printed Materials for Older Adults.* East Lansing, Mich. Michigan Health Council Health Promotion Project; 1981:1–4.

6. McKenzie, S. *Aging and Old Age.* Glenview, Ill. Scott, Foresman & Co; 1980:96–115.

7. Morsey S. Communicating with and treating the blind child. *Dent Hygiene.* 1980; 54(6): 288–290.

8. Wolcott LE. Rehabilitation and the aged. In: Reichel W, ed. *Clinical Aspects of Aging.* Baltimore, Md. Williams & Wilkins; 1983: 182–204.

9. Schwartz AN, Snyder CL, Peterson JA. *Aging and Life: An Introduction to Gerontology.* New York, NY. Holt, Rinehart and Winston; 1984.

10. Grob D. Prevalent joint diseases in older persons. In: Reichel W, ed. *Clinical Aspects of Aging.* Baltimore, Md. Williams & Wilkins; 1983:182–204.

11. Eigen B. Improving communications with the physically disabled. *Am Pharmacol.* 1982; NS22(10):37–40.

12. Horn JD. Dental management of the impaired individual. *Okla Dent Assoc J.* 1981; 71(3):12–14.

13. Rupp RR, Vaughn GR, Lightfoot RK. Nontraditional "aids" to hearing: Assistive listening devices. *Geriatrics.* 1984; 39(3):55–73.

14. Sanger RG, Casamassimo PS. The physically and mentally disabled patient. *Dent Clin North Am.* 1983; 27(2):363–385.

15. Price LL, Snider RM. The geriatric patient: Ear, nose, and throat problems. In: Reichel W, ed. *Clinical Aspects of Aging.* Baltimore, Md. Williams & Wilkins; 1983:489–497.

16. Hunt TE. Rehabilitation of the aged patient. In: Ham RJ, Holtzman JM, Marcy ML, et al., eds. *Primary Care Geriatrics: A Case-based Learning Program.* Boston, Mass. John Wright/PSG Inc.; 1983:89–111.

17. Entwistle B. Private practice preventive dentistry for the special patient. *Special Care Dent.* 1984; 4(6):246–252.

18. Burkhart N. Understanding and managing the autistic child in the dental office. *Dent Hygiene.* 1984; 58(2):60–63.

19. Nagel JA. Dental awareness for mentally handicapped children. *Dent Health.* 1987/88; 26(6):8–11.

20. Mulligan R, Wilson S. Design characteristics of floss-holding devices for persons with upper extremity disabilities. *Special Care Dent.* 1984; 4(4):168–172.

21. Ettinger R, Lancial L, Peterson L. Toothbrush modifications and the assessment of hand function in children with hand disabilities. *J Dent Handicapped.* 1980; 5(1):7–12.

22. Crespi PV, Ferguson FS. Approaching dental care for the developmentally disabled: A guide for the dental practitioner. *NYS Dent J.* 1987; 53:29–32.

23. Dwyer B. Professional tips for the nonhandicapped: Measuring expectations. *Dent Assist.* 1984; 53(1):21–23.

24. Udin R, Kuster C. The influence of motivation on a plaque control program for handicapped children. *J Am Dent Assoc.* 1984; 109(10):591–593.

25. Boneham L, Earl S, Holsapple C. Dental prevention for the patient with a disability. In: Margon C, Stiefel DJ, eds. *Self Instructional Series in Rehabilitation Dentistry.* Seattle, Wash. Project DECOD; 1985:Module 3:5–34.

26. Napierski G, Danner M. Oral hygiene for the dentulous total care patient. *Special Care Dent.* 1982; 2(6):257–259.

27. Napierski G. Positioning wheelchair patients for dental treatment. *Prosthet Dent.* 1982; 47(2):217–218.

28. Hylin D. Positioning of the cerebral palsy patient to facilitate dental treatment. *Texas Dent J.* 1984; 101:4–5.

29. Sklebinski G. Different strokes. *Dent Assist.* Jan/Feb 1984; 53:26–27.

30. Giles D, Murphy W. Dental treatment of the elderly inpatient. *J Dent.* 1980; 8(4):341–348.

31. Sroda R, Plezia RA. Oral hygiene devices for special patients. *Special Care Dent.* 1984; 4(6):264–266.

32. Arblaster DG, Rothwell PS, White GE. A toothbrush for patients with impaired manual dexterity. *Br Dent J.* 1985; 159:219–220.

33. Soncini JA, Tsamtsouris A. Individually modified toothbrushes and improvement of oral hygiene and gingival health in cerebral palsy children. *J Pedodontics.* 1989; 13(4):331–344.

34. Gratzer P. Elektrische zahnpflege beim mehrfachbeninderten kind. *Rehabilitation.* 1982; 21:73–75.

35. Mulligan R. Design characteristics of electric toothbrushes important to physically compromised patients. *J Dent Res.* 1980; 59:A731.

36. Fitchie JG, Reeves GW, Comer RW, et al. Oral hygiene for the severely handicapped: Clinical evaluation of the Mississippi dental care system. *Special Care Dent.* 1988; 8(6):260–264.

37. Fitchie JG, Comer RW, Hanes PJ, et al. The reduction of phenytoin-induced gingival overgrowth in a severely disabled patient: A case report. *Compend Contin Educ Dent.* 1989; Vol. X, No.6:316–319.

38. Bratel J, Berggren U, Hirsch JM. Electric or manual toothbrush? A comparison of the effects on the oral health of mentally handicapped adults. *Clin Prev Dent.* 1988; 10(3):23–26.

39. Mulligan R. Preventive care for the geriatric dental patient. *Calif Dent Assoc.* 1984; 12(1):21–32.

40. Addems A, Dip DH, Epstein JB, et al. The lack of efficacy of a foam brush in maintaining gingival health: A controlled study. *Special Care Dent.* 1992; 12(3):103–106.

41. Kambhu P, Levy S. An evaluation of the effectiveness of four mechanical plaque-removal devices when used by a trained care-provider. *Special Care Dent.* 1993; 13(1):9–14.

42. Spratley MH. A toothbrushing aid for a quadriplegic patient. *Special Care Dent.* 1991; 11(3):114–115.

43. Kritsineli M, Venetikidou A, Grigorakis G. The Myo as an oral prophylactic device used by motor skill functionally disabled patients. *J Clin Pediatr Dent.* 1992; 16:159–161.

44. Lizaire AL, Borkent A, Toor V. Dental health status of nondependent children with handicapping conditions in Edmonton, Alberta. *Special Care Dent.* 1986; 6(2):74–79.

45. Nowak AJ. Dental disease in handicapped persons. *Special Care Dent.* 1984; 4(2):66–69.

46. Swallow J, Swallow B. Dentistry for physically handicapped children in the International Year of the Child. *Int Dent J.* 1980; 30(1):1–15.

47. Shannon IL, Edmunds EJ. Reactions of tooth surfaces to three fluoride gels. *NY Dent J.* 1980; 46:426, 428–430.

48. Brayer L, Goultschin J, Mor C. The effect of chlorhexidine mouth rinse on dental plaque and gingivitis in mentally retarded individuals. *Clin Prev Dent.* 1985; 7(1):26–28.

49. Lang N, Brecx M. Chlorhexidine digluconate—an agent for chemical plaque control and prevention of gingival inflammation. *J Perio Res Supp.* 1986; 21:74–89.

50. Burtner AP, Low DW, McNeal DR, et al. Effects of chlorhexidine spray on plaque and gingival health in institutionalized persons with mental retardation. *Special Care Dent.* 1991; 11:97–100.

51. Kalaga A, Addy M, Hunter B. The use of 0.2% chlorhexidine spray as an adjunct to oral hygiene and gingival health in physically and mentally handicapped adults. *J Periodontol.* 1989; 60:381–385.

52. Francis JR, Addy M, Hunter B. A comparison of three delivery methods of chlorhexidine in handicapped children. *J Periodontol.* 1987; 58:456–459.

53. Persson RE, Truelove EL, LeResche L, et al. Therapeutic effects of daily or weekly chlorhexidine rinsing on oral health of a geriatric population. *Oral Surg Oral Med Oral Pathol.* 1991; 72:184–191.

54. Barnes GP, Parker WA, Lyon TC, et al. Clinical evaluation of three sanguinarine delivery systems for use in a psychiatric hospital preventive dentistry program. *Clin Prev Dent.* 1988; 10:25–30.

55. Wathen W. Geriatric dentistry. *Tex Dent J.* 1984; 101(6):3.

56. Thornton J. Dentistry and the handicapped child. *Ala J Med Sci.* 1983; 20(1):22–27.

57. American Association of Dental Schools. Curriculum guidelines for the person with a handicap. *J Dent Educ.* 1985; 49:118–122.

58. Thomas AM, Ship IJ. Current status of geriatric education in American dental schools. *J Dent Educ.* 1981; 45(9):589–591.

59. Fuerstenau K, Hawley D, Pitney B. Dental care in the nursing home. *J Oregon Dent Assoc.* 1983; 53(1):20–21.

60. Quinn MJ. Establishing a preventive dentistry program in a long term health care institution. *Gerodontics.* 1988; 4:165–167.

61. Shaw MJ, Shaw L. The effectiveness of differing dental health education programmes in improving the oral health of adults with mental handicaps attending Birmingham adult training centres. *Community Dent Health.* 1991; 8(2):139–145.

62. Dicks JL, Banning JS. Evaluation of calculus accumulation in tube-fed mentally handicapped patients: The effects of oral hygiene status. *Special Care Dent.* 1991; 11(3):104–106.

Chapter 20

Primary Preventive Dentistry in a Hospital-Based Setting

Michael T. Montgomery
Arden G. Christen

Objectives

At the end of this chapter it will be possible to

1. Discuss the scope of dental inpatient and outpatient services available at federal hospitals as compared with those in civilian hospitals.
2. List eight categories of patients seen on a hospital service who are in need of primary preventive dentistry services, and cite specific problems related to the care of each of these groups.
3. Explain how an inpatient with dentures should be cared for, including how the dentures should be cleaned.
4. Name four conditions for which prophylactic antibiotic coverage is necessary before performing a scaling.
5. List the minimum number of personal oral hygiene items that each hospitalized patient should possess and that should be stocked in the hospital's central supply.
6. Cite several oral side effects of cancer therapy that require dental intervention.
7. Summarize key concepts that should be imparted to parents and potential parents at the time of prenatal and postnatal oral health counseling sessions.

Introduction

The idea of providing dental services in a hospital setting is not new.[1] The first dentist to practice in an American hospital was Richard Courtland Skinner, who immigrated to Philadelphia in 1788.[2] Later he was the first dentist to ask for and receive an official appointment to a medical institution. In the 1790s he created the first hospital dental clinic in the Dispensary of the City of New York to treat the indigent. In 1901, the Philadelphia General Hospital developed the first dental intern-training program. Approximately 200 years later, in 1987, it was reported that about 40,000 dentists had hospital privileges.[3] In spite of the fact that about 60% of all hospitals have dental programs, not all hospitals presently extend staff privileges to dentists.[4] In 1983, hospital dental practice faced a serious challenge when the Joint Commission on Accreditation of Hospitals Organization (JCAHO) revised its accreditation guidelines for medical staffs by deleting all references to dentists and other nonphysicians. Although this was not the intent of the revision, some hospitals used the revised standards to exclude dentists from the medical staff. Presently, the appointment of dentists to a hospital staff and dental privileges is a determination made by each individual hospital.

Dentistry is integrated into the hospital system on three levels: *education, service,* and *administration.*[3] The majority of the dental care rendered in many hospitals is focused on the diagnostic and treatment care necessary to support the recovery of the medically compromised patients or patients admitted for serious head and neck diseases, infection, and trauma.[5] The medical profession has realized that the background training needed by dentists and dental auxiliaries can be incorporated into the care provided by the hospital. To support this continual need for training professional dental personnel, medical centers have rotated dental students and residents through hospital dentistry and other services of the teaching hospitals, such as emergency medicine, internal medicine, and anesthesiology. Every year more than 2000 American dentists receive training in hospitals.[6] At the same time, dental hygiene students and dental assistants have provided dental hygiene services for both ambulatory and non-ambulatory patients.[5] The scope of the dental services within a hospital varies greatly, depending on such factors as bed capacity, economic support, level of specialty expertise, and proximity to medical and research centers. As a result of these factors, the dental services of hospitals can be placed in one of two categories: (1) those that treat and maintain the total oral health of the individual during the hospitalization period, as is the case in federal hospitals[7]; and (2) those nonfederal hospitals (private and community) that provide acute therapies to support the recovery of the medically or surgically compromised patient.[5]

Military hospitals provide full dental service for their active duty personnel. These services include diagnosis, treatment planning, all restorative and rehabilitative services, primary preventive dentistry procedures, and counseling, as well as recall. Similarly, Veterans Administration and U.S. Public Health Service hospitals provide complete care to eligible inpatients and outpatients.[7,8]

In contrast, private, community, and general hospitals have only short-term commitments to patients; the dental care is rendered for acute, primary complaints. To support this limited objective, the dental services of many of the larger hospitals have emphasized oral surgery. In smaller hospitals the dentist may serve on a part-time basis or simply be on call for facial injuries arriving in the emergency room.[1] In these hospitals patients requiring dental care, other than that pertaining to head and neck trauma, are usually referred to a private dentist following the hospitalization.

In the 1990s and beyond, dentistry's presence in a hospital setting will increase in long-term facilities, acute care hospitals, home care programs, ambulatory care facilities, and hospice programs. This will accompany the expected move of hospitals into the community and anticipated changes in dental care reimbursement.[3]

PRIMARY PREVENTIVE DENTISTRY IN A HOSPITAL SETTING

The use of *specific* primary preventive dentistry procedures is *essential* in the treatment and posthospitalization maintenance of many patients, although the use of *routine* primary preventive dentistry procedures is *desirable* for all patients. The hospital dentist and the dental auxiliaries are the promoters of this total patient care concept. A shortage of funds and personnel, however, has hampered the achievement of this objective. As a result, patients have often been neglected and their dental needs have been left to their own resources.[9]

Dental Needs of Hospitalized Patients

Dentists as well as other health professionals realize that oral health cannot be divorced from the general health of the hospitalized patient. Many oral conditions are intimately related to systemic diseases. Optimally, total health care requires the combined efforts of the medical and dental professions. Two factors have focused attention on the prevention of oral disease in the hos-

pital patient. First is the poor oral health concepts and practices embodied by these patients. Second is the growing population of infection-prone patients, to whom oral disease poses a serious health risk. Such patients include organ transplant patients, diabetics, and AIDS patients. Maintaining a healthy oral environment alleviates the need to extract and replace teeth, which is cost-effective and minimizes a significant threat to the patient's systemic health. Tooth replacement and restoration often require special adjunctive treatments for these patients and many are poor candidates for sophisticated dental care.

Several surveys indicate that long-term hospitalized or chronically ill patients have many significant dental needs.[10–12] The Council on Hospital Dental Services' American Dental Association (ADA) survey of 1634 individuals estimated that about 80% of all patients admitted to the hospital had some form of oral pathology that required treatment.[10] The majority of these patients were unaware of dental problems and typically did not have a family dentist. The six greatest dental treatment needs, in descending order, were dental caries, periodontal disease, prophylaxis, dentures, missing teeth, and extractions. Harvey and coworkers[12] in their survey of a group of hospitalized, chronically ill patients in two hospitals reported almost identical findings. They also discovered that adequate, functional, fixed, and removable prosthetic devices were nearly nonexistent and that the level of dental care previously provided was very low. Poor oral hygiene, gingival inflammation, and papillary hyperplasia were the most prevalent problems. Almost all of the dentures examined were inadequate with gross amounts of materia alba present on the denture and in the buccal vestibule. About 57% of patients with acute dental pain had not received palliative care. In addition to these findings, dentists are being increasingly called on to provide care for growing numbers of patients with acquired immune deficiency syndrome (AIDS).

Several categories of patients are prime candidates for primary preventive dentistry programs, including

1. Patients with head and neck cancer, (those receiving head and neck radiation and chemotherapy)
2. AIDS patients
3. Renal failure patients
4. Patients in need of prophylactic antibiotics
5. Comatose patients
6. Paraplegics and amputees
7. Diabetic patients
8. Psychiatric cases
9. Obstetric patients
10. Organ transplant patients.

Patients in each of these categories require specialized care and counseling. Guidelines for managing the oral health care needs for the medically compromised patients discussed in this chapter are intended to provide the framework for making sound decisions. Recognizing the diversity of potential individual factors, the guidelines are only designed to assist the practitioner in making individual judgments. Strict adherence to these recommendations is not intended. Consultation with medical services and practitioners is encouraged, both as a form of courtesy to the referring physician and to ensure that patient treatment is appropriate.

In dental services providing complete dental care, administrative planning is necessary to ensure adequate funds, facilities, and personnel support to care for these patients. In smaller hospitals patient therapy needs should be ranked so that the more essential care is available and the remaining treatment areas are covered to the extent

possible within existing resources. In many instances the required preventive tasks can be assigned to dental hygienists or dental assistants. Such duties consist of daily ward rounds during which patient needs can be assessed, routine and palliative care administered, and more comprehensive needs referred to the dental staff.[13]

Personality Characteristics of Patient Treatment Personnel

Individuals selected to perform patient treatment functions should possess certain essential personality characteristics.[14] The individual must be psychologically prepared to work with short-term acutely ill, long-term chronically ill, and terminally ill patients. Empathy, tolerance, sensitivity, common sense, flexibility, and efficiency are required personality traits. Formal education in patient treatment is also desirable.[15]

The dentist or the auxiliary is often confronted by patients going through difficult psychologic stages after being informed of the seriousness of an illness, such as shock, anger, fear, bargaining, apathy, or acceptance. The dental care provider needs to show flexibility and tolerance to give psychologic support while carrying on the primary preventive functions.[15] These individuals must also foster continuous, effective, and amicable professional relationships with other members of the health team, such as physicians, nurses, dietitians, social workers, psychologists, and chaplains. Following patient discharge, the dental practitioner should communicate with the community health nurse as part of the posthospitalization care.[13]

Administrative Requirements

Participation of dentists or dental auxiliaries in an expanded hospital primary preventive dentistry program requires the agreement of the hospital administrator and the support of the medical and nursing staff. Unfortunately, the subject of dental care is not emphasized in the formal training of the majority of these nondental health professionals.[9] This education usually must come through continuing personal relationships between dental and medical personnel and through continuing education programs.

In hospitals offering complete dental care, consultation requests are routinely received from the various services to examine newly admitted patients. To ensure that the primary preventive dentistry services are rendered, a preventive dentistry officer is usually designated by the chief of the dental service. In turn, the preventive dentistry officer works closely with the dental hygienist and other auxiliaries in delegating preventive care duties for ambulatory and nonambulatory patients. As part of the dental clinic routine, regulations are established to ensure the effective and safe delivery of primary preventive dentistry procedures to meet the needs of the various levels of medically, physically, and mentally compromised patients. As with all procedures contemplated for hospitalized patients, consent for the dental treatment must be obtained from the service responsible for the patient's care.

THE SELF-SUFFICIENT PATIENT

Each self-sufficient patient admitted to the hospital should have a small container of fluoride rinse, along with a toothbrush and floss to carry out personal oral hygiene procedures.[15] The hospital's central supply should stock these dental products, along with dentifrices, floss threaders, disclosants, antimicrobial mouth washes, topical anesthetics, oral antifungal and antiviral agents, and denture cleaners. Dental hygiene counseling should be part of the total health care

of all patients. Daily ward rounds made by the dental auxiliary should similarly emphasize the need for and the most effective techniques for plaque control and topical fluoride therapy to nonambulatory patients. Cleaning the mouth after meals should be encouraged, and at least one thorough brushing and flossing should be accomplished in every 24-hour period. If a dental auxiliary is not available, another specifically designated ward person should assume this essential supportive task.[15]

GENERAL CONSIDERATIONS

If dental personnel are not employed in the hospital setting, others, such as nurses or nurses' aides, can be taught to provide the essential postoperative dental procedures as well as to initiate and to supervise the more routine personal oral hygiene techniques. The ward personnel providing patient dental care should receive in-service training on a regular and repeated basis. Most of the functions of oral care do not need to be performed during the time of peak morning activity on the ward, when baths, linen changes, routine therapy, or x-ray treatments are being carried out by the day shift. Instead, the afternoon can be used for oral care programs. Patient plaque control programs can be accomplished by the patient any time during the day.

A preventive dentistry kit should be available on each floor or ward in the hospital. Such a kit should include disposable plastic mouth mirrors, a pocket flashlight, a hand mirror for patient viewing, soft toothbrushes, dental floss, a fluoride dentifrice, sterile tongue blades and cotton applicator sticks, mouth props, and seizure sticks (double tongue blades wrapped in 4 × 4 gauze and taped securely). Additional aids include a high-volume, low-vacuum suction unit;

aspirator tips; 2 × 2 gauze squares; disclosing tablets; bridge cleaners; proxabrushes; fluoride gel; saliva substitute; and petroleum jelly for the lubrication of patients' lips with angular cheilosis. Alkaline mouth rinses can be made up in quantity by the pharmacy. Sufficient numbers of sterilized universal scalers, mirrors, explorers, and cotton forceps should also be available.

HEAD AND NECK CANCER

In 1993, the American Cancer Society estimated that more than 1.2 million new cases of cancer were discovered in the United States. Of these, 29,600 were diagnosed in the oral cavity, with 7,925 deaths occurring in patients having oral cancer.[16] Tobacco smoking accounts for about 30% of all cancer deaths and about 434,000 premature deaths in the United States annually.[17] Cancer is also the leading cause of death in children between the ages of 1 and 14 years. Despite the fact that the incidence of cancer is increasing, early diagnosis and significant advances in therapy have resulted in a much longer and more productive life for the cancer victim.[18]

Cancer Prevention

A tragedy associated with head and neck cancer deaths is that the death could have been prevented by modifying the victim's lifestyle. The great majority of head and neck cancers arise from three causes: *smoking* and the use of *smokeless tobacco* as agents of intraoral cancer and *exposure to the sun* as a medium for cancer of the lips and face. The decision to forsake tobacco in any of its forms and to shield the face is sufficient to return the risk of these head and neck cancers to near zero. Those ignorant of or ignoring the admonitions by the American Cancer Society concerning smoking and sun exposure frequently have a second chance. Slow, nonhealing, precancerous changes usually occur in the oral cavity or on the face prior to the development of cancer that should alert an individual to seek professional care. Stopping the use of tobacco or avoiding excessive exposure to the sun at this point usually returns the tissues to normal. Finally, in the early stages of cancer, immediate treatment is usually followed by cure, provided the patient does not return to the initiating habit. Rarely is an individual afforded so many life or death decisions about his or her personal behaviors.

Tobacco Education and Cessation Programs

All forms of tobacco cause significant damage to hard and soft tissues in and around the mouth.[17–19] These conditions include oral cancer, leukoplakia, sinusitis, delayed wound healing, miscellaneous tissue changes, discoloration of teeth and dental prostheses, abrasion, periodontal disease (with attendant bone loss, tooth mobility, tooth loss, acute necrotizing ulcerative gingivitis, and gingival recession), dental calculus, hairy tongue, dulled senses of taste and smell, and bad breath.

The National Cancer Institute (NCI) has initiated an ambitious, nationwide, community-based smoking cessation program that involves all physicians and dentists (and the American Cancer Society).[17] This program targets heavy smokers, and its goal is to effect a 50% reduction in the U.S. cancer death rate by the end of the next decade.

Many oral health teams are already working effectively on smoking cessation in the dental office.[17–19] An eight-step office-based smoking cessation plan for dental patients has been developed at the Indiana University School of Dentistry.[19] Preparatory steps include the selection of a smoking cessation office coordinator, the creation of a smoke-free office environment, the identification of all smoking patients in the practice, and the development of patient-targeted smoking cessation plans. The program involves the use of the "four A's" (eg, ASK patients about their smoking behaviors at every appropriate opportunity. ADVISE all smokers to quit. ASSIST patients in stopping, and ARRANGE for supportive follow-up procedures). The steps of this program dovetail with the NCI's nationwide program designed for all health care providers. The use of dentist-prescribed FDA-approved pharmaceutical agents (nicotine-containing gum and transdermal patches) are an important part of this progarm.[19]

The Cancer Patient

Head and neck cancer therapies can include surgery, chemotherapy, radiation therapy, bone marrow transplantation, or a combination thereof. Head and neck surgery is generally used to obliterate small tumors or to debulk large tumors. Chemotherapy involves the use of alkylating, antibiotic, and antimetabolite agents to kill cells undergoing mitosis, of which cancer cells are some of the most rapidly dividing. Unavoidably, rapidly dividing host cells, including hematopoietic cells in the bone marrow, epithelial cells of the oral mucosa and gastrointestinal tracts, and endothelial cells of terminal arterioles, are also affected. Like chemotherapy, radiation therapy also disrupts the nucleotide sequencing of nuclear genetic material in cells undergoing mitosis. Approximately one half of all head and neck tumors are treated with radiation therapy. The typical radiation dose is 5000 to 7000 cGy (centigrays equal rads) delivered in fractionations of 200 cGy/day, five days a week, for 5 to 7 weeks. *Host damage from radiation therapy is generally localized to the irradiated tissue, but the side effects of*

chemotherapy are systemic.[20] Bone marrow transplantation (BMT) entails the autolgous or allogeneic transplantation of marrow into a cancer patient following total body irradiation and near lethal doses of chemotherapy. This procedure affords the delivery of higher chemotherapy doses because transplantation of the bone marrow obviates the concern for destruction of the bone marrow. With isolated chemotherapy, the associated immunosuppression is generally less severe and less prolonged than with BMT. This therapy is routinely administered on an outpatient basis with patients being admitted for serious complications and more aggressive drug regimens. In contrast, BMT involves profound immunosuppression requiring patient hospitalization. The difference in immunosuppression also accounts for the *greater* incidence and severity of oral complications in BMT patients.[21,22] For patients undergoing chemotherapy or BMT the major oral complications are mucositis; immunosuppression (neutropenia); hemorrhage (thrombocytopenia); malnutrition; and infections secondary to periodontal disease, caries, and pericoronitis. Facial paresthesias have also been reported with use of such chemotherapeutic plant alkaloids as vinblastine and vincristine.[20] Oral complications of radiation therapy can include mucositis, infections, xerostomia, accelerated caries and periodontal disease, dysgeusia (altered taste), dysphonia (altered speech), malnutrition, trismus, osteoradionecrosis, and developmental disturbances. As for most of the patients discussed in this chapter, it is critical that potential sources of oral infection are alleviated *prior* to immunosuppression, organ transplantation, and radiation therapy. Systemic infections are responsible for *70% of the patient deaths* from chemotherapy. In addition, 75% of the patients have oral infections during chemotherapy, and oral infections account for 25% to 30% of all septicemias.[20–25] As such, infection is a significant source of morbidity and mortality, and oral infections are a prominent contributor to the incidence of infection in these patients. Therefore, these patients should have a thorough clinical (head, neck, and oral) and radiographic examination (at least a screening image) as soon as possible in the course of their hospital care.

A mutually respectful working relationship must exist between the dental service and other involved medical (oncology/hematology/radiation therapy) and surgical services (general surgery/otolaryngology) to afford a coordinated and timely approach to patient care. Generally, the approach to dental therapy is aggressive in the acute phase and more conservative in the chronic phase. Because many of the cancer therapy side effects cannot be avoided, *the best approach to patient care is prevention.* Preventive measures should begin with patient education that enhances the patients' awareness of the relationship between their oral health and their systemic disease. Future oral hygiene efforts must be detailed verbally and in writing, and these measures should be encouraged at follow-up appointments during and following the cancer therapy.[26,27] Research to date has clearly shown that routine oral hygiene measures combined with the use of a fluoridated dentifrice and regular dental monitoring, significantly reduce the incidence of caries and the progression of periodontal disease.[28] Recognizing that patient compliance with oral care following radiotherapy is reported to be less than 50%, *frequent recalls are essential.*[29] Teeth with a questionable prognosis should be extracted, such as those with moderate to severe periodontal disease, extensive decay, impacted third molars, and irreversible pulpitis. In addition to the patient's restorative needs and periodontal

disease status, the aggressiveness of the dentist's approach depends on the patient's present level of oral hygiene, prognosis, desires, functional and esthetic needs, and financial status. For most patients, the initial dental therapy should entail thorough scaling and prophylaxis, along with oral hygiene instructions. When providing dental care, it is important to remain cognizant of the psychologic and physical strain placed on patients by their illness and treatment. As such, patients may not be receptive to dental care, and their pain reaction threshold may be depressed. Education, patience, and a compassionate demeanor will facilitate care for most patients. Use of sedatives or anxiolytics may be advisable should the delivery of dental care be impaired by patient anxiety or uncooperative behavior.[20,26,30,31]

Essential information to obtain from the oncologist or radiotherapist includes the type of chemotherapeutic agents used, the degree of immunosuppression anticipated, the total radiation dose administered, the tissue fields (or ports) to be irradiated, and the patient's prognosis. Anticaries measures can include a fluoridated dentifrice, chlorhexidine rinsing, and the use of daily fluoride gels. Efforts to combat periodontal disease can include brushing and flossing and chlorhexidine rinsing. Needed dental care can be completed in the operating room during panendoscopy, which is performed on most head and neck cancer patients. This must be coordinated with the surgical oncology service and requires a close working relationship with the head and neck cancer team.[20,26,27,29–31]

Caries and Periodontal Disease

Chlorhexidine is presently the most effective antimicrobial mouth rinse available to combat periodontal disease and caries (Appendix 20–1). The drug is most effective against Gram-positive organisms and has been shown to decrease both plaque and oral inflammation.[32] Chlorhexidine is also effective against oral candidiasis in patients undergoing bone marrow transplantation.[33] Because the drug is not absorbed by the gastrointestinal tract, systemic toxic reactions are minimal. Noteworthy side effects are taste intolerance and staining of the teeth. The staining is unesthetic and tenacious, though reversible with professional prophylaxis. In normal patients, chlorhexidine is released for up to 24 hours in the oral cavity, and no significant differences have been shown between 0.1% and 0.2% concentrations. Patients should rinse with 15 mL of the drug three times a day, once after each meal. In patients undergoing head and neck radiation, the substantivity of the chlorhexidine diminishes after 4 hours, therefore more frequent rinsing is required to achieve the desired effect.[34,35] Chlorhexidine's effect on plaque and gingivitis improves if preceded by scaling and prophylaxis.[36] Although the drug is commercially available only as a 0.12% rinse, aerosol sprays, varnishes, and gels have been evaluated with favorable results in scientific investigations. The gel formulation appears to be the most effective method for decreasing caries and gingival inflammation.[37] *Fluoride* is the most effective anticaries drug available and is indicated for all medically compromised patients for whom caries poses a threat to systemic health. Systemic fluoride is important during tooth calcification, but is only modestly effective thereafter, hence this route of administration is not recommended for adult patients.[38,39] In contrast, topical fluoride is incorporated into tooth surfaces and plaque, providing reservoirs for sustained drug release. The effectiveness of fluoride depends on the availability of free fluoride ions in plaque during a cariogenic challenge. The duration of fluoride release from the teeth is weeks to months at a neutral pH,

though the release is accelerated at an acidic pH common to caries. The availability of free fluoride also varies over time and among regions within the mouth.[38-41] Recent research efforts have focused on various sustained-release techniques, attemping to achieve a more uniform and sustained release over time (Chapter 11). Technologic obstacles have thwarted this development, however.[38] As such, frequent exposure to topical fluoride appears to be the single most effective means of fluoride administration in caries-prone patients today. The cariostatic efficacy of fluoride improves with increased concentrations, multiple routes of administration, and frequency of use.[42] Fluoride rinsing is recommended twice a day following brushing, during which the fluoride should be held in the mouth for 30 to 60 seconds before expectoration. The fluoride should remain undisturbed (no rinsing, eating, or drinking) for 30 minutes thereafter. Acidulated fluoride should be avoided in patients suffering from mucositis to minimize mucosal irritation. Fluoride gel is applied once or twice a day via brushing or in custom application trays. The tray is preferred because of more uniform application and better distribution of fluoride into interproximal areas where caries is more likely to develop (Fig 20–1). Following brushing, 5 to 10 drops are applied to each tray, and the trays are left in place for 5 minutes. The fluoride should remain undisturbed (no rinsing, eating, or drinking) for 30 minutes thereafter. 0.4% stannous fluoride (SnF) or 1% sodium fluoride (NaF) are most commonly suggested, and stannous fluoride is sometimes preferred because of its modest advantage in antimicrobial activity.[20] Although these applications are effective alone, research has shown that without simultaneous routine oral hygiene measures, the cariostatic and periodontal effect is significantly diminished.[36] Various studies have

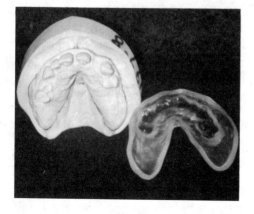

Figure 20–1. A polyvinyl fluoride gel tray of the maxillary arch prepared from a dental stone model. A ribbon of fluoride gel has already been placed in the teeth indentations.

also examined the efficacy of combining chlorhexidine and fluoride in a single rinse, showing an improved effect on gingivitis and plaque that is superior to either agent alone.[43,44]

Xerostomia

Direct irradiation of the parotid glands causes destruction of glandular tissue (acinar and ductal cells), which is responsible for an increase in salivary viscosity, xerostomia, and a drop in salivary pH from 7.0 to between 5.0 and 5.5. The xerostomia is generally irreversible, although some authors report some partial recovery (Fig 20–2). These salivary changes diminish saliva's buffering capacity, cause a shift towards more cariogenic organisms, such as mutans streptococci and lactobacillus (and away from less cariogenic organisms, such as *Streptococcus mitus* and *S sanguis*), and diminish the efficacy of fluoride therapy.[20,45–47] Cariogenic activity is rampant and accelerated under these conditions, with lesions developing at a rate six times that seen in normal individuals. The resultant radiation caries is distinctive, displaying a cervical and incisal predilection that amputates the crown over time (Fig 20–3). Because the salivary changes are permanent, the threat of radiation caries exists for all teeth throughout the patient's life.[20] The effects of xerostomia on periodontal disease are poorly documented; however, a few studies report a minimal relationship between the two.[47] Preventive therapy involves strict attention to oral hygiene, a low-carbohydrate diet, frequent dental check-ups (every 3 months), administration of topical fluoride

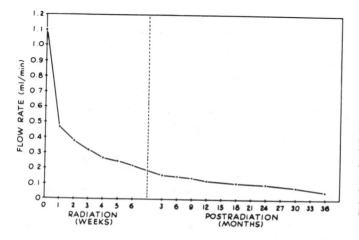

Figure 20–2. Mean flow rates of stimulated whole saliva in 42 patients with cancer before, during, and after radiotherapy. (*From Dreizen S, Brown LR, Daly TE, et al. Prevention of xerostomia-related dental caries in irradiated cancer patients. J Dent Res. 1977; 56:99–104.*)

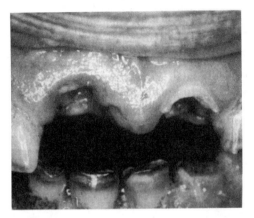

Figure 20–3. Severe radiation caries in the maxillary and mandibular anterior region of an adult treated for head and neck cancer. (*Courtesy of the late Dr Simon Katz, Indianapolis, Indiana.*)

gel, and rinsing with chlorhexidine.[48] Following head and neck radiation, chlorhexidine reduces the concentration of mutans streptococci but has little effect on lactobacillis.[35,37] In the restorative phase, the use of a fluoride-releasing material such as glass ionomer is suggested.

Salivary stimulants and saliva substitutes are used to combat xerostomia. Generally, saliva substitutes consist of a wetting agent (carboxymethylcellulose or sorbitol), electrolytes, fluoride, and flavoring. Saliva substitutes are poorly tolerated by patients because of their lack of substantivity and subsequent short duration of action (10–15 minutes). As such, the majority of xerostomic patients prefer frequent sips of water to the saliva substitutes.[49,50] Lemon drops, sugarless gum, and pilocarpine are recommended as methods of increasing salivary output.[20,51] Pilocarpine, a parasympathomimetic agent, increased salivary output both objectively and subjectively in studies involving a variety of xerostomic populations. The drug salagen has recently been

approved for the treatment of xerostomia following head and neck radiation therapy.[52]

Mucositis

Mucositis is the result of direct tissue toxicity from anticancer therapy, either drug-induced (chemotherapy) or radiation-induced. The rapidly dividing oral epithelium is a prime target for cancer therapy. Signs that include erythematous changes and ulcerations usually appear *1 to 2 weeks* following the onset of treatment and completely resolve in a similar period after treatment's end. All oral tissues can be affected, and the latency period reflects the time required for maturation of epithelial cells in the basal cell layer. The associated pain is debilitating, profoundly affecting patients' ability to speak and swallow, their diet and nutrition, and oral hygiene efforts.[20] For toxicity-induced mucositis, the *treatment is palliative* and includes alkaline *irrigating and debriding agents* and *topical anesthetics* (Appendix 20–2). Unfortunately, the accompanying relief is brief for most agents, though appreciated by the patient with significant mucositis. Oratect Gel (MGI Pharma) provides extended relief for 4 to 6 hours that is not affected by eating, although the application of the gel is technique-sensitive. Most commonly, the topical anesthetics are combined with an adhering agent (sucralfate, kaolin, magnesium hydroxide, or milk of magnesia), in a 50:50 ratio that coats the oral mucosa to provide the mixture with substance. One of the most common combinations is "triple mix," which combines diphenhydramine, viscous lidocaine, and magnesium hydroxide. For severe mucositic pain, *systemic analgesics* should be administered ad lib.[53–55] Chlorhexidine rinsing has been shown to decrease the incidence, severity, and duration of mucositis following chemotherapy but has little effect on radiation-induced mucositis.[33,56–58] Patients should also avoid substances that aggravate the mucositis pain, such as alcohol, tobacco, and over-the-counter mouth washes.

In addition to toxicity-induced mucositis, *oral pathogens*, such as *Candida albicans* and herpes simplex virus (HSV) can also be responsible for these lesions or secondarily infect them. In the immunocompromised host, these lesions are atypical in appearance and location, requiring laboratory testing for an accurate diagnosis. A positive history of yeast infections, cold sores, and fever blisters can be used to predict susceptibility, along with HSV antibody titers.[20] *Candidiasis is the most common infection* and can be quickly diagnosed via a Gram's stain or potassium hydroxide wet prep. Generally, *Candida* appears as either a white, raised, cottage-cheese-like lesion that leaves a bleeding surface when removed (*pseudomembranous* candidiasis) or as an erythematous ulceration (*erythematous* candidiasis). Candidiasis can also occur at the corners of the mouth as erythematous fissures termed angular cheilitis. Treatment consists of topical or systemic antifungal agents listed in Appendix 20–1 for a 2-week period.[20,59–62] In denture patients, candidiasis can be perpetuated by the continual wear of contaminated dentures. The dentures should be left out at night and soaked in an antifungal agent to decontaminate them.[63,64] In addition to the antifungal agents, chlorhexidine has also been effective in reducing the incidence of mucositis and candidal infections in BMT patients.[33,56,57,65] As such, an antifungal agent and chlorhexidine are commonly prescribed prophylactically in BMT patients.

Herpes is also a problem for the severely immunocompromised patient; however, HSV reactivation does not appear to be a problem for patients undergoing head and neck radiation therapy.[20] The incidence of HSV reactivation in BMT patients is reported to be between 68% and 90% from numerous studies.[66–68] With chemotherapy, the incidence of HSV reactivation is reduced to around 40%. Herpetic lesions are typically described as small vesiculi that erupt into nondescript ulcerations with erythematous borders, which can reside on any oral tissue. Because the time spent in the vesiculous stage is short, it is uncommon for lesions to have this appearance when discovered. When the lesions occur on the lips or around the nares, the lesions can be seen to progress through the classic stages of vesiculi, ulceration, and crusted lesion.[20] Rapid diagnosis can be made using an enzyme-linked immunosorbent assay (ELISA), but the most accurate diagnostic method is culturing.[69,70]

Intravenous acyclovir (5 mg/kg tid), can significantly decrease viral shedding time, healing time, and pain duration and is the recommended therapy to prevent HSV reactivation in immunocompromised patients. For severely immunosuppressed patients (ie, BMT), prophylactic acyclovir is commonly prescribed. In nonimmunosuppressed patients acyclovir ointment or tablets may be successful in preventing HSV recurrence if administered during the prodromal period; however, the oral and topical regimens are not helpful once lesions appear. A drawback to acyclovir therapy is the rapid recurrence of an HSV infection following cessation of the drug.[20,71,72] Because the chance of septicemia with significant morbidity or mortality is a real concern in immunocomprised patients, early detection, accurate diagnosis, and treatment are critical. Predicting HSV recurrence has been the focus of numerous scientific investigations. Relationships have been suggested between HSV reactivation and the chemotherapeutic conditioning regimen (greater incidence with total body irradiation), the type of cancer (greater incidence with leukemia), the HSV antibody titer (greater with more than a 1:4 dilution), and lymphocyte and monocyte counts (greater with less than 600 cells/mm[3] and 250 cells/mm[3], respectively).[66,67,72–74] The preferred predictor is yet to be established.

Nutrition

Nutritional counseling is essential as patients eat sparingly and resort to cool, soft, high-carbohydrate foods that promote caries development, potentially blunt host resistance, and contribute to dehydration. The mucositis, xerostomia, dysgeusia, and nausea and vomiting are responsible for these dietary changes. Patients must be encouraged to take vitamin supplements and eat balanced and creative diets that minimize mucositic pain, yet promote the desire to eat. Having the patient consult a dietitian is recommended to combat this side effect.[20]

Osteoradionecrosis

Osteoradionecrosis (ORN) is a radiation-induced wound repair deficit that predisposes bony wounds to secondary infection. The destruction of alveolar vascularity secondary to radiation-induced endarteritis is responsible for the host's inability to heal the wound. Osteoradionecrosis has been defined as an area of exposed bone in the field of radiation that persists for 3 months. Any surgical trauma to tissue in the radiation field following radiotherapy is prone to ORN. The potential for ORN increases as the time from radiotherapy increases because the blood supply to the affected tissues declines over time. As such, the risk of ORN is perpetual but exists only for tissue within the field of radiation.[75–77] The risk of ORN also depends on the delivered radiation dose; ORN is uncommon at doses below 6000 cGy. Osteoradionecrosis occurs

mainly in the mandible, although cases in the maxilla have been reported. The predilection for the mandible is a reflection of the more modest blood supply and denser bone compared with the maxilla. Initial signs and symptoms include constant, throbbing pain; soft-tissue breakdown with exposed bone; and irregular radiographic radiolucencies (Fig 20–4). Late signs and symptoms include suppuration, a fetid oral odor, pathologic fractures, and orocutaneous fistulas. Attention to subtle oral changes is required for an early diagnosis. The incidence of ORN following head and neck irradiation is estimated at 10%, but the consequences of treatment are so debilitating that prevention is the essential therapy. Conservative treatment of ORN involves some combination of oral rinsing, professional irrigation and debridement, antibiotics, analgesics, and hyperbaric oxygen therapy (HBO). This last method increases tissue oxygenation by driving oxygen into the tissues under pressure (3 atm). The increase in tissue oxygenation promotes the healing process by encouraging the formation of a connective tissue matrix and capil-

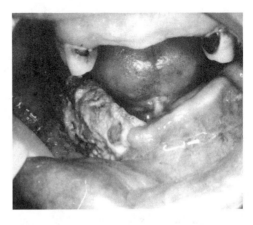

Figure 20–4. Massive mandibular osteoradionecrosis secondary to heavy x-ray irradiation for epidermoid carcinoma in the jaw. (*Courtesy of Dr Robert P. Johnson, San Antonio, Texas.*)

lary budding. Unfortunately, HBO is ineffective alone, is time-consuming, and expensive. Alveolar resection is the definitive therapy for refractory ORN, which can be physically disfiguring and disabling. To prevent or minimize the risk of osteoradionecrosis, 14 to 21 days is desired between oral surgery procedures and the initiation of head and neck radiation. A 21-day waiting period is associated with minimal risk of ORN, and the risk increases with shorter latency periods. Radical alveolectomy, primary closure, and antibiotic therapy (Appendix 20–1) are suggested with extractions to accelerate the healing process and minimized postsurgical complications. If possible, needed dental surgery should be accomplished *prior* to radiotherapy because 90% of all ORN is associated with oral surgery following radiotherapy. Dental care postradiation therapy should be conservative, emphazing root canal therapy and other tooth retention measures instead of extraction. If oral surgery is required following radiotherapy, adjunctive HBO therapy should be considered to improve host healing.[20] A recent study, however, found that no ORN developed following tooth extractions in the field of radiation after a median dose of 5000 cGy (median follow-up was 5 years). The authors attributed this outcome to minimizing surgical trauma, antibiotic coverage, and the avoidance of a vasocontrictor in the local anesthetic.[78]

In the immunosuppressed patient, the use of adjunctive systemic antibiotics should be considered when oral surgery is needed and neutrophil counts are below 500/mm³. Broad-spectrum antibiotics can be administered prophylactically for 7 to 10 days following surgery. Similarly, some authors recommend stopping or minimizing mechanical oral hygiene measures (brushing and flossing) when patients are neutropenic. Foam toothbrushes have been suggested during this time; however, the literature has shown that these devices are ineffective in removing plaque and disliked by patients.[79,80] Because signs and symptoms of infection are manifestations of an immunocompetent host, *these markers of infection may be absent or blunted with immunosuppression.* As such, the practitioner should not rely solely on these clinical parameters to determine the presence of infection. With chemotherapy, bleeding secondary to thrombocytopenia must also be considered. Signs and symptoms of bleeding tendency include ecchymotic and petechial lesions (commonly on the palate), epistaxis and gingival bleeding. With platelet counts less than 50,000/mm³, prolonged bleeding should be anticipated. Local hemostatic measures are indicated for such patients, including some combination of direct pressure, primary closure, gelfoam, topical thrombin, microfibrillar collagen, and tranxemic acid. *Platelet transfusions* should be considered for patients with platelet counts below 30,000/mm³ before dental care is rendered.[20]

Question 1. Which of the following statements, if any, are correct?

A. The three most commonly used cancer therapies are surgery, chemotherapy, and radiation therapy.

B. Meticulous plaque control and fluoride therapy should be instituted as soon as possible after radiation therapy to prevent the onset of radiation caries.

C. Opportunistic oral infections, such as candidiasis and HSV, have characteristic appearances in BMT patients and thus can be diagnosed based on clinical examination.

D. Salivary substitutes are well accepted by patients with xerostomia.

E. Systemic immunosuppression is a common side effect of radiation therapy for head and neck cancer.

ACQUIRED IMMUNODEFICIENCY SYNDROME

Acquired immunodeficiency syndrome (AIDS) is an infectious disease in which lymphocytes, specifically T helper cells (T4), are invaded and impaired by a retrovirus, the human immunodeficiency virus (HIV). The subsequent decline in the T4 cell population results in immunosuppression, placing the host at risk for opportunistic infections and cancers. The virus is bloodborne and is transmitted through body fluids either via sexual contact or from exposure to a significant amount of blood, i.e. by the sharing of contaminated needles. Initially, the disease was most prevalent in the homosexual population; however, the incidence is increasing in the heterosexual and female populations.[81] Acquired immunodeficiency syndrome is projected to infect between 5 and 6 million persons worldwide by the year 2000.[82] Following initial infection with the virus, patients remain asymptomatic for years during a viral dormancy. Nearly all patients eventually develop symptoms that classically consist of opportunistic infections, such as *Pneumocystis carinii* pneumonia, candida esophagitis, toxoplasmosis, mycobacterial infections, and viral infections (HSV and CMV).[83–89] Patients with AIDS appear to be at risk for opportunistic infections when the T4 count drops *below 400* cells and the T4 to T8 ratio drops below 0.9. The most common malignancies associated with AIDS are *Kaposi's sarcoma* and *lymphoma.*[90] Patient mortality is nearly 100% and is the result of an opportunistic infection.[81]

Most of the opportunistic infections and cancers are manifested orally, allowing dental practitioners to play a major role in diagnosis, patient monitoring, and treatment. The immunosuppression in these patients is similar to that seen in BMT patients, and AIDS patients are victims of similar oral infections. *The most common oral infection is candidiasis,* which affects 75% of all AIDS patients at least once in the course of the disease. The appearance, diagnosis, and management of this infection was presented earlier in this chapter in the Cancer Treatment section. The high frequency of candidal infections in AIDS patients suggests that AIDS should be on the differential diagnosis of all patients with oral candidiasis. Although much less frequent, histoplasmosis is the next most common fungal infection among AIDS patients.[91–94] Herpes simplex infections affect 24% of all AIDS patients, presenting with the same atypical appearance described for chemotherapy patients.[95] The diagnosis and treatment of these lesions was also described previously. Other viral infections, such as cytomegalovirus (CMV) and varicella zoster (VZ), can occur and appear as indistinct ulcerations from which the virus can be cultured.[96] Antiviral agents, such as acyclovir and gancyclovir, are appropriate therapies. *Hairy leukoplakia* is a corrugated, white, raised lesion located on the ventral and lateral surfaces of the tongue. The leukoplakia cannot be wiped off and is thought to be caused by Epstein-Barr virus (EBV). The presence of this lesion appears to be an *accurate predictor of AIDS* as approximately 83% of patients who develop hairy leukoplakia are diagnosed with AIDS within 30 months. This benign lesion does not require treatment and can usually be diagnosed based on clinical appearance without the need for biopsy.[97] Aphthous ulcers are also common in AIDS patients and range from small, discrete lesions to large denuded areas. No etiologic agent can be identified on cytology or culture, and treatment is palliative (topical anesthetics).[98–101] Kaposi's sarcoma appears as a flat or raised, purple-to-brown lesion and occurs orally in 50% of all AIDS patients. The lesions are most commonly seen on the hard palate and when indicated, biopsy is suggested for definitive diagnosis. Treatment of these lesions is only needed when they interfere with patient function.[90]

Acute periodontal infections are also common in AIDS patients. HIV gingivitis appears as an erythematous band of inflammation on the marginal gingiva that does *not improve with oral hygiene measures.* HIV periodontitis is a rapidly progressive infection characterized by soft-tissue ulceration and necrosis, and loss of periodontal attachment. Clinically, the disease mimics acute necrotizing ulcerative gingivitis (ANUG). Present treatment recommendations include aggressive scaling and root planing combined with chlorhexidine therapy and antibiotics (Appendix 20–1). Early treatment of HIV gingivitis may prevent the development of HIV periodontitis.[102–104] The immunocompromised status of these patients requires the same aggressive preventive approach to caries and periodontal disease suggested for cancer patients. Potential sources of oral infection should be definitively treated to prevent the development of an oral infection that threatens the patient's systemic health.[105]

Question 2. Which of the following statements, if any, are correct?

A. Thrombocytopenia is a concern for dental practitioners treating AIDS patients.

B. Patients with AIDS need not worry about their periodontal health.

C. Hairy leukoplakia is a premalignant lesion in AIDS patients that requires aggressive treatment.

D. The most commonly occurring oral malignancy in AIDS patients is Kaposi's sarcoma.

E. The use of chlorhexidine is contraindicated in AIDS patients.

Renal Disease

Renal disease affects 3% of the U.S. population, of which more than 150,000 patients require routine renal dialysis and more than 40,000 are recipients of renal transplantations. Renal disease is divided into acute (ARF) and chronic renal failure (CRF), the causes of which include diabetes, hypertension, drug reactions, and obstruction. Because ARF is a medical emergency, patients with this problem are rarely encountered by the dental service. The two major treatments for CRF are *dialysis* and *kidney transplantation.* Dialysis is a palliative means of treatment in which metabolic waste is mechanically removed. This can be accomplished by either *hemodialysis* or *peritoneal dialysis.* Hemodialysis involves passing the patient's blood through a machine that extracts the waste using filters and osmotic gradients created by a dialysate (hyperosmolar solution). A surgical anastamosis of a *vein and an artery* in the forearm is created to provide a reusable, high-volume, vascular access to the dialysis unit. Three to 6 hour appointments, three times a week is required for hemodialysis, and the annual mortality rate is 10% to 15%. As such, hemodialysis is *not* a long-term solution to renal failure but is rather a maintenance therapy until renal transplantation is available. With peritoneal dialysis, the waste is extracted through the peritoneal capillaries by placing the dialysate in the peritoneum. Peritoneal dialysis is reserved for emergency situations, hemodynamically unstable patients, and for patients with poor vascular access. In contrast to dialysis, renal transplantation normalizes kidney function. The donor source for renal transplantation can be either cadavers or from a living relative (allogeneic). Allogeneic transplants are much more successful (80% compared with 30%), and immunosuppression is required following *all* organ transplantations to minimize organ rejection.[106]

Oral manifestations of renal failure and dialysis can include developmental disturbances, halitosis, stomatitis, dysesthesias, renal osteodystrophy, pallor from anemia, and signs of hemorrhage. The developmental disturbances can be enamel hypoplasia or intrinsic brown staining of the teeth secondary to uremia during tooth development. As such, these signs are expected only with congenital or early-onset renal failure. Halitosis and stomatitis are also uncommon findings because they result from elevations in salivary urea that occur with uncontrolled disease. Renal osteodystrophy is a florid display of bony irregularities including altered trabeculation, multilocular radiolucencies, areas of radiopacities, and loss of the lamina dura. This benign condition reflects irregularities in calcium and phosphate metabolism that results from renal failure. Anemia is caused by a decrease in red blood cell (RBC) production (erythropoietin is produced in the kidney) and from the destruction of RBCs during dialysis. The oral manifestation of anemia is mucosal pallor. The hemorrhagic tendency displayed by these patients reflects the *destruction of platelets* during dialysis, the *inhibition of platelet aggregation* by uremia, and the *anticoagulation* of the blood required during dialysis (heparin). Ecchymotic and petechial lesions or spontaneous gingival bleeding may be recognized. The incidence of caries and periodontal disease appears reduced in these patients secondary to an increase in salivary pH and the bacteriocidal effects of elevated urea levels in saliva.[106,107]

For the CRF patient on dialysis, dental care is recommended on the day *between* dialysis treatments. This avoids potential bleeding problems induced by heparin during dialysis. The duration of effect for heparin is 2 to 4 hours; therefore, dental care could also be administered 4 hours following the cessation of dialysis. Platelet counts and bleeding times are usually not needed prior to care because the hemorrhage tendency is usually controllable with local measures (hemostatic agents, pressure, and primary closure). With scaling and prophylaxis, it is important to remember that the intrinsic staining secondary to uremia cannot be removed. Hepatitis (HBV and HCV) is common among dialysis patients because of the need for repeated transfusions (RBCs or platelets) and the inability to completely sterilize the dialysis unit. Approximately 17% of all dialysis patients are HBV carriers. Hepatitis and AIDS profiles are routinely performed by the nephrologist, so a consultation is recommended to determine the patient's status. The use of universal infectious disease precautions should preclude the need to modify treatment relative to the infectiousness of these medical problems.[107–113]

Infection is the major cause of morbidity and mortality in CRF and renal transplant patients. For the CRF patients, 60% to 70% of the infections arise at the *access port,* and the access port is the patient's lifeline to dialysis. Therefore, care must be exercised by the practitioner to avoid traumatizing or infecting this vital structure. Recommendations include not using this arm to place the sphygmomanometer cuff and avoiding drawing blood from or injecting any parenteral fluids into this arm. Antibiotic prophylaxis has been suggested in these patients to avoid seeding of the access port by bacteremias during dental care. To date, only empirical support exists for this recommendation, and the American Heart Association (AHA) no longer stresses coverage for these patients. As such, the decision concerning antibiotic prophylaxis should be jointly made between the dental practitioner and the nephrologist. If antibiotic prophylaxis is desired, then the AHA guidelines (Appendix 20–3) should be followed. A simple way of achieving antibiotic coverage is to have the nephrologist give the patient intravenous vancomycin at the time of dialysis. In dialysis patients, the duration of parenteral vancomycin is approximately 5 to 7 days, giving the practitioner ample time to perform the needed dentistry. Potentially nephrotoxic drugs to avoid are tetracycline, streptomycin, gentamicin, phenacetin, meperidine, and nonsteroidal antiinflammatory agents.[106]

Infection remains the major concern in renal failure patients following renal transplantation because of the immunosuppressive drugs used to minimize organ rejection. Although the degree of immunosuppression is not as severe as that seen with chemotherapy and BMT, the concerns about oral infection, candidiasis, and recurrent HSV infection are the same. The incidence of HSV infection recurrence following renal transplantation is reported to be between 15% and 50% in seropositive patients. Patient education should ensure that the patient understands the relationship between oral disease and their immunosuppression. These patients should be followed on a short recall schedule, and attention to routine oral hygiene measures should be frequently encouraged. White blood cell counts are routinely maintained by the nephrologist for reference. Antibiotics are recommended following oral surgery to minimize the chance of an oral infection developing. Because renal function is normalized following

transplantation, treatment concerns reviewed in the CRF patient are not an issue. A new concern in the posttransplantation patient is *gingival hypertrophy* secondary to use of certain immunosuppressive medications (ie, cyclosporine) and calcium channel blockers (verapamil, diltiazem, nifedipine). The incidence of gingival hypertrophy for patients on cyclosporine is 30%. This side effect can be minimized with scrupulous oral hygiene, and a gingivectomy can be performed in cases of marked hypertrophy.[114] Finally, because glucocorticoids are frequently used as immunosuppressive agents following organ transplantation, adrenal insufficiency and stress management must be considered with invasive procedures and anxious patients. Doubling of the glucocorticoid dose is recommended prior to treatment in the aforementioned cases.[106–115]

Question 3. Which of the following statements, if any, are correct?

A. Thrombocytopenia is a concern for dental practitioners treating renal failure patients on hemodialysis.
B. Accelerated caries and periodontal disease are manifestations of renal failure.
C. Antibiotic prophylaxis should be considered prior to treatment of hemodialysis patients.
D. Dialysis normalizes renal function.
E. The prominent concern for patients following renal transplantation is their enhanced susceptibility to infection due to immunosuppression.

The Patient with Cardiovascular Disease

Cardiovascular disease (CVD) embraces a varied array of cardiac pathologies. Generally, CVD can be subdivided into ischemic heart disease (IHD) and myocardial infarction (MI), hypertension, valvular and congenital heart disease, dysrhythmias, congestive heart failure (CHF), and cardiac transplantation. Cardiovascular disease is the *leading cause of death* in the United States, responsible for twice as many deaths as cancer. It is also the most frequent cause of sudden death, of which dysrhythmias are the major contributor. Irrespective of the underlying cardiovascular problem, understanding the patient's stress tolerance is essential prior to dental care. Assessing the need for antibiotic prophylaxis and additional measures of hemorrhage control are also important concerns. Stress tolerance is a gauge of a patient's cardiac reserve, or the ability of the heart to sustain additional stress. Patients with poor cardiac reserve include those with severe hypertension, uncontrolled CHF, severe dysrhythmias, unstable angina, those having suffered a myocardial infarction within 6 months and persons experiencing cardiac instability following cardiac transplantation. Severe hypertension is characterized by a diastolic blood pressure greater than *115* mm Hg or a systolic blood pressure greater than *200* mm Hg. Poorly controlled CHF is defined by the presence of tachycardia, tachypnea, or hemodynamic instability (blood pressure). Severe dysrhythmias include any ventricular dysrhythmias (frequent or multiformed premature ventricular contractions, ventricular tachycardia, and third-degree heart block) and hemodynamically unstable, supraventricular dysrhythmias (atrial flutter, atrial fibrillation, or atrial tachycardia associated with hypotension or hypertension). Unstable angina is defined by either new-onset angina, pain at rest, pain that is poorly controlled with medication, or pain that has recently changed character.[116,117]

For patients with poor cardiac reserve, a vasoconstrictor should be avoided in the local anesthetic, electrocardiography and vital signs monitoring are essential, and the dental care should be delivered in a controlled environment such as an operating room. All other CVD patients are considered stable or to have a good cardiac reserve in the absence of critical signs and symptoms or a confluence of cardiovascular problems. Electrocardiography and vital signs monitoring in these patients is left to the practitioner's discretion; however, a vasoconstrictor is appropriate in patients with stable CVD because the effect of exogenous epinephrine on vital signs is minimal. *Prophylactic nitroglycerin* given prior to the dental appointment can help prevent an angina attack in patients who experience frequent angina.[116,117]

Stress management is also an essential consideration for cardiovascular patients who are anxious about dental visits. Effective stress management begins with patient rapport, although oral, inhalational, or parenteral sedation is commonly indicated. Supplemental oxygen is also suggested for the anxious patient. The appropriate stress management approach should be determined by the stressfulness of the procedure and the patient's level of anxiety. Dental practitioners should encourage all CVD patients to maintain behaviors that minimize disease risk factors, such as smoking, high-fat diets, lack of exercise, and stress.[116,117]

Patients with valvular heart disease, prosthetic valves, and unrepaired congenital defects, and those who have undergone cardiac transplantation are candidates for antibiotic prophylaxis prior to dental procedures involving bleeding.[118] The American Heart Association's (AHA) recommendations concerning candidates for antibiotic prophylaxis and suggested antibiotics are listed in Appendices 20–3 and 20–4.[119] These recommendations are based on the recognition that dental care can cause transient bacteremias and that some of the oral microorganisms have been identified in infections of the heart endothelium (this infection is termed bacterial endocarditis). The standard regimen (Appendix 20–3) can be used for all high-risk patients, although alternative parenteral regimens are available when deemed necessary. When the need for antibiotic prophylaxis cannot be accurately determined, empirical prophylaxis is recommended until the necessity can be confirmed.

Gingival hyperplasia is an additional concern in CVD patients who are taking calcium channel blockers and in posttransplantation patients taking certain immunosuppressants. Patients at risk for this development need to exercise more fastidious oral hygiene, and gingivectomies should be performed if the gingival hyperplasia becomes clinically significant. For patients on multiple agents known to cause this side effect, gingival hyperplasia can develop rapidly, requiring a gingivectomy every 3 to 6 months.[114]

Bleeding is an additional concern for CVD patients on anticoagulant therapy (warfarin). Anticoagulants are needed to prevent clotting in patients prone to blood stasis from such conditions as atrial fibrillation, but this type of medication is needed predominantly by patients with prosthetic heart valves. Generally, prothrombin times (PT) are routinely (monthly) performed on these patients and can be obtained from the patients' cardiologists. Patients with PT values within $1\frac{1}{2}$ to 2 times normal can be treated using the local hemostatic measures previously listed. Higher PT values require either a decrease in warfarin (Coumadin) dosage, stopping warfarin administration, or converting the warfarin to heparin. This decision must be made in conjunction with the patient's cardiologist. An aggressive approach to preventive dental care that re-

duces oral sources of infection and minimizes the need for dental treatment is recommended for patients prior to and after heart valve replacement and for heart transplant candidates. Both types of patients are at risk for endocarditis from oral infections, and the patient with a prosthetic heart valve requires modulation of the anticoagulant before invasive dental care.[116]

As with other organ transplant patients, the cardiac transplant patient is prone to oral infections and opportunistic infections, such as candidiasis and recurrent HSV infection. The incidence of HSV recurrence following cardiac transplantation is reported to be around 25% in seropositive patients. *Patient education* should ensure that patients understand the relationship between the presence of oral disease and their immunosuppression. These patients should be followed on a *short recall schedule* and attention to routine *oral hygiene* measures should be frequently encouraged. White blood cell counts are routinely maintained by the cardiologist for reference. Antibiotics are recommended following oral surgery to minimize the chance of an oral infection developing. Cardiac function may or may not be normalized following transplantation, therefore treatment concerns reviewed in the cardiac patient cannot be ignored. As with the renal transplant patient, gingival hypertrophy from *immunosuppressive medications* and *calcium channel blockers* and *adrenal insufficiency* from gluocorticosteroids are new concerns. Patient care should follow the guidelines listed following renal transplantation.[116]

In the past, patients with prosthetic joints were considered candidates for antibiotic prophylaxis for dental care associated with bleeding. This recommendation is based on retrospective case reports in the absence of investigations confirming a causative relationship between oral bacteremias and joint infections. The AHA no longer suggests antibiotic coverage for these patients. Because the offending organism (*Staphylococcus aureus*) in joint infections is not a common oral inhabitant and in the face of scientific evidence that fails to show a relationship between dental care and joint infections, antibiotic prophylaxis cannot be recommended for these patients. Practitioners concerned about this advice should consult the patient's orthopedic surgeon.[116]

Question 4. Which of the following statements, if any, are correct?

A. Patients needing subgingival scaling and curettage are priority candidates for antibiotic prophylaxis.

B. It is recommended that the glucocorticoid dose be halved prior to dental treatment on an anxious cardiac transplant patient who is taking a glucocorticosteroids.

C. Opportunistic infections are a concern for dental patients with ischemic heart disease.

D. Vasoconstrictors are contraindicated in patients with unstable angina and in patients with poorly compensated congestive heart failure.

E. Patients with prosthetic joints should be treated with antibiotic prophylaxis prior to dental care involving gingival bleeding.

Diabetics

Approximately 15 million Americans are estimated to be afflicted with diabetes, and only half of these individuals have an established diagnosis. Although a common disorder, the multiple and protean symptoms associated with diabetes hinder an early diagnosis. Nevertheless, every health care worker must remain alert to the disease's manifestations because an early diagnosis is

associated with less severe disease complications. Dentists and hygienists should be especially alert because they regularly encounter a large segment of the population.[120,121]

Diabetes mellitus, the *most common endocrine disorder*, is an abnormality in glucose metabolism associated with either a decrease in insulin production, a deficit in insulin receptors, or an error in insulin metabolism. Whatever the cause, the result is an inadequate supply of insulin to meet physiologic needs. *Type I* diabetes, also termed *insulin-dependent diabetes mellitus* (IDDM), results from the destruction of pancreatic beta cells. The pathophysiology is thought to involve autoimmune and virally mediated processes that lead to inadequate insulin production. This type of diabetes mellitus is one tenth as common as type II and develops early in life. Patients are generally physically thin, and ketosis is a common finding. By definition, supplemental insulin therapy is required to manage this type of diabetes. *Type II* diabetes, also termed *non-insulin-dependent diabetes mellitus* (NIDDM), results from defects in either the insulin molecule or the insulin receptors. As such, glucose metabolism is impaired due to insulin dysfunction rather than underproduction. This type of diabetes develops later in life, is associated with obesity, and does not result in ketosis. Patient treatment commonly requires dietary modifications, oral hypoglycemic agents or both. Supplemental insulin can also be required in the treatment of type II diabetes, although this is uncommon.[120,121]

The oral signs and symptoms of diabetes can include xerostomia, parotid gland enlargement, gingival hyperplasia, rapid alveolar bone loss, burning or numbness of the oral tissues, and oral infections (ie, multiple or recurrent periodontal abscesses and facial cellulitis). In addition, the caries rate may be increased and wound healing may be delayed following surgery or trauma. Generally these symptoms occur more quickly and are more severe in IDDM than in NIDDM cases. The xerostomia may result from the basic disease process or be a manifestation of systemic osmotic diuresis. As with radiation caries, the xerostomia can predispose patients to both caries and periodontal disease by enhancing plaque accumulation, increasing the glucose content in saliva and crevicular fluid, and decreasing the saliva's buffering capacity. Microangiopathies in the periodontal tissue, decreased collagen synthesis, nephropathy-induced hyperparathyroidism, and blunted polymorphonuclear leukocyte (PMN) chemotaxis and phagocytosis may also contribute to accelerated periodontitis by reducing the host's resistance to infection. Although numerous case reports have suggested that undiagnosed and uncontrolled diabetes makes patients susceptible to accelerated periodontal disease, investigations in known diabetic populations have been conflicting. On balance, the evidence suggests that the incidence and severity of marginal gingivitis increases in young patients with IDDM, especially those with severe systemic complications or poor metabolic control. Severe periodontal destruction appears to be more common in adult diabetics with advanced systemic complications. Conversely, meticulous control of infections (including periodontal disease) can be essential to establishing adequate metabolic control of diabetes in some patients. It has been demonstrated that insulin requirements can be reduced in some diabetic patients following periodontal therapy and after the extraction of hopeless teeth. As such, proper patient motivation and compliance with oral home care regimens may be important in the control of both oral diseases and diabetes mellitus.[120–124]

Dental care of the diabetic patient encompasses both the detection of undiagnosed disease and the treatment of patients once disease has been diagnosed. Detection of undiagnosed or poorly controlled diabetes can be made based on elicited signs and symptoms from a medical history, patient observation, and on a blood glucose screening test. In the hospital and in the dental office, the use of dry reagent strips with a reflectance meter is an adequate method for screening occult diabetes and for monitoring known diabetes prior to dental procedures. The procedure is simple and accurate, and the equipment is inexpensive. When evidence arises of undiagnosed or poorly controlled disease, dental practitioners should refer the patient to a physician for evaluation.

Intraoffice blood glucose monitoring is also recommended for controlled diabetes prior to and following dental procedures that impair or restrict such patients' oral intake. The most common examples include diabetic patients who are required to have nothing by mouth (NPO) prior to pharmacosedation and patients who are having surgical procedures that restrict postoperative eating.[120]

Irrespective of the type of diabetes, it is important to communicate the interrelationship between patients' systemic disease and their oral health. Patients should understand that the diabetes may increase the severity of oral diseases and thereby require that closer attention be paid to oral hygiene measures. In addition, patients should comprehend that inattention to oral health and subsequent development of oral infections can complicate the management of their systemic disease.[120,121]

Patients with NIDDM and with well-controlled IDDM can be treated essentially the same as nondiabetics for routine dental procedures. *Early morning appointments are preferred* because endogenous corticosteroid levels are highest at this time, allowing patients to be more stress-tolerant. In addition, this timing allows patients to eat a normal breakfast and is least likely to interfere with medication regimens. At this time, patients are also more likely to be hyperglycemic than hypoglycemic, which is the preferred deviation from the norm. Concerning the use of local anesthetics, epinephrine release is associated with inducing hyperglycemia, and epinephrine-containing local anesthetics have been shown to elevate blood glucose levels by 30 to 40 mg/dL. The amount of epinephrine in local anesthetics is small, however, compared with the quantity available for endogenous release. Because stress promotes the endogenous release of both catecholamines and glucocorticoids, both of which induce hyperglycemia, patient anxiety is of greater concern than is the exogenous administration of epinephrine. As such, it is not necessary to avoid the use of a vasoconstrictor in the local anesthetic.[120]

If pharmacosedation is indicated, short midmorning appointments are advised. When patients are required to be NPO prior to the sedation or when eating will be hampered following the dental procedure, the patient's diet and medication requires special attention. Consultation with the patient's endocrinologist is advised to determine the preferred method of drug and diet modification[120].

Hospitalization should be considered for patients with "brittle" diabetes (ie, hyperglycemia poorly controlled by insulin) and for all diabetics requiring insulin or oral hyperglycemic agents, whose oral intake will be reduced for a prolonged period. Both of these groups of patients are at a high risk for hyperglycemia and may be best treated in an environment allowing close monitoring and adjustment of blood glucose levels.

The following guidelines are suggested for the use of antibiotics and glucocorticoids. Antibiotic recommendations are based on the presence of infection, the severity of the patient's diabetes, and the invasiveness of the dental procedure. Antibiotics should accompany definitive management of cellulitic infections in all diabetic patients. Antibiotics are also recommended following invasive surgery for all patients with IDDM. Antibiotic type, dosage, and administrative regimen are the same as those recommended for nondiabetic patients (Appendix 20–1). These empirical recommendations reflect the diabetic patient's susceptibility to infections, the relationship between infections and the systemic disease, and the patient's propensity for delayed healing. The use of glucocorticoids to control postoperative swelling (ie, following third-molar surgery) is contraindicated in IDDM secondary to the hyperglycemic effects of steroids. In addition, dental practitioners should avoid using intramuscular injections of any medication in diabetics with significant peripheral disease. The impaired peripheral vascularity predisposes these patients to peripheral infections, which can be induced by intramuscular injections.[120]

Xerostomia in diabetic patients is usually secondary to the dehydrational effects of the disease process itself. As such, xerostomia suggests that the patient's hyperglycemia is out of control, and the appropriate therapy is to better manage the patient's systemic disease. Recognized dental therapies for xerostomia (ie, replacement and stimulation therapy) in these patients are not indicated. The management of advanced periodontal disease or a high caries incidence in diabetic patients is similar to that in nondiabetic patients. Patient education, short recall visits, and the use of supplemental fluoride and chlorhexidine are potential treatment modifications. These suggestions are in addition to routine therapies for caries and periodontal disease.[120–124]

Question 5. Which of the following statements, if any, are correct?

A. Diabetes mellitus renders patients more susceptible to oral infection.
B. The use of systemic glucocorticoids to reduce postoperative swelling following oral surgery is contraindicated in diabetic patients.
C. Dental practitioners have a significant role to play in the recognition of undiagnosed diabetes.
D. Periodontal disease may be accelerated in certain diabetics.
E. The use of a vasoconstrictor in a local anesthetic is contraindicated in diabetics because of the drug's potential for inducing hyperglycemia.

Physically and Mentally Handicapped Patients

An estimated 150,000 paraplegics and quadriplegics live in the United States, with about 11,000 new cases of spinal cord injury occurring every year.[12,125] These and other handicapped individuals, including those who suffer strokes, often have difficulty learning how to care for their mouths.[126] These patients also suffer from a significantly higher prevalence of oral disease risk factors, such as poorer dietary habits, increases in plaque and calculus, and a greater incidence of mucosal lesions. Gingival hypertrophy is also a common oral finding in these patients because many are taking antiseizure medications (phenytoin) known to cause this complication. Should oral hygiene efforts fail to control gingival growth, a gingivectomy may be performed to correct the problem. The use of chlorhexidine and fluoride oral sprays have been assessed in physically and mentally handicapped patients and in the elderly. The sprays usually consisted of 0.2% chlorhexidine and 0.2% stannous fluoride applied twice a day without other oral hygiene measures. Results have been mixed; however, most investigations suggest a decrease in plaque and gingivitis and in oral bacterial counts.[127–132] A 1% chlorhexidine gel has also been evaluated and showed a decrease in cariogenic bacterial counts for 3 weeks following a 1-week application. The gel may also be more effective than chlorhexidine rinses and sprays at decreasing plaque and gingivitis.[133] For many of these patients (moderate to severely handicapped), daily oral hygiene measures must be completed for the patient. The mild to moderately handicapped can usually perform tooth brushing with assistance. Commonly, a toothbrush with a modified handle that allows a full palm grip, gives the patient better control and improves brushing efficacy.

The paraplegic in a Stryker frame should receive oral hygiene care in an upright position. Suction and an assistant should be available to help in the cleaning process. The patient in such a frame may also take water through a straw and expectorate through the straw into an emesis basin. It is desirable to use a toothbrush fitted with a saliva ejector attached to a hole bored in the brush head and connected to a suction device. An ingestible toothpaste may be used to minimize the need for expectoration. If the auxiliary is working alone or the patient is only partially disabled, an electric toothbrush is helpful. As recovery progresses, the patient should be encouraged to participate in personal oral health care, with support and encouragement provided by the auxiliary, who may be needed to complete the task. Patience on the part of the auxiliary is *essential* during this recovery phase.

Staff members of the University of Mississippi School of Dentistry have developed and tested a dental care unit with an automatic toothbrushing apparatus that can be operated by people unable to control their hands[125] (Fig 20–5). This device allows handicapped people, such as C-3 quadriplegics, stroke victims, arthritic patients, and motor-impaired individuals, to independently dispense fluoride, toothpaste and water, look in a mirror, brush their teeth, clean their mouths, and expectorate. All of these components are clustered in an arrangement that permits unsupervised use with minimal motion. The toothbrushes, bent in several angles, can be selected by an individual from a foam block and inserted into the head of the power unit. A head-operated toggle switch activates the automatic brush.

Patients with double or single amputations can use the electric toothbrush with or without modifications to fit into the patient's prosthesis. For patients with a single hand or arm amputation, every encouragement should be given to developing a suitable dexterity in the other hand. For those patients who have lost fingers or who have severe arthritis or sclerotic disease of the hand, modified devices can provide a better handgrip for a toothbrush or floss holder (Fig 20–6). A hair dryer or an optical-shop glass-bead bath may be used to alter the angle of the plastic toothbrush shaft to suit individual needs.[125] The nylon bristles, however, must be shielded from the heat to prevent deformation. Other modifications can range from a bicycle handgrip to a simple styrofoam Christmas ball in which toothbrush handles are inserted or attached by adhesives.

Frequent recalls for prophylaxis are necessary to ensure interproximal cleaning. Frequent fluoride rinses are indicated to help remove food debris as well as to aid in caries control.

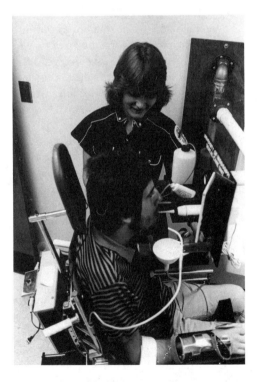

Figure 20–5. A paraplegic receiving initial instructions in the use of the University of Mississippi Dental Care Unit. The wall-mounted unit features custom-angle toothbrushes, adjustable mirror, and easily accessible head-activated switch. (*Courtesy of Eric H. Rommerdale, Jackson, Mississippi.*)

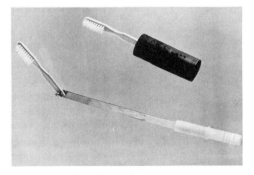

Figure 20–6. Improvised toothbrushes—one for limited arm motion and one for limited finger motion.

Facial Fractures and the Comatose Patient

Maxillary and mandibular fractures are commonly encountered on otolaryngology, oral and maxillofacial surgery, plastic surgery, and orthopedic services. Many of these cases are still managed with intermaxillary fixation, in which the maxilla is wired to the mandible to maintain the correct occlusion and assist in fracture reduction. This therapy lasts for weeks and is a great barrier to oral hygiene efforts.[134] Interproximal tooth surfaces are at greatest risk for caries, because flossing is prohibited by the intraoral hardware. Preventive self-care consists of restricting the intake of sugar products and the use of a fluoride mouth rinse prior to and following meals. Increasing the frequency of fluoride rinsing elevates the fluoride concentration in interproximal plaque, thereby better protecting the teeth against demineralization. A soft toothbrush should be used, employing the Johnson "pick-and-poke" brushing method. This technique uses the bristles of the toothbrush, especially those on the toe, like a toothpick to probe and disturb the plaque.[135] Irrigating devices can also assist in removing the larger interproximal debris.

Comatose patients present an unusual challenge to dental practitioners because of their inability to communicate or follow commands. Caution should be observed in performing oral hygiene for these patients because they are unable to voluntarily control their oral movements. Many of these patients engage in repetitive oral dyskinesias consisting of bruxism and lip biting. A padded tongue blade or, preferably, a mouth prop is essential to keep the patient's mouth open while performing oral hygiene. Such patients can be made to open their mouth by either pinching their nostrils or by placing significant bilateral pressure on the masseter muscles. Conversation should be maintained with all comatose patients because they can be aware of external events. Comatose patients do possess pain reflexes, therefore, a yawn or a groan may signify discomfort. All of these patients should have an oral exam at bedside, with special attention paid to opportunistic infections such as candidiasis. Scaling should be completed by the practitioner, and nurses or nurses aides should follow up with daily brushing. Chlorhexidine and fluoride applications should also be performed to minimize gingival inflammation and caries development. In cases of lip biting, oral appliances can be fabricated that protect the lip and tongue from mutilation.

Psychiatric Patients

The average general hospital does not normally retain patients for long periods who have mild or moderate psychologic disorders. Those admitted for evaluation of psychologic dysfunction are usually treated with appropriate psychotropic or neuroleptic drugs. Therefore, motivation of any kind, especially toward preventive dentistry, is practically nonexistent. Eating and sleeping take precedence over personal hygiene, and oral hygiene is almost always lacking. The challenge to the dental practitioner is to stimulate patient motivation often under hostile circumstances. With some of these patients, a childlike relationship can be established. A child is not interested in how plaque is formed, nor the techniques of brushing and flossing needed for its removal. As is true with children, some psychiatric patients can be helped to understand that oral hygiene is something that needs to be done every day. The *need* for clean teeth can sometimes be developed by emphasizing a better, fresher taste, a nicer smile, or a better appreciation for food. The first visit should be kept short and the practitioner should offer a great deal of verbal encouragement and extend a reward, such as a new toothbrush, sugar-free treats, or a colorful poster. The patient's first impression may be the only one remembered, because such patients are usually transferred to a permanent facility for extended treatment for the underlying mental condition. Xerostomia is a common oral finding in the mentally ill secondary to antipsychotic, antidepressant, and anticholinergic medications. Substance abuse and medicolegal competency represent additional concerns for the dental practitioner.[136]

Once an individual is admitted to a psychiatric institution, the two most effective and realistic approaches to caries control are (1) *water fluoridation* and (2) *curtailment of sugar intake by careful planning of the master diet.* These two methods of caries control are relatively easy and economical to implement throughout the institution, regardless of patient cooperation.

PRENATAL AND POSTNATAL MATERNAL COUNSELING

All hospital obstetric services should develop a positive referral system to ensure that expectant mothers receive a dental examination, preventive dentistry counseling, and necessary treatment. The referral may be to the hospital dental service or, in the event that such a service is not available for outpatient care, the patient's private dentist should be asked to provide feedback to the obstetrician, indicating completion of the primary, secondary, and tertiary preventive dentistry treatment plans.

At the time the pregnancy is established an expectant mother is exposed to a barrage of information about her health and that of her unborn child. At the time of the primary preventive dentistry counseling session, a knowledgeable dental professional should be the source of the essential information. Major education and counseling emphasis for the mother-to-be should focus on meticulous plaque control, dietary discipline, and fluoride therapy. The purpose of this emphasis is to reduce the risk and progression of caries and periodontal disease throughout gestation. This risk also appears to carry over into the postnatal period. Mothers with mouths highly infected with mutans streptococci tend to have children with mouths that are also highly infected, and mothers with minimal infection have children with a similar pattern.[137,138]

Dental counseling should come early, because the first trimester of pregnancy is a critical time. All organ systems, including bones and teeth, are formed during this period. Tooth buds begin formation at the 4th to 5th week of gestation followed by initial mineralization from the 9th to 12th week. Stress applied to the fetus at this time can produce dental and oral deformities. For example, a cleft lip or palate results when the maxilla fails to unite between the fourth to sixth weeks. This can be caused by a variety of factors, such as genetics, the stress of an injury, severe viral infections, or alcohol toxicity. Excessive stress to the fetus at any crucial time in development can result in a *temporary but irreparable arrest* in cellular growth.

Proper nutrition during pregnancy is essential. Although nutritional deficiencies in the mother must be severe to affect the unborn child, a daily balanced diet containing basic proteins, fats, carbohydrates, vitamins, and minerals is necessary. This requirement can usually be met by adequate intake from the six basic foods in the U.S. Department of Agriculture's Food Guide Pyramid, although the obstetrician may prescribe nutritional supplements.

A pregnant woman is often at greater risk for caries development. The mother's teeth do not lose calcium because the mother's bones and the calcium she ingests in her diet form the reserve of calcium for use by the developing child. Instead, tooth decay may increase because of changes in eating habits during pregnancy. For example, the sucking of hard candy to reduce nausea, dietary cravings, and frequent between-meal snacks of refined carbohydrates can raise the caries potential of the dental plaque. In addition, the mother often experiences nausea or "morning sickness," causing vomiting or a regurgitation of stomach acid with a resultant acid erosion or demineralization on the *lingual surfaces* of the teeth. Many times only a toothbrush or a sudsy dentifrice is needed to trigger the gag reflex.

Avoiding bad eating habits and snacking, as well as exercising sugar discipline can greatly minimize the possibility of caries development. If the mother is living in a non-fluoride area, fluoride supplements should be considered during gestation. Several studies have shown a beneficial systemic effect on the teeth of the developing child from the mother drinking fluoridated water. These studies report a decrease in caries incidence in children born to mothers taking fluoride compared with siblings born during periods when the mother was not taking a fluoride supplement.[139] Because fluoride supplements only bring the level of fluoride intake to 1 ppm (a level ingested daily by more than 100 million Americans), no danger of excessive dosage exists. In addition, the expectant mother should be provided with professional topical fluoride applications at appropriate treatment and recall appointments during the pregnancy. These topical applications should be supplemented daily by home use of fluoride dentifrices and mouth rinses. These measures both *prevent demineralization* of teeth and *facilitate remineralization*.

As the obvious physiologic changes of pregnancy take place, less obvious but important changes in the woman's metabolism are often reflected in changes in the oral soft tissues. Gingival tissues may become red and swollen, bleed easily, and lead to *pregnancy gingivitis*. This type of gingivitis cannot be differentiated from that induced by plaque. During pregnancy, a woman's gingival tissues appear to have an exaggerated response to dental plaque. Suggested reasons for this are an increase in gingival estrogen metabolism or an increase in the production of gingival prostaglandins.[140] Pregnancy gingivitis can be prevented and controlled by adequate plaque control measures. Unfortunately, once a slight amount of bleeding occurs, many patients are reluctant to use a toothbrush or dental floss to avoid further bleeding.

After the first trimester of pregnancy some women develop a well-defined soft-tissue swelling adjacent to the necks of the teeth. The mass, sometimes called a *pregnancy tumor* (Fig 20–7), is a benign, exuberant overgrowth of highly vascular connective

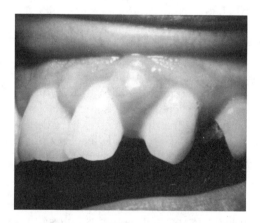

Figure 20–7. "Pregnancy tumor" (pyogenic granuloma) occurring in the interproximal gingival tissues between the maxillary left lateral incisor and cuspid. The woman was in her third month of pregnancy.

tissue, more accurately termed a *pyogenic granuloma.* The lesion is frequently sore, and the pain increases with chewing. Pregnancy tumors do not spontaneously heal after delivery unless the oral hygiene practices established throughout the pregnancy are continued following childbirth.[141] Lesions that do not resolve should be excised by a dentist.

An early appointment for dental examination and possible treatment is indicated when the pregnancy is confirmed. Many pregnant women are already long overdue for dental care and postponement for 9 additional months could cause severe problems. Dental x-ray films taken for emergencies may be necessary but should be avoided whenever possible during the first trimester. If x-ray films are taken at any time, careful gonadal and abdominal shielding is required (as with all dental patients). Emergency dental care is appropriate at any point during pregnancy, although nonemergency care should be completed in the second trimester. Teratogenetic effects are the major concern during the first trimester, and the risk of spontaneous delivery and discomfort associated with the position of the baby are concerns during in the third trimester.[140]

INFANT ORAL CARE

Some research studies have demonstrated that caries incidence is lower in breast-fed children, whereas other investigations have come to the same conclusion for children who were bottle-fed.[142] Either position can be adequately defended. One of the first major hazards to the child's primary dentition is *"baby-bottle tooth decay"* (BBTD).[143] This condition, which is also called *nursing-bottle caries, nursing-bottle mouth, baby-bottle syndrome,* and *bottle-mouth caries,* is

highlighted by rampant dental caries of the maxillary incisors.[143–146] This problem results from continual, prolonged exposure of the primary teeth to milk, sugar- and carbohydrate-containing infant formula, fruit juices, or soft drinks placed in the nursing bottle. This type of caries can also occur in some breast-fed children who are fed every time the infant indicates a desire for feeding (demand feeding); however, the lactose contained in breast milk does not act as rapidly as refined sugars in producing dental caries. The loss of teeth from nursing-bottle caries can have far-reaching effects on the child's facial growth.[147]

Because none of the primary teeth erupt before the first year, the acidogenic capabilities of the oral bacteria prior to that time are of only academic interest. Once the teeth erupt, however, the dental plaque forms, and all acidogenic bacteria pose a threat. It is at this time that the ingestion of any sugar-containing fluids, especially at nap or bedtime, is especially deleterious, because salivary flow and the frequency of swallowing decrease with drowsiness and sleep. This permits a pooling of the fluids around the upper maxillary teeth, which are the teeth most affected by this behavior.[144,145,147] During suckling of the nipple (either bottle or breast), the tongue lies over the lower incisors, which diverts the sweetened liquid against the upper incisors and back over the palate. The lower incisors often are either completely intact or only slightly affected, whereas the upper incisors bear the brunt of the repeated acid attacks. The other primary teeth are involved to various degrees, depending on the sucking habits of the infant.

The BBTD begins with the appearance of white areas of demineralization around the gingival third of the teeth. With time these incipient lesions begin to turn brown as active caries progresses. Eventually, the carious lesions that ring the cervical areas of the teeth can result in entire crowns being lost, either by fracture of the undermined enamel or by the continuous action of the caries. In either event, only the exposed root is left in the alveolus (Fig 20–8).

According to a joint policy statement issued by the American Academy of Pediatric Dentistry and the American Academy of Pediatrics, nursing-bottle caries can be avoided if (1) milk in a bottle is not used as a pacifier at nap or bedtime, (2) milk bottle feeding is discontinued as soon as possible after the first birthday, and (3) juice is always offered from a cup.[146,148]

Unfortunately, most children don't usually visit the dentist until about age 3, when primary prevention of baby bottle caries is no longer possible. Many parents, when informed of the cause of the condition, express dismay that they were unaware of the dangers of unregulated intake of sugar solutions.[149,150] Most parents believe they are showing love and affection by offering their child sweet drinks. The main problem is one of ignorance, as very few parents would knowingly cause their children's teeth to be damaged.

A pacifier is preferable to putting a baby to bed with a bottle, but if the bottle is used, it should be filled with water. As a safety consideration, the pacifier should be of one-piece construction, so that parts cannot separate and possibly cause choking. Furthermore, the pacifier's shape should anatomically duplicate the mother's nipple, which avoids malformation of the dental arches. For this reason, any pacifier is preferable to children sucking their thumb or fingers. Weaning the child from a pacifier should not be a major concern as peer pressure usually discourages continued use.

The educational process can probably best begin with the obstetrician and pediatrician explaining to the expectant or recent parents, the cause and consequences of continued intake of sugared fluids. The physician can further aid in reducing the problem by prescribing those bottle formulas that contain the least sugar. The amount of sugar found in the various commercially available baby foods varies considerably. Finally, the dental profession should emphasize the need for high school and community based dental education programs to alert would-be parents of their dental responsibilities in infant care. In 1986, the American Academy of Pediatric Dentistry stated, "*Infant dental care begins with dental health counseling for the newborn, which should include a dental office visit for preventive oral health counseling no later than 12 months of age.*"[146]

Early Dental Care

The newborn should become accustomed to oral care as early as possible.[146] After feeding, the ridges where the teeth will later appear and the palate should be gently wiped with gauze or a soft washcloth. This

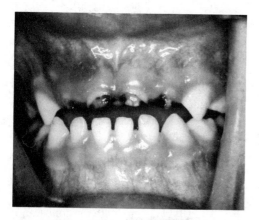

Figure 20–8. Nursing bottle caries in a child affecting the maxillary primary anterior teeth. (*Courtesy of Dr James E. McIlwain, Tampa, Florida.*)

removes leftover food and establishes a routine for the mother to clean inside the child's mouth. Throughout childhood, parents should directly supervise oral hygiene care. It is recommended that a child visit the dental office as early as possible after the first year of life. The purpose of this initial visit is to evaluate the mouth and jaws for proper formation and alignment of structures. A secondary but equally important objective is to allow the child to become familiar with the dental office under pleasant circumstances and to prevent any future apprehension.

If water fluoridation is not available, parents should be informed that small daily dosages of fluoride, starting at birth, are beneficial to the child's teeth. Following birth, the child should receive fluoride drops to bring the daily intake to 1 ppm, corrected for both weight and the average annual temperature of the area (Table 20–1). Around the age of 3 years, the drops can be replaced by fluoride tablets, which are swallowed. Later, as the child gains skill in chewing the tablet, the fluoride-laden saliva can be swished around the mouth to provide topical as well as systemic benefits. The practice of using a tablet a day should continue until the child is at least 12 years old. When primary teeth begin to erupt, a parent can moisten a small gauze with a commercial fluoride mouth rinse to provide a daily topical application. Later, the child can use a small toothbrush to clean the teeth and mouth. In one study almost half the parents started toothbrushing programs for their infants at 12 months and 75% by 18 months. At this age only a small amount of a dentifrice with a low-fluoride content, (approximately *the size of a small pea*,) should be used to avoid the possibility of ingesting an excess of fluoride. There is mounting concern about the possibility of increasing the

TABLE 20–1. DAILY FLUORIDE (F) DOSAGE RECOMMENDATIONS*

Fl° Content of Drinking Water	0–2 Years	2–3 Years	3–14 Years
0.0–0.3 ppm	0.25 mg	0.50 mg	1.00 mg
0.3–0.7 ppm	0.00 mg	0.25 mg	0.50 mg

*Approved by the Council on Dental Therapeutics of the American Dental Association. *Accepted Dental Therapeutics,* 40th ed. 1984:401.
Note: Research and dental public health officials are currently discussing the desirability of lowering the dosage of daily fluoride supplements to curtail the increasing prevalence of *mild* fluorosis. (Chapter 8)

incidence of fluorosis by the use of toothpastes with higher fluoride concentrations. Around the age of 6 years, daily use of fluoride mouth rinses should be initiated as part of the total, life-long oral health program.

Question 6. Which of the following statements, if any, are correct?

A. Caries infection is transmissible from mother to child.

B. Malnutrition in the form of excess sucrose intake by the mother is probably responsible for the folklore expression of "one tooth for every pregnancy."

C. Baby-bottle caries affects the lower anterior teeth the most.

D. Fluoride tablets up to *1 ppm* should not be recommended for a pregnant woman.

E. The dentist is the person most available to impart prenatal and postnatal preventive dentistry counseling for a woman.

DENTURE CARE IN THE HOSPITAL

The American Dental Association (ADA) has published guidelines concerning the importance and mechanisms of denture care.[151,152] Ill-fitting and improperly cleaned dentures are important causes of denture stomatitis (inflammation), which is present in as many as two thirds of denture wearers. Denture stomatitis is related specifically to the yeast organism, *Candida albicans*.[153] Dirty dentures provide growth sites for both bacteria and fungi that may cause unpleasant odors and localized or systemic infections.[19]

Denture cleaning "home remedies" and other agents that traditionally have been used to clean dentures are hand soap, bicarbonate of soda, precipitated calcium carbonate, chlorine-containing solutions such as hypochlorite NF (half a teaspoonful to half a tumbler of water), an alkaline solution of hydrogen peroxide mixed with sodium perborates or percarbonates, full-strength vinegar, and abrasive denture pastes. Ideally, all of the agents should be applied using a brush that closely adapts to the denture's contour.

The "perfect" denture cleaning product does not yet exist.[153] In general, however, the ADA makes the following recommendations: (1) rinse the denture thoroughly before and after applying the cleaning agent; (2) brush the denture thoroughly, but carefully, so as not to bend the clasps or abrade the denture; (3) have the denture cleaned by a dentist with an ultrasonic device at least once a year; (4) because of the chemical nature of these cleaning agents, keep them out of the reach of children; and (5) avoid harsh abrasives or strong caustic agents for cleaning dentures because they can lead to pitting and improper fit.

Consumers should also be aware of the warning labels that accompany alkaline denture cleaners. If ingested, caustic and acidic denture cleaners can produce mucosal or oropharyngeal burns. One death has been attributed to the inadvertent swallowing of a denture-cleaning tablet.[153] If denture cleansers are used as directed by the manufacturer, they are considered completely safe. Hypochlorite and acidic solutions are a hazard to the metal components of removable prostheses (framework and clamps) and to the pins by which porcelain denture teeth are retained. Acidic solutions are strictly contraindicated for metal-containing prostheses, and hypochlorites should be used only for 15-minute soaks and not overnight.[153] A more detailed list of denture cleaners to be used with different denture frames and bases is contained in the same advisory.

All dentures should be removed and cleaned after eating. The cleaning and scrubbing of dentures should be accomplished over a sink in which a towel or washcloth has been placed and covered with a few inches of water. This provides a cushion in case the denture is accidentally dropped. The denture is held with a 4 × 4 gauze square and brushed thoroughly with a denture brush and cleaner or with a handbrush and water if necessary. Dentures left out overnight should be *completely* immersed in water to prevent partial desiccation.

All full and partial dentures should be removed before surgery and kept in water. Ideally, the dentures should remain outside the mouth during early convalescence. The patient might need the denture to take nourishment, however, or may want them for psychologic support. Once the effects of the anesthesia have disappeared and the patient is mentally alert, the dentures may be returned.

Many patients are concerned about their appearance and are reluctant to remove dentures when they are expecting visitors or when they are in a semiprivate room or a public setting. These patients should be advised that the oral tissues under dentures become easily inflamed and that these tissues require periods of recovery. If the patient is completely edentulous, all soft tissues, including the tongue, should be cleaned with a soft brush or with a 2 × 2 gauze sponge held with a hemostat. Whenever a patient is unable to adequately clean either the dentures or the mouth, the dental auxiliary or the designated member of the ward staff should provide the service.

SUMMARY

Some hospitals have dental services that provide complete dental care, including primary preventive care; others provide only the care that supports the medical treatment for which the patient was admitted. In either event, several conditions occur in which a hospitalized patient *must* receive primary preventive dental care as a part of total patient care. For many hospitalized patients, oral health is intimately connected to systemic health. Ignorance of this link in organ transplant patients, chemotherapy and radiation therapy patients, autoimmune disease syndrome (AIDS) patients, patients with insulin-dependent diabetis mellitus (IDDM), and patients with significant cardiovascular disease (CVD) poses a threat to the systemic health of these individuals. Serious conditions occur for which primary preventive dentistry is required in conjunction with prophylactic antibiotic therapy. In other cases, primary preventive procedures must be accomplished for patients who cannot help themselves, such as comatose or mentally and physically handicapped individuals, and infants. In hospitals with obstetric services, mothers and mothers-to-be need to be counseled on primary preventive dentistry procedures for themselves and their babies. The majority of the preventive dentistry functions can be accomplished by a dental auxiliary working in a hospital dental clinic for ambulatory patients and on the wards for nonambulatory patients.

In some of the conditions affecting hospital patients, meticulous plaque control programs, rigid sugar discipline, effective fluoride therapy, and tobacco cessation programs are essential for extending both the length and quality of life. In other patients a more routine preventive program can be established to promote patient comfort, improve appearance, and extend the retention of the dentition. This expanded primary preventive dentistry program in a hospital can be accomplished with a minimal expansion of dental personnel and space. Usually the responsibility for the delivery of these services can be delegated to a dental auxiliary under the supervision of a preventive dentistry officer.

ANSWERS AND EXPLANATIONS

1. A
   B—incorrect. The entire preventive program should be planned, demonstrated, and in use before radiation therapy begins.
   C—incorrect. The clinical appearance of HSV and candida infections are atypical in BMT patients and require culturing and Gram's staining (or KOH), respectively, for accurate diagnoses.
   D—incorrect. Saliva substitutes are poorly accepted by patients who generally prefer frequent sips of water.
   E—incorrect. Head and neck radiotherapy is a localized treatment and does not cause systemic immunosuppression.
2. D
   A—incorrect. AIDS is associated with neutropenia but not thrombocytopenia.
   B—incorrect. AIDS is associated with causing an aggressive form of periodontal disease termed HIV periodontitis.

C—incorrect. Hairy leukoplakia is a benign lesion that does not require treatment.

E—incorrect. Chlorhexidine is not contraindicated in AIDS patients.

3. A, C, E

B—incorrect. Caries and periodontal disease do not appear to be increased in renal failure patients.

D—incorrect. Renal transplantation, not dialysis, normalizes renal function. Patients on dialysis continue to have thrombocytopenia, anemia, accelerated atherosclerosis, and renal osteodystrophy.

4. A, D

B—incorrect. The glucocorticosteriod dose should be doubled to correct for adrenal suppression secondary to chronic dosing.

C—incorrect. Patients with ischemic heart disease are not immunosuppressed and therefore are not at risk for opportunistic infections.

E—incorrect. Acceptable data does not exist to suggest that prosthetic joint infections are caused by dental bacteremias.

5. A, B, C, D

E—incorrect. The dose of epinephrine in a local anesthetic is too small to induce significant hyperglycemia.

6. A, B,

C—incorrect. Because of the position of the tongue over the nipple, the greatest effect is on the maxillary anterior teeth.

D—incorrect. Pregnant women should be given up to 1 ppm of fluoride.

E—incorrect. It is the obstetrician. The dentist never sees the child until the mother brings the child in for treatment, which is too late for prevention.

SELF EVALUATION QUESTIONS

1. The three most frequent causes of head-and-neck cancer are _____, _____, and _____; these can easily be prevented by _____.

2. Five general categories (10 are listed in the text) of patients needing dental care as an integral part of their hospitalization are _____, _____, _____, _____, and _____.

3. The source of dental education of most hospital administrators and staff is usually from _____.

4. As part of a self-care effort, all patients should have the following three primary preventive items at the time of admission to the hospital: _____, _____, and _____.

5. To prevent breakage of a denture when cleaning over a basin, the following precaution should be taken: _____.

6. The best agent for the *chemical* control of radiation caries is _____.

7. The dental caries seen following head and neck radiation is known as _____; the dental caries seen following chemotherapy is known as _____; and the bone necrosis that sometimes follows head and neck radiation is termed _____.

8. The whitish membrane often seen in the mucositis caused by *Candida* is called _____ membrane.

9. Appointments for dental care of hemodialysis patients should be scheduled at least _____ (time) after dialysis because of _____.

10. Prophylactic antibiotic coverage (even for simple primary preventive procedures that might cause bleeding) are required for patients with the following conditions: _____, _____, and _____.

11. The "Four A's" used in smoking cessation programs are _____, _____, _____, and _____.

12. Two reasons, one self-imposed and the second physiologic, for the high caries incidence for pregnant women are _____ and _____.

13. Nursing-bottle caries can be prevented if the following three recommendations of the American Academy of Pediatric Dentistry are followed: _____, _____, and _____.

14. Fluoride usage should be from "womb to tomb"; it should start with the mother having _____ ppm as part of her daily intake. Once the child is given bottled water, fluoride should be administered daily as _____ (method used to administer). Topical fluoride applications should begin when teeth erupt; they may be applied by use of a small toothbrush with a small amount of dentifrice containing _____, the parent applying a _____ with a *slightly* moistened cloth; or by the dentist at the early "get-acquainted" visits. Fluoride _____ should replace the fluoride around the age of _____, with the swish-and-swallow technique being preferable to ensure a _____ application as well as systemic benefits. Finally, around the age of _____ the use of commercially available _____ mouth rinses should become a part of the lifetime oral hygiene program.

15. Two effective means to reduce caries on an institutionwide basis are _____ and _____.

REFERENCES

1. Salley JJ, Van Ostenberg PR, Gump ML. Dentistry and its future in the hospital environment. *J Am Dent Assoc.* 1980; 101:236–239.

2. Asbell MB. Hospital dental service in the United States—A historical review. *J Hosp Dent Pract.* 1969; 3:9–11.

3. Giangrego E. Dentistry in hospitals: Looking to the future. *J Am Dent Assoc.* 1987; 115:545–555.

4. Rafal S. The dentist in a hospital setting. *Special Care Dent.* 1983; 3:200.

5. Caveny M. The dental hygienist in hospital practice. *Dent Hygiene.* 1976; 50:205–209.

6. Taylor JA. Dentists and hospitals. *ADA News.* February 14, 1983; 14:4.

7. Thornton MA. Preventive dentistry in the Veterans Administration. *Dent Hygiene.* 1979; 53:121–124.

8. Gravois SL. Inpatient preventive dentistry within a Veterans Administration Medical Center. *Dent Hygiene.* 1979; 53:513–517.

9. Benson CM, Mailbusch R, Zimmer SE. An overview of oral hygiene nursing care. Part I. Oral health of hospitalized patients. *Dent Hygiene.* 1980; 54:384–386.

10. American Dental Association, Council on Hospital Dental Service. Oral evaluation of hospitalized patients. *J Am Dent Assoc.* 1966; 72:911–912.

11. Emery CA Jr. Evaluation of oral hygiene in a hospitalized population. *Gen Dent.* 1980; 28(1):54–57.

12. Harvey HS, Truelove EL, Stiefel DJ, et al. Survey of dental needs in hospitalized chronically ill patients. *J Hosp Dent Pract.* 1980; 14:123–127.

13. Zimmer S, Maibusch R. Oral health of hospitalized patients. Part II. A clinical study. *Dent Hygiene.* 1980; 54:423–425.

14. Dwyer B. Professional tips for the non-handicapped: Measuring expectations. *Dent Assist.* 1984; 53:21–23.

15. Block PL. Dental health in hospitalized patients. *Am J Nurs.* 1976; 76:1162–1164.

16. American Cancer Society. *Cancer Facts and Figures 1994.* Atlanta, Ga. American Cancer Society. 1994:1–30.

17. Christen AG, Klein JA, Christen JA, et al. "How-To-Do-It" quit-smoking strategies for the dental office team: An eight step program. *J Am Dent Assoc.* 1990; 120 (Supplement):20–27.

18. Christen AG, McDonald JL, Christen JA. *The impact of Tobacco Use and Cessation on Nonmalignant and Precancreous Oral and Dental Diseases and Conditions.* Indianapolis In. Indiana University School of Dentistry. 1991: 1–73.

19. Christen AG, McDonald JL, Klein JA et al. *A Smoking Cessation Program for the Dental Office.* Indianapolis, In: Indiana University, School of Dentistry. 1994:1–51.

20. Redding SW. Hematologic and Oncologic Disease. In: Redding SW, Montgomery MT, eds. *Dentistry in Systemic Disease.* Portland, Ore. JBK Publishing; 1990:81–118.

21. Lockhart PB, Sonis ST. Relationship of oral complications to peripheral blood leukocyte and platelet counts in patients receiving cancer chemotherapy. *Oral Surg.* 1979; 48:21–28.

22. Dreizen S, Menkin DJ, Keating MJ, et al. Effect of antileukemia chemotherapy on marrow, blood, and oral granulocyte counts. *Oral Surg Oral Med Oral Pathol.* 1991; 71:45–49.

23. McElroy TH. Infection in the patient receiving chemotherapy for cancer: Oral considerations. *J Am Dent Assoc.* 1984; 109: 454–456.

24. Nguyen A-M H. Dental management of patients who receive chemo- and radiation therapy. *Gen Dent.* 1992; 40:305–311.

25. Naylor GD, Terezhalmy GT. Oral complications of cancer chemotherapy: Prevention and management. *Spec Care Dent.* 1988; 150–156.

26. Greene SL. Treating the head and neck cancer patient. *Dent Hygiene.* 1980; 54:23–24.

27. Miller CE, Vergo TJ Jr, Felman MJ. Dental management of patients undergoing radiation therapy for cancer of the head and neck. *Compend Cont Educ Dent.* 1981; 2: 350–356.

28. Axelsson P, Lindhe J, Nyström B. On the prevention of caries and periodontal disease. Results of a 15-year longitudinal study in adults. *J Clin Periodontol.* 1991; 18:182–189.

29. Cacchillo D, Barker GJ, Barker BF. Late effects of head and neck radiation therapy and patient/dentist compliance with recommended dental care. *Special Care Dent.* 1993; 13:159–162.

30. Allard WF, El-Akkad S, Chatmas JC. Obtaining pre-radiation therapy dental clearance. *J Am Dent Assoc.* 1993; 124:88–91.

31. Wright WE, Haller JM, Harlow SA, et al. An oral disease prevention program for patients receiving radiation and chemotherapy. *J Am Dent Assoc.* 1985; 110:43–47.

32. Caton JG, Blieden TM, Lowenguth RA, et al. Comparison between mechanical cleaning and an antimicrobial rinse for the treatment and prevention of interdental gingivitis. *J Clin Periodontol.* 1993; 20:172–178.

33. Ferretti GA, Raybould TP, Brown AT, et al. Chlorhexidine prophylaxis for chemotherapy and radiotherapy-induced stomatitis: A randomized double-blind trial. *Oral Surg Oral Med Oral Pathol.* 1990; 69:331–338.

34. Toljanic JA, Hagen JC, Takahashi Y, et al. Evaluation of the substantivity of a chlorhexidine oral rinse in irradiated head and neck cancer patients. *J Oral Maxillofac Surg.* 1992; 50:1055–1059.

35. Epstein JB, Loh R, Stevenson-Moore P, et al. Chlorhexidine rinse in prevention of dental caries in patients following radiation therapy. *Oral Surg Oral Med Oral Pathol.* 1989; 68:401–405.

36. Bergmann OJ, Ellegaard B, Dahl M, et al. Gingival status during chemical plaque control with or without prior mechanical plaque removal in patients with acute myeloid leukaemia. *J Clin Periodontol.* 1992; 19:169–173.

37. Epstein JB, McBride BC, Stevenson-Moore P, et al. The efficacy of chlorhexidine gel in reduction of *Streptococcus mutans* and *Lactobacillus* species in patients treated with radiation therapy. *Oral Surg Oral Med Oral Pathol.* 1991; 71:172–178.

38. Ekstrand J, Spak CJ, Vogel G. Pharmacokinetics of fluoride in man and its clinical relevance. *J Dent Res.* 1990; 69:550–555.

39. Margolis HC, Moreno EC. Physicochemical perspectives on the cariostatic mechanisms of systemic and topical fluorides. *J Dent Res.* 1990; 69(special issue):606–613.

40. Chow LC. Tooth-bound fluoride and dental caries. *J Dent Res.* 1990; 69(special issue):595–600.

41. Rolla G, Øsgaard B, De Almeida Cruz R. Topical application of fluorides on teeth. New concepts of mechanism of interaction. *J Clin Periodontol.* 1993; 20:105–108.

42. Marthaler TM. Cariostatic efficacy of the combined use of fluorides. *J Dent Res.* 1990; 69:797–800.

43. Jenkins S, Addy M, Newcombe R. Evaluation of mouth rinse containing chlorhexidine and fluoride as an adjunct to oral hygiene. *J Clin Periodontol.* 1993; 20:20–25.

44. Joyston-Bechal S, Hernaman N. The effect of a mouth rinse containing chlorhexidine and fluoride on plaque and gingival bleeding. *J Clin Periodontol.* 1993; 20:49–53.

45. Liu RP, Fleming TJ, Toth BB, et al. Salivary flow rates in patients with head and neck cancer 0.5 to 25 years after radiotherapy. *Oral Surg Oral Med Oral Pathol.* 1990; 70:724–729.

46. Sreebny LM. Salivary flow in health and disease. *Compend Contin Educ Dent.* 1989; (Suppl 13):S461–S469.

47. Markitziu A, Zafiropoulos G, Tsalikis L, et al. Gingival health and salivary function in head and neck irradiated patients. *Oral Surg Oral Med Oral Pathol.* 1992; 73:427–433.

48. Driezen S, Brown LR, Daly TE, et al. Prevention of xerostomia-related dental caries in irradiated cancer patients. *J Dent Res.* 1977; 56:99–104.

49. Epstein JB, Stevenson-Moore P. A clinical comparative trial of saliva substitutes in radiation-induced salivary gland hypofunction. *Spec Care Dent.* 1992, 2:21–23.

50. Shannon IL, McCrary BR, Starcke EN. A saliva substitute for use by xerostomic patients undergoing radiotherapy to the head and neck. *Oral Surg.* 1977; 44:656–661.

51. Aguirre-Zero O, Zero DT, Proskin HM. Effect of chewing xylitol chewing gum on salivary flow rate and the acidogenic potential of dental plaque. *Caries Res.* 1993; 27:55–59.

52. LeVeque FG, Montgomery MT, Potte D, et al. A multicenter, randomized, double-blind, placebo-controlled, dose-titration study of oral pilocarpine for treatment of radiation-induced xerostomia in head and neck cancer patients. *J Clin Oncol.* 1993; 11:1124–1131.

53. Rothwell BR, Spektor WS. Palliation of radiation-related mucositis. *Spec Care Dent.* 1990; 10:21–25.

54. Hurt WC. Pharmacologic management of stomatologic problems. *Dent Clin North Am.* 1984; 28:545–554.

55. Barker G, Loftus L, Cuddy P, et al. The effects of sucralfate suspension and diphenhydramine syrup plus kaolin-pectin on radiotherapy-induced mucositis. *Oral Surg Oral Med Oral Pathol.* 1991; 71:288–293.

56. Epstein JB, Vickars L, Spinelli J, et al. Efficacy of chlorhexidine and nystatin rinses in prevention of oral complications in leukemia and bone marrow transplantation. *Oral Surg Oral Med Oral Pathol.* 1992; 73:682–689.

57. Meurman JH, Murtomaa H, Lindqvist C, et al. Effect of antiseptic mouthwashes on some clinical and microbiological findings in the mouths of lymphoma patients receiving cytostatic drugs. *J Clin Periodontol.* 1991; 18:587–591.

58. Brown AT, Shupe JA, Sims RE, et al. In vitro effect of chlorhexidine and amikacin on oral gram-negative bacilli from bone marrow transplant recipients. *Oral Surg Oral Med Oral Pathol.* 1990; 70:715–719.

59. Fotos PG, Vincent SD, Hellstein JW. Oral candidiasis. Clinical, historical, and therapeutic features of 100 cases. *Oral Surg Oral Med Oral Pathol.* 1992; 74:41–49.

60. Wahlin YB, Odont. Salivary secretion rate, yeast cells, and oral candidiasis in patients with acute leukemia. *Oral Surg Oral Med Oral Pathol.* 1991; 71:689–695.

61. Epstein JB. Antifungal therapy in oropharyngeal mycotic infections. *Oral Surg Oral Med Oral Pathol.* 1990; 69:32–41.

62. Bissell V, Felix DH, Wray D. Comparative trial of fluconazole and amphotericin in the treatment of denture stomatitis. *Oral Surg Oral Med Oral Pathol.* 1993; 76:35–39.

63. Budtz-Jorgensen E. The significance of *Candida albicans* in denture stomatitis. *Scand J Dent Res.* 1974; 82:151–190.

64. Schneid TR. An in vitro analysis of a sustained release system for the treatment of denture stomatitis. *Spec Care Dent.* 1992; 12:245–250.

65. Thurmond JM, Brown AT, Sims RE, et al. Oral *Candida albicans* in bone marrow transplant patients given chlorhexidine rinses: Occurrence and susceptibilities to the agent. *Oral Surg Oral Med Oral Pathol.* 1991; 72:291–295.

66. Schubert M, Peterson DE, Flournoy N, et al. Oral and pharyngeal herpes simplex virus infection after allogeneic bone marrow transplantation: Analysis of factors associated with infection. *Oral Surg Oral Med Oral Pathol.* 1990; 70:286–293.

67. Epstein JB, Sherlock C, Page JL, et al. Clinical study of herpes simplex virus infection in leukemia. *Oral Surg Oral Med Oral Pathol.* 1990; 70:38–43.

68. Woo SB, Sonis ST, Sonis AL. The role of herpes simplex virus in the development of oral mucositis in bone marrow transplant recipients. *Cancer.* 1990; 66:2375–2379.

69. Flaitz CM, Hammond HL. The immunoperoxidase method for the rapid diagnosis of intraoral herpes simplex virus infection in patients receiving bone marrow transplants. *Spec Care Dent.* 1988; 8:82–85.

70. Laga EA, Toth BB, Rolston KV, et al. Evaluation of a rapid enzyme-linked immunoassay for the diagnosis of herpes simplex virus in cancer patients with oral lesions. *Oral Surg Oral Med Oral Pathol.* 1993; 75:168–172.

71. Park N-H, Park JB, Min B-M, et al. Combined synergistic antiherpetic effect of acyclovir and chlorhexidine in vitro. *Oral Surg Oral Med Oral Pathol.* 1991; 71:193–196.

72. Epstein JB, Scully C. Herpes simplex virus in immunocompromised patients: Growing evidence of drug evidence. *Oral Surg Oral Med Oral Pathol.* 1991; 72:47–50.

73. Peterson DE, Minah GE, Reynolds MA, et al. Effect of granulocytopenia on oral microbial relationships in patients with acute leukemia. *Oral Surg Oral Med Oral Pathol.* 1990; 70:720–723.

74. Childers NK, Stinnett EA, Wheeler P, et al. Oral complications in children with cancer. *Oral Surg Oral Med Oral Pathol.* 1993; 75:41–47.

75. Morrish R, Chan E, Silverman S, et al. Osteonecrosis in patients irradiated for head and neck carcinoma. *Cancer.* 1981; 47: 1980–1983.

76. Marx RE, Johnson RP. Studies in the radiobiology of osteoradionecrosis and their clinical significance. *Oral Surg Oral Med Oral Pathol.* 1987; 64:379–390.

77. Marx RE. A new concept in the treatment of osteoradionecrosis. *J Oral Maxillofac Surg.* 1993; 41:351–357.

78. Maxymiw WG, Wood RE, Liu FF. Postradiation dental extractions without hyperbaric oxygen. *Oral Surg Oral Med Oral Pathol.* 1991; 72:270–274.

79. Kambhu PP, Levy SM. An evaluation of the effectiveness of four mechanical plaque-removal devices when used by a trained care-provider. *Spec Care Dent.* 1993; 13:9–14.

80. Addems A, Epstein JB, Damji S, et al. The lack of efficacy of a foam brush in maintaining gingival health: a controlled study. *Spec Care Dent.* 1992; 12:103–106.

81. Ferretti GA, Redding SW. Infectious disease. In: Redding SW, Montgomery MT, eds. *Dentistry in Systemic Disease.* Portland, Ore. JBK Publishing; 1990:1–27.

82. Pindborg JJ. Global aspects of the AIDS epidemic. *Oral Surg Oral Med Oral Pathol.* 1992; 73:138–141

83. Silverman S. AIDS update: Oral findings, diagnosis, and precautions. *J Am Dent Assoc.* 1987; 115:559–563.

84. Little JW, Falace DA. Therapeutic considerations in special patients. *Dent Clin North Am.* 1984; 28:455–469.

85. Greenspan JS, Barr CE, Sciubba JJ, et al. The U.S.A. Oral AIDS Collaborative Group: Oral manifestations of HIV infection. Definitions, diagnostic criteria, and principles of therapy. *Oral Surg Oral Med Oral Pathol.* 1992; 73:142–144.

86. Scully C, Laskaris G, Pindborg J, et al. Oral manifestations of HIV infection and their management. I. More common lesions. *Oral Surg Oral Med Oral Pathol.* 1991; 71:158–166.

87. Scully C, Laskaris G, Pindborg J, et al. Oral manifestations of HIV infection and their management. II. Less common lesions. *Oral Surg Oral Med Oral Pathol.* 1991; 71:167–171.

88. Gicarra G. Oral lesions of iatrogenic and undefined etiology and neurologic disorders associated with HIV infection. *Oral Surg Oral Med Oral Pathol.* 1992; 73:201–211.

89. Leggot PJ. Oral manifestations of HIV infection in children. *Oral Surg Oral Med Oral Pathol.* 1992; 73:187–192.

90. Epstein JB, Silverman S Jr. Head and neck malignancies associated with HIV infection. *Oral Surg Oral Med Oral Pathol.* 1992; 73:193–200.

91. McCarthy GM. Host factors associated with HIV-related oral candidiasis. *Oral Surg Oral Med Oral Pathol.* 1992; 73:181–186.

92. Samaranayake LP. Oral mycoses in HIV infection. *Oral Surg Oral Med Oral Pathol.* 1992; 73:171–180.

93. Franker CK, Lucartorto FM, Johnson BS, et al. Characterization of the mycoflora from oral mucosal surfaces of some HIV-infected patients. *Oral Surg Oral Med Oral Pathol.* 1990; 69:683–687.

94. Redding SW, Farinacci GC, Smith JA, et al. A comparison between fluconazole tablets and clotrimazole troches for the treatment of thrush in HIV infection. *Spec Care Dent.* 1992; 12:24–27.

95. Eversole LR. Viral infections of the head and neck among HIV-seropositive patients. *Oral Surg Oral Med Oral Pathol.* 1992; 73:155–163.

96. Epstein JB, Sherlock CH, Wolber RA. Oral manifestations of cytomegalovirus infection. *Oral Surg Oral Med Oral Pathol.* 1993; 75:443–451.

97. Greenspan D, Greenspan JS. Significance of oral hairy leukoplakia. *Oral Surg Oral Med Oral Pathol.* 1992; 73:151–154.

98. MacPhail LA, Greenspan D, Feigal DW, et al. Recurrent aphthous ulcers in association with HIV infection. Description of ulcer types and analysis of T-lymphocyte subsets. *Oral Surg Oral Med Oral Pathol.* 1991; 71:678–683.

99. Phelan JA, Eisig S, Freedman PD, et al. Major aphthous-like ulcers in patients with AIDS. *Oral Surg Oral Med Oral Pathol.* 1991; 71:68–72.

100. Glick M, Muzyka BC. Alternative therapies for major aphthous ulcers in AIDS patients. *J Am Dent Assoc.* 1992; 123:61–65.

101. Vincent SD, Lilly GE. Clinical, historic, and therapeutic features of aphthous stomatitis. Literature review and open clinical trial employing steroids. *Oral Surg Oral Med Oral Pathol.* 1992; 74:79–86.

102. Glick M, Pliskin ME, Weiss RC. The clinical and histologic appearance of HIV-associated gingivitis. *Oral Surg Oral Med Oral Pathol.* 1990; 69:395–398.

103. Winkler JR, Robertson PB. Periodontal disease associated with HIV infection. *Oral Surg Oral Med Oral Pathol.* 1992; 73:145–150.

104. Winkler JR, Murray PA, Grassi M, et al. Diagnosis and management of HIV-associated periodontal lesions. *J Am Dent Assoc.* 1989; 119(Supplement):25–34.

105. Scully C, McCarthy G. Management of oral health in persons with HIV infection. *Oral Surg Oral Med Oral Pathol.* 1992; 73:215–225.

106. Montgomery MT. Renal disease. In: Redding SW, Montgomery MT, eds. *Dentistry in Systemic Disease.* Portland, Ore. JBK Publishing; 1990:249–271.

107. Heard E Jr, Staples AF, Czerwinski AW. The dental patient with renal disease: Precautions and guidelines. *J Am Dent Assoc.* 1978; 96:792–795.

108. Levy HM. Dental considerations for the patient receiving dialysis for renal failure. *Spec Care Dent.* 1988; 8:34–36.

109. Kirkpatrick TJ, Morton JB. Factors influencing the dental management of renal transplant and dialysis patients. *Br J Oral Surg.* 1971; 9:57–64.

110. Westbrook SD. Dental management of patients receiving hemodialysis and kidney transplants. *J Am Dent Assoc.* 1978; 96: 464–468.

111. Bottomley WK, Cioffi RF, Martin AJ. Dental management of the patient treated by renal transplantation: Preoperative and postoperative considerations. *J Am Dent Assoc.* 1972; 85:1330–1335.

112. Chow MH, Peterson DS. Dental management for children with chronic renal failure undergoing hemodialysis therapy. *J Oral Surg.* 1979; 48:34–38.

113. Ziccardi VB, Saini J, Demas PN, et al. Management of the oral and maxillofacial surgery patient with end-stage renal disease. *J Oral Maxillofac Surg.* 1992; 50: 1207–1212.

114. Seymour RA, Smith DG. The effect of a plaque control program on the incidence and severity of cyclosporin-induced gingival changes. *J Clin Periodontol.* 1991; 18: 107–110.

115. Greenberg MS, Cohen G. Oral infections in immunosuppressed renal transplant patients. *Oral Surg.* 1977; 54:23–24.

116. Montgomery MT. Cardiovascular disease. In: Redding SW, Montgomery MT, eds. *Dentistry in Systemic Disease.* Portland, Ore. JBK Publishing; 1990:169–213.

117. Brooks SL, Millard HD. The damaged heart. Part I. *Dent Clin North Am.* 1983; 27:303–311.

118. Little JW. Prevention of bacterial endocarditis in dental patients. *Gen Dent.* 1987; 35:382–387.

119. Dajani AS, Bisno AL, Chung KJ, et al. Prevention of bacterial endocarditis. Recommendations by the American Heart Association. *J Am Med Assoc.* 1990; 264:2919–2922.

120. Montgomery MT, Rees TD, Moncrief JW. *The Diagnosis and Management of the Diabetic Patient: Implications for Dentistry.* Monograph. Texas Department of Health, Bureau of Dental and Chronic Disease Prevention. 1992.

121. Hicks JL. Endocrinologic disease. In: Redding SW, Montgomery MT, eds. *Dentistry in Systemic Disease.* Portland, Ore. JBK Publishing; 1990: 119–167.

122. Katz PP, Wirthlin MR, Szpunar SM, et al. Epidemiology and prevention of periodontal disease in individuals with diabetes. *Diabetes Care.* 1991, 14:375–385.

123. Anil S, Remani P, Vijayakumar T, et al. Cell-mediated and humoral immune responses in diabetic patients with periodontitis. *Oral Surg Oral Med Oral Pathol.* 1990; 70:44–48.

124. Miller LS, Manwell MA, Newbold D, et al. The relationship between reduction in periodontal inflammation and diabetes control: A report of 9 cases. *J Periodontol.* 1992; 63:843–848.

125. Rommerdale EH. Toothbrushing for the handicapped. *Spec Care Dent.* 1983; 3: 108–109.

126. Stiefel DJ, Truelove EL, Menard TW, et al. A comparison of the oral health of persons with and without chronic mental illness in community settings. *Spec Care Dent.* January-February 1990; 10:6–12.

127. Chikte UM, Pochee E, Rudolh MJ, et al. Evaluation of stannous fluoride and chlorhexidine sprays on plaque and gingivitis in handicapped children. *J Clin Periodontol.* 1991; 18:281–286.

128. McKenzie WT, Forgas L, Vernino AR, et al. Comparison of 0.12% chlorhexidine mouth rinse and an essential oil mouth rinse on oral health in institutionalized, mentally handicapped adults. One-year results. *J Periodontol.* 1992; 63:187–193.

129. Stiefel DJ, Truelove EL, Chin MM, et al. Efficacy of chlorhexidine swabbing in oral health care for people with severe disabilities. *Spec Care Dent.* 1992; 12:57–62.

130. Burtner AP, Low DW, McNeal DR, et al. Effects of chlorhexidine spray on plaque and gingival health in institutionalized persons with mental retardation. *Spec Care Dent.* 1991; 11:57–62.

131. Stiefel DJ, Truelove EL, Chin MM, et al. Efficacy of chlorhexidine swabbing in oral health care for people with severe disabilities. *Spec Care Dent.* 1992; 12:57–62.

132. Burtner AP, Low DW, McNeal Dr, et al. Effects of chlorhexidine spray on plaque and gingival health in institutionalized persons with mental retardation. *Spec Care Dent.* 1991; 11:57–62.

133. Clark DC, Morgan J, MacEntee MI. Effects of a 1% chlorhexidine gel on the cariogenic bacteria in high-risk elders: A pilot study. *Spec Care Dent.* 1991; 11:101–103.

134. Phelps-Sandall BA. Effectiveness of oral hygiene techniques on plaque and gingivitis in patients placed in intermaxillary fixation. *Oral Surg.* 1983; 56(5):487–490.

135. Johnson W. "Pick-and-Poke"—a supplement to the Bass method. *J Tex Dent Hygien Assoc.* 1981; 18(2):16–18.

136. Friedlander AH, Liberman RP. Oral health care for the patient with schizophrenia. *Spec Care Dent.* 1991; 11:179–183.

137. Kohler B, Bratthall D. Intrafamilial levels of *Streptococcus mutans* and some aspects of the bacterial transmission. *Scand J Dent Res.* 1978; 86:35–42.

138. Kohler B, Andreen I, Jonsson B. Proceedings, annual meeting. *Scand Res.* 1983.

139. *Perspectives on the Use of Prenatal Fluorides: A Symposium.* Moderator, H. Horowitz, Annual Session American Dental Association; October 1980. New Orleans, La.

140. Gier RE, Janes DR. Dental management of the pregnant patient. *Dent Clin North Am.* 1983; 27:419–428.

141. Boundy SS, Reynolds NJ. Current concepts in dental hygiene. Randolph PM, ed. *The Role of Diet and Nutrition in Pregnancy and Lactation,* Vol. 2. St. Louis, Mo. Mosby; 1979:179–191.

142. Fass EN. Is bottle feeding of milk a factor in dental caries? *J Dent Child.* 1962; 29: 245–251.

143. Ripa LW. *Baby Bottle Tooth Decay (Nursing Caries): A Comprehensive Review.* Dental Health Section. Washington, DC. American Public Health Association; 1988: 1–13.

144. American Dental Association. *Pamphlet: Nursing Bottle Mouth,* Chicago, Ill. 1985.

145. Knoll RG, Stone JH. Nocturnal bottlefeeding as a contributory cause of rampant dental caries in the infant and young child. *J Dent Child.* 1967; 29:454–459.

146. Moss SJ. The year 2000 health objectives for the nation. *Pediatr Dent.* 1988; 10:228–233.

147. McIlwain JE, Matis BA, Christen AG. Pre- and postnatal dental counseling. *USAF Med Serv Dig.* 1979; 30:28–31.

148. American Academy of Pedodontics. *Pediatric Dental Care Update for the Dentist and for the Pediatrician.* New York, NY. MEDCO; 1978:6–48.

149. Goose DH. Infant feeding and caries of the incisors. An epidemiologic approach. *Caries Res.* 1964; 1:167–173.

150. Pitts AT. Some observations on the occurrence of caries in very young children. *Br Dent J.* 1927; 48:197–214.

151. American Dental Association. Denture Cleaning Agents. *Dentist's Desk Reference,* 2nd ed. Chicago, Ill. American Dental Association; 1983:424–425.

152. American Dental Association. Council on Dental Materials, Instruments and Equipment. Denture cleansers. *J Am Dent Assoc.* 1983; 106:77–70.

153. Abelson DC. Denture plaque and denture cleansers: Review of the literature. *Gerodontics.* 1985; 1:202–206.

Appendix 20–1. Treatment Options for Oral Infections

Agent	Dose/Administration
ANTIMICROBIAL RINSES	
0.12% Chlorhexidine	Rinse with 15 mL for 30 s and expectorate; bid
ORAL SYSTEMIC ANTIBIOTICS	
Penicillin	1 g stat followed by 500 mg q6h
Erythromycin	1 g stat followed by 500 mg q6h
Metronidazole	1 g stat followed by 500 mg q6h
Clindamycin	300 mg stat followed by 150 mg q6h
Cephalexin	1 g stat followed by 500 mg q6h
ANTIFUNGAL AGENTS	
Nystatin pastille (200,000 units)	1–2 pastilles, 4–5 times/day
Chlotrimazole troche (10 mg)	5 times/day
Ketaconazole (200 mg)	1/day
Fluconazole (100 mg)	200 mg loading dose followed by 100 mg/day
Amphotericin B (IV)	0.25 mg/kg/day to a maximum of 1–1.5 mg/kg/day
ANTIVIRAL AGENTS	
Acyclovir (IV)	5 mg/kg tid for 1 week
Acyclovir (PO)	200 mg 5 times a day for 1 week

Appendix 20–2. Palliative Treatments for Oral Mucositis

Agent	Dose/Administration

IRRIGATION/DEBRIDEMENT

0.5% Hydrogen peroxide	1 tbp in 8 oz of water
Saline	
Sodium bicarbonate	½ tsp in 8 oz of water

ADHERING AGENTS

Sucralfate
Kaolin
Magnesium hydroxide
Milk of magnesia (MOM)

TOPICAL ANESTHETICS

Diphenhydramine	1 tsp q2h
2% Viscous lidocaine	1 tbp q2h; rinse and expectorate
1% Dyclonine	1 tsp q2h; rinse and expectorate
15% Oratect Gel benzocaine and cellulose	Dry tissue and keep dry for 60 s after application; qid

COMBINATION RINSES

Topical anesthetic + Adhering agent
Topical anesthetic + Adhering agent + Corticosteroid or Antibiotic or Antifungal

Appendix 20–3. Antibiotic Prophylaxis Regimens Recommended by the American Heart Association

Patient Type	Drug	Dosing Regimen
STANDARD REGIMEN*		
Not allergic to penicillin	Amoxicillin	3 g orally, 1 h prior to procedure. 1.5 g 6 h after initial dose
Allergic to amoxicillin or penicillin	Erythromycin	Initially erythromycin ethylsuccinate 800 mg or erythromycin stearate 1 g orally 2 h prior to procedure followed by half the initial dose 6 h later; or
	Clindamycin	300 mg orally 1 h prior to procedure and 150 mg 6 h after the initial dose
ALTERNATIVE REGIMENS†		
Cannot take oral medications	Ampicillin	2 g IV/IM, 30 min prior to procedure, followed by 1 g IV/IM 6 h after initial dose
Allergic to amoxicillin or penicillin or ampicillin and cannot take oral medications	Clindamycin	300 mg IV 30 min prior to procedure, followed by 150 mg IV 6 h after initial dose
High-risk patients	Ampicillin, gentamicin, and amoxicillin	2 g IV/IM, Ampicillin 30 min prior to procedure with 1.5 mg/kg of gentamicin not to exceed 80 mg, followed by 1.5 g orally of Amoxicillin, 6 h after initial dose; alternately, the parenteral regimen may be repeated 8 h after the initial dose.
High-risk patients who are allergic to amoxicillin or penicillin or ampicillin	Vancomycin	1 g IV, administered over 1 h prior to the procedure; a follow-up dose is not needed.

*For pediatric patients, the initial doses are amoxicillin 50 mg/kg, erythromycin ethylsuccinate or stearate 20 mg/kg, and clindamycin 10 mg/kg. The total pediatric dose should not exceed the adult dose. All follow-up doses are half of the initial dose.
†For pediatric patients, the initial doses are ampicillin 50 mg/kg, gentamicin 2 mg/kg, vancomycin 20 mg/kg, and clindamycin 10 mg/kg. The total pediatric dose should not exceed the adult dose. All follow-up doses are half of the initial dose. The recommended follow-up dose for amoxicillin is 25 mg/kg.
(*Source:* Committee on Rheumatic Fever, Endocarditis, and Kawasaki Disease of the Council on Cardiovascular Disease in the Young of the American Heart Association. *J Am Med Assoc.* 1990; 264:2919–2922.)

Appendix 20–4. American Heart Association Recommendations Concerning Candidates for Antibiotic Prophylaxis

ANTIBIOTIC PROPHYLAXIS RECOMMENDED

Prosthetic cardiac valves
Most congenital cardiac malformations
Surgically constructed systemic pulmonary shunts
Rheumatic heart disease and other acquired valvular pathology
History of endocarditis
Mitral valve prolapse with insufficiency
Hypertrophic cardiomyopathy

ANTIBIOTIC PROPHYLAXIS NOT RECOMMENDED

Physiologic, functional, or "innocent" heart murmurs
Isolated secundum atrial septal defect
Surgical repair of congenital heart defects, without residua beyond 6 months
Previous coronary artery bypass graft surgery
Mitral valve prolapse without insufficiency
Previous Kawasaki disease without valvular dysfunction
Cardiac pacemakers and implanted defibrillators
Dental procedures not likely to induce gingival bleeding (ie, adjustment of orthodontic appliances and supragingival restorations)
Intraoral local anesthetic injections except for intraligamentary injections
Shedding of primary teeth

Source: Committee on Rheumatic Fever, Endocarditis, and Kawasaki Disease of the Council on Cardiovascular Disease in the Young of the American Heart Association. J Am Med Assoc. 1990; 264:2919–2922.)

Chapter 21

Clinical Procedures for Controlling Plaque Diseases

Norman O. Harris
Marsha A. Cunningham-Ford

Objectives

At the end of this chapter it will be possible to

1. List seven caries activity indicators (CAI) and four periodontal disease activity indicators (PAI) that should aid the dental practitioner in determining the *probability* of, as well as the *existence* of, either caries or periodontal disease or both.
2. Explain why the detection of incipient carious lesions and subsequent appropriate use of chemical and mechanical plaque control, sealants, and remineralization strategies can greatly reduce the need for restorations.
3. Name two plaque control measures (one home-based and the other office-based), and state why these procedures are *essential* in the control of incipient caries or gingivitis or both.
4. Discuss the various roles of a dental hygienist in optimal caries and periodontal disease preventive programs.
5. Propose an individualized "fail-safe" examination, primary preventive care regimen, and recall schedule that would enable a clinical practice to rapidly change from mainly a treatment orientation to one emphasizing the prevention, arrest, or reversal of incipient carious lesions and gingivitis.
6. On the basis of what you have learned throughout the book, contrast what you think *can* be done to prevent the plaque diseases with what is *being accomplished*.

Introduction

It is the goal of the dental profession to help individuals achieve and maintain maximum oral health throughout their lives. Success in attaining this objective is highlighted by the decline of caries throughout the Western world[1,2] and the dramatic reduction of tooth loss in U.S. adults.[3] This progress has been mainly due to the use of water fluoridation and fluoride products and acceptance of primary preventive dentistry procedures.

Untold millions of research hours and money have been invested in reaching our present capability to control the ravages of the plaque diseases. Effective strategies that can markedly reduce the toll of teeth resulting from caries and periodontal disease *are now* available. They need only be used.

The onset of caries and periodontal disease may be either acute or chronic. In one study, it took an average of 12 months for a carious lesion to progress through the outer half of the enamel and an average 10 to 12 months for the lesion to progress through the inner half.[4] In another study only 56% of the incipient lesions became overt, indicating that *the end point of the caries process can be modified by remineralization.*[5]

For periodontal disease periods of quiescence and exacerbation usually occur, probably related to changes in metabolism of the plaque microorganisms or reduction in host resistance or both. Many times the plaque diseases require years to develop. During this time, routine caries activity tests and visual examination of the mouth should alert the health professional of impending problems. For caries, deep, "sticky" pits and fissures; a change in the microbial caries activity test scores; an excessively high plaque index; and the presence of incipient or overt caries or both are signs of impending or actual caries. For periodontal disease, mar-

ginal gingivitis, bleeding, the presence of excessive plaque and calculus, and the existence of spirochetes in deep pockets are evidence of actual or impending periodontal problems. If any of these signs are noted prior to reaching the irreversible points in either the caries or the periodontal disease process, the progress of the plaque diseases can often be arrested and reversed by primary preventive procedures.

WHY PREVENTION?

In the last two decades, prevention has become an integral part of a patient's treatment plan. Fewer patients seek professional dental help only when they have obvious pain, infection, trauma, or malformation. Most oral health professionals recognize the need to emphasize that patients should seek entry into well-planned preventive programs. With such programs, the possibility exists of a near 100% control of caries and periodontal disease; without them the only future is restorations, periodontal care, extractions, and dentures. The changeover in priority from treatment to prevention requires active leadership in health promotion[a] by the dental profession, consumer advocates, public health educators, and health policy makers.[6,7]

Public health delivery systems, such as the military and industrial organizations that provide employee benefits, have usually been at the forefront of such change because of the economic benefits to the provider and the health benefits to the recipients. In 1989, a report by Malvitz and Broderick[8] recounts the results following the change of focus toward a maximum em-

---

[a] Health promotion can be defined as "the process of advocating health to enhance the probability that personal, private, and public support of positive health practices will be a society norm."

phasis on prevention for dental services in the Oklahoma City Area of the Indian Health Service. Total visits increased by 10% but the number of dental personnel remained constant. The percentage of preventive services increased and the number of restorative procedures concomitantly decreased. Most dramatically, the number of occlusal amalgams required and the number of pit-and-fissure sealants placed was reversed. The changeover to provide comprehensive primary preventive care mandated administrative planning, support, and guidance.[8] In private practice it is the dentist who must provide the same leadership.

Benefits of Primary Preventive Dentistry to the Patient

For the patient who thinks in terms of economic benefits, prevention pays. If preventive programs are started early enough by the patient—or by the parents of young children—long-range freedom from plaque diseases is possible—a sound cost-benefit investment. The teeth are needed over a lifetime for *eating,* and *speech* is greatly improved by the presence of teeth. Also, a pleasant *smile greatly enhances personality expression* (Fig 21–1). Natural teeth also contribute to good *nutrition* for all ages. An absence of teeth, or presence of poor teeth results in a loss of self-esteem and minimizes employment possibilities where continual public contact is required.

Benefits for the Dentist

The dentist, through ethics and training, should derive a deep sense of satisfaction from helping people to maintain their teeth in a state of maximum function, comfort, and esthetics. A well-balanced practice that actively seeks to prevent disease but is available to care for those cases where prevention has failed is highly competitive with other dental practices. Patients can be outstanding public relations advocates if they

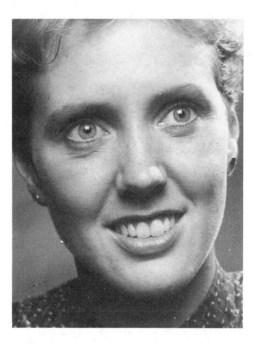

Figure 21–1. Vibrant dental health enhances personality expression.

are convinced that their dentist and staff are truly interested in preventing disease. Appendix 21–1 illustrates a letter used in one dental practice to emphasize their interest in disease prevention for the patient.

If for no other reason, a dentist should consider prevention to avoid possible legal problems. Long-term patients and the courts are taking a more unsympathetic attitude toward dentists who have permitted a disease to progress over many years without having taken some primary preventive actions to have slowed or halted its progress. Patients no longer tolerate supervised professional neglect.

THE DENTAL EXAMINATION

The initial dental examination is probably the most important event in the entire oral health program. At this point, a person seeking dental care has the opportunity to have his or her current oral status carefully assessed by a professional, a treatment plan prepared, restorative care accomplished, and a *comprehensive preventive dentistry plan* initiated that will help prevent future plaque disease, as well as forestalling a recurrence of the present problems.[9] This *baseline* examination is one against which all future examinations will be compared so as to evaluate temporal deviations from normal health.[10] Assuming that prophylaxis is scheduled following the initial examination, the examination should possibly be separated into two parts with the dentist and the dental hygienist functioning as a team. Part 1 of the examination by the *dentist* should include as a minimum

- A *medical history* that provides information about possible systemic problems that might be important etiologic cofactors in caries or periodontal disease development. At each subsequent recall prophylaxis, the dental hygienist or dentist should update the medical history
- A *mouth mirror examination* of *all* the teeth for incipient[b] and overt coronal and root caries and an explorer examination for ditched amalgams and secondary (ie, recurrent) caries
- A periodontal *probe examination* of all gingival crevices and a concurrent recording of a *bleeding index,* this probing will be performed at *each recall prophylaxis* by the dentist or dental hygienist
- A set of *bite wing* and *periapical* radiographs as part of the examination for interproximal caries and loss of supporting bone by the teeth.

Part 2 of the examination can be delegated to the *dental hygienist* as part of the prophylaxis appointment. This phase of the examination should include a plaque index (Appendix 21–2), a carbohydrate intake score (Appendix 21–3), a calculus site recording, a saliva flow rate notation, and appropriate caries activity tests. All can be easily accomplished in the dental office to furnish valuable *baseline* information for comparison in future examinations.

A carbohydrate intake score, such as shown in Appendix 21–3, provides an estimate of sugar intake by the patient. It also serves as a basis for discussion in later education sessions to emphasize the key role of sucrose in the caries process.

The plaque index, which is discussed later, provides a means of evaluating at sequential appointments whether recommended plaque control techniques are adequately maintaining a satisfactory 10% or lower plaque level. The calculus sites can be recorded on the same form, thus providing further means of identifying areas of stagnation where toothbrushing and flossing have been inadequate.

All microbiologic caries activity tests—plate counts, Alban's test, or dip slides—provide a good assessment of caries risk, especially if the results are compared with previous baseline results.[11] Dip-slide kits are commercially available for evaluating the salivary levels of mutans streptococci and lactobacilli, respectively.[c] The salivary levels of mutans streptococci and lactobacilli found in either plate counts or by dip-slide evaluation are significantly correlated.[12] Of the two, the dip slide is easier to

---

[b] Incipient lesions are those white spots that have not reached the irreversible point in the demineralization process. Overt lesions are those with frank cavitation.

[c] Ivoclar North America
 Dentocult SM—mutans streptococci
 Dentocult LB—lactobacilli
 175 Pineview Drive
 Amherst, NY 14228

perform. An added advantage is that it can be kept for up to 6 months for a later comparison and for counseling.[12]

A *negative test* is highly indicative of caries *inactivity.* If each increase in the activity test score is viewed as indicating a greater potential for disease, it is prudent to take action to return the test score to as near zero as possible. Microbiologic test scores also serve as tools for assessing patient *compliance* with recommended measures to reduce the bacterial challenge (ie, sucrose).[13] The importance of bacteriologic testing is summarized by Krasse, "To run a caries preventive program without using microbiological methods, is like running a weight control program without scales."[14]

Because the saliva must be collected for the microbiologic caries activity tests, the flow per minute is easy to determine. This latter data provides additional valuable information needed to establish an integrated office and home preventive dentistry routine.

It should be noted that *all* the various components of part 1 and part 2 of the dental examination are either part of present examination routine or can be easily added.

Use of Examination Data

The medical history should be carefully perused. For example, a patient taking antihypertensive medication, tranquilizers, or many other drugs often has xerostomia as a side effect. This can contribute to caries development,[15] whereas a blood dyscrasia might indicate the need for medical as well as dental intervention to forestall periodontal involvement. A Finnish study of 368 subjects, ages 71 to 86, found 23% were unmedicated, 47% required between one and three medications daily, and 30% used more than four.[16] In this population, the saliva flow rate was significantly greater in the unmedicated patients than in those who took

from four to six or more medications. The medical history also helps identify conditions, such as Crohn's disease[17] or diabetes mellitus, that are background factors for caries or periodontal disease, respectively.

It should be noted that the data recorded for part 1 of the initial dental examination are those that are usually required for eventual treatment and should be completed by the dentist. *The data also identify conditions that can be used as caries activity indicators (CAI) needed to establish treatment procedures and prepare an individualized preventive dentistry plan.* For caries, the CAI are

1. Anatomic status of the pits and fissures
2. Number and location of incipient, overt, and recurrent coronal and root lesions
3. Plaque index
4. Saliva flow
5. Refined carbohydrate intake
6. Caries activity testing

The periodontal activity indicators (PAI) are addressed later.

The items included in part 2 of the examination—the carbohydrate intake score, plaque index, calculus site location, saliva flow, and appropriate microbiologic tests (ie, dip slide test[s])—are means of monitoring oral health status as a function of time. There is little difference between the data needed for the treatment phase and the data needed for prevention. Instead, the difference is in how the information is *collected,* how it is *recorded,* and how it is to be *used.*

Perhaps the greatest contrast between treatment needs and prevention requirements is in the decision-making process. The treatment examination concentrates on the presence or absence of overt pathology. If lesions are identified, the urgency of treatment and the type of restorations must be decided.

On the other hand, an emphasis or prevention using the same examination data should focus on the possible presence of *subclinical* and *visible* incipient lesions for which remineralization strategies or sealants are indicated. Thus, decisions must be made about whether to institute *remineralization therapy and use sealants* or *to restore*—and *in that order*. With this policy, the arsenal of preventive dentistry concentrates on reducing tooth demineralization during the subclinical state and intensifies remineralization therapy once the incipient lesion is identified. The objective is to prevent, arrest, or reverse *all* incipient lesions by remineralization strategies *before* they become overt.[d]

The second major difference between how the treatment and preventive aspects of the examination are carried out lies with office time priorities. In the usual treatment plan, the time commitments emphasize disease eradication and prophylaxis. Presently, there is relatively little use of sealants[18,19] and even less consideration given to applying remineralization therapy, partially because of lack of information.[20] In an ideal preventive program, optimal time is allowed for *both* primary and secondary prevention.

Another critical difference is that the treatment plan ends when the recorded pathology is successfully treated. In the preventive examination, the information can be arrayed in a manner that permits better development of reasoned therapeutic strategies that can be used to prevent future plaque disease development.

---

[d] For planning purposes, an incipient smooth-surface lesion should remain under observation and remineralization treatment for at least 6 months. At that time, if the plaque index and microbiologic caries activity test scores are low, the lesion can be tentatively considered as remineralized.

Question 1. Which of the following statements, if any, are correct?

   A. All overt carious lesions were once incipient lesions.

   B. It is necessary for the dentist to accomplish the *entire* dental examination.

   C. An examination for a patient's preventive dentistry plan requires totally different data from that for a treatment plan.

   D. Neither sealant placement nor remineralization strategies are used extensively in the United States.

   E. Private practitioners presently feature a *balance* in *time* and *diagnostic effort* devoted to primary preventive practices *compared* with secondary prevention.

THE PROBLEM

The Incipient Lesion

Every day, *multiple* instances of microscopic demineralization of areas on the tooth occur.[21] Only a few of these in situ demineralized areas progress to become incipient lesions, and even fewer go on to overt cavitation—mainly because of the physiologic remineralization potential of the saliva. Other more advanced "white spots" can be returned to normal by intensified remineralization therapy, diet alteration, and mechanical and chemical plaque control. Incipient lesions occur (1) *interproximally*, apical to the contact point, (2) as *cervical white spots* on the buccal and lingual surfaces or even as a white band of decalcification circling the crown, and (3) on the walls of the deep *occlusal fissures*—all areas of plaque accumulation and bacterial stagnation.

Because of the critical importance of remineralization of incipient lesions, the use of the explorer to search for carious lesions is being questioned both in Europe and the United States.[22] This concern is generated by the fact that explorer examinations damage the *surface zone* of subsurface lesions and negate the possibility of remineralization. They also transfer organisms from one tooth to another.[23–25] To avoid this problem of iatrogenic damage, several studies have suggested that *visual examinations* and *professional judgment* equal the value of the explorer in the diagnosis of smooth-surface lesions and root caries.[23,24] The one exception is the need for an explorer to search for secondary (ie, recurrent) caries and ditched margins of existing faulty restorations.[26]

This changeover to an *explorerless examination* should be greatly facilitated and possibly improved in accuracy by the increasingly frequent use of the intraoral video camera (IVC), which greatly magnifies the structures being scrutinized (Fig 21–2).

The IVC has the advantage of allowing an area to be freeze-framed to study a questionable site better or, if desired, to make high-quality color photographs by outputting an image to a high-resolution color printer. Cracked or fractured amalgams are easy to identify using this technique. Because the camera has its own light source, each of the frames has the same high-quality color. The presentation of the examination on the high-resolution television screen is an outstanding means of educating and motivating patients. Because the entire examination is on video tape, it is possible to restudy previous treatment decisions and to compare a patient's clinical progress over time.

Interproximal Incipient Lesions

Many interproximal R1 smooth-surface lesions[e] detected on bite wing radiographs should be considered as candidates for re-

---

[e] An R 1 interproximal radiolucency is one that that has not progressed past the midpoint in the enamel.

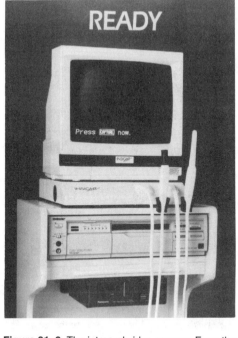

Figure 21–2. The intraoral video camera. From the top: High-resolution monitor on top of computer processing unit (CPU), high-quality color photograph printer (on shelf), and a video tape deck (at bottom). In front are two video cameras, with the intraoral camera to the right (white), and the straight-on camera to the left (black top). In use, the image from either camera is recorded to the tape in the video processor and, if desired, sent to the monitor. The tape recording can be kept for record purposes or for single "freeze frames" which can be downloaded to the monitor for review or to the printer for photographic prints. The straight-on camera is used for facial views or for photographing radiographs for computer storage. (*Courtesy of Insight Imaging Systems, Inc., 981 Industrial Road, San Carlos, CA 94070.*)

mineralization therapy. Once the interproximal incipient lesions are diagnosed from the radiograph, there should be *no need* to use the explorer to probe the site further. If these radiolucent areas are probed for explorer "stickiness," many of the white spots, which could otherwise be remineralized, immediately become overt lesions that must be restored. As an example, when probing incipient (white spot) interproximal lesions of recently extracted teeth, 0.5- to 2.0-mm overt lesions were created with an explorer.[27]

The value of considering remineralization as a priority approach to care for radiolucent interproximal lesions is seen in a study in Denmark.[28] The radiographs of 1080 proximal radiolucencies, which were used as the basis for *restorations* by 263 Danish dentists, were examined after treatment. The lesions that had been restored varied from barely visible radiolucencies to overt cavitation. The most frequent lesion demonstrated demineralization that had not progressed to obvious cavitation; frank cavitation accounted for *less than 10%* of the inserted restorations. It was concluded that the dentists could distinguish between sound and carious teeth but needed to identify better those lesions that were amenable to remineralization.[28]

Buccal and Lingual Incipient Lesions

For buccal and lingual smooth-surface lesions, a well-dried tooth and a good light are the main requisites for a visual examination. *No explorer is needed.* As early as 1970, von der Fehr and coworkers in a study involving multiple sugar water mouth rinses per day, *visually* observed the development of white spots over 23 days. Remineralization of the white spots was accomplished by use of oral hygiene and a fluoride mouth rinse.[29]

The importance of *not* penetrating the surface zone of incipient lesions with the tine of an explorer is illustrated by a 2-year study of 2767 free-standing smooth-surface lesions in the teeth of Scottish school children.[30] At the end of the 2 years of observing the status of buccal and lingual incipient lesions, 1543 (56%) remained the same, 505 (18%) had regressed *without any profes-*

sional intervention, 171 (7%) had progressed, 90 (3%) were restored, and 80 (3%) had been extracted. An observation was also made that the white spots that required restoration were accompanied by a greater plaque presence. Another possibly more important observation was that individuals having decalcification on free smooth surfaces had a greater incidence of caries on fissure walls and interproximal surfaces.[30] This appears to indicate that *once an incipient lesion is identified, it portends the development or presence of other sites of smooth-surface demineralization.* It also implies that once a *single* incipient lesion is identified, any remineralization procedures that are instituted should benefit *all* in situ sites that have not progressed to the point of visibility.

Pit-and-Fissure Lesions

The deep pits and fissures harbor bacteria and food debris. They are the privileged sanctuaries from which the contained bacteria can seed neighboring sites. Deep occlusal pits and fissures have a much greater caries risk than those with smooth, rounded fossae. Approximately 95% of all the carious lesions of children occur in occlusal pits and fissures.[31] Many already contain histologic (but not clinically discernible) caries involvement of the dentin. The correct diagnosis of occlusal pit-and-fissure caries is *precarious* by either visual or explorer techniques.[32] Reinforcing this conclusion is a study by 34 dentists who were asked to examine 61 extracted teeth for the presence of caries.[24] Histologic serial sections of the teeth were then made to provide the "correct" diagnoses. The results demonstrated that dentists were more likely not to treat decayed teeth than to restore sound teeth. Forty-two percent of all the teeth were correctly diagnosed. One of the teeth was diagnosed correctly by 70% of the dentists, and two lesions were never correctly diagnosed.[24] Another similar study using teeth extracted for orthodontic purposes found that 15% of the diagnoses were false-positives, which would normally have subjected such sticky fissures to unnecessary restorations.[33,34] The sensitivity of an explorer examination can decrease from 80% for wide fissures to 52% for those that are narrow.[34] It has also been suggested that the sharp explorer can even damage the nonmature occlusal surface of a recently erupted noncarious tooth, as well as the walls of the fissures.[23]

Sealants provide a perfect solution to the dilemma of the apparent probability of restoring fissures with a false-positive diagnosis, neglecting teeth with false-negative designations, or waiting indefinitely for a lesion to finally occur. First, sealants should be placed in *all* vulnerable fissures. The sealing of the fissures can be easily, quickly, and painlessly accomplished. The sealant serves to interdict the nutrient supply of the fissure microorganisms, leading to their extinction and the *hardening* of the underneath dentin.[35,36] As pointed out in Chapter 10, the placement of a sealant is probably the most conservative solution to arresting the caries process (if present), thereby saving tooth structure and avoiding the future probability of recurrent caries.[37] The placement of a sealant should be followed by a topical application of fluoride to help protect the *whole* tooth.

Traditionally, the majority of sealants were placed on the occlusal surfaces of children's teeth. The risk-assessment and *not the age* of the individual, however, should guide the decision to place or not to place a sealant. For every occlusal restoration present at any age, *a sealant was indicated previous to the development of overt cavitation.*

Despite the proven benefits of sealants, only 6.4% of children between ages 5 and 8, and 11.5% of those 9 to 11 years old exhibited occlusal surfaces covered with sealant in 1988.[18,19] Contrast this limited use of sealants with the fact that up to 95% of the caries experience for U.S. children are occlusal fissure lesions.[31,38]

The Remineralizable Cervical Lesion

The presence of an overt lesion is an indisputable sign of caries activity. Each lesion shelters acidogenic organisms that serve to maintain high mutans streptococcal and lactobacilli populations. Eliminating active, overt caries usually requires secondary preventive procedures, although some exceptions exist. Nyvad, Billings, and Markitzui each separately studied different chemotherapeutic approaches, using small numbers of subjects. RJ Billings and associates,[39] as well as A. Markitzui[40] and his colleagues *used topical fluorides.* Nyvad and Fejerskove[41] found that *where root lesions were accessible to brushing with a fluoride dentifrice,* it was possible to convert active root caries to an inactive status. Their reported success rates in arresting the caries after a year or more were 70%, 91%, and 100%, respectively.

Schaeken and associates found that the use of chlorhexidine causes a *hardening* of root caries as well as markedly suppressing the mutans streptococci over several months.[42] Zichert and coworkers also reported that chlorhexidine had a valuable suppressive effect on mutans streptococci in highly infected children.[43]

With the difficulty experienced in cavity preparation and retaining cervical restorations, either of the above mentioned options, (ie, use of fluoride or chlorhexidine) is preferable to restorations.

A Rational Approach to Caries Prevention

In previous chapters it was pointed out that

1. Caries only occurs if episodes of acid-induced demineralization are of *greater frequency* and *duration* as a *function of time,* than is the capacity of the host *defenses* to meet the acidogenic bacterial challenge and to *repair* the damage through *remineralization.*

2. Three different stages occur in the caries process: the initial microscopic in situ demineralization of rod ends in contact with the subsurface pellicle and plaque, the *incipient subsurface lesion* characterized by the white spot, and finally, overt cavitation.

3. The caries process can be prevented, arrested, and reversed in the in situ and incipient (white spot) stages on all surfaces of the teeth by use of sealants for pit and fissures and remineralization regimens for incipient smooth-surface lesions.

4. At the time of the dental examination it is necessary for the dentist to reasonably *anticipate in situ demineralization on the basis of tests and indices* and *to recognize and record the presence of white spot lesions* as well as overt lesions.

5. Once the mouth is restored to maximum health, the period till the next prophylaxis recall should be inverse to the level of the present treatment urgency.

It is the purpose of this chapter to enlarge on the above mentioned rational in order to point out how the profession can move from traditional emphasis on restorative dentistry to a preventive focus requiring appropriate sealant placement and re-mineralization strategies. Such a change-over requires no change in dental office routine, except for a much greater emphasis on the identification and care of teeth *needing sealants or remineralization therapy.*

PREVENTING CARIOUS LESIONS

Selecting Treatment Strategies

The caries activity indicators (CAI) recorded for parts 1 and 2 of the dental examination—incipient and overt coronal, root, and recurrent caries, and deep pits and fissures in part 1 of the examination; and the bacterial population found in the microbiologic caries activity test(s), saliva flow, plaque index, carbohydrate intake score found in part 2—can all be assigned ascending scores to reasonably indicate increasing levels of presumed caries activity (Table 21–1).

To use Table 21–1 begin at the upper left following the Treatment Urgency *column.* The next six columns represent clinical diagnostic findings that if positive, represent a threat to a tooth. If the finding for each of the caries categories is negative, a zero is placed in the appropriate block of the 0 Treatment Urgency *row.* If however, incipient or overt lesions are identified, enter the number found for each caries category in the Treatment Urgency 4 row. There is no intermediate possibility between Treatment Urgency 0 and 4 for the diagnostic entities—either a tooth is at risk due to impending or actual lesions and should be given priority treatment, or it is at no immediate risk.

The next four columns reflect the level of *risk* of incipient or overt caries. Circle the most appropriate number of bacteria found with the dip-slide results, the amount of saliva flow, and the plaque index. Because no standard has been established for the carbohydrate index, the score can only be arbitrarily placed at the treatment urgency level deemed most appropriate by the examiner.

TABLE 21–1. PATIENT'S CARIES ACTIVITY INDICATOR (CAI) "SCORECARD"

Treatment Urgency	Caries						Caries Activity Test	Saliva Flow	Plaque Index	Carbohydrate Intake
	Incipient		Overt							
	Proximal	Bucco-lingual	Coronal	Root	Recurrent	Deep Fissures				
0	0		0	0	0		100	<1.0/min	<10%	
1							1,000	1.0	10%	
2							10,000	0.5–1.0	20%	
3							100,000	0.5–1.0	30%	
4		1				2	1,000,000	,0.5/min	40%	

Note: Circle the highest notation in any of the columns to establish treatment urgency, 4 being most urgent.

Table 21–1 illustrates a typical patient profile. To determine the Treatment Urgency, select the highest Treatment Urgency row in which there is a number or a circle. In this case it is Treatment Urgency 4 because of the one incipient buccal lesion and two deep fissures. The level 4 rating will be retained until the two fissures are covered with pit-and-fissure sealants and fluoride remineralization strategies completed for the incipient lesion. If these two entries had been 0, the Treatment Urgency would have been 3 because of the bacterial counts.

Table 21–2 provides a *guide to* matching appropriate preventive dentistry options to the level of Treatment Urgency established in Table 21–1. To use Table 21–2, select the Treatment Urgency level determined in Table 21–1 and move horizontally across the row for suggested options to be used in a combination of office, home, and recall program directed to reducing present and future caries risk. Note that with each increase in treatment urgency from 0 to 4, the treatment response is escalated. Generally, these responses require education sessions in addition to the treatment regimen, to raise the patient's knowledge of dental health and to motivate the individual to comply better with recommended mechanical and chemical plaque control techniques.

Once the CAI primary preventive dentistry "score card" has been completed for the office record, a copy should be given to the patient as part of the education and counseling process. The written preventive plan should be well thought out to *match* the treatment intensity to the cariogenic challenge.

Remineralization Strategies

The evidence is now conclusive that physiologic remineralization occurs.[44] The remineralization includes nucleation and growth of the crystal. If fluoride is in the oral environment, the remineralized tooth structure is more resistant to demineralization than it was previously.[45] Theoretically, to curtail caries development and best accomplish remineralization of microscopic in situ, as well as *visible* incipient lesions, it is necessary to (1) reduce the population of cariogenic bacteria in the environment, (2) maintain low plaque index scores, (3) minimize the intake of sugar, and (4) utilize remineralization strategies to enhance the normal

TABLE 21–2. GUIDE FOR ESTABLISHING PRIMARY PREVENTIVE PLAN TO MATCH THE SEVERITY OF CAI CHALLENGE

Treatment Urgency	Prophy-laxis	Plaque Control	Nutrition Counseling	Office	Home	Restor-ation	Sealants	Recall Interval
0	P			F G	F, O			6
1	P	E	E	F G	F, O			6
2	P	E	E	F G	F, O			6
3	P	C	C,D	F G	F, R$_x$			3
4	P	C	C,D,M	F G	F, R$_x$	R	S	3

Key: P = Prophylaxis; E = Education if needed; C = Counseling session; D = 3-day diary; M = Medical referral, if necessary; FG = Fluoride gel of choice; F = Fluoride products (dentifrices and mouth rinses); O = Over-the-counter mouth rinses (Listerine); R$_x$ = Prescription chlorhexidine mouth rinse (Peridex); R = Restoration(s) needed; S = Sealant(s) needed.

salivary-driven tooth remineralization. The first of these objectives can be accomplished using two approaches.

The first step following the examination is to restore all overt lesions, thus preventing further progress of disease as well as eliminating bacterial seeding sites for infecting other vulnerable tooth surfaces. Restorative procedures alone, however, do not affect the mutans streptococci population for any length of time until the overt caries-seeding sites are eliminated. To overcome this problem, daily chlorhexidine rinses should be prescribed to suppress the mutans streptococci population.[46–49] The use of mutans streptococci and lactobacilli dip-slide tests at the end of the treatment phase can provide guidance in determining the need for a longer utilization of chemical plaque control.

Fluorides provide the basis for remineralization strategies. Water fluoridation, the "halo" effects of fluoridated water (in processed food and drink), and the use of fluoride-containing dentifrices all help to both curtail demineralization and enhance remineralization. Until recently, the consensus has been that fluoride tablet supplementation should be *discontinued* during the teenage years. Horowitz questions this practice on the basis of our present knowledge,

which indicates that fluoride continues to benefit dentate persons throughout life.[50] Thus, in fluoride-deficient areas, a high CAI score at *any* age should be the basis for considering fluoride supplementation.

Question 2. Which of the following statements, if any, are correct?

A. Smooth-surface white spots represent a potential carious lesion unless reversed by remineralization.

B. An explorer can produce iatrogenic damage to incipient lesions of the smooth surfaces or fissures.

C. Physiologic remineralization of teeth can occur without professional intervention.

D. The arraying of the caries activity indicators identifies the priority of actions needed for both preventive and treatment plans.

E. The strategies necessary to prevent overt caries are the same as those used to reverse incipient lesions.

Fluorides and Remineralization

Two times when a tooth is especially vulnerable to caries are (1) immediately after eruption and before maturation of the enamel, and (2) at any time in life following bacterial acid-induced demineralization. To meet the first of these dual challenges, several fluoride applications should be made from the time the first tip of the erupting cusp appears until the tooth is in occlusion. Even after full eruption is attained, fluoride should be applied several times professionally during the first year of intraoral maturation. The daily use of a fluoride dentifrice can help in attaining this objective.

In the second incidence, the many cycles of demineralization and remineralization at different periods throughout life are usually subclinical and are not possible to detect. Probably the best way to ensure enamel protection from caries progression during such periodic negative mineral balances is by a daily self-application of fluoride. The daily home application of topical fluoride by use of products, such as fluoride dentifrices and over-the-counter rinses (Fluorigard, Act) is easy to accomplish, effective, economical, and readily accessible to most consumers (Fig 21–3).

The *office* application of fluoride for the purpose of reducing demineralization or encouraging remineralization may take several forms. It may be a 4-minute tray application of a neutral fluoride or an APF gel.*f* Once the white spot is diagnosed, more urgent action is indicated. Here, a series of fluoride applications is indicated, much as advocated by Stookey for teeth that are erupting and seriously at risk due to their immature surface (Chapter 9). The extreme importance of remineralization therapy, as well as that of sealant placement, is that *they both help to maintain an intact tooth.* Once a restoration is inserted, experience indicates that because of the relatively short

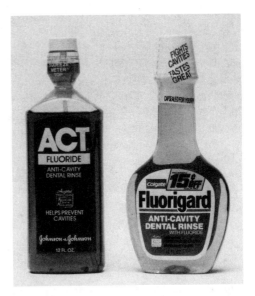

Figure 21–3. These readily available over-the-counter fluoride mouth rinses offer an effective and economical approach of reducing caries.

life span of the average filling, another restoration will be needed in its place in less than a decade.[51] Several studies have demonstrated a longevity of amalgam restorations of only a few years to as many as 10 years.[52–56] Thus, preventing *one* new cavity engenders a lifetime multiplier effect of preventing several recurrent lesions.

With the present knowledge on how to arrest the progression of incipient lesions without operative intervention, the present goal for the profession and the public should be the preservation—not the restoration—of teeth wherever possible without invasive treatment.[57]

EDUCATION PROGRAM

The educational process should begin with an interview to identify what the patient already knows about oral health and personal oral hygiene skills. This interview period

---

f The Council of Dental Materials, Instrument and Equipment of the ADA cautions that acidic preparations (APF) can cause surface roughening of porcelain teeth and composite restorations.

provides an opportunity to discuss the broad concepts of the relationship of caries and periodontal disease to individual personal oral hygiene habits. Specific attention should be directed to the patient's own problems, as well as to learning more about his or her aptitude for and attitudes about prevention.

In a primary prevention program that places priority on remineralization and sealant use, it is necessary to focus on the actions needed for success. To accomplish this, it is essential to enlist the patient as a "cotherapist" with the dentist and the dental hygienist in developing an integrated office virgule home self-care program. For patients to assume this role, they need to know *what* they are expected to do, *how* it is to be done, and *why* it is to be accomplished. They need to understand the interrelated roles of sugar, bacteria, and plaque in causing demineralization and eventual cavitation. Finally they need to understand the roles of prophylaxis, toothbrushing, and flossing; of fluoride and remineralization; and chemical plaque control in meeting the cariogenic and gingivitis challenges. At this time it is critical that the patient be informed of the advantage of a *prevention-oriented* dental program compared with a treatment-oriented one. This only can be accomplished as part of the office education plan.

If possible, one individual from the office should be selected to carry out the main thrust of the education program. The person selected can be an assistant or a dental hygienist. The main attributes desired are that the person be mature, intelligent, and compassionate; has leadership ability; likes people; can persuade; has the patience to accept and to improve on the daily presentations; and has the flexibility *to adapt presentations to meet patients' needs.*

At the end of the educational sessions, *it is exceedingly important that patients fully*

realize that they are at risk, but that the disease can be overcome as a result of the recommended therapy.* As a part of the medicine's "one third rule," one third of all patients with chronic disease can be expected to comply with instructions, one third comply erratically, and one third do not comply at all.[58,59] It is also necessary to inform the patient that all treatment eventually fails without a wholehearted and effective self-care commitment. Only the patient can decide whether she or he wants to pay to *prevent* disease or to accept—and pay for—*more extensive treatment.* If the patient continually fails to comply with instructions, it is prudent to document a warning advisory in the dental record to forestall any possible later legal repercussions.[60]

The Learning Environment

This discussion is tempered by the realization that not all dental offices have the necessary patient flow or the office space to support a separate *preventatory* (Fig 21-4).[g] Several ideas are suggested, however, that are applicable to supporting an intensified preventive thrust in a practice.

The preventatory should be a cheerful, well-lighted, and comfortable room. It is desirable to have floor benches and wall cabinets around the room to store necessary supplies. Appropriate nutrition and other oral health posters can be displayed.

A table is needed around which individuals can comfortably sit while listening to the dental hygienist or assistant. If possible, the spouse of a patient should be included in the educational programs conducted in the preventatory to provide desirable peer

---

[g] The preventatory is a separate room in the dental office where patients learn how to help prevent *their* dental problems. In the same way that an operatory is equipped to treat a patient efficiently, the preventatory should be equally well equipped to teach prevention.

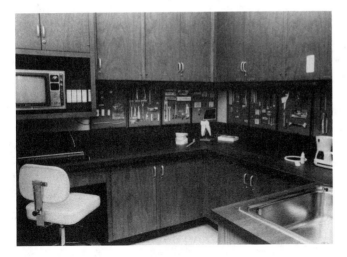

Figure 21–4. The preventatory includes facilities for video presentations, display boards, and all necessary equipment and facilities to explain, demonstrate, and involve patient participation in self-care instruction.

support.[61] The fee for additional individuals can be waived as a public relations gesture because no financial loss is attributable to such a practice (see Appendix 21–1).

Because plaque and bacterial control are to be the main focus of any education program, training aids can be used that illustrate the different procedures needed to attain this objective. Emphasis should be on the use of those training aids specifically applicable to the patient's problem. Slides, photographs, and hand-outs relating to the subjects being discussed are some examples. A video cassette player and high-resolution monitor should be available to review the intra oral video camera examination. The slides and software selected for use with the other audio–visual equipment should be short, interesting, well prepared, and directly related to the education program of the office or clinic. The material should, if possible, be acceptable to the age, ethnic, or racial group represented by the patient.

Instructions in the use of fluoride products requires an additional set of supplies. Mouth rinses, such as Fluorigard and Act, should be available for demonstration purposes and as samples for the patient to take home and use. A mouth rinse is easy to use. If used before bedtime, its action continues throughout the night; if applied before breakfast, it probably provides a reservoir of fluoride in the plaque that is protective during the high sugar-consuming period known as the breakfast hour. A daily mouth rinse can be included in the busy morning bathroom schedule of any patient. For instance, it is so easy to accomplish a several-minute mouth rinse while taking a shower.

Other fluoride products, such as fluoride dentifrices, gels, and fluoride supplements, should be available so the hygienist or assistant can discuss their relative merits, as well as the need for care in handling (See Chapter 8). The tablets and drops are prescription items, but the dental hygienist should be able to reinforce any instructions by the dentist (Table 21–3).

Plaque Control

Dental plaque is *always* present at the interface between the saliva and the tooth surface. A shift within the plaque environment in the colonization by acidogenic bacteria in combination with a cariogenic

TABLE 21–3. DAILY FLUORIDE (F) DOSAGE RECOMMENDATIONS

F Content of Drinking Water (ppm)	0 to 2 Years (mg)	2 to 3 Years (mg)	3 to 14 Years (mg)
0.0–0.3	0.25	0.50	1.00
0.3–0.7	0.0	0.25	0.50

Approved by the Council on Dental Therapeutics of the American Dental Association, *Accepted Dental Therapeutics*, 40th ed. 1984:401.

substrate causes demineralization. As increasing amounts of plaque accumulate at different locations, the probability for caries activity increases. If oral hygiene has been inadequate, the prudent practitioner, as a precautionary measure, should assume that subclinical in situ precarious lesions are *in progress* particularly in the interproximal areas.[62] The presence of more than a minimal amount of plaque in any area should be considered an infectious site in need of plaque control.

Plaque control is usually associated with the daily use of a toothbrush and floss. In this situation, plaque removal must be accomplished by the individual; the dental health professional can only help by providing guidance. Brushing and flossing can be taught to those who are motivated to learn and who have no physical disability.

The majority of the public regard a routine prophylaxis as simply a "cleaning"; few consider it as an essential part of an integrated dental office/home self-care plaque control program. Often the cosmetic effects are more important to the patient than the fact that it removes the plaque that is the underlying cause of both caries and periodontal disease. Remedying this misinformation is a teaching task for the dental hygienist. Also, the fact that dental insurance plans usually reimburse the policy owner for only a twice yearly prophylaxis places a restraint on the number of prophylaxes accomplished during the year, whatever the need.

Probably the most underused and one of the most effective methods of reducing the mutans streptococci population is chemical plaque control. Because of its effect on the plaque population chlorhexidine, a prescription item, is extremely effective in reducing caries, as well as in aiding the treatment of gingivitis. Listerine has less substantivity, but costs less and is available over the counter.

Brushing and Flossing

The brushing and flossing techniques used by the patient can be observed by providing a model on which procedures can be performed; the method used on the model can later be verified in the mouth. The Bass method of brushing should be demonstrated, as outlined in Chapter 5, making appropriate modifications to accommodate the individual patient's teeth, such as malaligned teeth, tight contacts, or any anatomic deviations that could lead to plaque formation. Individuals who use a powered brush should be advised prior to the appointment to bring it to the teaching sessions. The methods of flossing are next explained and demonstrated.

The Plaque Index

The plaque index is used to evaluate the extent of plaque on the teeth. First, all teeth are stained with a disclosing solution (Fig 2–1). After a short rinse, the still stained *smooth surfaces* of all teeth are recorded on a form (Appendix 21–2). The number of smooth surfaces showing disclosing agent are then divided by the total number of smooth surfaces available to give a plaque index as a percentage. For instance, if 20 surfaces are stained out of 80 possible smooth surfaces, the plaque index is 25%.

The patient is then asked to proceed to brush under supervision, going from tooth to tooth in a patterned sequence. Corrections are made as the patient proceeds from one quadrant to the next. Once brushing is complete, another disclosing tablet is used to develop a new plaque index, which is then compared with the one made before brushing. If both the plaque index and the specific sites of plaque accumulation are compared with previous plaque indices, it is possible to identify areas where oral hygiene efforts need to be reinforced. If the plaque index is not down to *10%, or less*, a second reinforcing session should be scheduled. A sufficient number of disclosing tablets should be dispensed to permit the patient to practice tooth brushing and flossing at home. This allows the patient to observe both successes and failures of his or her brushing techniques. At the second appointment, the patient brushes and flosses *prior to* completing a plaque index. The purpose of the use of the disclosing tablet *after* brushing is to determine the effectiveness of the habit patterns the patient has developed.

NUTRITION APPLICATION

Although most individuals entering the dental office appear outwardly healthy and do not seem to be suffering from overt malnutrition, such appearances provide insufficient information for determining whether a patient needs diet assessment and counseling. Patients who benefit from nutrition interventions in the dental office fall into several categories:

- Those who have incipient or overt caries, gingivitis, or periodontitis
- Those who may be at risk for developing dental disease as a result of physiologic deficiencies (ie, xerosto-

mia) or habit factors (ie, cracking open watermelon seeds with the anterior teeth)
- Those who are at risk for developing nutritional problems as a result of their oral or dental condition (eg, oral cancer patients)
- Those for whom medical or psychosocial factors (ie, bulimia) may impair nutritional status or those whose nutritional status may affect their medical or psychologic state.

The first two of these groups benefit from appropriate counseling by dental team members. Those in the latter two groups should be referred to the patient's physician or to a registered dietitian for more indepth nutrition care. In all cases, however, the patient's dietary status cannot be determined without some form of nutritional screening. Thus, it can be argued that all patients should be screened for nutrition risk, with the results of the screening dictating any further action.

Three-day Food Diary

The most common approaches to diet screening involve a nutrition history questionnaire and some form of food intake report. This information is then evaluated to determine whether the patient needs further nutrition intervention.

The 3-day food intake record is a special form (Appendix 21–4) on which the patient enters all the foods, beverages, and snacks he or she has consumed over a 3-day period. Also included are such items as medications, vitamins, and breath fresheners. The patient must understand that the diary is employed to determine what is typically eaten. For purposes of example, the health professional should aid the patient in completing the entries for the previous day. This helps ensure that the patient understands the correct procedure and the necessary detail desired. In addition to the kind of food eaten, the amount (ie, one large apple, 4 oz steak [barbecued], ½ cup of carrots [raw], etc.) and method of preparation (baked, fried, etc.) should also be recorded. Because eating habits often differ on the weekends, at least one weekend day should be included in the record.

Evaluation of General Diet Adequacy

When the 3-day record is complete, the evaluator must review the entries with the patient. An analysis of the patient's diet is made at this time. This can be facilitated by using a green pencil to circle the acceptable foods that fall within the various compartments of the USDA Food Guide Pyramid. Then a red pencil is used to circle the fermentable carbohydrates. The next step for the evaluator requires a separate worksheet (Appendix 21–5). Each item circled in green on the food intake record is assigned to the appropriate Pyramid food group and a chit mark made in the column for that particular day and group. At the end, the number of chit marks for each group is totaled and divided by 3 to obtain the average number of daily servings. This average is compared with the daily recommended averages for the Food Pyramid groups (Fig 15–1) which are:

- Fats, Oils, and Sweets: Use sparingly
- Milk, Yogurt, and Cheese: 3–5 servings
- Meat, Poultry, Fish, Dry Beans, Eggs, and Nuts: 2–3 servings
- Vegetables: 3–5 servings
- Fruit: 2–4 servings
- Bread, Cereal, Rice, and Pasta: 6–11 servings.

The plus or minus differences between the average for the 3 days and the recommended number of servings is recorded in the column marked "adequacy."

The use of the 3-day record can be carried one step further. The food items and the quantity of the food servings can be entered on a computer software program to provide a printout listing the patient's estimated intake of key nutrients in relation to the RDA. In this way possible inadequacies or excesses of nutrients can be assessed.

If at this time a nutritional problem is still suspected, medical referral is indicated.

Assessment of Cariogenic Potential

The frequency of intake and the consistency of refined carbohydrates are key factors in the initiation and continuation of the caries process. Any patient who demonstrates a higher than average risk, as demonstrated by the caries activity indicators, needs an evaluation of refined carbohydrate intake. This can be accomplished on a screening basis by having the patient complete a short carbohydrate intake form (Appendix 21–3). This form can be used as a basis for discussion in the counseling session. All nutritional guidance that is directed to reducing sugar intake should be paralleled by microbiologic testing to monitor streptococci and lactobacilli saliva levels.[18]

Nutrition Counseling

The nature of the counseling is mainly determined on the basis of the information contained in the medical history, the nutrition questionnaire, and the 3-day record. From the beginning of the counseling session, it should be emphasized that it is the patient, and not the counsellor, who bears the responsibility for making any needed changes in eating habits.

Throughout the counseling period, the key concept advanced for caries control should be that the bacterial challenge factor can be minimized by reducing the intake of fermentable carbohydrates. This discussion can include suggestions for noncariogenic alternatives or the use of the noncariogenic sugar substitutes. The host's tooth defense factors can be maximized by the availability of fluoride and through the intake of a *well-balanced diet* that provides the nutrients necessary for maintaining the immune and nonimmune defenses of the body.

Diet Plan

A plan to deal with any nutritional deficiency is then developed. This specific plan should be individualized according to the patient's food preferences, habits, and environment. It can be based on the nutrition assessment sheet prepared by both the counselor and the patient (Appendix 21–4). Initial efforts should be to reduce the cariogenic potential and to ensure a nutritious diet. In this way, any changes in dietary behavior agreed to by the patient are realistic. The active involvement and participation of the patient's family can often be helpful in motivating and encouraging the patient to adhere to a selected dietary regimen.

On return visits, patient adherence to the dietary plan can be reevaluated and, if necessary, more assistance and relevant information provided. For those needing more in-depth nutritional care, referral to the patient's physician or a nutritionist is essential. The use of microbiologic caries activity testing is helpful in corroborating adherence with the reduced fermentable carbohydrate diet recommended in the oral hygiene plan.

Question 3. Which of the following statements, if any, are correct?

A. The daily use of a fluoride mouth rinse or use of a fluoride dentifrice can enhance remineralization.

B. In using the various CAI to develop the preventive response to meet the

bacterial challenge, it is desirable to use the indicator that has the *maximum,* rather than the minimum, severity level.

C. To learn whether a patient has mastered mechanical plaque control techniques, it is better to disclose *before* brushing.

D. A high plaque index score should trigger an evaluation of remineralization options.

E. In the Food Pyramid, more daily servings are recommended from both the vegetable and fruit groups than from the pasta group.

PERIODONTAL DISEASE AND PRIMARY PREVENTION

A Rational Approach to Preventing Gingivitis

In previous chapters it has been emphasized that

1. A high gingival plaque index score or the presence of supragingival calculus (or both) usually accompanies a gingivitis; as a result, bleeding on probing is a reasonable indicator of gingivitis.

2. Gingivitis can be reversed by office-instituted and home oral hygiene measures that remove or severely disturb the dental plaque.

3. Once the gingiva is restored to maximum health, the next recall interval should be based on the *present* treatment urgency rating, that is, the higher the "score," the shorter the time interval between appointments.

Periodontal activity indicators and guidelines for appropriate therapy, counseling, and recall schedules can be developed

TABLE 21–4. A PATIENT'S PERIODONTAL DISEASE ACTIVITY INDICATOR (PAI) "SCORECARD"

Treatment Urgency	Plaque Index*	Calculus Level†	Pocket Depth	Bleeding on Probing Number Sites
0	0%	0	<3 mm	0
1	10%	A	<3 mm	0
2	20%	B	<3 mm	0
3	30%	C	3 mm	0
4	40%	D	>3 mm	1

Note: Circle appropriate entry in each column.
* Plaque index = Number of stained smooth surfaces/Total number of smooth surfaces
† Calculus level: 0 = Insignificant; A = Slight; B = Moderate supragingival with isolated subgingival calculus; C = Moderate supragingival and moderate subgingival calculus; D = Heavy supra- and/or subgingival calculus.

in the same way as the previously discussed caries activity indicator guidelines (Tables 21–4 and 21–5). Four accepted indicators are the plaque index, calculus severity, number of bleeding sites on probing, and pocket depth. Unlike the CAI laboratory tests in which caries risk is related to mutans streptococci and lactobacilli levels, no parallel acceptable *screening* tests are available for periodontopathogens. A number of tests for *Actinobacillus actinomycetemcomitans, Bacteroides gingivalis,* and *B intermedius* are used as guidelines for *treatment* decisions, but their cost-benefit as microbiologic periodontal activity indicator tests has not been adequately assessed (see Chapter 13 for details).

Plaque and Plaque Control

As a general rule, *no treatment nor any preventive measures designed to arrest and reverse the periodontal disease process can be successful without the constant and effective daily removal of the bacterial plaque.* Initially, a marginal gingivitis of local origin occurs as a result of bacterial metabolic end products in the *supra*gingival plaque. The resultant gingivitis may or may not eventually progress to periodontitis. If it does, the supragingival plaque can serve as an initial source of microorganisms for the *subgingival* plaque.[63,64] It is essential that starting at an early age a person use plaque control measures that remove or severely disturb plaque at least once a day. The toothbrush-

TABLE 21–5. GUIDE FOR ESTABLISHING PRIMARY PREVENTIVE PLAN TO MATCH THE SEVERITY OF PAI CHALLENGE

Treatment Urgency	Prophylaxis Education Counseling	Chemical Plaque Control		Recall Interval
		Office	*Home*	
0	P,E	FG	Hf,O	6
1	P,E	FG	Hf,O	6
2	P,E	FG	Hf,O	6
3	P,C	FG	Hf,R$_x$	3
4	P,C	FG	Hf,R$_x$	3,PS

Key: P = Prophylaxis; E = Education if needed; C = Nutrition and plaque control counseling; FG = Fluoride gel of choice; H = Home fluorides (fluoride dentifrices and mouth rinses); O = Over-the counter antiplaque agents (Listerine); R$_x$ = Prescription antiplaque agent (Peridex); PS = Referral to periodontal specialist if necessary.

ing and flossing accomplished while the periodontium is healthy are intended to prevent marginal gingivitis.

If unsuccessful in this objective, the preventive effort should immediately be directed to reversing the disease process before permanent changes occur in the periodontium that signal the onset of inflammatory periodontitis. Once pocket formation has commenced, the daily plaque control program becomes increasingly difficult and time-consuming.

In August 1986, the U.S. Food and Drug Administration approved the *prescription* sale of Procter and Gamble's Peridex, a 0.12% chlorhexidine gluconate solution as a mouth rinse. This action was soon followed by the American Dental Association approving the product as a plaque control agent, useful in the control of gingivitis. Peridex provides a potent new adjunctive agent for the primary prevention of *both* caries and gingivitis. In controlled mouth rinse test programs, chlorhexidine has both prevented a buildup of plaque and reduced plaque accumulations with the use of brushing. These qualities are due to the *substantivity* of the agent; that is, (1) it adsorbs to the tissues in the target area, (2) it is released slowly, and (3) it is released in an active form. The variable amount of tooth staining that occurs with the use of chlorhexidine can often be removed at home by some of the powered rotary toothbrushes or by office prophylaxis. Philosophically, the staining might be advantageous inasmuch as it is a positive signal for patients to participate in recall programs, which in turn enhances the probability for a "fail-safe" plaque disease control program.

Following the approval of chlorhexidine as a *prescription* item, Listerine was approved as an *over-the-counter* antiplaque product that does not have the same substantivity of chlorhexidine and hence must be used more often. The widespread use of Listerine, however, could have a considerable effect on the prevalence and severity of gingivitis if used by large portions of the U.S. population.

Calculus is an indicator of impending gingivitis mainly because its porous surface permits the plaque to accumulate on its roughened surface (Fig 21–5). The presence of calculus should connote the need for an appointment for prophylaxis. If an undue amount of calculus rapidly accumulates, more effective plaque control procedures and more frequent prophylaxes are indicated. The rapid accumulation of calculus indicates a deficiency in the patient's current daily toothbrushing and flossing routines. Other factors that are harbingers of periodontal problems are overhanging restorations, ill-fitting crowns and bridges, orthodontic appliances, and prosthetic devices.

Gingivitis Evaluation

The progression from gingival health to gingivitis is indicated by changes in tissue color, contour, consistency, and bleeding. The bleeding accounts for the "pink tooth brush" first noticed by the individual. Probably the most objective, sensitive, reproducible, and reliable indication of the pres-

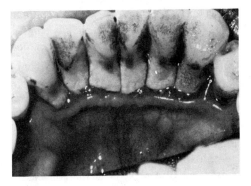

Figure 21–5. The heavy calculus must be removed by a professional to assist the patient's plaque control effort.

ence of gingivitis is the bleeding of the gingiva that follows gentle probing. The number and location of such bleeding sites should be entered on the patient's "score card" (Table 21–4). The apical migration of the epithelial attachment, gingival recession, furcation exposure, tooth mobility, and exudation that characterize inflammatory periodontitis all require secondary preventive dentistry treatment before primary preventive procedures can again be used to maintain oral health.

With the great importance of plaque control for periodontal disease prevention or maintenance programs, a patient with any level of periodontal involvement should complete the same educational and plaque control program as recommended for the patient at high risk for caries.

Periodontal Management with Primary Prevention

In the treatment of periodontal disease, the judgment must always be made about whether the patient is sufficiently motivated to participate in daily time-consuming routines of plaque control. If the patient cannot accomplish the desired level of control, gingival surgery is often necessary to provide a better access to the subgingival plaque. *It should be noted that gingival surgery is not a cure for periodontal disease;* the patient must still master effective plaque control techniques to avoid a recurrence of epithelial attachment loss.

The Recall Appointment

Although Table 21–6 is intended as a guide, its use must be moderated by professional judgment. The recall appointment permits a reevaluation of past treatment and the establishment of a new recall interval based on the new CAI and PAI findings. Essentially, the recall appointment provides an opportunity for a screening examination

TABLE 21–6. MINIMAL COMPONENTS OF A RECALL APPOINTMENT IN AN INTEGRATED PREVENTIVE DENTISTRY PLAN

Recall Appointment
1. Check integrity of previous sealants and progress of remineralization of white spots (visual check).
2. Check restorations for ditching or recurrence of caries (explorer).
3. Complete a plaque index for previous CAI and PAI treatment urgency scores of 2, 3, or 4.
4. Dip-slide tests for all previous CAI treatment urgency scores of 3 or 4.
5. Complete a periodontal screening and recording examination for pocket depth (Chapter 13, (PSR)).
6. Evaluate calculus extent, and determine the bleeding index for previous PAI treatment urgency scores of 3 and 4.
7. Accomplish a prophylaxis.
8. Establish next recall appointment on basis of severity of above findings.

Annual Dental Examination
Repeat parts 1 and 2 of original dental examination.

and a prophylaxis that can be accomplished by the dental hygienist. Shallhorn and Snider[65] and Pfeifer and Pfeifer[66] found that it took approximately 53 and 57 minutes, respectively, to complete such a recall routine.

If compliance with mechanical and chemical plaque control instructions have been adequate during the interim between recalls, the treatment urgency level should have dropped to the 0 or 1 level. This should reduce the time needed for education, except to point out minor problem areas of plaque accumulation.

The practice of mechanical and chemical plaque control at home, coupled with the prophylaxis at recall is beneficial for the prevention of both caries and periodontal problems. Axelsson and Lindhe, in a study of the benefits of a 3-month prophylaxis schedule found that *both* caries and periodontal disease could be well controlled over a 6-year period.[67] Ramfjord and colleagues also noted that professional toothcleaning at 2- to 3-month intervals could compensate for *imperfect* patient plaque control.[68] This success is attributed to the fact that the professional cleaning interrupts (ie, removes) the stable, pathogenic plaque, converting it to a temporary nonpathogenic state.[69] Approximately 3 months are required before the pathogenic plaque reforms.[60] Thus, for those with a record of past rampant caries or gingivitis, the 3-month recall is salient. Those with a severity index from 0 to 2, can be placed on 12- or 6-month recall intervals. In view of Axellson and Lindhe's success, however, all patients should be offered the shorter periodic prophylaxis as a "fail safe" option for preventing both caries and periodontal disease. For those undergoing maintenance therapy following periodontal surgery, the 3-month recall should be considered *mandatory.*[60]

In addition to the recall appointments, an annual dental examination should be scheduled with a repeat of the part 1 and part 2 dental examinations, comparable to an annual medical examination.

Question 4. Which of the following statements, if any, are correct?

A. A "pink toothbrush," (due to gingival bleeding) is one of the first signs of gingivitis.

B. Chlorhexidine is an *over-the-counter* agent used for gingivitis and for control of mutans streptococci.

C. The *same* plaque control methods used for caries prevention are applicable for controlling gingivitis and periodontitis.

D. Periodontal surgery is a *cure* for periodontitis.

E. Prophylaxes to control accumulation of plaque following periodontal surgery are indicated at *6-month intervals.*

The Computer

The computer is now a standard piece of equipment in the dental office. It is useful for appointment making, stock control, billing, correspondence, diagnosis, and charting. In this last area, the computer is rapidly becoming essential. Computerized charting systems are available that enable direct chairside entry of examination data by voice entry or by touch screen technique. The latter technique allows the assistant to touch the screen at the appropriate point and key in a code to indicate the type of lesion or restoration. The same can be done for a periodontal examination by use of another screen activated from the keyboard (Fig 21–6).

Concomitant with the increased need for charting the multiple findings of the caries and periodontal examinations is a need for expanded software to facilitate much of the recording now made on paper forms. To help in this effort periodontal probes are now available that automatically signal the computer to record the pocket depth when encountering a given resistance at the base of the gingival sulcus. It has already been mentioned that diet analysis can be rapidly and probably more effectively accomplished using computer programs now available for the purpose. Another valuable program is available for determining the indications, contraindications, and incompatibilities of available drugs. If desired, software can be developed to take the data of the dental examination and format it into CAI and PAI arrays, such as portrayed in Tables 21–1, 21–2, 21–4, and 21–5. Even the differences between examinations can be placed on a graph to show progress or decline.

In addition to the advantages for professional and administrative uses, recall programs can be easily handled. With very little instruction, an office manager or dental as-

578   PRIMARY PREVENTIVE DENTISTRY

Total Chart - Gates, Coral D [perio comparison]

Patient Teeth Perio Tplan Print Undo Exit

Date																		
10/25/91	·	·	2-2-2	3-3-3	3-3-3	3-2-3	3-2-3	2-2-2	3-3-3	2-3-2	3-3-3	3-3-3	3-3-3	3-3-3	4-3-4	4-4-4	·	·
11/15/92	·	·	3-4-3	3-3-3	3-4-3	3-3-3	3-4-3	3-3-3	3-3-3	2-3-2	3-3-3	3-3-3	3-4-3	3-4-3	3-4-3	3-3-3	·	·
11/16/93	·	·	5-4-4	5-4-4	3-4-4	4-4-4	5-4-4	4-4-4	5-4-4	5-4-4	3-3-3	4-3-3	3-3-4	4-4-5	4-4-5	5-5-5	·	·

Teeth: 1 2 3 4 5 6 7 8 9 10 11 12 13 14 15 16

Date																	
10/25/91	·	3-3-3	2-3-3	3-4-3	4-3-3	4-3-4	3-2-3	2-3-3	3-4-3	2-3-2	3-2-3	2-3-2	3-2-3	4-4-4	4-3-4	·	·
11/15/92	·	4-4-4	3-3-3	2-3-2	3-3-3	3-4-3	4-3-4	2-2-2	4-4-4	3-4-3	3-4-3	4-4-4	3-4-3	4-4-5	4-4-5	·	·
11/16/93	·	4-4-5	4-3-3	3-4-4	5-5-3	3-3-5	4-4-3	5-5-4	5-5-5	3-3-3	4-4-4	5-5-5	4-4-4	5-5-5	7-6-6	·	·

Date																	
10/25/91	·	3-3-2	4-4-3	4-4-3	3-3-2	3-3-2	3-3-2	3-3-2	3-3-2	3-3-3	3-2-3	3-3-2	3-3-3	4-4-4	3-3-4	·	·
11/15/92	·	3-3-4	2-3-3	4-3-4	2-3-2	3-3-3	3-3-3	3-3-3	3-3-3	3-3-3	4-4-4	3-4-3	3-3-4	4-4-4	3-4-3	·	·
11/16/93	·	5-4-5	5-5-3	4-3-4	3-4-3	3-3-3	4-3-3	3-3-4	5-4-4	4-4-5	4-4-3	4-3-3	3-3-4	4-3-5	5-4-5	·	·

Teeth: 32 31 30 29 28 27 26 25 24 23 22 21 20 19 18 17

Date																	
10/25/91	·	4-3-3	2-3-3	4-3-3	2-3-2	3-3-3	3-3-3	3-3-3	3-3-3	3-3-3	3-3-3	3-3-3	4-3-3	4-4-4	3-3-3	·	·
11/15/92	·	3-3-3	4-3-3	3-3-3	3-4-3	4-3-4	3-3-3	3-3-3	3-3-3	4-3-4	4-4-4	3-4-3	3-3-3	4-3-4	3-4-3	·	·
11/16/93	·	5-4-5	5-4-5	4-5-4	4-4-4	4-3-4	4-4-4	4-4-4	4-4-4	3-3-3	3-3-3	3-3-5	4-4-5	5-6-6	4-4-5	·	·

	Teeth	Bleed	Pus	Both	Furc	Mob	1 - 3 mm	4 - 5 mm	6+ mm
10/25/91	28	0	0	0	1	1	139	29	0
11/15/92	28	8	9	7	6	5	115	53	0
11/16/93	28	11	11	9	7	6	44	119	5

Figure 21–6. A computer-generated record that permits easy comparison of the findings of any past three periodontal examinations. Color coding (not possible on this black and white photo) allows easy detection of differences in gingival sulcus probing depths of 1–3 mm (black), 4–5 mm (yellow), and 6+ mm (red). The tooth icons are used to indicate (by use of different colored dots) the location of calculus, bleeding, exudation, mobility, and furcations. A total summary of the findings of the three compared examinations is automatically presented in the bottom score box. The data can be presented on a monitor, or they can be printed. (*Courtesy of Professional Systems Plus, Inc., 7030 S. Yale, Tulsa, OK 496-0042.*)

sistant can easily enter changes in appointments and generate programmed recall notices that are automatically printed out for mailing on scheduled dates. Such time savings and improved administration are essential, even in small private dental practices.

One recent advance in dental technology that should be important in conducting future caries prevention programs is *computed dental radiography (CDR)*. A key feature is its use of intraoral sensors *instead* of film, onto which the x-rays are beamed (Fig 21–7). This activation of the sensors by the x-ray beam requires only approximately 10% to 50% of the radiation required for ultraspeed film. The resulting digitalized image can then be fed into a computer for instant record *storage* and *retrieval* (Fig 21–8). Alternatively, the digitalized image, which is stored either on the computer hard drive or on a floppy disc, can be fed into a printer to produce a photograph for comparison with past radiographs. These photographs can be used for patient education or for insurance company verification. The automatic exposure compensation results in

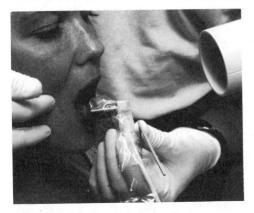

Figure 21–7. A demonstration of the insertion of the sensor into the mouth. The electronic sensor and exit wires from the mouth to the computer cable are covered with a plastic sheath. The present office x-ray unit can be utilized as the energy source for the image. (*Courtesy of New Image Industries, Inc., 21218 Vanowen Street, Canoga Park, CA 91303.*)

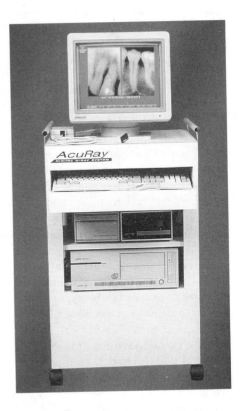

Figure 21–8. After the intraoral sensor is activated, the image is sent to the computer processor, thence it can be directed to (1) a high-resolution 13-inch monitor, (2) storage on a hard or floppy disc, or (3) to a high-resolution printer for a printout. The recessed keyboard, along with appropriate software, permits control of density, size, and points of entry of superimposed notations and patient identification. (*Courtesy of New Image Industries, Inc., 21218 Vanowen Street, Canoga Park, CA 91303.*)

a uniform density over a wide range of exposure values. It is possible to zoom in on parts of the image on the computer screen to examine the smallest details, and enhancement techniques can be used to lighten or darken areas of the screen for better diagnosis.

The above capabilities of CDR enable radiographs to be made that are much more uniform in contrast than those now possible. Also, CDR allows evaluation of density changes before and after remineralization therapy. It permits radiographs to be made without exposing the patient to excessive doses of radiation—a problem that until now prompted the American Dental Association to recommend that all radiographs be accomplished *only* if clinical signs indicated a need.[70] The abovementioned applications are but a few of the wonders to come.[71] Electronic media are even now used to transmit medical and oral health records around the world. The era of the computer has arrived in the dental office to the benefit of both the dental profession and the patient.

Financial Realities of Prevention

Like treatment regimens, primary preventive dentistry often necessitates multiple appointments. Individualized recall schedules are required to reinforce plaque control effectiveness and to monitor the success of self-care programs. For a patient to achieve optimal oral health within a preventive program, the health professional's time and expertise *must be reimbursed with a fair and equitable fee*—one based on preventing disease, just as a fair and equitable fee is now paid for treating disease.

The idea of purchasing good oral health is alien to Americans who have traditionally purchased restorations, extractions, and prosthetic devices as a means to cope with disease. Thus, public expectations of dental care must change if the profession is to move into an era in which prevention replaces the amalgam restoration. The profession must prepare the *public* and *itself* for their new roles in this rapidly approaching epoch of oral disease prevention and full dentulism.

In 1989, in an editorial in the *Journal of Dental Research*, Thylstrup identified two major reasons that the benefits of prevention are not universally available. First, dental school curricula do not emphasize the importance of preventing disease. The second, and probably the most important reason, points out that "No reward is given for the arrest of ongoing disease by nonoperative techniques. No wonder then that dentists are performing operative dentistry the majority of the time."[72] As a more optimistic viewpoint of preventive dentistry, Moss, in another editorial in the same journal, pointed out that a group of pediatric dentists have established an office in California that specializes only in prevention and refers all restorative dentistry to others.[73]

In most cases, dental hygienists and assistants can provide the staffing to deliver the majority of primary preventive procedures considered as effective in the control of plaque diseases. This should reduce the cost to the patient and permit the dentist to increase the number of patients he or she cares for who have treatment needs. Oral health maintenance and enhancement, not just disease treatment, should be the hallmark of the dental profession.

Question 5. Which of the following statements, if any, are correct?

A. A 3-month interval between prophylaxes greatly decreases the incidence of *both* caries and gingivitis.

B. Patients should be given a copy of their CAI and PAI so they can monitor their progress.

C. Bite wing radiographs should be used *routinely* at 6-month intervals to detect interproximal caries.

D. Dental hygienists can supply the personnel needed to develop CAI and PAI indices to monitor caries and periodontal disease progress.

E. Dental examination information can be entered into the computer from chairside for use in primary, secondary, and tertiary preventive procedures.

SUMMARY

Every overt carious lesion that has occurred in the mouth started as a microscopic in situ demineralization and progressed through the subsurface lesion (white spot) stage prior to frank cavitation. If these incipient lesions on the smooth surfaces—interproximal, buccal, lingual—had been identified during routine office dental examinations, they could probably have been easily and economically returned to normal by remineralization therapy. In the case of the occlusal surface, the easy and painless placement of a sealant would have prevented the need for later restorations. Unfortunately, sealants are little used in children, even more rarely in adults, and seldom placed with the idea of their being considered as a conservative treatment for early fissure caries. Every deep fissure not showing frank cavitation should be considered for sealant placement. In practice, remineralization strategies are used to an even lesser extent than sealant placement.

The dental examination should not be solely focused on a search for pathology. Much more valuable is the search for and the recordings of caries and periodontal disease activity indicators—the CAI and PAI. Such an examination for caries should search for both overt and incipient lesions. It should include a plaque index, a carbohydrate intake score, and microbiologic test(s) to help in quantifying the number of cariogenic organisms. In searching for periodontal problems, the plaque index is associated both with gingivitis and inflammatory periodontitis. An examination of pocket depth can be used to determine epithelial attachment loss and the number of gingival bleeding sites. All these CAIs and PAIs provide evidence of impending or actual hard- and soft-tissue disease, which should trigger a series of treatment procedures for office or home application.

An examination focusing on primary prevention uses the same recorded data differently from its use as a basis for treatment. The various CAIs and PAIs can be arrayed according to severity. Then, based on the severity, a therapeutic response can be devised to match the bacterial challenges. By giving the highest priority to the remineralization of incipient lesions and placement of sealants in vulnerable fissures, *the disease chain from in situ demineralization to cavitation can be broken.* For those individuals at high risk for caries and gingivitis, more frequent recalls and closer monitoring of the CAIs and PAIs are possible.

At the end of the first treatment cycle, all overt lesions should be restored, all incipient lesions should be undergoing remineralization therapy, all the necessary sealants should be in place, and all gingivitis should be under control. Also, by this time, the patient should have the knowledge and understanding to participate with the oral health professionals in a team effort of prevention. At each future recall period, only reinforcement and a prophylaxis should be needed—at most, more remineralization procedures and sealant use may be indicated. For those dental practitioners and concerned patients with a commitment to optimal oral health, the time is NOW to enter the dawning new age of total plaque disease prevention.

ANSWERS AND EXPLANATIONS

1. A, D
   B—incorrect. The dental hygienist can share the task, including completion of the plaque index, microbiologic tests, and probing.
   C—incorrect. The difference is mainly in the way the same data are used.
   E—incorrect. Routine private practice patient care plans are heavily weighted in favor of disease control.
2. A, B, C, D, E
3. A, B, D
   C—incorrect. To learn if correct habits have been acquired, it is best to follow brushing with disclosing.
   E—incorrect. The pasta group, with 6 to 11 daily servings is the highest intake group, with the vegetable group requiring 3 to 5 servings and the fruit group, 2 to 4.
4. A, C
   B—incorrect. In the United States chlorhexidine is available by prescription only.
   C—incorrect. Periodontal surgery only removes the pockets to make plaque control possible.

E—incorrect. A 3-month interval is rec-ommended.

5. A, B, D, E

C—incorrect. Radiographs are not to be used routinely; they are to be used only when a clinical situation dictates their use. (This situation may change with the advent of computerized dental radiography with its minimal x-ray dosage.)

SELF-EVALUATION QUESTIONS

1. Health promotion may be defined as _____.

2. Four benefits of having teeth are _____, _____, _____, and _____.

3. The three stages from crystal dissolution to overt caries are (1) in _____ demineralization, which is microscopic; (2) visible demineralization, which is referred to as an _____ lesion; and (3) the overt carious lesion, which is not reversible.

4. Name at least five caries activity indicators that should be evaluated as part of the dental examination: _____, _____, _____, _____, and _____.

5. Name three conditions that are used to construct the PAI "score card." _____, _____, and _____.

6. Two differences between a treatment and a preventive examination are _____ and _____.

7. The main thrust in caries dietary counseling for caries control is limiting the intake of _____; in periodontal disease the best advice is to eat a balanced diet that provides sufficient nutrients to potentiate the immunologic and nonimmunologic defenses of the body.

8. The initial manifestation of periodontal pathology is _____ (name the condition) that is due to the (supra) (sub) gingival plaque.

9. If a gingival crevice is over _____ mm in depth, it should be considered for periodontal therapy.

10. Name at least two information forms used routinely in nutrition counseling.

11. A patient's CAI or PAI "score card" is an aid for educating and motivating the patient; it also is a document that can protect the dentist from a _____ suit due to alleged long-term neglect in instituting preventive actions.

12. An agent has substantivity if it can be adsorbed onto a tissue at the target site, _____ and _____. (Characteristics which define substantivity)

13. If identified in a routine dental examination, the appropriate use of _____ strategies for managing smooth-surface incipient lesions and the placement of _____ in deep fissures would probably eliminate the need for a great majority of restorations.

14. Iatrogenic damage can be caused by the dentist using the explorer to probe _____(s) (name of visible incipient lesions) of the smooth surfaces and fissures.

15. A high-tech device which will probably replace the explorer without causing iatrogenic damage to white spots is the _____.

REFERENCES

1. Bohannan HM, Graves RC, Disney JA, et al. Effect of secular decline in caries on the evaluation of preventive dentistry demonstrations. *J Public Health Dent.* 1985; 45:83–89.

2. Graves RC, Bohannan HM, Disney JA, et al. Recent dental caries and treatment patterns in US children. *J Public Health Dent.* 1986; 46:23–29.

3. *Oral Health of United States Adults, The National Survey of Oral Health in U.S. Employed Adults and Seniors: 1985–86, National Findings.* U.S. Department of Health and Human Services, Public Health Service, National Institutes of Health, NIH Publication No. 87-2868, August 1987.

4. Schwartz M, Grondahl HG, Pliskin JS, et al. A longitudinal analysis from bite-wing radiographs of the rate of progression of approximal carious lesions through human dental enamel. *Arch Oral Biol.* 1984; 29:529–536.

5. Loesche WJ, Straffon LH. Longitudinal investigation of the role of *Streptococcus mutans* in human fissure decay. *Infect Immunity.* 1979; 26:498–507.

6. Bok S. Truth-telling: ethical aspects. In: Reich WT, ed. *Encyclopedia of Bioethics.* New York, NY: Macmillan; 1978: 1683.

7. Dwore RB, Kreuter MW. Update: Reinforcing the case for health promotion. *Fam Community Health.* 1980; 2:103–109.

8. Malvitz DM, Broderick EB. Assessment of a dental disease prevention program after three years. *J Public Health Dent.* 1989; 49: 54–57.

9. Shallhorn RG, Snyder LE. Preventive maintenance therapy. *J Am Dent Assoc.* 1981; 103:227–231.

10. McFall WT Jr, Bader JD, Posier RB, et al. Presence of periodontal data in patient records of general practitioners. *J Periodontol.* 1988; 59:445–449.

11. Emilson CG, Krasse B. Comparison between a dip-slide test and plate count for determination of *Streptococcus mutans* infection. *Scand J Dent Res.* 1986; 94:500–505.

12. Davenport ES, Day S, Hardie JM, et al. A comparison between commercial kits and conventional methods for enumeration of salivary mutans streptococci and lactobacilli. *Community Dental Health.* 1992; 9:261–271.

13. Stecksen-Bicks C. Lactobacilli and *Streptococcus mutans* in saliva, diet and caries increment in 8- and 13-year old children. *Scand J Dent Res.* 1987; 95:18–26.

14. Krasse B. Can microbiological knowledge be applied in dental practice for the treatment and prevention of dental caries? *J Can Dent Assoc.* 1984; 50:221–223.

15. Sreebny LM, Schwartz SS. A reference guide to drugs and dry mouth. *Gerodontology.* 1986; 5:75–99.

16. Närhi TO, Merrman JH, Ainamo A, et al. Association between salivary flow rate and the use of systemic medication among 76-81- and 86-year-old inhabitants in Helsinki, Finland. *J Dent. Res.* 1992; 71:1875–1880.

17. Benvenius J. Caries risk for patients with Crohn's disease: A pilot study. *Oral Surg Oral Med Oral Pathol.* 1988; 65:304–307.

18. Ripa LW. A half-century of community water fluoridation in the United States: Review and commentary. *J Public Health Dent.* 1989; 53:17–44.

19. Simonsen RJ. Why not sealants. *J Publ Health Dent.* 1993; 53:211. Guest editorial.

20. Gonzalez CD, Frazier PJ, Messer LB. Sealant use by general practitioners. *Dent Child.* 1990; 57:38–45.

21. Silverman LM. Significance of remineralization in caries prevention. *J Can Dent Assoc.* 1984; 50:157–166.

22. Bader JD, Brown JP. Dilemmas in caries diagnosis. *J Am Dent Assoc* 1993; 124:48–50.

23. Ekstrand K V, Thylstrup A. Light microscope study of the effect of probing in occlusal surfaces. *Caries Res.* 1987; 21:368–374.

24. Lussi A. Validity of diagnostic and treatment decisions of fissure caries. *Caries Res.* 1991; 25:296–303.

25. Loesch WJ, Svanberg ML, Pape HR. Intra oral transmission of *Streptococcus mutans* by a dental explorer. *J Dent Res.* 1979; 58: 1765–1770.

26. Osborne JW. Five-year clinical assessment of 14 amalgam alloys. *Oper Dent.* 1990; 15: 20–26.

27. Bergmann G, Lindén LA. The action of the explorer in incipient caries. *Svensk Tandläkar Tidsskrift.* 1969; 62: 625–634.

28. Thylstrup A, Bille J, Qvist V. Radiographic and observed tissue changes in approximal carious lesions at the time of operative treatment. *Caries Res.* 1986; 20:75–84.

29. von der Fehr, Löe H, Theilade F. Experimental caries in man. *Caries Res.* 1970; 4: 131–138.

30. Neilson A, Pitts NB. The clinical behavior of free smooth surface carious lesions monitored over 2 years in a group of Scottish children. *Br Dent. J.* 1991; 171:313–318.

31. Mertz-Fairhurst EJ. Pit-and-fissure sealants; A global lack of science transfer? *J Dent Res.* 1992; 71:1543–1544. Editorial.

32. van Dorpe CSE, Exterkate RAM, ten Cate JM. The effect of dental probing on subsequent demineralization. *J Dent Child.* 1988; 55:343–347.

33. Downer MC, O'Mullane DM. A comparison of the concurrent validity of two epidemiological diagnostic systems for caries evaluation. *Community Dent Oral Epidemiol.* 1975; 3:20–24.

34. Downer MC. Validation of methods used in dental caries diagnoses. *Inter Dent J.* 1989; 39: 241–246.

35. Mertz-Fairhurst EJ, Call-Smith KM, Shuster GS, et al. Clinical performance of sealed composite restorations placed over caries compared with sealed and unsealed amalgam restorations. *J Am Dent Assoc.* 1987; 115:689–694.

36. Handlemann SL, Jensen OE. The effect of an autopolymerizing sealant on the viability of the microflora in occlusal dental caries. *Scand J Dent Res.* 1980; 88:382–388.

37. Mertz-Fairhurst EJ, Shuster GS, Fairhurst CW. Arresting caries by sealants: Results of a clinical study. *J Am Dent Assoc.* 1986; 112: 194–203.

38. Gift H, Newman J. Oral health activities of U.S. children: Results of a National Health Interview Survey. *J Am Dent. Assoc.* 1992; 123:96–106.

39. Billings RJ, Brown LR, Kaster AG. Contemporary treatment strategies for root surface dental caries. *Gerodontics.* 1985; 1:20–27.

40. Markitziu A, Rajstein, Deutsch D, et al. Arrest of incipient cervical caries by topical chemotherapy. *Gerodontics.* 1988; 4:293–298.

41. Nyvad B, Fejerskov O. Active root surface caries converted into inactive caries as a response to oral hygiene. *Scand J Dent Res.* 1986; 94:281–284.

42. Schaeken MJ, Keltjens HM, Van Der Hoeven JS. Effects of fluoride and chlorhexidine on the microflora of dental root surfaces and progression of root-surface caries. *J Dent Res.* 1991; 70:150–153.

43. Zickert I, Emilson CG, Krasse B. Effect of caries-preventive measures on children highly infected with the bacterium *Streptococcus mutans. Arch Oral Biol.* 1982; 27: 861–868.

44. Liefde B de. Dental caries: Diagnosis and treatment planning. *NZ Dent J.* 1980; 76: 12–15.

45. Koulourides TI, ed. *Proceedings of Symposium on Incipient Lesions of Enamel.* NO Rowe, University of Michigan, November 11–12, 1977: 51–68.

46. Emilson CG. Susceptibility of various organisms to chlorhexidine. *Scand J Dent Res.* 1977; 85:225–265.

47. Persson RE, Truelove EL, Le Resch L, et al. Therapeutic effects of daily or weekly chlorhexidine rinsing on oral health in a geriatric population. *Oral Surg Oral Med Oral Pathol.* 1991; 72:184–191.

48. Emilson CG, Lindquist B, Wennerholm K. Recolonization of human tooth surfaces by *Streptococcus mutans* after suppression by chlorhexidine treatment. *J Dent Res.* 1987; 66:1503–1508.

49. Hildebrandt GH, Pape HR Jr, Syed SA, et al. Effect of slow-release chlorhexidine mouthguards on the levels of selected salivary bacteria. *Caries Res.* 1992; 26:268–274.

50. Horowitz HS. The future of water fluoridation and other systemic fluorides. *J Dent Res.* 1990; 69(special issue); 760–764.

51. Qvist J, Qvist V, Mjor IA. Placement and longevity of amalgam restorations in Denmark. *Acta Odont Scand.* 1990; 48:297–303.

52. Cecil JC, Cohen ME, Schroeder DC, et al. Longevity of amalgam restorations: A retro-

spective view. *J Dent Res.* 1982; 61:185. Abstract 1956.

53. Lavell CL. A cross-sectional, longitudinal survey into the durability of amalgam restorations. *J Dent Res.* 1976; 4:139–143.
54. Hunter B. The life of a filling. *Br Dent J.* 1982; 61:537. Abstract 18.
55. Elderton RJ. Longitudinal study of dental treatment in the general dental service in Scotland. *Br Dent J.* 1983; 155:91–96.
56. Elderton RJ. Clinical studies concerning re-restoration of teeth. *Adv Dent Res.* 1990; 4:4–9.
57. Silverstone LM. Experimental caries models and their clinical implications. In: Guggenheim B, ed. *Cariology Today.* Basel, Switzerland. Karger; 1984:237–244.
58. Levine RA, Wilson TG. Compliance as a major risk factor in periodontal disease progression. *Compendium.* 1992; 13:1072–1079.
59. Podell RN, Gary L. Compliance: A problem in medical management. *Am Fam Physician.* 1976; 13:74–80.
60. Greenwell H, Bissada NF, Wittwer JW. Periodontics in general practice: Professional plaque control. *J Am Dent Assoc.* 1990; 121:642–646.
61. Frazier RL Jr. Austin, TX; 1981. Personal communication.
62. Brown LR. In: *Symposium on Dental Caries,* San Diego, Professional Division, Procter & Gamble, Cincinnati, Ohio. 1982.
63. Darwish S, Hyppa T, Socransky SS. Studies of the predominant cultivable microbiota in early periodontitis. *J Periodont Res.* 1978; 13:1–16.
64. Siegrist B, Kornman KS. The effect of supragingival plaque control on the composition of the subgingival microbial flora in ligature-induced periodontitis in the monkey. *J Dent Res.* 1982; 61:936–941.
65. Shallhorn RG, Snider LE. Preventive maintenance therapy. *J Am Dent Assoc.* 1981; 103:227–231.
66. Pfeifer MR, Pfeifer JS. Dental prevention: The oral prophylaxis. *Clin Prevent Dent.* 1988; 10:18–24.
67. Axelsson P, Lindhe J. Effect of controlled oral hygiene procedures on caries and periodontal disease in adults. Results after six years. *J Clin Periodontol.* 1981; 8:239–248.
68. Ramfjord SP, Morrison EC, Burrgett FG, et al. Oral hygiene and the maintenance of periodontal support. *J Periodontol.* 1982, 53:26–30.
69. Barrington EP, Nevins M. Diagnosing periodontal disease. *J Am Dent Assoc.* 1990; 121:460–464.
70. American Dental Association. Council on Dental Materials, Instruments and Equipment, American Dental Association. Recommendations in radiographic practices. *J Am Dent Assoc.* 1989; 118:115–117.
71. Waigmann P. What is an electronic patient record. *Texas Dent J.* 1993; 110:21–26.
72. Thylstrup A. Mechanical vs. disease-oriented treatment of dental caries: Educational aspects. *J Dent Res.* 1989; 68:1135. Editorial.
73. Moss SJ. A cavity-free generation. *J Dent Res.* 1991; 70:158.

Appendix 21–1. Open Letter to New Patients

Dear _____:

For myself and on behalf of my staff, I would like to extend a warm welcome to our dental practice. As we all readily admit, going to the dentist is not exactly our favorite pastime. Unfortunately many of us have had experiences in the past that have caused us to avoid dental visits. Although we cannot promise you that you will never have an uncomfortable moment while in our office, we can promise you to do all in our power to make your dental experience a pleasant one.

We believe that it is the right of every patient to know the cause of his or her dental disease and how he or she can prevent it. Ninety-five percent of dental disease is preventable, and it is our intention that the dental treatment we perform for you will last a lifetime. We believe that we should make every effort to preserve every natural tooth for life (with the possible exception of some wisdom teeth). We have organized a series of appointments with the express purpose of stopping your dental disease (tooth decay and gum disease). We believe that anyone with active dental disease should receive this counseling as the first phase of his or her treatment, after we relieve any emergency condition, of course. If we were to repair the damages of disease without stopping the disease, our treatment would eventually fail. If you accept and practice good home care, you should need little more than an annual checkup. This means low dental costs over the years. As you will find out, however, the only person who can truly stop dental disease is you, and we acknowledge that every person reserves the right to remain sick if they so choose.

I hope that you have more of an insight into how I practice and thus you can decide if I am the right dentist for you. I hope that this will mark the beginning of an enjoyable experience and continued good dental health.

Courtesy of Dr. R L Frazier, Jr.[61] Austin, TX. 1981.

Appendix 21–2. Plaque Index Form

Name _____

	Date _____ Day Month Year		Date _____ Day Month Year		Date _____ Day Month Year	
	Upper Tooth M B D L	Lower Tooth M B D L	Upper Tooth M B D L	Lower Tooth M B D L	Upper Tooth M B D L	Lower Tooth M B D L
Before After	2	18	2	18	2	18
Before After	3	19	3	19	3	19
Before After	4	20	4	20	4	20
Before After	5	21	5	21	5	21
Before After	6	22	6	22	6	22
Before After	7	23	7	23	7	23
Before After	8	24	8	24	8	24
Before After	9	25	9	25	9	25
Before After	10	26	10	26	10	26
Before After	11	27	11	27	11	27
Before After	12	28	12	28	12	28
Before After	13	29	13	29	13	29
Before After	14	30	14	30	14	30
Before After	15	31	15	31	15	31

	1st Period	2nd Period	3rd Period
Before After	Plaque Index _____	Plaque Index _____	Plaque Index _____

Instructions: Place a RED X through the tooth number if tooth is missing
Before brushing, place red X in proper block if plaque seen
After brushing, place blue X in proper block if plaque seen

$$\text{Plaque Index} = \frac{\text{Number of smooth surfaces WITH plaque}}{\text{Total number of smooth surfaces}}$$

Appendix 21–3. Carbohydrate Intake—Short Form

Name: _____ Date: _____

Patient: Please check the column that best describes your consumption of the following foods.

Instructor: To derive score, multiply group number by column number.
(*Example*: If check is in second column (2) × group 3, score = 6).

	Group	1 Seldom (1 or 2 times monthly)	2 Not often (1 or 2 times weekly)	3 Often (1 or 2 times daily)	Score
Group 1	Tea or coffee with sugar				
	Chocolate milk, or hot chocolate				
	Soft drinks, (regular, NOT diet)				
	Milk shakes				
	Dessert wines and cordials				
	Fruit drinks				
	Lemonade				
Group 2	Custards, puddings				
	Whipped cream				
	Ice cream, sherbert, popsicles				
	Flavored yogurt				
	Applesauce				
	Canned fruit in syrup				
Group 3	Jams and jellies				
	Whipped cream				
	Cakes, coffee cakes				
	Bananas				
	Doughnuts				
	Cookies				
	Cereals, sugar-coated				
	Pies				
	Dried fruits				
Group 4	Candy bars				
	Hard candy				
	Chocolate candy				
	Caramels				
	Cough drops				

*Group 1 = Liquids
Group 2 = Liquid to soft
Group 3 = Slowly dissolve
Group 4 = Sticky

Total score:

Appendix 21–4. Food Intake Record, 3 Day

PATIENT NAME _____

DATE _____   DATE _____   DATE _____

BEFORE BREAKFAST	AMOUNT	BEFORE BREAKFAST	AMOUNT	BEFORE BREAKFAST	AMOUNT
BREAKFAST		BREAKFAST		BREAKFAST	
BETWEEN MEALS		BETWEEN MEALS		BETWEEN MEALS	
LUNCH		LUNCH		LUNCH	
BETWEEN MEALS		BETWEEN MEALS		BETWEEN MEALS	
SUPPER		SUPPER		SUPPER	
AFTER SUPPER		AFTER SUPPER		AFTER SUPPER	

Appendix 21–5. Nutrition Assessment Sheet, 3-Day Record

Name: _____ Date: _____

Food Groups	Evaluation of Intake			Average Intake	
	Day 1	Day 2	Day 3	Average	Adequacy
Fats, oils, & sweets: Use sparingly					
Milk, yogurt, and cheese: 2–3 servings					
Meat, poultry, fish, dry beans, eggs, and nuts: 2–3 servings					
Vegetables: 3–5 servings					
Fruit: 2–4 servings					
Bread, cereal, rice, and pasta: 6–11 servings					

Chapter 22

"Hot Topics"
Geriatric Dentistry

Janet A. Yellowitz

With more people living to older ages and the older population itself getting older, the 20th century is experiencing an unprecedented "graying of America." Since 1980, the percentage of the population aged 65 years and older increased by 24%, whereas the population younger than 65 increased by only 9%.[1] In 1991, about one in every eight Americans was 65 or older, with 10% of this population (85+ years) accounting for the fastest growing age segment. By the year 2030, the percentage of the population 65 and older is expected to increase to 22% of the population.[1] Likewise, minority populations are projected to represent 25% of the elderly population in 2030, an increase from 14% in 1990. These dramatic population changes will continue to alter the availability and delivery of oral health care.[2] To be best prepared for the future practice of dentistry, oral health professionals need to be knowledgeable about the trends in oral disease prevalence, patterns of dental utilization, and changing characteristics of the elderly.

During the past 25 years, one of the major changes in oral disease patterns in the United States has been a steady decrease in the rate of edentulism. Compared with almost 30% edentulism in people between 65 and 74 years old in 1986, it is estimated that in 2024 only 10% of this group will be edentulous.[3] The decline in edentulism appears as a result of water fluoridation, increased public awareness of preventive approaches, improved access to services, and a decrease in early tooth loss.[4] Although the prevalence of edentulism increases in the older age groups (10% of 45–54 years, 28.4% of 65–74 years, and 52.5% of 85+ years), these rates have steadily decreased over time.[5] Although these numbers do not include institutionalized persons, it is likely that for the first time in recorded history more older adults now have their teeth than do not have their teeth. This continuous decline in tooth loss will result in more natural teeth being at risk for caries (coronal, recurrent, and root) and a greater incidence of periodontal disease. As these trends continue, it appears that fewer prosthodontic replacements and more restorative and preventive services will be provided in future dental practices.

Although dental caries has not traditionally been perceived as a problem for the elderly, decay rates have recently been found to be higher in some adult groups than in children. A survey of Iowa's population found 30% of dentate elderly had untreated coronal decay, with 77% having either a new coronal or root lesion in the last 3 years.[6] Root caries, a problem in many older adults, was found (either a decayed or filled root surface) in 65% of the males and 53% of the females in the 1985–1986 National Institute of Dental Research study.[7] With the implementation of new preventive approaches and new restorative materials (some of which leach fluoride), the dilemma of restoring root carious lesions is expected to diminish in the future.

It is estimated that 90% of adults 65 years old and older need periodontal treatment, with 15% needing complex treatment.[8] The apparent increase of prevalence of periodontal disease with age may be due to the character of the disease being long-standing and chronic, with its onset much earlier in adulthood. Because the rate of periodontal disease progression is related partly to the mass and composition of the microbiota and the host's ability to respond to this microbial population, research has focused on new diagnostic and treatment modalities, such as DNA diagnostic probes, enzymatic assays and bacterial analyses, the use of lasers, new pharmaceutical preparations, and subtraction radiography. With new diagnostic methods complementing traditional clinical techniques, earlier identification of periodontal disease and risk factors will be possible, as well as early treatment to help reduce disease progression and the subsequent loss of teeth.

Like most cancers, oral cancer occurs in the older segments of the population, with the majority of cases diagnosed after age 65, and more than 95% occurring after age 45.[9] The central problem in oral cancer is the need for an early and effective diagnosis. Risk factors for the development of oral squamous cell carcinoma have traditionally included alcohol abuse and use of tobacco products. As the multifactorial etiology of oral cancer becomes evident, other factors, including alterations in cellular oncogenes[a] and the role of microbial and viral infections, may be found to be important in the pathogenesis of premalignant lesions and oral squamous cell carcinoma.[10] Given that early diagnosis of oral cancer greatly improves the prognosis of the disease and that many factors influence the timing at which oral cancers are diagnosed (lack of access to care and patient delay in seeking treatment[11]), health professionals must encourage routine comprehensive intra- and extraoral examinations of their patient populations.

It is essential to recognize that no broad, generalized decremental changes in oral health occur simply because of age. Healthy older people can expect to keep their teeth, secrete adequate levels of saliva, and accurately taste their food with few significant differences from their younger counterparts.[12] In the presence of one or more medical conditions or their treatments, however, oral functions may be directly or indirectly altered, thus affecting the patients' general and oral health status.

The three leading causes of death of the elderly are diseases of the heart, malignant neoplasms, and cerebrovascular disease. Although great strides in health care have reduced the morbidity and mortality of many chronic conditions, and many dollars are spent on research to reduce disease prevalence, if cancer as a cause of death were eliminated, the average life span would

---

[a] Oncogene = A gene having the potential to cause a normal cell to become cancerous.

be extended by less than 2 years. Eliminating deaths due to heart disease, however, would add an average of 5 years to life expectancy at age 65 and would lead to a marked increase in the proportion of older persons in the population.[13]

For most older Americans, chronic disease is a fact of life. Eighty percent of senior citizens have one or more chronic medical conditions, with the most common ones being hypertension, arthritis, hearing and vision loss, and heart disease. Because the average individual 65 years old or older consumes four to five medications at a time and up to 20 medications annually, the risk for drug interactions is great—a fact of which both the medical and dental health team need to be aware.[14] Oral health professionals must constantly update their patients' medical history and need to be aware of the continually changing medications and their side effects. Because adverse drug reactions increase with age and with the number of medications consumed, health professionals need to be knowledgeable about adverse drug reactions common to the elderly, as well as potential interaction of currently consumed drugs with those they may prescribe. New computerized programs and drug data bases designed for in-office use are now available to provide health care providers with current drug information, side effects, and contraindications.

Functional status is commonly defined in terms of an individual's ability to perform basic and instrumental activities of daily living (ADLs, IADLs). Functional limitations serve as key indicators of an older person's ability to remain independent in the community, his or her quality of life, and his or her active life expectancy. Approximately 72% of the population aged 65 years and older reported having no difficulty with ADLs and IADLs, and about 10% had difficulty with three or more ADLs.[2] As age increases, the percentage of the population having no difficulty with ADLs or IADLs decreases. The two most common IADLs identified by the elderly are difficulty walking and getting outside.[2] These common conditions may require dental health professionals to alter the individual's treatment plan.

To provide optimal care to the aging population, a dentist must remain current on oral medicine, pharmacotherapeutics, and changing technologies. Oral health care professionals must address how this aging population will manage in the dental facility, and, at a minimum, have accessible offices, large-type medical history forms, and easy to read signs and appointment cards.

The majority of the people aged 65 and older are able to continue living in the community; only 5% are in nursing homes.[15] Not surprisingly, the older a person is, the greater the risk for institutionalization. Of those institutionalized in 1990, 1% were aged 65 to 74 years, 6% were aged 75 to 84, 19% were aged 85 to 89, 33% were aged 90 to 94, and 47% were aged 95 years and older.[2] Given the growth of the population aged 85 and older, a substantial increase in the future use of nursing homes appears inevitable.[16]

For the first time, the provision of oral health care is mandated in long-term care institutions. The Omnibus Budget Reconciliation Act (OBRA) of 1987 (Public Law 100-203) requires all Medicaid- and Medicare-certified facilities to provide an oral examination to all residents within 48 hours of admission and requires all residents to be regularly examined not less than once per year. Although these services need not be completed by a dental professional, dentists or dental hygienists need to be identified as part of the health care team of the long-term care facility. Given a rapidly growing population of dentally aware older adults, future population growth patterns and technologic advances in portable and mobile dental equipment, oral health care programs in long-term care facilities will become feasible and common locations for providing dental care.

One major influence on dental utilization is having dental insurance. Because dental insurance is generally provided as an employee benefit, the elderly frequently do not have this benefit. According to the National Center for Health Statistics,[17] 50% of the population between 35 and 54 years old, 37% of those age 55 to 64, and 15% of those age 65 and older had private dental insurance in 1989. Dental benefits are not included in Medicare, and very few states provide dental service to adults through the Medicaid program. In 1990, nearly 75% of edentulous persons 35 years old and older did not have private dental insurance compared with about half of the dentate population.[16] Because edentulous persons are less likely to have visited a dentist for the past 5 years, routine examinations for and early treatment of oral soft-tissue diseases are precluded.[16] Thus, the elderly edentulous population may be identified as one of the major underserved populations of this country.

Question 1. Which one of the following statements, if any, are correct?

A. It is expected that by the year 2024 there will be more dentulous than edentulous Americans over age 65.
B. Approximately 50% of all oral cancers are diagnosed after age 75.
C. If cancer was eliminated as a cause of death, the life span of Americans would be extended by less than 2 years.
D. Federal law requires than an oral examination be completed within 2 days after admittance to a long-term care institution.

E. Only about *15%* (± *5%*) of people older than 65 have dental insurance.

SUMMARY

With more older adults and more teeth per older adult, the composition of services rendered to this population will change dramatically in the next decade. Advances in materials and technology in combination with the changing patterns of oral diseases will continue to have dramatic effects on the practice of dentistry. The role of the oral health care professional will focus more on the diagnosis and treatment of oral diseases and disorders, using new aids and devices such as lasers, CAD/CAM,[b] and molecular probes. As diseases of the hard tissues are resolved, more emphasis will be placed on the diagnosis and treatment of soft-tissue lesions. With new and improved diagnostic skills, the older adult, the group identified as having the highest risk of oral cancer, may no longer require the extensive and often disfiguring surgical remedies currently in place. Oral disease preventive approaches need to be maintained throughout the life span.

REFERENCES

1. American Association of Retired Persons. *A Profile of Older Americans: 1992.* Administration on Aging, U.S. Department of Health and Human Services. PF 3049 (1292) D996; 1992.
2. Vital and Health Statistics. *Health Data on Older Americans: U.S. 1992.* The Centers for Disease Control and Prevention, Na-

---

[b] CAD/CAM = An application of computer technology used to design and fabricate dental restorations, often within the same office.

tional Center for Health Statistics, Series 3 (27), January 1993.

3. Weintraub JA, Burt BA. Tooth loss in the United States. *J Dent Educ.* 1985; 49:368.

4. National Center for Health Statistics. *Dental Services and Oral Health: U.S. 1989.* Dec. 1992, NCHS Series 10, no. 183.

5. Vital and Health Statistics. *Dental Services and Oral Health: United States, 1989.* The Centers for Disease Control and Prevention, National Center for Health Statistics, December 1992.

6. Hand JS, Hunt RJ, Beck JD, Coronal and root caries in older Iowans: 36 month incidence. *Gerodontics.* 1988; 4:136.

7. National Institute of Dental Research. *Oral Health of United States Adults: National Findings.* NIH Publ NO 87-2868. Washington DC, Government Printing Office, 1987.

8. Berg RL, Cassells JS, eds. *Oral Health Problems in the 'Second Fifty' Years: Promoting Health and Preventing Disability.* Washington, DC. National Academy Press; 1990: 120–125.

9. Berkey DB, Shay K. Geriatric dental care for the elderly in clinics in geriatric medicine. Baum B, ed. *Oral Dent Prob Elderly.* 8(3):1992; 579.

10. Greer RO. "Recent clinical and molecular biological advances in diagnosis and treatment of oral cancer." Abstract presented at the symposium *Scientific Frontiers in Clinical Dentistry, An Update.* National Institute of Dental Research, April 1993, Rockville, MD.

11. Sadowsky D, Kunzel C, Phelan J. Dentists' knowledge, case-finding behavior and confirmed diagnosis of oral cancer. *J Cancer Ed.* 1988; 2:127–134.

12. Baum BJ. Oral and dental problems in the elderly. *Clin Geriatr Med.* 1992; 8(3): Preface. xi–xii.

13. U.S. Senate Special Committee on Aging. *Aging in America: Trends and Projections.* Washington, DC: U.S. Dept. of Health and Human Services 91-28001:1991.

14. Haas DA, Grad HA, Sumney DL, et al. Pharmacology and therapeutics: The older periodontal patient. In: Ellen RP, ed. *Periodontal Care for Older Adults.* Toronto, Canadian Scholars' Press; 1992:199.

15. Yamagata PAB, Sue C, Stiefel D. Use of dental service in a nursing home. *Spec Care Dent.* 1985; 5:64–67.

16. Brody JA, Brody DA, Williams TF. Trends in the health of the elderly population. *Ann Rev Public Health.* 1987; 8:211–234.

17. Vital and Health Statistics. *Dental Services and Oral Health: United States, 1989.* The Centers for Disease Control and Prevention, National Center for Health Statistics, December 1992.

Smoking (Tobacco) Cessation

Arden G. Christen

Today, dental professionals are addressing treatment issues by placing a stronger emphasis on disease prevention, oral health research, and more highly developed clinical abilities. As oral care options continue to evolve and expand, other health care arenas are also becoming professionally relevant. One new focus of interest is the dental professional's role in smoking cessation.[1-5] Since the mid-1980s, oral health providers have been helping their patients to quit smoking by providing dental office-based tobacco cessation programs. What has prompted these positive changes within dentistry?

The first surgeon general's report which related to the systemic hazards of tobacco was issued in 1964.[6] This publication and over 20 subsequent reports from the surgeon general continue to motivate and educate health care providers and tobacco cessation advocates throughout the world. (The 1986 report deals exclusively with the health consequences of *smokeless tobacco* usage.[7]) There is a growing realization that tobacco not only threatens systemic health

(for example, it produces lung cancer, chronic bronchitis, emphysema, heart disease, and damage to the fetus during pregnancy), but it also causes a number of significant dental problems. Scientifically sound evidence documents that smoked and smokeless tobacco have profound ill effects on tissues in and around the oral cavity. A recent, extensive review of the literature (800 scientific articles) has revealed that the use of tobacco products causes a wide range of oral conditions, including oral cancer, leukoplakia, various forms of periodontal disease, stained teeth, halitosis, and dental calculus.[8] Moreover, tobacco usage increases and complicates the dentist's treatment management risks by compromising the prognosis for periodontal therapy, producing a greater likelihood of the occurrence and recurrence of oral cancers, and retarding wound healing.

Conversely, the cessation of tobacco usage greatly improves oral health. For example, quitting smoking or stopping the use of smokeless tobacco significantly decreases the development of periodontal disease and reduces the rate and incidence of alveolar bone and tooth loss.[8]

From 1984 to 1991, nine scientifically validated published studies documented the usefulness of dentally oriented smoking cessation programs that utilize nicotine withdrawal therapy (ie, a prescribed usage regimen for FDA-approved nicotine-containing gum and patches) in conjunction with a comprehensive behavioral program.[4-5] These reports showed that oral health team members can be effective tobacco interventionists and health advisors. Additionally, these studies concluded that[1-5]

- Approximately 80% of all smokers would like to quit.
- Dentists and hygienists are in an ideal position to assess the oral ill effects of tobacco use.
- Brief "teachable moments" occur for dental professionals during contact with their patients. At these times, they can address the cause and effect relationship between the patients' tobacco use and their resulting oral disease.
- Even simple quitting advice given by health care professionals is an effective smoking cessation strategy. Therefore, during routine office visits, the oral health team members need to give brief smoking cessation advice to their tobacco-using patients. These consciousness-raising efforts generally involve only 3 to 5 minutes of office time.

Since the early 1970s, the American Dental Association has produced and distributed increasing amounts of tobacco cessation and educational audio–visual materials, including wall plaques, posters, pamphlets, signs, package libraries, videos, and slide sets. Today, virtually all major dental organizations have issued official policy resolutions and position statements concerning tobacco usage. Additionally, these groups acknowl-

edge the need for more thorough tobacco education activities and for cessation programs within the dental office setting.[4]

Recently published dental school curricular guidelines for the American Association of Dental Schools support these ideas and mandate that students learn to recognize and treat tobacco-related conditions that they have diagnosed in their patients.[9-10] Additionally, students are taught to develop and employ smoking cessation counseling methods as part of their treatment plans.

At present, practicing oral health team members are being taught how to use nicotine withdrawal therapy. These teaching programs are offered either by dental educators or by trainers from the National Cancer Institute (NCI), who sponsor these full- or half-day smoking cessation events.[2] The proper use of nicotine patches and gum offers recovering smokers some important advantages over "cold-turkey" quitting.[5] Appropriate usage of these prescription items greatly reduces withdrawal symptoms. Withdrawal is one of the primary factors that deters or prevents recovery. During this treatment process, the body is not suddenly and completely deprived of nicotine but gradually "weaned" from nicotine over time. The use of nicotine-containing therapeutic products also enables quitters to split their nicotine addiction into two treatable segments: (a) physiologic dependency and (b) psychologic–sociocultural addiction. As a result, individuals learn to deal sequentially with this complex addiction. It is absolutely vital to address all of these components of cigarette usage to achieve smoking cessation.

The cessation of cigarette use immediately eliminates the ingestion of the 4000 harmful chemicals and gases contained in cigarette smoke and routinely inhaled by smokers. This detoxification process is extremely important in helping the body repair the ravages caused by smoking.

For the past 10 years, multifaceted plans developed at the Indiana University School of Dentistry and the NCI have been used to teach students and practitioners how to implement an office-oriented smoking cessation program.[1-5] These strategies are now being taught to dentists, hygienists, and assistants throughout the country.[2] Although these steps can be modified to fit individual dental practices, they should include the following basic guidelines:[c]

- Select a smoking cessation coordinator. In a dental office, this role is logically assumed by the dental hygienist. All office workers need to have some involvement in the overall program in order to project a consistent and unified effort.
- Create a nonsmoking office atmosphere. It is imperative that all employees serve as nonsmoking role models who provide a smoke-free environment.
- Identify all smoking (or smokeless tobacco users) in the practice. The tobacco use of all patients should be noted on their records and updated regularly.
- Collect teaching materials and develop patient-targeted smoking cessation plans.
- Follow prescribing instructions carefully when using nicotine gum or patches.[5]

---

[c] To receive a free monograph entitled "A Smoking Cessation Program for the Dental Office," write to the Department of Oral Biology, The Indiana University School of Dentistry, Room B-19, 1121 West Michigan Street, Indianapolis, Indiana 46202. This monograph explains all aspects of an eight-step program in detail. For the NCI program manual, write to The National Cancer Institute, Building 31, Room 10A24, Bethesda, Maryland 20892 and ask for NIH Publication 91-3191 entitled, "How to Help Your Patients Stop Using Tobacco."

- Provide supportive follow-up to those who show interest in quitting.

It is recommended that the *"four A's"* be used in office smoking cessation programs, as defined by the NCI protocol: *ASK* patients about their smoking behaviors at every appropriate opportunity; *ADVISE* all smokers to stop and to set a quit date; *ASSIST* them in stopping by using multiple-pronged approach; and *ARRANGE* for supportive follow-up procedures.[2,5] Patients can also be referred to formal, community-based smoking cessation programs, such as those offered by the American Cancer Society, American Lung Association, or Seventh Day Adventists. Course leaders also teach coping skills, stress reduction methods, quitting techniques, and strategies that help the quitter maintain successful recovery.

Although no smoking cessation formula is universally accepted and easily applied, many effective strategies exist to help a dental patient become smoke-free. Although some individuals are able to succeed alone via "cold turkey" quitting, others need the support and encouragement provided by a supportive health care provider or by an organized cessation group. Have the individual quitter select a quit date in the near future, for instance a time that is far enough in the future to allow for mental preparation but not so distant that it results in procrastination. Perhaps the individual can consider quitting when life stressors are relatively low and select a quit date that is memorable, such as a birthday, anniversary, or holiday. The clinician must not be discouraged by setbacks. The quitting process continues over an extended period. Many smokers try three to eight times before they are successful, and research shows that chances for success increase with each attempt. If relapse occurs, smokers should be urged to reuse those strategies that worked before and to discard those that were ineffective.

Remember, tobacco use intervention services are among the most important health services that oral health team members can provide for their patients!

Question 2. Which of the following statements, if any, are correct?

A. Patients seen in the dental office with oral disease of smokeless and smoking tobacco origin, should be advised of the risk of systemic cancers.

B. Nicotine gum and patches better suppress the physiologic dependence on tobacco than they affect the psychosocial desire to smoke.

C. A dentist is authorized to prescribe nicotine gum and nicotine patches.

D. The four *aids* that a dentist can offer a patient as part of an office smoking cessation program are *ask, advise, assist,* and *arrange* for supportive follow-up procedures.

E. Multiple smoking relapses are not uncommon in a serious smoking cessation program.

REFERENCES

1. Christen AG, McDonald JL, Klein JA, et al. How-to-do-it quit-smoking strategies for the dental office team: An eight-step program. *J Am Dent Assoc.* 1990; 120:(suppl) 20–27.

2. Mecklenburg RE, Christen AG, Gerbert B, et al. *How to Help Your Patients Stop Using Tobacco: A National Cancer Institute Manual for the Oral Health Team.* Bethesda, Md. U.S. Public Health Service; 1990.

3. Christen AG, McDonald JL, Klein JA, et al. *A Smoking Cessation Program for the Dental Office.* Indianapolis, In. Indiana University School of Dentistry, 1993.

4. Christen AG, Christen JA, Klein JA. Nicotine withdrawal therapy in dental practice: Cessation strategies. *Health Values.* 1993; 17:59–68.

5. Christen AG, Christen JA. The prescription of transdermal nicotine patches for tobacco-using dental patients: Current status in Indiana. *J Indiana Dent Assoc.* 1992; 71:12–18.

6. U.S. Public Health Service. *Smoking and Health.* Report of the Advisory Committee to the Surgeon General of the Public Health Service. Washington, DC. U.S. Dept of Health, Education and Welfare. Centers for Disease Control. PHS Publication No. 11–3, 1964.

7. U.S. Department of Health and Human Services. *The Health Consequences of Using Smokeless Tobacco.* A Report of the Advisory Committee to the Surgeon General. Washington, DC. Public Health Service. PHS Publication No. 86-2874, 1986.

8. Christen AG, McDonald JL, Christen JA. *The Impact of Tobacco Use and Cessation on Nonmalignant and Precancerous Oral and Dental Diseases and Conditions.* Indianapolis, In. Indiana University School of Dentistry; 1991.

9. American Association of Dental Schools. Curriculum guidelines for predoctoral preventive dentistry. *J Dent Educ.* 1991; 55: 746–750.

10. American Association of Dental Schools. Curriculum guidelines for education in substance abuse, alcoholism, and other chemical dependencies. *J Dent Educ.* 1992; 56: 405–408.

The New Zealand School Dental Service

F. Morell MacKenzie
Mirren Peterson

At the time of the writing of this edition a national debate ensues in the United States on health care reform. One of the objectives is a desire to ensure equal and accessible dental care for all children. The following is a summary account of how one nation approached this same challenge. Editors' note

The 70th year of the existence of the New Zealand School Dental Service was marked in 1991. The Service arose from the pressure put on the government of the day *by the dental profession,* which had long been concerned about the poor state of the teeth of New Zealand children. Since 1921, the Service has made New Zealand a world leader in the provision of organized state-funded dental care for children, a model which has been copied in several other countries. Young women, known as *dental nurses*, were trained specifically in the de-livery of basic dental care for children—not as a partially trained or as a lower grade of dentist—but as auxiliaries to the dental profession with a professional status in their own right.[1] At the present time dental nurses may be employed only in state-run institutions. There is no right of private practice.

Initially, caries was controlled solely by fillings and extractions of unsaveable teeth, but as time passed the Service began to concentrate more on preventive measures and health education.[2] The Service is based on sound principles and provides an organized program of dental health education, preventive dentistry, and dental care tailored to the *needs* of children without concern for their ability to pay for care. The Service is based in larger schools and brings care to most children, thus saving classroom time and parents' time and effort in transporting their children long distances for dental care.

CARING FOR THE CHILDREN

Preschool, primary, and intermediate schoolchildren (aged from 2½) receive basic oral health care from the dental nurse. Dental nurses (a term used interchangeably with *dental therapist*) work under the direction and supervision of public health dentists, who are assisted in management and supervision by one or more of the senior supervising dental nurses. In 1988, more than 1350 school dental clinics were staffed by 900 dental nurses. Regular dental care, based on a 6-monthly examination, was provided for 512,000 children.

The enrollment rate is 96% of all schoolchildren aged 5 to 13 years. Previously, all children were examined semiannually, but now recalls are needs-based. Those who are classified as high risk—about 25%—are seen at 6-month intervals, whereas those classified as low risk are recalled annually.

The guidelines for classifying children as high risk are

- *Over 6 and under 9 years of age:* Four or more deciduous teeth with full occlusal or compound fillings or new carious lesions other than buccal or lingual pits in deciduous or permanent teeth after age 5
- *Over 9 years of age (permanent teeth only):* A full occlusal restoration or carious lesion on a first permanent molar or an interproximal cavity before age 9 or a new lesion in the previous 12 months, other than a buccal or lingual pit

The professional judgment of the dental nurses is also important when assessing risk because it takes into account their knowledge of the patient and previous family dental histories.

ROLE OF FLUORIDES

The preventive program is likewise geared more to those in need. Emphasis is placed on the use of a 0.2% sodium fluoride mouth rinse for very high risk children to arrest (ie, remineralization therapy) early decalcification of enamel (ie, incipient lesions). For instance, R1 interproximal lesions[d] detected on radiographs of permanent molars are treated with Duraphat (fluoride) varnish. Fissure sealants are placed on all newly erupted vulnerable fissures of permanent molars to prevent occlusal caries. Finally, the school dental service advocates fluoridation of water supplies (or tablets in unfluoridated areas) and fluoride toothpaste for all.

Figures 22–1 and 22–2 show the very favorable trend that has occurred towards better oral health over the past years, as reported by the New Zealand Department of Health.[3] Concurrent with this reduction in the prevalence of dental caries has been a parallel drop in the number of extractions of deciduous teeth from 18.20 per 100 children in 1966, to 4.00 in 1992. This trend is due to the School Dental Service's emphasis on oral health education and prevention; to the timely screening, remineralization, and restoration of incipient and carious lesions; and to the introduction of water fluoridation in most main towns, the availability of fluoride tablets, and the widespread use of fluoride toothpastes. As a result of these efforts, approximately one half of all 5-year-old children now have decay-free mouths. About a third of form (grade) 11 also are free from dental decay and on the average have had only 2.5 or fewer filled teeth.[3]

---

[d] An R1 radiographic lesion is an initial lesion of a proximal surface extending less than halfway through the enamel. This type of lesion can be remineralized by the use of Duraphat applications.

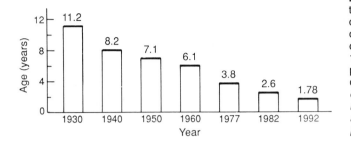

Figure 22–1. New Zealand Dental Service. Average def of 5-year old children. 1930–1991. Fluoridation caused a nationwide decline in caries during the late 1960s. Over the 62 years of reporting, the average dft decreased by 84%. (*From Internal data of the New Zealand Department of Health, generated from annual returns prepared by principal dental officers.*)

OTHER CONTRIBUTORY FACTORS

The Dental Health Education programs undertaken by the dental nurses continue to target the parent or caregiver of the child patients for dietary advice. Part of this program is done by dental nurses in cooperation with the Plunket Society[e] child health centers for mothers of infants. Here, mothers learn the correct use of feeding bottles to prevent "baby-bottle caries." They also talk to preschool parent groups as well as to the school-age patients themselves. Education is seen as a very important part of the Service although with the increase in pa-

tient numbers, the availability of dental nurses is more limited.

Schools are becoming more diet conscious, with the National Heart Foundation advocating a program for healthy foods served in school canteens. Dental nurses have had input into some of these programs, especially in intermediate schools (11- to 13-year-olds).

CHANGES IN THE SCHOOL DENTAL SERVICE

The Service *is* controlling dental decay in children. It has adapted to many changes from the late 1970s. As caries declined, the Dental Service has undergone restructuring and as a result the patient–nurse ratio in the School Dental Service has increased quite considerably from about one nurse to 450 children to one nurse to between 750 and

---

[e] The Plunket Society dates from 1920 and promotes the health of new mothers and their babies by regular checking of the newborn to 4 years of age by specially trained infant health nurses who also educate in child rearing, breast feeding, and correct nutrition.

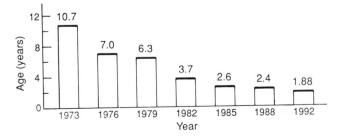

Figure 22–2. New Zealand Dental Service. Average DMF, ages 12–14 years, 1973–1991. Caries in permanent teeth has declined 78% in 18 years. (*From Internal data of the Department of Health, New Zealand, generated from annual returns prepared by principal dental officers.*)

1000, depending on the fluoridation status of her area.[3] As a result of the success of the program, the number of dental nurses is now only half that in 1975 (Fig 22–3).

Dental nurses have had to adapt to advances introduced into the dental delivery system: compressed-air equipment and higher standards of hygiene involving autoclaves, gloves, face masks, and eye protection. Also, newer techniques, such as the use of fissure sealants, fluoride varnish, and light-cured glass ionomer cement fillings, have been adopted.

In view of the decline in the prevalence of decay, the need to continue the School Dental Service has been questioned. Yet, it is undeniable that half the 5-year-olds still have decayed teeth and still require treatment care. Tooth decay among the

lower socioeconomic stream is frequently severe and appears to be increasing. Nearly 70% of children age 12 to 13 still have decayed teeth, although the extent of the decay is much less.

A MODERN HEALTH SERVICE

Until recently, the New Zealand School Dental Service was a national service controlled and directed by the Department of Health in Wellington, the seat of government. As part of the restructuring of the health services, however, administrative control devolved to local area health boards in 1989, and to Crown Health Enterprises in 1992.[3] Throughout all the years of change, the School Dental Service has con-

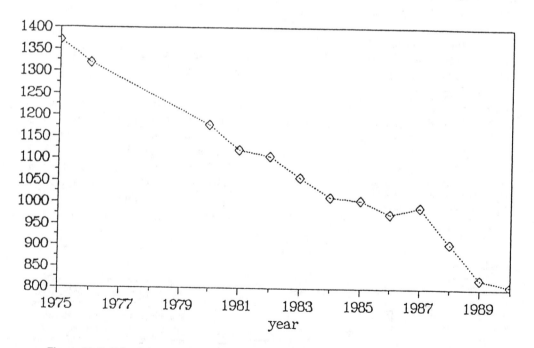

Figure 22–3. School dental nurse population: Number of practicing dental nurses 1975–1990. ◊ represents the actual number at the year in question. (*From Dental Health Unit, Department of Health, Area Health Board Survey, November 1990. Workforce Development Section, New Zealand Department of Health.*)

tinued to meet the required criteria of a modern health service, that is, it is

- Accessible, being based in schools
- Equitable, with all children able to enroll
- Affordable, with no charges being levied
- Acceptable, with 96% of primary pupils being enrolled

Question 3. Which of the following statements, if any, are correct?

A. The New Zealand School Dental Service was instigated 70 years ago at the recommendation of the nation's *dental profession.*

B. Approximately 75% ($\pm$5%) of all of New Zealand's children are enrolled in the New Zealand School Dental Service.

C. Sealants and fluoride remineralization strategies are featured in the New Zealand School Dental Service.

D. The New Zealand School Dental Service requires a minimum copayment for dental insurance for enrollment in the New Zealand School Dental Service.

E. Children from ages 12 to 14 have, on the average, fewer than 2.00 DMF in New Zealand.

REFERENCES

1. Walsh JP. International patterns of oral care—the example of New Zealand. *N Z Dent J.* 1970; 66:143–147.
2. Hunter PBV, Hollis MJ, Drinnan HB. The impact of the WHO/DD International Collaborative Study of dental manpower systems on the New Zealand School Dental Service. *J Dent Res.* 1980; 59:2268–2273.
3. Hunter PB, Kirk R, de Liefde B. *The Study of Oral Health Outcomes.* The 1988 New Zealand Section of the WHO second international collaborative study. Te Tara Ora Health Department of Health Research Services. New Zealand Department of Health. Wellington, New Zealand 1992.

Antiplaque Agents

Kichuel K. Park

The oral cavity has a great variety of bacteria that can produce oral diseases. It is logical to believe that if the appropriate oral pathogens could be eliminated or their metabolism moderated, the plaque diseases could be prevented, arrested, or reversed. Even now, several antiplaque agents are available that are effective in aiding to help control gingivitis. To develop yet *more effective* agents, the specific plaque pathogen(s) need to be identified more precisely. Enhanced specificity would achieve the optimal antibacterial effect, determine the most effective and safest concentration of agents, and minimize any adverse side effects.

In December 1985, the Council on Dental Therapeutics of the American Dental Association (ADA) adopted guidelines for manufacturers of products intended for the chemical control of the microbial plaque. To be granted the ADA's *Seal of Acceptance,* any new antiplaque agent must have been successfully tested in a *minimum of two* independent clinical studies, each having a *minimum duration of 6 months;* be

proven effective in *inhibiting or reducing plaque formation;* be associated with *significant clinical disease (gingivitis) reduction;* be *safe* for all oral tissues; and engender *no overgrowth of opportunistic or resistant microorganisms.*[1] Based on these guidelines, approximately 100 products have been granted full acceptance by the Council.[2]

In recent years attention has been focused on the following antibacterial compounds: chlorhexidine, phenolic compounds, quaternary ammonium agents, oxygenating agents, sanguinarine, and stannous fluoride. Those that have received the most attention during the past decade are listed in Appendix 22–1.

Chemotherapeutic antiplaque agents can also be categorized into five areas by their type(s) or mechanism(s) of action,[3] which include (1) antiseptics; (2) antibiotics; (3) single, or combinations of enzymes; (4) agents that interfere with bacterial attachment; and (5) a miscellaneous group, including nonenzymatic, dispersing, denaturing, or modifying agents.

Although all the antiplaque agents exhibit some degree of antimicrobial activity, not all antimicrobial agents are necessarily antiplaque agents. To qualify as a potential antiplaque agent, the agent must exhibit *substantivity* in the mouth after use, that is it must adsorb to the tissues in the target area, exhibit a slow release, and be released in an active form.

CHLORHEXIDINE DIGLUCONATE

Extensive research efforts have yet to produce an equal to chlorhexidine in effectiveness and substantivity.[4] Chlorhexidine is more potent against *Gram-positive* than Gram-negative bacteria. *Mutans streptococci (MS) are particularly sensitive* to the agent, whereas lactobacilli are less susceptible. *Lactobacillus* organisms usually survive in concentrations of chlorhexidine that are normally bactericidal to MS.[5,6] Chlorhexidine attaches to the bacterial cell membrane, where it increases permeability, thereby initiating outward leakage of vital cytoplasmic constituents. In turn, this leakage causes a precipitation of intracellular proteins and the ultimate death of the bacteria. Chlorhexidine also has the ability to bind strongly to many sites in the oral cavity. It is gradually released over a period of *8 to 12 hours* after a mouth rinse to maintain a high sustained level of antiplaque activity (ie, substantivity). The strong cationic effect of chlorhexidine can interfere with fluoride adsorption into tooth and root surfaces. At present, it is recommended that fluoride and chlorhexidine treatments be *separated in time* by at least 1 hour to attain the optimal benefits of the fluoride products.

A limited number of promising longitudinal studies of the effects of chlorhexidine on approximal and root caries have been accomplished, using various protocols. The results of 2 to 3-years' duration have yielded *reductions in caries* ranging from 26% to 68%.[7] In schoolaged children at high risk for caries, the best effect was achieved when subjects had high levels of colonized MS. In cases in which the MS were *suppressed* to low or undetectable levels by chlorhexidine gel treatment, it usually took *2 to 6 months* for the MS to reach pretreatment levels.[8] Unfortunately, following irradiation for oral cancer, reccurrence of MS in patients at high risk for caries is very rapid.[9] Chlorhexidine containing *varnish* has promise for the prevention of caries. Some studies have shown that varnish treatment has resulted in reduced root demineralization, with a decreased level of new root caries lesions.[6,10] The slight ecologic changes in plaque composition produced by the chlorhexidine varnish treatments do not increase any opportunistic infections by pathogenic microorganisms.[5] Chlorhexidine mouth rinse is the most effective *adjunctive* product for the treatment and prevention of gingivitis when coupled with other mechanical methods of plaque control.

Its routine use has also been suggested as a 30-second rinse *before* clinical procedures to minimize the risk of operator infection from handpiece-generated aerosol production. The rinse procedure has also become a part of the *standard protocol* for before-and-after implants and guided-tissue regeneration procedures. Preoperative and postoperative use of a chlorhexidine mouth rinse usually enhances wound healing; improves the success of bone marrow transplants; minimizes the oral side effects of head and neck irradiation; and helps reduce opportunistic bloodborne infections of oral origin in endocarditis, cancer chemotherapy, and in AIDS.

The intraoral problems accompanying the routine use of chlorhexidine include the *staining* of the teeth, tongue, composite resins, and artificial teeth. Increased calculus formation is sometimes noted because dead bacteria tend to calcify more rapidly than the living.

Since the Food and Drug Administration's approval to market a chlorhexidine containing antiplaque mouthrinse in 1986, this agent has only been available in the United States by *prescription*. It is marketed in a 0.12% concentration under the brand name of *Peridex*. The mouth rinse contains 11.6% alcohol and has a pH of 5.5. In Europe, chlorhexidine is available as an over-the-counter (OTC) product in a variety of concentrations, with 0.2% concentration being the most popular.

PHENOLIC COMPOUNDS

An average 35% reduction of plaque and gingivitis has been documented by using a mouth rinse containing phenolic compounds.[11] Listerine is the first ADA-approved phenol-containing mouth rinse to be used to control plaque and gingivitis. Its substantivity is *less* than that of chlorhexidine, hence, it must be used more frequently. This mouth rinse can be purchased *without* a prescription.

The mechanism of action of Listerine (and other phenolic compounds) may result from an alteration of the bacterial cell wall caused by the mixture of the mouth rinse's essential oils: thymol, menthol, eucalyptol, and methylsalicylate. Reported adverse side effects include the production of a burning sensation, bitter taste, and possible staining of teeth. It is available in either a 26.9% or 21.6% alcohol vehicle and has a pH of 4.3.

TRICLOSAN

Triclosan (2,4,4'-trichloro-2'-hydroxydiphenylether) is a noncationic, *broad-spectrum* antibacterial agent. It has been used widely in the cosmetic and hygiene industry for a number of years, including in toothpaste and mouth rinse products available *outside* of the United States. When Triclosan is combined with a copolymer of vinylmethyl ether and maleic acid (PVM/MA) and used as a dentifrice, it is effective against oral pathogens. In long-term clinical studies, Triclosan prevents or reduces both plaque and gingivitis.[4]

ANTIMICROBIALS COMBINATION THERAPY

In the search to develop more effective antiplaque agents, combinations of different antimicrobial agents and delivery methods have been evaluated. Under certain conditions, suitable combinations of antimicrobial agents can produce synergistic antiplaque effects.[1] These systems often consist of antiplaque agents in combination with certain metals such as zinc salts. For example, *zinc acetate* combined with chlorhexidine has been used as a mouth rinse.[12]

Triclosan is also being used in mouth rinses or toothpastes at a concentration of 0.2 to 0.3%. Interestingly, the copolymer incorporated in the product formulation appears to increase the uptake of Triclosan on enamel surfaces. The use of Triclosan combined with *zinc* citrate has a substantial amount of long-term clinical data with respect to plaque and gingivitis reduction. Significant reductions have occurred in the amount of plaque (up to 50%), calculus (up to 52%), and gingivitis (up to 66%), as well as improved gingival health following brushing with a dentifrice containing Triclosan and zinc salts. Both of these compounds are retained in the mouth for considerable periods between applications, and they produce multiple complementary modes of action.[13,14] To increase its clinical efficacy, Triclosan has also been combined with a compatible and complementary antimicrobial agent, zinc citrate.[14,15]

The results from another combination system using Triclosan and Gantrez, a PVM/MA polymer, are positive, with significant reductions being demonstrated in both plaque and calculus over periods from a few weeks to a few months. Of interest is the fact that neither the Triclosan–zinc combination, nor Triclosan and Gantrez had any effect on the plaque salivary microorganisms.

The combination of chlorhexidine with fluoride has been shown to be particularly effective against MS. This effect appears to be synergistic.[10] Considerable work is underway to establish the potential clinical benefits of using a compatible combination of agents, including a mixture of 1.0% chlorhexidine, stannous fluoride, and zinc citrate.

Oxygenating Agents

The efficacy of oxygenating agents such as peroxide in oral hygiene practices has long been recognized. Such compounds have proven effective in treating gingivitis, oral lesions, and periodontitis, and in combatting plaque bacteria. Additionally, peroxide compounds have been utilized for oral cosmetic purposes such as the bleaching and cleansing of tooth surfaces (ie, tooth whitening).

When peroxide compounds are used in combination with most conventional dentifrice formulations or oral hygiene preparations, the compounds tend to react with other ingredients. This at times has presented significant problems in achieving expected benefits. Abrasive constituents in dentifrices containing peroxide compounds may irritate the gingival tissues, and the peroxide may react with the abraded tissue surfaces. Mouth rinses containing peroxide have demonstrated encouraging results, however.[16] Recently, a more stable form of peroxide, tetrapotassium peroxydiphosphate, has been incorporated in a dentifrice formulation.[16] Recently, the Council on Dental Therapeutics awarded a Seal of Acceptance to *Mentadent,* a toothpaste containing peroxide, sodium bicarbonate, and fluoride.

An enzyme combination system consisting of amyloglucosidase and glucose oxidase, which is capable of generating the antibacterial *hypothiocyanite,* has been proposed. Early clinical studies with these enzyme systems have produced considerable favorable antiplaque results,[17] although confirmatory studies have failed to duplicate the positive earlier results.[18]

The great advantage of the majority of the population using effective antiplaque agents in dentifrices and mouth rinses is to reduce the prevalence of the plaque diseases and their sequelae—much as has been seen with fluoride products and the reduction of dental caries.

Question 4. Which of the following statements, if any, are correct?

A. All antiplaque agents are antimicrobial agents, but not all antimicrobial agents are antiplaque agents.
B. Chlorhexidine has a potent effect in suppressing mutans streptococci and lactobacilli.
C. The duration of chlorhexidine substantivity is approximately 3 to 6 hours.
D. Triclosan is an antiplaque agent but not an antigingivitis agent.
E. The peroxide in Metadent makes it an anticariogenic dentifrice.

EPILOGUE

Throughout the years the grand strategy for the conquest of any disease has been (1) surgery to arrest, treat, or repair the ravages of disease; (2) development of chemicals (drugs) for the prevention and the treatment of disease; and (3) immunization directed toward the complete elimination of disease. To these three a fourth potent strategy can be added—*behavior control*. Caries would be much less of a problem if individuals disciplined their sugar intake. Intraoral cancer would be a rare disease if people stopped smoking and using smokeless tobacco. Face and lip cancer would also decrease markedly if sun worshipping—and sunburning—was not practiced in excess. These self-inflicted orofacial diseases have major consequences for the individual and society.

In the last half century, the science of dentistry has made tremendous advances in the area of primary prevention. With the fluoridation of the water supply in Grand Rapids, Michigan, dentistry took its first faltering steps to use chemistry to control dental caries. S. Arnim demonstrated that plaque control was one of the keys to reducing the bacterial challenge to the teeth and to the supporting structures. B. E. Gustafson, in the Vipeholm study, established that the frequency of intake and the consistency of sugar products were probably more important than the total intake of sugar. M. Buonocore provided the initial studies that indicated that pit-and-fissure sealants could provide an effective physical barrier between occlusal defects and the hostile oral environment.

F. J. Orland and P. H. Keys opened up a completely new concept of plaque disease control with their classic animal studies, which demonstrated that both dental caries and periodontal disease were *infectious* diseases. These findings provide the promise that basic research in the area of immunology might eventually culminate with vaccines to combat first caries and then periodontal disease.

With the great reduction of caries prevalence in the past decade due to fluoridation of water, the extensive use of fluoridated dentifrices and mouth rinses, the increasing substitution of noncariogenic and possibly anticariogenic sweeteners for sucrose, and the increasing use of sealants, the research focus is now rapidly shifting from caries to periodontal disease. The search for the microorganisms responsible for the different periodontal disease processes has been intensified, much like the earlier research that linked mutans streptococci to smooth-surface caries, the lactobacilli to pit-and-fissure lesions, and the actinomyces to root caries. Already, *Actinobacillus actinomycetemcomitans* (Aa), *Bacteroides gingivalis*, and *B intermedius* are prime suspects as periodontopathogens. Now a search is also underway for an antiplaque agent that will provide the same "magic bullet" for periodontal disease control as fluoride has for caries. Chlorhexidine is a drug that now has the promise of being a potent drug in the combat against caries *and* gingivitis. Finally, as the causal organisms for periodontal disease are identified, the search for a vaccine for periodontal disease can be accelerated.

Despite these great scientific advances, dentistry is still characterized as a profession that treats disease and not one that maintains oral health. Part of this is due to the fact that the public has been educated to see the dentist twice a year for a checkup, with the implication that if disease is found, it will be treated. No fault can be found with this response to the presence of disease. However, if each recall appointment could be expanded to look for the indicators of impending caries (ie, white spots) and periodontal disease (ie, gingivitis) and then the appropriate primary preventive responses be taken when indicated, there would be much less need for treatment at the next appointment.

New diagnostic techniques such as *computed dental radiography* promises to replace x-ray film with electronic sensors. The resultant images, which are stored in a computer, allow several electronic enhancement techniques to be used in achieving greater use of the radiographs. Another high tech instrument, the *oral video camera,* allows a much clearer and much more magnified view of the oral structures than is possible with the mouth mirror. It also allows the examination to be stored on tape for careful future review. Each of these additions to the dental armamentarium will permit the *earlier identification* of incipient carious lesions, probably in time to accomplish therapy *before the need for restorations.*

By training and experience, the dentist should be able to use the routine clinical and x-ray examination as a vehicle to evaluate the *probability* for the development of, as well as the existence of, disease. As the probability of plaque disease increases, so should the primary treatment response escalate. Much of the responsibility for implementing a prescribed preventive program can be delegated to the dental hygientist, who is superbly trained to (1) provide patient education, (2) instruct in plaque control measures, (3) counsel on nutrition and the need for sugar discipline, (4) apply topical fluorides and demonstrate prescribed topical fluoride therapy programs, and (5) place pit-and-fissure sealants in all vulnerable fissures.

This book has attempted to provide the basic science background for each of the clinical applications used to prevent, arrest, and reverse the caries and periodontal disease processes. It has also provided explanations about how primary preventive dentistry programs can be accomplished by, or for, normal and handicapped individuals at home, in school, or in institutional or hospital settings.

Given the present state of the dental art, the two plaque diseases—caries and periodontal disease—can be largely controlled by the average motivated individual who has the average amount of guidance and support from health sciences personnel. With this possibility, the litmus test for the dental professional should be based on how well the original state of oral health is maintained—*not* on how well dental disease is treated.

ANSWERS AND EXPLANATIONS

1. A, C, D, E
   B—incorrect. The majority (over 50%) of cancer cases have been diagnosed by 65 years of age.
2. A, B, C, D, E
3. A, C, E
   B—incorrect. Approximately 95% of New Zealand's children are enrolled in the school dental service program.
   D—incorrect. Care for children by the New Zealand School Dental Service is gratis.
4. A, B
   C—incorrect. The substantivity of chlorhexidine is approximately 8 to 12 hours.
   D—incorrect. Any agent that is an antiplaque agent helps to reduce gingivitis.
   E—incorrect. The fluoride is the anti-caries agent.

SELF-EVALUATION QUESTIONS

1. The risk of contracting oral cancer is increased by the consumption of _____ and the use of _____.

2. It is not unusual for senior citizens to routinely take _____ to _____ (number of) medications; in fact, at times they may be taking up to _____.

3. The *Omnibus Budget Reconciliation Act of 1987* requires that all nursing home residents receive a dental examination every _____ (time period).

4. Smoking is a dual addiction—an addiction to _____ (drug) and a _____ addiction (habit and pleasure).

5. The use of nicotine _____ and _____ are effective in reducing nicotine dependence during a smoking cessation program.

6. The four A's to be used in a dental office nonsmoking program to help addicted tobacco users to quit smoking are A _____, A _____, A _____, and A _____.

7. The title of the New Zealand auxiliaries who staff the school dental service is dental _____ or dental _____.

8. An interproximal x-ray lucency without otherwise overt signs of caries, is considered as a candidate for remineralization if it has not progressed past ($\frac{1}{4}$) ($\frac{1}{2}$) ($\frac{3}{4}$) through the enamel.

9. Proportionately (more)(fewer) children are enrolled in the New Zealand School Dental Service program than is the case for school dental programs in the United States.

REFERENCES

1. Council on Dental Therapeutics of the American Dental Association. Guidelines for acceptance of chemotherapeutic products for the control of supragingival dental plaque and gingivitis. *J Am Dent Assoc.* 1986; 112:529–532.

2. American Dental Association. *Clinical Products in Dentistry—A Desktop Reference,* January, 1993.

3. Mandel ID. Chemotherapeutic agents for controlling plaque and gingivitis. *J Clin Periodontol.* 1988; 8:488–498.

4. Stephan KW, Saxton CA, Jones CL, et al. Control of gingivitis and calculus by dentifrice containing a zinc salt and Triclosan. *J Periodontol.* 1990; 61:674–678.

5. Cleghorn B, Bowden GH. The effect of pH on the sensitivity of species of *Lactobacillus* to chlorhexidine and the antibiotics minocycline and spiramycin. *J Dent Res.* 1989; 68:1146–1150.

6. Sandham HJ, Nadeau L, Phillips HI. The effect of chlorhexidine varnish treatment on salivary mutans streptococcal levels in child orthodontic patients. *J Dent Res.* 1992; 71:32–35.

7. Emilson CG. Potential efficacy of chlorhexidine against mutans streptococci and human dental caries. *J Dent Res.* 1994; 682–691.

8. Ostela I, Tenovuo J, Soderling E, et al. Effect of chlorhexidine–sodium fluoride gel applied by tray or by toothbrush on salivary mutans streptococci. *Proc Finn Dent Soc.* 1990; 85:9–14.

9. Epstein JB, McBride BC, Stevenson-Moore, et al. The efficacy of chlorhexidine gel in reduction of *Streptococcus mutans* and *Lactobacillus* species in patients treated with radiation therapy. *Oral Surg Oral Med Oral Pathol.* 1991; 71:172–178.

10. Schaeken MJM, deHaan P. Effects of sustained release chlorhexidine acetate on the human dental plaque flora. *J Dent Res.* 1989; 68:119–123.

11. Fine DH, Letisia J, Mandel ID. The effect of rinsing with Listerine antiseptic on the properties of developing dental plaque. *J Clin Periodontol.* 1989; 12:660–666.

12. Giertsen E, Svatun B, Saxton CA. Plaque inhibition by hexitidine and zinc. *Scand J Dent Res.* 1987; 95:49–54.

13. Bradshaw DJ, Marsh PD, Watson GK, et al. The effects of Triclosan and zinc citrate, alone and in combination, on a community of oral bacteria grown in vitro. *J Dent Res.* 1993; 72:25–30.

14. Cummins D. Mechanisms of action of clinically proven anti-plaque agents. In: Embery G, Rolla G, eds. *Clinical and Biological Aspects of Dentifrices.* Oxford, Oxford Medical Publications; 1992; 204–228.

15. Saxton CA, van der Ouderaa FJG. The effect of a dentifrice containing zinc citrate and Triclosan on developing gingivitis. *J Periodont Res.* 1989; 24:75–80.

16. Afflitto J, Gaffar A, Marcus EC. Effects of tetrapotassium peroxydiphosphate on plaque—gingivitis in vivo. *J Dent Res.* 1988; 67:401.

17. Rotgans J, Hoogendoorn H. The effect of toothbrushing with toothpaste containing amyloglucosidase and glucose-oxidase on plaque accumulation and gingivitis. *Caries Res.* 1979; 13:144–149.

18. Midda M, Cooksey MW. Clinical uses of an enzyme-containing dentifrice. *J Clin Periodontol.* 1986; 13:950–956.

Appendix 22–1. Antiplaque Agents Showing Chemotherapeutic Potential

Chlorhexidine digluconate
Phenolic compounds
Triclosan
Pyrimidines (hexetidine)
Quats (quarternary ammonium compounds)
Bispyridines (octenidine)
Iodine, iodophores, and fluorides (halogens)
Metal salts (silver, mercury, zinc, copper, tin)
Plant alkaloids (sanguinaria)
Oxygenating agents (peroxide, K_4-peroxidiphospate, and perborates)
Plaque pH regulators (urea, lysyl-arginine)
Others (sodium borate, taroulin, kamillosan, allopurinol, cyclosporin)

Index

A

Abrasives. *See* Dentifrices
  tooth damage from, 112, 112*f*
Abutment teeth, brushing, 99
Accurate empathy, 402–403
Acesulfame K, 9, 353–354
Acid
  damage caused by, reduction of, 265
  in plaque development, 50
Acidic solutions, for denture cleaning, contraindications to, 150, 540
Acidulated phosphate fluoride. *See* Fluoride, topical therapy
Acquired immunodeficiency syndrome
  and gingivitis, 524
  patients with
    dental care of, 434–435, 523–524
      in hospital setting, 511–512
    nutrition in, 379
    periodontitis in, 524
Actinobacillus, 26
Actinobacillus actinomycetemcomitans, 574, 611
  and periodontal disease, 67, 330, 331
Actinomyces, 54

Actinomyces naeslundi, 48
Actinomyces odontolyticus, 48
Actinomyces viscosis, 298
Actinomycetes, 22
Activities of daily living cuffs, 493
ACT mouth rinse, 567, 567*f*
ADA. *See* American Dental Association
Adherence, 400
Alabama probe, 334
Alban's test, 12–13, 299*f*, 299–300
Alcohol, in mouth rinses, lethal potential of, 118
Alitame, 354
Alkaline cleaners, for dentures, 149
  dangers of, 540
Aluminum sulfate, for defluoridation of water, 176
Alveolar bone, 62
Amalgams, versus sealants, 248–249
American Association of Public Health Dentistry, 431
American Dental Association, 423
  guidelines for therapeutic agents for gingivitis, 108, 108*t*
  acceptance of dental products, 106–109
American Public Health Association, Oral Health Section, 431

Also from Appleton & Lange

Essentials of Dental Radiography for
Dental Assistants and Hygienists, 5/e
Wolf R. de Lyre, BA, DDS; Orlen N. Johnson, MS, DDS
1995, 448 pp., 222 illus., case, ISBN 0-8385-2025-1, A2025-3

Periodontal Instrumentation, 2/e
Anna Matsuishi Pattison, RDH, MS; Gordon L. Pattison, DDS
1992, 485 pp., illus., spiral, ISBN 0-8385-7804-7, A7804-6

Appleton & Lange's Review for the
Dental Hygiene National Board Examination, 4/e
Caren M. Barnes, RDH, MS; Margaret B. Waring, RDH, MS, EdD
1995, 272 pp., illus., paperback, ISBN 0-8385-0230-X, A0230-1

Medical Terminology With Human Anatomy, 3/e
Jane Rice, RN, CMA-C
1995, 616 pp., illus., spiral, ISBN 0-8385-6268-X, A6268-5

Human Diseases
A Systemic Approach, 4/e
Mary Lou Mulvihill, PhD
1995, 496 pp., illus., paperback, ISBN 0-8385-3928-9, A3928-7

Available at your local health science bookstore
or call 1-800-423-1359 (in CT 838-4400).